Clinical Neuropsychiatry

Clinical Neuropsychiatry

Editor: Otis Thompson

MURPHY & MOORE
www.murphy-moorepublishing.com

www.murphy-moorepublishing.com

MURPHY & MOORE

Cataloging-in-Publication Data

Clinical neuropsychiatry / edited by Otis Thompson.
p. cm.
Includes bibliographical references and index.
ISBN 978-1-63987-767-6
1. Neuropsychiatry. 2. Mental illness. 3. Nervous system--Diseases.
4. Neuropsychology. I. Thompson, Otis.
RC341 .C55 2023
616--dc23

Murphy & Moore Publishing
1 Rockefeller Plaza,
New York City,
NY 10020, USA

ISBN 978-1-63987-767-6

Contents

Preface

This book has been an outcome of determined endeavour from a group of educationists in the field. The primary objective was to involve a broad spectrum of professionals from diverse cultural background involved in the field for developing new researches. The book not only targets students but also scholars pursuing higher research for further enhancement of the theoretical and practical applications of the subject.

Psychiatry is a specialty of medical science that is concerned with the diagnosis, prevention and treatment of mental disorders. Some of the subspecialties within this area of medicine are neuropsychiatry, addiction psychiatry, sleep medicine, child and adolescent psychiatry and social psychiatry. Neuropsychiatry studies psychiatry from a neurological perspective, in order to attribute and understand the behavior and its interaction with social psychology and neurobiology factors. It considers mind to be a part of the brain, while in neurological and behavioral specialties they are considered distinct entities. It is especially important for the treatment of medical conditions which are classified as both neurological and mental. The objective of this book is to give a general view of neuropsychiatry and its applications. It strives to provide a fair idea about this discipline and to help develop a better understanding of the latest advances within this field. This book is a vital tool for all researching and studying this field.

It was an honour to edit such a profound book and also a challenging task to compile and examine all the relevant data for accuracy and originality. I wish to acknowledge the efforts of the contributors for submitting such brilliant and diverse chapters in the field and for endlessly working for the completion of the book. Last, but not the least; I thank my family for being a constant source of support in all my research endeavours.

Editor

1

Chronic Depression Alters Mothers' DHEA and DEHA-to-Cortisol Ratio: Implications for Maternal Behavior and Child Outcomes

Yael Apter-Levy, Orna Zagoory-Sharon and Ruth Feldman*

The Center for Developmental Social Neuroscience, Interdisciplinary Center Herzliya, Herzliya, Israel

***Correspondence:**
Ruth Feldman
feldman.ruth@gmail.com

Maternal depression is a major public health problem that typically occurs in the period surrounding childbirth. The neurobiological mechanisms underlying maternal depression have been the focus of increasing research and studies pointed to the crucial role of the HPA axis in this disorder. However, most studies focused on cortisol expression and regulation while recent attention has shifted to include the sulfate steroids DHEA and DHEA-S. A community cohort of 1,983 women with no comorbid risk was recruited at birth and depression was assessed periodically across the first postpartum year. At 6 years, 156 families were re-visited: 46 mothers were defined as chronically-depressed and 103 controls reported no depression from birth to six years. Mothers and children were diagnosed by structured psychiatric interviews and mother-child interactions were observed. Maternal diurnal cortisol (CT) and dehydroepiandrosterone (DHEA) were assessed. Depressed mothers had lower levels of DHEA (AUCg), flattened DHEA diurnal variability (AUCi), and smaller DHEA-to-CT Ratio. Regression analysis demonstrated that maternal sensitivity during mother-child interaction was independently predicted by maternal depression, DHEA levels, child CT, and child social withdrawal. Results underscore the need for multi-level understanding of the dynamic interplay between maternal psychopathology, mother-child relationship, and pituitary–adrenal-cortex-to-medulla balance in studying the cross generational transfer of psychiatric vulnerability from depressed mothers to their children.

Keywords: HPA, maternal depression, cortisol, dehydroepiandrosterone, longitudinal studies

INTRODUCTION

Maternal Depression is a common condition and constitutes a major public health problem. During pregnancy and the postpartum period the body is more vulnerable to many different disorders including hypertension, diabetes, and cardiovascular disease, in addition to high stress and psychopathology (1). One of the most investigated mechanisms of depression is dysfunction of the

HPA Axis. The functioning of the HPA system is thought to be shaped in prenatal and early neonatal life through a variety of proximate conditions, including maternal stress physiology, contextual conditions, and parenting quality (2–4). Additionally, the HPA axis is thought to play a crucial role in the initiation and maintenance of depressive illness. The most thoroughly investigated aspect of the HPA axis are variations in the secretion of the stress hormone Cortisol (CT). During the days and weeks after birth, there is a fall in cortisol and CRH (Cortisol Releasing Hormone), which is especially marked in women suffering from postpartum depression (5, 6). Glynn et al. proposed that depressive postpartum symptoms may be due to prenatal HPA axis dysregulation (7, 8).

However, CT is not the only stress-related hormone associated with depression and malfunctioning and its potential impact on offspring psychopathology. The adrenal androgen dehydroepiandrosterone (DHEA) plays a critical role in controlling mood and anxiety, and changes in DHEA levels have been reported in conditions pertaining to increased stress and psychiatric disorders (9, 10). It had been recognized as early as 1952, that lower DHEA/DHEAS in adult life is associated with neuropsychiatric disorders (eg schizophrenia, depression). However, the mechanistic role for DHEA/DHEAS in any of these domains remains speculative, not the least because the presence of these androgens in the adrenal gland and brain is largely confined to humans and a few non-human primates. DHEA and DHEAS are dynamically regulated from before birth and before the onset of puberty, and therefore an understanding of the synthesis, regulation, and functions of this important androgen pathway warrants attention. Davies (11) has stressed the important role of the steroid sulfate axis for maternal mental health and there evidence suggesting that maternal caregiving may affect the psychological adjustment of offspring *via* these hormonal mechanisms. Furthermore, these hormones seem to have some therapeutic value (11). In a recent meta-analysis, there seem to be a significant treatment effect for these hormones in depression when compared to placebo (12) and DHEA and DHEA-s were found to influence basic electrophysiological processes. An interest finding in this regard is that depression is accompanied by an attenuated DHEA and DHEA-S response to acute psychosocial stress, which may help elucidate the relationship between the HPA axis and stress (13). Thus, higher DHEA-to-cortisol and DHEAS-to-DHEA ratios are hypothesized to be involved in negative stimuli processing, preventing the interference of negative stimuli in cognitive tasks. DHEA-S may play important roles in cortical development and plasticity, protection against negative affect and depression, and might even enhance attention and overall working memory (14). Alterations in DHEA activity seem to be trait rather than state phenomena and are predictive of future depressive episodes (15–17). Additionally, there is evidence of anatomical structural changes in the brain related to these findings. Thus, both pituitary (18) and hippocampal volume appears to be reduced in depressive patients (16).

Maternal depression, both antenatal and postnatal, is associated with reduced maternal sensitivity to offspring (19). In a recent prospective study, it was found that the presence of depressive symptoms augmented deficits in maternal sensitivity in mothers who suffer from personality disorders (20). Moreover, poor quality mother-infant interactions in the perinatal period predicted is associated with suicidal ideation in pregnancy (21). In a recent meta-analysis, the association of reduced maternal sensitivity to maternal depression was clearly demonstrated, and it may be that the pernicious influence of maternal depression on child development is mediated by maternal sensitivity (22). The HPA Axis appears to play a seminal role in maternal sensitivity (7). For example, results from the Alberta Pregnancy Outcomes and Nutrition Study, (a prospective longitudinal cohort of pregnancy), suggested that maternal HPA axis is a means by which early life stress in mothers is transmitted to their children. The authors point out that their results show that the HPA axis is sensitive to social stimuli (23). However, although much research has been devoted to study mechanisms by which cortisol changes are associated with depression (1), very little research has been devoted DHEA and no study, to our knowledge, has focused on DHEA in the context of maternal depression and the mother's observed caregiving.

Thus, the overall goal of this prospective longitudinal study was to examine the vicissitudes of DHEA/CT ratio in depressed mothers of preschoolers in a community cohort followed from birth to six years. Two hypotheses were proposed; First, depressed mothers will have lower DHEA levels than mothers without depression in combination with a less dynamic DHEA system (24), and that DHEA-to-CT ratio will be smaller for the depressed group (16). Second, interactions between depressed mothers and their children would be expected to be less optimal, marked by lower maternal sensitivity and greater child social withdrawal during social contact. Consistent with ecological models on the determinants of sensitive parenting (25), which suggested that both child biological factors and parental characteristics contribute to the development of sensitive parenting, in addition to recent evidence that child and maternal cortisol are inter-correlated in the context of maternal depression (26) we expected that maternal hormones and depression will predict the degree of maternal sensitivity during naturalistic interactions with her child.

METHODS

Methods of the study have been reported extensively in our previous publications, and are summarized here briefly (27, 28). We included **Figure 1**, which details the five ways of sample recruitment and follow-up from birth to six years, including the exact number of participants at each wave and numbers lost to attrition.

Participants

Participants were recruited in five waves of data collection utilizing an extreme-case design as follows: 1,983 consecutive admissions to maternity ward were included in the initial sample. Inclusion criteria were physically healthy mothers, a healthy,

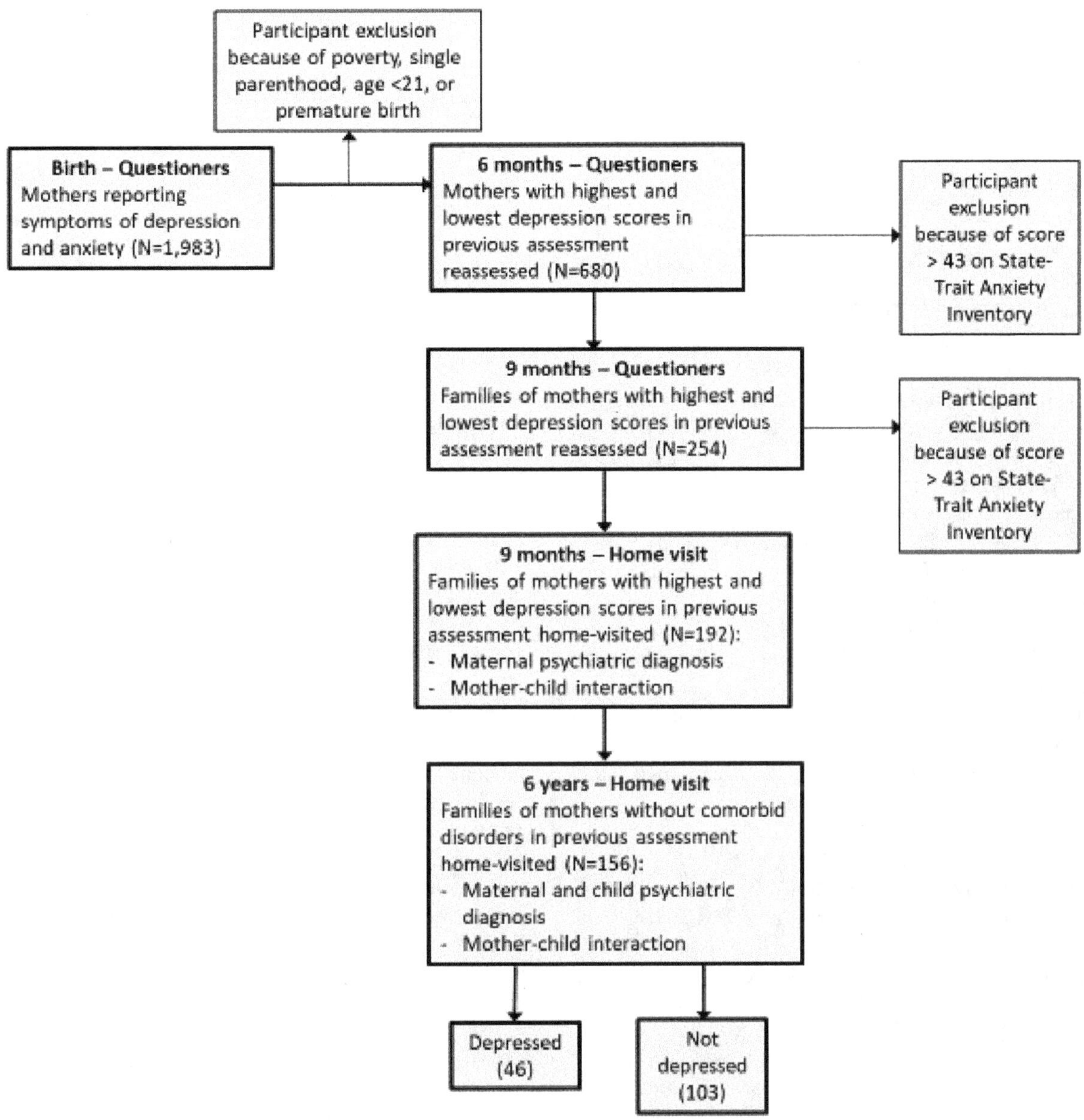

FIGURE 1 | Flow chart depicting sequence of assessments.

term, and singleton infant, and stable family situations with low-risk socio-economic status: mother age above 21 years, completed high-school education, cohabitating with infant father, and family above poverty line. The initial assessment included demographic questionnaires, BDI [Beck Depression Index (29)] and STAI [State-Trait Anxiety Inventory (STAI) (30)]. Six months later the mothers were reassessed and divided to those with high BDI scores (>11) and low scores (0–5), respectively. At nine months, we approached 350 mothers for reassessment, of which 254 responded. Of the 254 mothers who responded at nine months, 210 were contacted who had high and low depressive symptomatology without high anxiety symptoms (STAI>43). Of those, 192 agreed to a home visit, which included the Structured Clinical Interview for DSM-IV Axis I Disorders (SCID-I; (31). At all stages of the evaluation there were no differences in the demographic characteristics between those who agreed or disagreed to participate in the study. At 6 years, 156 mothers and children were revisited. At this stage, two final study groups of mothers remained: those with high depressive symptoms from birth (n=46), and those with no psychiatric diagnosis from 9 months to 6 years. No differences in demographic factors were found between these two groups (**Table 1**). The study was approved by the Institutional Review Board and all participants signed an informed consent.

TABLE 1 | Demographics information for depressed and non-depressed groups.

	Non-depressed		Depressed		Statistics
	Mean	SD	Mean	SD	*T* value
Mother education	14.24	2.54	13.97	2.78	0.54, ns
Mother age (years)	37.05	4.12	35.74	4.9	1.76, ns
Child age (months)	76.51	24.69	71.33	13.46	1.84, ns
Child gender					$\chi^2(5) = 0.25$, ns
Male%	52.7%		57.5%		54.2%
Child birth order					$\chi^2(1)=3.50$, ns
Firstborn%	36.2%		54.1%		41.1%

Procedure and Measures

All interviews were conducted at home, in the afternoon, after 3:00PM. Mothers were administered the DAWBA (32) and then the SCID (31), and the child was evaluated with a neuropsychological test, the NEPYS and Vocabulary part and Block sub-test from the WIPPSI. In addition, the children underwent emotion regulation and empathy paradigms. Mother and child were videotaped in a 10-min interaction with age-appropriate pre-selected toys. Mothers were given 12 tubes for diurnal salivary samples collection from themselves and the child (3 per day) by passive drool on two consecutive weekend days of the same week.

Maternal Psychiatric Diagnosis was by SCID-I (31), 46 mothers (29.6%) were defined as chronically depressed. These mothers showed high depressive symptoms (BDI >11) at birth, six, and nine months, received a clinical diagnosis of MDD at both nine months and 6 years, and reported being depressed throughout most of the child's first six years. One hundred and three mothers (66%) non-symptomatic mothers formed the control group,

Hormone Collection and Analysis

Cortisol and DHEA Diurnal Collection

Participants were provided with detailed instructions for collecting saliva. Samples were collected upon wakening, 30 min after wakening, and before going to bed. Mothers and children were asked to chew on salivates (Sarstedt, Rommelsdorft, Germany) until saturation on two consecutive days. Mother received salivates for cortisol and DHEA assays, and the children for cortisol alone. Participants kept a collection diary in which they noted exact awakening and sampling times for each sampling day. Salivates were stored at −20°C until analysis. Child results are reported elsewhere (28).

Cortisol Analysis was done using standard procedures and described in our original paper (27).

DHEA Analysis was done using standard procedures described by our group elsewhere (33): In order to precipitate the mucus, samples underwent several freeze-thaw cycles. After the fourth cycle the tubes were centrifuged at 1,500 x g (@3,000 rpm) for 20 min. Supernatants were collected and stored at -20°C until assayed. Determination of DHEA was performed using a commercial DHEA ELISA kit (Salimetrics, USA). Salimetrics DHEA kit is a competitive immunoassay specifically designed for the quantitative measurement of salivary DHEA. On the day of assay, samples were thawed, and 50 micro-liters were pipette into the appropriate well of the kit. Measurements were performed in duplicate and the concentrations of samples were calculated by using MatLab-7 according to relevant standard curves. The intra-assay and inter-assay coefficients are 20.9 and 22.7 percent, respectively.

Two measures were calculated for diurnal CT and DEHA: area under the curve with respect to ground (AUCg) and area under the curve with respect to increase (AUCi) (34). The AUCg is an estimate of the total diurnal CT or DHEA secretion over six measurements (3 times a day, for two consecutive days: waking, noon and evening) (28). The AUCi is a measure of the dynamic increase of diurnal secretion, associated with the variability and sensitivity of the system and emphasizing changes over time during the days (34).

Mother-Child Interaction

10 min of mother-child interaction with a set of pre-selected toys were filmed and coded with the Coding Interactive Behavior (CIB) manual [for review: (35)], a coding system that has shown good psychometric properties and have been utilized across the world in research spanning infancy to adulthood. We have described this procedure in previous reports (36). In brief, interactions are coded offline on 52 scales that are combined into eight theoretically-determined maternal, child, and dyadic constructs. In the current study, we focused on the construct of maternal sensitivity, which includes codes related to the expression of maternal behavior (e.g, positive affect, warm vocalizations, continuous social gaze), adaptation to the child's state and signals (e.g., appropriate range of affect, resourcefulness), and the provision of a secure base (e.g., maternal supportive presence). Maternal sensitivity is the key construct that describes the mother's growth-promoting style in attachment research. The CIB maternal sensitivity construct has been shown to be individually stable from infancy to adolescence, associated with a host of positive child outcomes, and compromised in multiple high-risk conditions (35). In addition, we used the CIB *Child Social Withdrawal,* which comprises codes related to child avoidance, distancing from mother, negative/withdrawn mood, and minimal social involvement and has shown to be altered in children of depressed mothers (37, 38).

Statistical Analysis

Differences between depressed and non-depressed mothers and their children in diurnal and reactive hormone levels and behavior were tested with ANOVA. Hierarchical multiple regression was used to predict maternal behavior by maternal depression and maternal and child hormonal profiles.

RESULTS

Group Differences in Hormonal Profiles and Interactive Behavior

Hormones

Depressed mothers showed significantly lower levels of total diurnal DHEA secretion, lower variability of DHEA, and smaller DHEA to CT Ratio compared to controls (**Table 2**, **Figures 2A–D**). We have reported elsewhere on child CT levels. In short diurnal cortisol secretion in mothers was associated with that of the child (39).

Interactive Behavior

Depressed mothers showed less sensitivity during mother-child interaction compared to non-depressed mothers. Children of depressed mothers were more withdrawn during interactions with their mother compared to children of non-depressed mothers (**Table 2**).

Maternal Sensitivity was negatively associated with Child Withdrawal during mother-child interaction, $r=-.381$, $p<.001$. Maternal Sensitivity correlated with higher mother's (AUCg) diurnal DHEA production, $r= 0.157$, $p<.05$ and diurnal DHEA variability (AUCi) $r=.187$, $p<.05$.

Predicting Maternal Sensitivity From Maternal Depression and Mother and Child Hormones

A hierarchical multiple regression was computed to predict maternal sensitivity from maternal and child stress-related hormones in the context of chronic maternal depression. Variables were entered in four theoretically-determined order to test the unique effect of neuroendocrine markers in mother and child above and beyond the effect of depression. In the first, step, maternal depression was entered to control for its effect on maternal sensitivity. In the second block, maternal DHEA level (AUCg) and variability (AUCi) were entered, and in the third block, child CT level (AUCg) and variability (AUCi) were entered. In the final block, child social withdrawal during mother-child interaction was entered to address the impact of child social involvement and withdrawal on the mother's sensitive behavior. Results regression model appear in **Table 3** and detail the four steps of the model. As seen, each step contributed meaningfully to the prediction of maternal sensitivity, indicating that maternal depression, maternal and child stress-related neuroendocrine markers, and child social behavior jointly impact the mother's sensitive style. In combination, the variables included in the model explained 43% of the variability in maternal sensitivity.

TABLE 2 | Differences in hormonal measures and maternal sensitivity according to maternal depression.

	Depressed Mothers		Non-Depressed Mothers		T
	Mean	**SEM**	**Mean**	**SEM**	
Maternal DHEA AUCg	279.35	24.38	391	48.29	2.07*
Maternal DHEA AUCi	-570.02	59	-903.89	187.25	1.701*
Maternal DHEA-CT	.03	.02	.09	.01	1.8*
Child CT AUCg	3777.85	227.95	2910.26	80.27	3.59**
Child CT AUCi	-3784.84	217.78	-3140.97	252.98	1.93*
Maternal Sensitivity	3.37	0.13	3.75	.06	2.65*
Child Withdrawal	1.5	.11	1.21	.03	-2.56*

*Differences between depressed mothers and non-depressed mothers, and their children in means and SEM of mother's and child's diurnal cortisol and DHEA secretion and variability and maternal sensitivity and child withdrawal CIB scores at 6 years *p < .05 **p < .01.*

DISCUSSION

The major novel finding of this study was the close association between maternal depression and maternal DHEA hormonal activity. It may be that elevated stress activates the HPA axis either as a result of maternal depression or alternatively as a cause of maternal depression. Our results point to dysregulation of maternal HPA functioning as expressed by disturbances in DHEA secretion and the DHEA-to-Cortisol ratio. As expected, mothers with a chronic history of depression showed flattened diurnal curves. The most common explanation for such flattened curve is that an "allostatic overload" of the HPA system from exposure to prolonged stress leads to exhaustion of the system, resulting in inflexible hormonal production (40). Interestingly, similar findings have been shown with patients suffering from "Burnout" (41), and also from a history of physical abuse in early life (42).

The concept of "allostatic load" has received increasing attention and some researchers have even recommended placing it alongside in importance to traditionally recognized cardinal factors such as genes and the environment (43). Although in the past interest in "allostatic load" has mainly been limited to CT expression, it now seems that the allostatic load story "is a tale of two axes" (44). The second axis being the sulfate steroid axis, and our mothers with a history of depression showed both lower levels and flatter diurnal curves of DHEA. There is much evidence to show that the DHEA to CT ratio has a pivotal role in depression particularly in a developmental context, as has been recently reviewed (45). The authors concluded that absolute and relative hormone levels of DHEA and CT may be relevant in understanding developmental psychopathology and the two hormones may have opposing effects, and speculate that these hormones may be the basis for developing biomarkers that are relevant when making a clinical diagnosis. Interestingly, CT to DHEA ratio have been found to be markers of emotional resilience in rats in animal models, independent of the presence or absence of depression (46). This ratio was altered following reproductive experience. Thus, this endocrine ratio may be particularly relevant for maternal depression (47).

Our findings also support Girdler et al. (24) suggestion that neuroactive steroids are mainly synthesized in the adrenals and that a history of depression may be associated with persistent adrenal suppression (24). Indeed, we show that the DHEA to

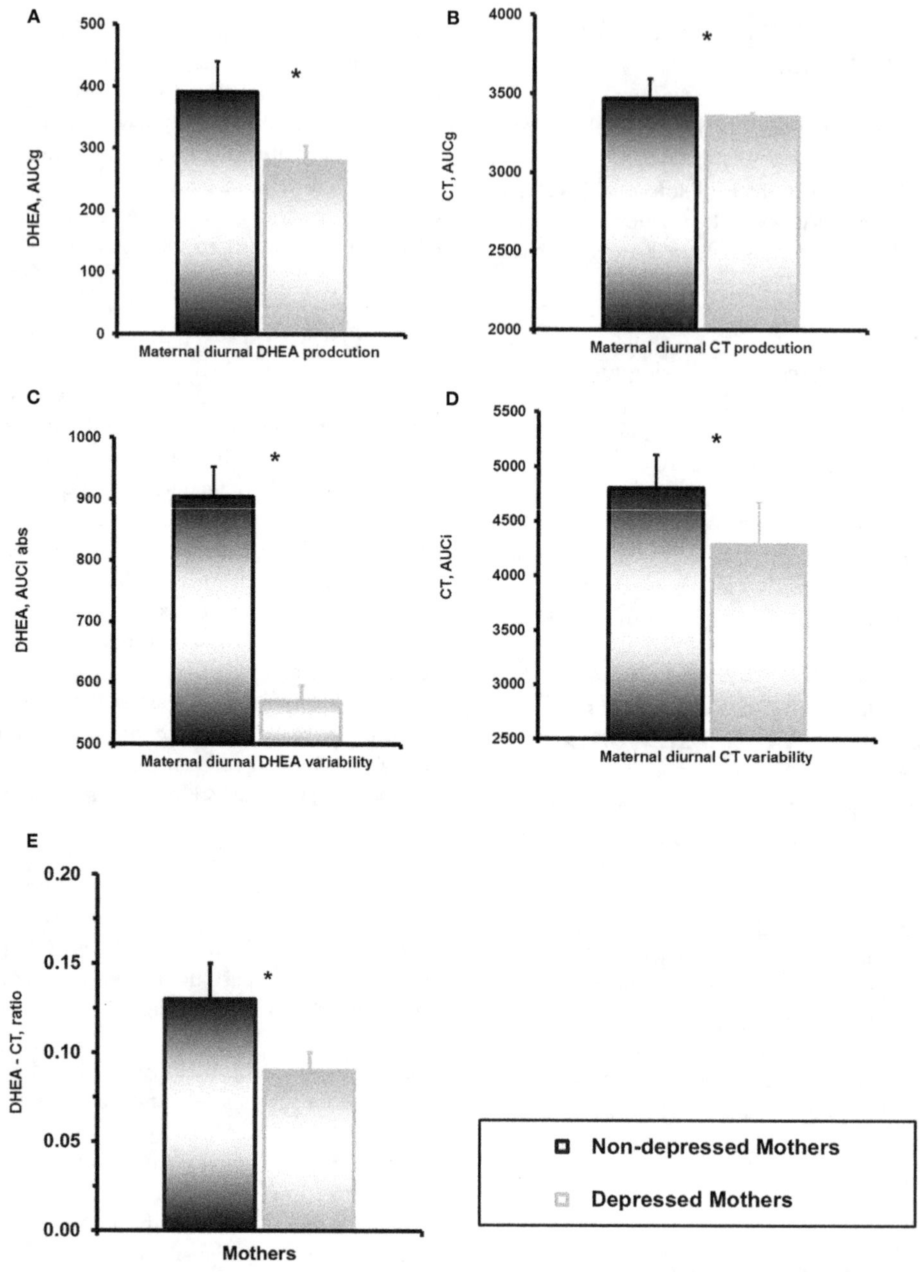

FIGURE 2 | (A) Mother's dehydroepiandrosterone (DHEA) diurnal secretion in depressed and non-depressed mothers at 6 years. *p<0.05. **(B)** Mother's and child's cortisol diurnal secretion in children of depressed and non-depressed mothers at 6 years. *p<0.05. **(C)** Mother's DHEA diurnal variability in depressed and non-depressed mothers at 6 years. *p<0.05. **(D)** Mother's and child's cortisol diurnal variability in children of depressed and non-depressed mothers at 6 years. *p<0.05. **(E)** DHEA-CT ratio in depressed and non-depressed mothers at 6 years. *p<0.05.

CT ratio was significantly lower in depressed mothers compared to controls; it seems that DHEA secretion was even more sensitive than CT to allostatic pressures in depressed mothers, a finding that may be of interest when developing new therapeutic strategies for chronic maternal depression (9, 12). There is some evidence that the beneficial effects of these agents are mediated by the regulation of the HPA axis (48). Depressed mothers tend to respond less sensitively to their infants' signals (49), which in turn may affect the infants' ability to regulate stress and negative emotions (38) and engage in social interactions (50). Results of the regression model from the current study may shed further light on this interplay among

TABLE 3 | Hierarchal regression analysis predicting maternal sensitivity correlates.

		B	SEB	β	Adjusted R^2
Step 1					
	Maternal Depression	-.64	.16	-.42**	.17
Step 2					
	Mother DHEA AUCg	-2.51	1.10	-.57*	
	Mother DHEA AUCi	.38	.29	.27	.23
Step 3					
	Child CT AUCg	-.48	.64	-.27*	
\	Child CT AUCi	.15	.09	.16	.28
Step 4					
	Child withdrawal	-.52	.15	-.35**	.38

R^2 *Total = .43* $F_{(6,65)} = 8.443$, $p < .001$.
*$p < .05$ **$p < .001$, sample size=137 mother and child.*

the different levels of functioning. Maternal sensitivity during interaction with her child was predicted by the mother's depression, her DHEA levels, and her child's withdrawal behavior and cortisol levels. Taken in conjunction with the association between low child cortisol secretion and variability and child withdrawal when interacting with the mother, we can surmise that the interplay between cross- generational HPA function, mother-child relationship, child behavior, and maternal depression are all inextricably intertwined leading to greater child psychiatric vulnerability (51, 52). A recent study, (3) showed an association between maternal depression and infant HPA axis sensitization. In this study, CT reactivity was increased and also magnified over time. This pattern of response predicted maternal depressive disorder, which in turn was related to poorer infant development. It has been reported that mothers' sensitivity is related to bonding and social and emotional behavioral problems (53). Thus, maternal factors impacting the quality of mother-child interaction are important for children's positive social-emotional development.

It is still uncertain as to whether hyperactive stress responsivity is associated with affective disorder *via* changes occurring overtime due to chronic stress response and whether these findings will fit a classic "allostatic load" model which indicates that elevated HPA activity results in accumulated "wear and tear" (54, 55). However, whereas studies report contradictory results with regards to hyper or hypo-cortisolism following early stress, it appears that the most consistent finding is reduction in the system's variability and flexible response to both daily states and momentary stressors (56). Overall, our findings highlight the complexity of HPA functioning in the face of acute or chronic stress and the need for an integrative multi-level understanding of the vicissitudes of maternal psychopathology, associated stress, mother-child relationships, pituitary–adrenal-axis, and medulla interplay when attempting to tease apart the bio-behavioral mechanisms underlying some of the well-known devastating effects of maternal depression on children.

Limitations include the decision to exclude mothers with comorbid anxiety disorder. This may limit the generalizability of our results, since anxiety is highly comorbid with depression. Thus, future studies may be needed to look at a group of mothers suffering from depression with comorbid anxiety. Furthermore, although salivary cortisol and DHEA are well accredited methodologies these are peripheral measures and may not reflect actual central nervous system activity. In addition, paternal psychopathology was not assessed. Finally, our findings remain to be integrated with the vast network of variables that act within the central nervous system and our knowledge and ability to understand and work with the multiple arrays of factors involved is necessarily limited (27). The current findings shed further light on these complex systems and future research is needed to advance our efforts to help children of depressed mothers already in the first years of life through the construction of more specifically targeted early interventions. These results raise the intriguing possibility that in the future vicissitudes of DHEA regulation may be used as a biological marker for maternal sensitivity and/or the quality of the mother-child dyadic relationship. Such a marker could prove invaluable in the assessment of techniques to improve the maternal sensitive caregiving.

AUTHOR CONTRIBUTIONS

RF designed the study and conducted the follow-up and wrote the paper. YA-L conducted the 6-year follow-up, analyzed the data, and wrote the paper. OZ-S conducted the hormonal analysis.

REFERENCES

1. Dickens MJ, Pawluski JL. The HPA axis during the perinatal period: Implications for perinatal depression. *Endocrinology* (2018) 159(11):3737–46. doi: 10.1210/en.2018-00677
2. Juster RP, Bizik G, Picard M, Arsenault-Lapierre G, Sindi S, Trepanier L, et al. A transdisciplinary perspective of chronic stress in relation to psychopathology throughout life span development. *Dev Psychopathol.* (2011) 23(3):725–76. doi: 10.1017/S0954579411000289
3. Laurent H. Early calibration of the HPA axis by maternal psychopathology. *Psychoneuroendocrinology* (2017) 78:177–84. doi: 10.1016/j.psyneuen.2017.01.034
4. Van den Bergh BRH, van den Heuvel MI, Lahti M, Braeken M, de Rooij SR, Entringer S, et al. Prenatal developmental origins of behavior and mental health: The influence of maternal stress in pregnancy. *Neurosci Biobehav Rev* (2017) 16:3074–5. doi: 10.1016/j.neubiorev.2017.07.003
5. Seth S, Lewis AJ, Galbally M. Perinatal maternal depression and cortisol function in pregnancy and the postpartum period: A systematic literature review. *BMC Pregnancy Childbirth* (2016) 16(1):016–0915. doi: 10.1186/s12884-016-0915-y
6. Szpunar MJ, Parry BL. A systematic review of cortisol, thyroid-stimulating hormone, and prolactin in peripartum women with major depression. *Arch Women's Ment Health* (2018) 21(2):149–61. doi: 10.1007/s00737-017-0787-9
7. Glynn LM, Davis EP, Sandman CA. New insights into the role of perinatal HPA-axis dysregulation in postpartum depression. *Neuropeptides* (2013) 47(6):363–70. doi: 10.1016/j.npep.2013.10.007
8. Glynn LM, Sandman CA. Evaluation of the association between placental

corticotrophin-releasing hormone and postpartum depressive symptoms. *Psychosom. Med* (2014) 76(5):355–62. doi: 10.1097/PSY.0000000000000066
9. Kurita H, Maeshima H, Kida S, Matsuzaka H, Shimano T, Nakano Y, et al. Serum dehydroepiandrosterone (DHEA) and DHEA-sulfate (S) levels in medicated patients with major depressive disorder compared with controls. *J Affect. Disord* (2013) 146(2):205–12. doi: 10.1016/j.jad.2012.09.004
10. Maninger N, Capitanio JP, Mason WA, Ruys JD, Mendoza SP. Acute and chronic stress increase DHEAS concentrations in rhesus monkeys. *Psychoneuroendocrinology* (2010) 35(7):1055–62. doi: 10.1016/j.psyneuen.2010.01.006
11. Davies W. The steroid sulfate axis and its relationship to maternal behaviour and mental health. *J Mol Endocrinol* (2018) 61(2):T199–210. doi: 10.1530/JME-17-0219
12. Peixoto C, Grande AJ, Mallmann MB, Nardi AE, Cardoso A, Veras AB. Dehydroepiandrosterone (DHEA) for Depression: A Systematic Review and Meta-Analysis. *CNS Neurol Disord - Drug Targets* (2018) 17(9):706–11. doi: 10.2174/1871527317666180817153914
13. Simmons JG, Byrne ML, Schwartz OS, Whittle SL, Sheeber L, Kaess M, et al. Dual-axis hormonal covariation in adolescence and the moderating influence of prior trauma and aversive maternal parenting. *Dev Psychobiol* (2015) 57 (6):670–87. doi: 10.1002/dev.21275
14. do Vale S, Escera C. Dehydroepiandrosterone and Dehydroepiandrosterone-Sulfate and Emotional Processing. *Vitamins Hormones* (2018) 108:413–41. doi: 10.1016/bs.vh.2018.01.022
15. Jiang X, Zhong W, An H, Fu M, Chen Y, Zhang Z, et al. Attenuated DHEA and DHEA-S response to acute psychosocial stress in individuals with depressive disorders. *J Affect. Disord* (2017) 215:118–24. doi: 10.1016/j.jad.2017.03.013
16. Ter Horst DM, Schene AH, Figueroa CA, Assies J, Lok A, Bockting CLH, et al. Cortisol/DHEA ratio and hippocampal volume: A pilot study in major depression and healthy controls. *Psychoneuroendocrinology* (2016) 72:139–46. doi: 10.1016/j.psyneuen.2016.06.017
17. ter Horst DM, Schene AH., Figueroa CA, Assies J, Lok A, Bockting CLH, et al. Cortisol, dehydroepiandrosterone sulfate, fatty acids, and their relation in recurrent depression. *Psychoneuroendocrinology* (2019) 100:203–12. doi: 10.1016/j.psyneuen.2018.10.012
18. Kaess M, Whittle S, O'Brien-Simpson L, Allen NB, Simmons JG. Childhood maltreatment, pituitary volume and adolescent hypothalamic-pituitary-adrenal axis – Evidence for a maltreatment-related attenuation. *Psychoneuroendocrinology* (2018) 98:39–45. doi: 10.1016/j.psyneuen.2018.08.004
19. Binda V, Figueroa-Leigh F, Olhaberry M. Antenatal and postnatal depressive symptoms: Association with quality of mother–infant interaction. *Infant Behav Dev* (2019) 57:101386. doi: 10.1016/j.infbeh.2019.101386
20. Nath S, Pearson RM, Moran P, Pawlby S, Molyneaux E, Howard LM. Maternal personality traits, antenatal depressive symptoms and the postpartum mother–infant relationship: a prospective observational study. *Soc Psychiatry Psychiatr Epidemiol* (2019) 55(5):621–34. doi: 10.1007/s00127-019-01790-y
21. Gordon H, Nath S, Trevillion K, Moran P, Pawlby S, Newman L, et al. Self-Harm, Self-Harm Ideation, and Mother-Infant Interactions. *J Clin Psychiatry* (2019) 80(5):18m12708. doi: 10.4088/JCP.18m12708
22. Bernard K, Nissim G, Vaccaro S, Harris JL, Lindhiem O. Association between maternal depression and maternal sensitivity from birth to 12 months: A meta-analysis. *Attach. Hum Dev* (2018) 20(6):578–99. doi: 10.1080/14616734.2018.1430839
23. Thomas JC, Letourneau N, Campbell TS, Giesbrecht GF. Social buffering of the maternal and infant HPA axes: Mediation and moderation in the intergenerational transmission of adverse childhood experiences. *Dev Psychopathol.* (2018) 30(3):921–39. doi: 10.1017/S0954579418000512
24. Girdler SS, Lindgren M, Porcu P, Rubinow DR, Johnson JL, Morrow AL. A history of depression in women is associated with an altered GABAergic neuroactive steroid profile. *Psychoneuroendocrinology* (2012) 37(4):543–53. doi: 10.1016/j.psyneuen.2011.08.004
25. Belsky J. of Parenting: A Process Model. *Child Dev* (1984) 55(1):83–96. doi: 10.2307/1129836
26. LeMoult J, Chen MC, Foland-Ross LC, Burley HW, Gotlib IH. Concordance of mother-daughter diurnal cortisol production: Understanding the intergenerational transmission of risk for depression. *Biol Psychol* (2015) 108:98–104. doi: 10.1016/j.biopsycho.2015.03.019
27. Apter-Levi Y, Pratt M, Vakart A, Feldman M, Zagoory-Sharon O, Feldman R. Maternal depression across the first years of life compromises child psychosocial adjustment; relations to child HPA-axis functioning. *Psychoneuroendocrinology* (2016) 64:47–56. doi: 10.1016/j.psyneuen.2015.11.006
28. Pratt M, Apter-Levi Y, Vakart A, Kanat-Maymon Y, Zagoory-Sharon O, Feldman R. Mother-child adrenocortical synchrony; Moderation by dyadic relational behavior. *Horm. Behav* (2017) 89:167–75. doi: 10.1016/j.yhbeh.2017.01.003
29. Beck AT, Ward CH, Mendelson M, Mock J, Erbaugh J. An Inventory for Measuring Depression. *Arch Gen Psychiatry* (1961) 4(6):561–71. doi: 10.1001/archpsyc.1961.01710120031004
30. Spielberger CD, Gorsuch RL, Lushene RE. *State-trait anxiety inventory.* Palo Alto. Cal.: Consulting Psychologists Press (1970).
31. First MB, Spitzer RL, Gibbon M, Williams JBW. The structured clinical interview for DSM-III-R personality disorders (SCID-II). Part I: Description. *J Pers Disord* (1995) 9(2):83–91. doi: 10.1521/pedi.1995.9.2.83
32. Mansbach-Kleinfeld I, Apter A, Farbstein I, Levine SZ, Ponizovsky AM. A population-based psychometric validation study of the strengths and difficulties questionnaire - hebrew version. *Front Psychiatry* (2010) 1:151. doi: 10.3389/fpsyt.2010.00151
33. Yirmiya K, Djalovski A, Motsan S, Zagoory-Sharon O, Feldman R. Stress and immune biomarkers interact with parenting behavior to shape anxiety symptoms in trauma-exposed youth. *Psychoneuroendocrinology* (2018) 98:153–60. doi: 10.1016/j.psyneuen.2018.08.016
34. Pruessner JC, Kirschbaum C, Meinlschmid G, Hellhammer DH. Two formulas for computation of the area under the curve represent measures of total hormone concentration versus time-dependent change. *Psychoneuroendocrinology* (2003) 28 (7):916–31. doi: 10.1016/S0306-4530(02)00108-7
35. Feldman R. Bio-behavioral Synchrony: A Model for Integrating Biological and Microsocial Behavioral Processes in the Study of Parenting. *Parenting* (2012) 12(2–3):154–64. doi: 10.1080/15295192.2012.683342
36. Pratt M, Apter-Levi Y, Vakart A, Feldman M, Fishman R, Feldman T, et al. Maternal depression and child oxytocin response; Moderation by maternal oxytocin and relational behavior. *Depress. Anxiety* (2015) 32(9):635–46. doi: 10.1002/da.22392
37. Dollberg D, Feldman R, Keren M, Guedeney A. Sustained withdrawal behavior in clinic-referred and nonreferred infants. *Infant Ment Health J* (2006) 27(3):292–309. doi: 10.1002/imhj.20093
38. Feldman R, Granat A, Pariente C, Kanety H, Kuint J, Gilboa-Schechtman E. Maternal Depression and Anxiety Across the Postpartum Year and Infant Social Engagement, Fear Regulation, and Stress Reactivity. *J Am Acad Child Adolesc Psychiatry* (2009) 48(9):919–27. doi: 10.1097/CHI.0b013e3181b21651
39. Pratt M, Apter-Levi Y, Vakart A, Kanat-Maymon Y, Zagoory-Sharon O, Feldman R. Mother-child adrenocortical synchrony; Moderation by dyadic relational behavior. *Horm. Behav* (2017) 89:635–46. doi: 10.1016/j.yhbeh.2017.01.003
40. Miller GE, Chen E, Zhou ES. If it goes up, must it come down? Chronic stress and the hypothalamic-pituitary-adrenocortical axis in humans. *Psychol Bull* (2007) 133(1):25–45. doi: 10.1037/0033-2909.133.1.25
41. Hintsa T, Elovainio M, Jokela M, Ahola K, Virtanen M, Pirkola S. Is there an independent association between burnout and increased allostatic load? Testing the contribution of psychological distress and depression. *J Health Psychol* (2016) 21(8):1576–86. doi: 10.1177/1359105314559619
42. Scheuer S, Wiggert N, Brückl TM, Awaloff Y, Uhr M, Lucae S, et al. Childhood abuse and depression in adulthood: The mediating role of allostatic load. *Psychoneuroendocrinology* (2018) 94:134–42. doi: 10.1016/j.psyneuen.2018.04.020
43. Duong MT, Bingham BA, Aldana PC, Chung ST, Sumner AE. Variation in the calculation of allostatic load score: 21 examples from NHANES. *J Racial Ethn. Heal Disparities* (2017) 4(3):455–61. doi: 10.1007/s40615-016-0246-8
44. Greaves RF, Wudy SA, Badoer E, Zacharin M, Hirst JJ, Quinn T, et al. A tale of two steroids: The importance of the androgens DHEA and DHEAS for early neurodevelopment. *J Steroid Biochem Mol Biol* (2019) 188:77–85. doi: 10.1016/j.jsbmb.2018.12.007

45. Kamin HS, Kertes DA. Cortisol and DHEA in development and psychopathology. *Hormones Behav* (2017) 89:69–85. doi: 10.1016/j.yhbeh.2016.11.018
46. Kent M, Bardi M, Hazelgrove A, Sewell K, Kirk E, Thompson B, et al. Profiling coping strategies in male and female rats: Potential neurobehavioral markers of increased resilience to depressive symptoms. *Horm. Behav* (2017) 95:33–43. doi: 10.1016/j.yhbeh.2017.07.011
47. Sullivan EDK, Kent M, Thompson B, Bardi M, Lambert K. Maternal-induced shifts in allostatic demands: Reproductive experience alters emotional and cognitive biobehavioral responses in rats (Rattus norvegicus). *Neurosci Lett* (2019) 701:1–7. doi: 10.1016/j.neulet.2019.01.048
48. Lopresti AL, Smith SJ, Malvi H, Kodgule R. An investigation into the stress-relieving and pharmacological actions of an ashwagandha (Withania somnifera) extract. *Med (Baltimore).* (2019) 98(37):e17186. doi: 10.1097/MD.0000000000017186
49. Field T. Infants of depressed mothers. *Dev Psychopathol.* (1992) 4(1):49–66. doi: 10.1017/S0954579400005551
50. Kaplan LA, Evans L, Monk C. Effects of mothers' prenatal psychiatric status and postnatal caregiving on infant biobehavioral regulation: Can prenatal programming be modified? *Early Hum Dev* (2008) 84(4):249–56. doi: 10.1016/j.earlhumdev.2007.06.004
51. Cicchetti D, Toth SL. The past achievements and future promises of developmental psychopathology: The coming of age of a discipline. *J Child Psychol Psychiatry Allied Discip.* (2009) 50(1–2):16–25. doi: 10.1111/j.1469-7610.2008.01979.x
52. Laurent HK, Leve LD, Neiderhiser JM, Natsuaki MN, Shaw DS, Harold GT, et al. Effects of prenatal and postnatal parent depressive symptoms on adopted child HPA regulation: Independent and moderated influences. *Dev Psychol* (2013) 49(5):876–86. doi: 10.1037/a0028800
53. Behrendt HF, Scharke W, Herpertz-Dahlmann B, Konrad K, Firk C. Like mother, like child? Maternal determinants of children's early social-emotional development. *Infant Ment Health J* (2019) 40(2):234–47. doi: 10.1002/imhj.21765
54. McEWEN BS. Stress, Adaptation, and Disease: Allostasis and Allostatic Load. *Ann N Y. Acad Sci* (1998) 840(1):33–44. doi: 10.1111/j.1749-6632.1998.tb09546.x
55. Strain JJ. The psychobiology of stress, depression, adjustment disorders and resilience. *World J Biol Psychiatry* (2018) 19(supl):S14–20. doi: 10.1080/15622975.2018.1459049
56. Apter-Levy Y, Feldman M, Vakart A, Ebstein RP, Feldman R. Impact of maternal depression across the first 6 years of life on the child's mental health, social engagement, and empathy: The moderating role of oxytocin. *Am J Psychiatry* (2013) 170(10):1161–8. doi: 10.1176/appi.ajp.2013.12121597

2

Sleep Problems and Social Impairment in Psychosis: A Transdiagnostic Study Examining Multiple Social Domains

Jack J. Blanchard[1], Christina L. G. Savage[1], Ryan D. Orth[1], Anyela M. Jacome[1] and Melanie E. Bennett[2,3]*

[1] Department of Psychology, University of Maryland, College Park, College Park, MD, United States, [2] Department of Psychiatry, University of Maryland, Baltimore, Baltimore, MD, United States, [3] Department of Psychiatry, Baltimore VA Medical Center, Baltimore, MD, United States

***Correspondence:**
Jack J. Blanchard
jblancha@umd.edu

Psychotic disorders are characterized by profound social impairment. An accumulation of research has explored the contribution of symptoms, cognitive functioning, and behavioral skills deficits to this social dysfunction. Recent research indicates that sleep disturbance has significant social implications in nonclinical populations—this research suggests that sleep problems may also be relevant to understanding social impairment in psychosis. This study adopted a symptom-oriented dimensional approach to examine how sleep disturbance and sleep-related impairment are related to multiple social domains within a transdiagnostic sample (N = 90). This sample included individuals with a variety of psychotic disorders (n = 75) along with healthy non-clinical participants (n = 15) to ensure sampling across the full range of sleep problems and social functioning. Social domains spanned self-reported perceptions of social relationships, social functioning in the community, and behavioral assessments of social competence. We hypothesized that greater sleep disturbance and sleep-related impairment would be associated with more negative or problematic perceptions of social relationships (i.e., less social support, less companionship, and greater distress), poorer social functioning in the community, smaller social networks, and poorer behavioral ratings of social competency. Results supported these hypotheses indicating that sleep disturbance and sleep-related impairment have widespread deleterious impacts on perceptions of social relationships, social functioning, and competence. Sleep disturbance retained associations with perceptions of social relationships, social functioning, and social competence even after controlling for total symptoms or cognitive functioning. These findings indicate that sleep problems may have important implications for fully understanding the causes of social impairment in psychosis.

Keywords: psychotic disorders, sleep disturbance, social functioning, social relationships, transdiagnostic, clinical symptoms

INTRODUCTION

Psychotic disorders, such as schizophrenia and bipolar disorder with psychosis, lead to profound and enduring social impairment (1–3). This impairment includes greater social isolation, lower rates of marriage, fewer friends, and strained family relationships (4, 5). When individuals with psychotic disorders do interact socially, they often have difficulty with the basic skills necessary to have a successful social interaction (6–8). This social impairment persists following stabilization of psychotic symptomatology with medication (9, 10). In a recent 20-year outcome study of individuals initially admitted with a first episode of psychosis, results indicated stable impairment in social functioning across psychotic diagnoses (11).

Social impairment in psychosis is determined by multiple factors. Findings in schizophrenia indicate that social impairment is a consequence of the combined effects of negative symptoms (12), cognitive impairment [e.g., (13, 14)], social cognitive impairment (15), and poor functional capacity or social skill (6–8). These factors have been shown to interact to result in social impairment in schizophrenia (16). A similar pattern of results has been obtained in bipolar disorder with negative symptoms, cognitive impairment, and poor functional capacity associated with poor community functioning (17).

Recent research suggests the novel idea that sleep may be an important consideration in understanding social impairment in psychosis. Sleep disturbances, such as insomnia, have been found to be related to a variety of mental disorders (18, 19). As a result, sleep disturbance has increasingly been viewed as a transdiagnostic factor contributing to psychiatric symptomatology and functional impairment (20, 21). Research indicates that sleep may be especially important in psychosis given that sleep disturbances and sleep disorders occur frequently in psychotic disorders [e.g., (22–24)] and are evident early in the course of psychosis (25, 26). Importantly, as reviewed below, sleep problems are tied to a variety of social difficulties.

Gordon et al. (27) have proposed a model outlining the bidirectional effects of sleep and social processes [also see review by Troxel (28) for a similar bidirectional perspective]. In this model, sleep has widespread impacts on social processes from social cognition to interpersonal behavior. Further, one's social environment and experiences can have both positive and negative implications for various sleep parameters (27). Evidence supporting these bidirectional models comes from a variety of sources. Poor sleep quality, including even mild insomnia, has adverse impacts on overall quality of life including reports of poorer social functioning (29, 30). Marital relationship quality has been found to be related to sleep disturbances [see (28)] and perceived better relationship quality with relatives and friends has been found to be associated with better sleep quality (31). Supportive social relationships have been shown to be related to better sleep quality while aversive or strained social ties are related to poorer sleep quality (32–34). Finally, loneliness has been shown to be associated with poorer sleep efficiency (35) and sleep-related daytime dysfunction (36).

Beyond cross-sectional findings showing an association between social relationships and sleep, other methods have been used to directly test the causal role that sleep may have in social outcomes. In a 3-year longitudinal study, Tavernier and Willoughby (37) found bidirectional effects of sleep problems and poorer social ties with a mediating role of affect regulation. Using daily sleep diaries, Gordon and Chen (38) demonstrated that relatively poorer sleep leads to greater interpersonal conflict the following day (even after controlling for prior conflict). Providing social rejection feedback has been shown to lead to poorer subsequent sleep (27). Within couples' interactions, poorer prior night sleep has been found to be related to a lower ratio of positive to negative affect, lower empathic accuracy, and less conflict resolution (38). Simon and Walker (39) have shown that experimental sleep deprivation can lead to social withdrawal and feelings of loneliness. Importantly, it was also demonstrated that when sleep deprived, individuals behave in ways that lead observers to perceive the individual as lonely and observers reported that they would be less willing to interact socially or collaboratively with the sleep deprived individual (39). Simon and Walker (39) concluded that sleep loss leads to a self-reinforcing cycle of social separation and withdrawal. Finally, sleep intervention for insomnia has been shown to improve self-reported social functioning [e.g., (40)], and treatments for obstructive sleep apnea have been shown to improve social functioning (41) and marital satisfaction (42).

Less is understood regarding the social implication of sleep in psychosis. In schizophrenia, poor sleep quality has been found to be associated with lower self-reported quality of life (43, 44) including less enjoyment and satisfaction with social relationships (45). Relationships between sleep quality and quality of life (including satisfaction with social relationships) have been shown to persist even after controlling for depression or medication side effects (45). Beyond ratings of satisfaction, lower sleep quality has been found to be related to poorer personal and social functioning in individuals with schizophrenia (46). Liu et al. (47) examined self-reported symptoms of obstructive sleep apnea (OSA; snoring, pauses in breathing during sleep, and disrupted sleep) within individuals with psychotic disorders and found that reports of pauses in breathing were associated with poorer overall health-related quality of life, including lower independent living and lower well-being (but not social relations). Findings from Liu et al. (47) are somewhat limited in that only single items were used to assess OSA-related symptoms and these symptoms were dichotomously scored as present or absent. In addition to research conducted on individuals with psychosis, other research indicates that sleep problems are related to poor role and social functioning in those at clinical high-risk for psychosis (48).

Consistent with the research in non-clinical populations, the existing literature suggests potential links between sleep disturbance and social impairment in psychosis. However, this sleep research in psychosis is limited in that few studies have examined objective indicators of social functioning [e.g., (46)] and most studies have examined social functioning at a very broad level focusing on quality of life or satisfaction with social functioning. Further, we are not aware of any study that has examined the impact of sleep on self-reports of social support (33, 34) or other perceptions of social relationships [e.g., loneliness (35)] that have been found to be associated with sleep quality. Finally, no study has examined how sleep is related to actual social behavior in psychotic disorders using assessments of social skill or competence—an important consideration given the clinical importance of skills deficits in determining functional impairment in psychosis (7, 8, 16, 17).

Guided by the NIMH research domain criteria (RDoC) framework (49–51), we adopted a symptom-oriented dimensional approach to examine how sleep disturbance and sleep-related impairment are related to multiple social domains within a transdiagnostic sample of individuals (N = 90). This sample included individuals with a variety of psychotic disorders (n = 75) along with healthy non-clinical participants (n = 15) to ensure sampling across the full range of sleep problems and social functioning. Social domains spanned self-reported perceptions of social relationships, functioning in the community, and behavioral assessments of social competence. We hypothesized that greater sleep disturbance and sleep-related impairment would be associated with more negative or problematic perceptions of social relationships (i.e., less social support, less companionship, and greater distress), poorer social functioning in the community, smaller social networks, and poorer behavioral ratings of social competency.

TABLE 1 | Sample characteristics (N = 90).

	Mean (SD) or n (percent)
Age (years)	44.44 (11.66)
Sex	
Male	55 (61.1%)
Female	35 (38.9%)
Race	
African-American	66 (73.3%)
White	19 (21.1%)
Asian	2 (2.2%)
More than one race	3 (3.3%)
Ethnicity	
Non-Hispanic or Latino	82 (91.1%)
Hispanic or Latino	7 (7.8%)
Unknown	1 (1.1%)
Marital Status	
Married	6 (6.7%)
Divorced/separated	13 (14.4%)
Never married/single	71 (78.9%)
Education (years)	12.78 (2.32)
Has a paying job	
Yes	29 (32.2%)
No	61 (67.8%)
Diagnosis	
Schizophrenia	34 (37.8%)
Schizoaffective Bipolar Type	13 (14.4%)
Schizoaffective Depressive Type	13 (14.4%)
Delusional disorder	1 (1.1%)
BP I w/ psychotic features	8 (8.9%)
MDD w/ psychotic features	6 (6.7%)
No diagnosis (healthy control)	15 (16.7%)

BP, Bipolar; MDD, Major Depressive Disorder.

MATERIALS AND METHODS

Participants

Participants were enrolled in a larger ongoing grant-funded project examining social affiliative deficits from an RDoC perspective (National Institutes of Health grant R01MH110462). The mixed sample (N = 90) included clinical (n = 75) and non-clinical community (n = 15) participants. Participants diagnosed with a psychotic disorder (e.g., schizophrenia/schizoaffective disorder, delusional disorder, major depression with psychosis) were recruited from outpatient mental health clinics in the Baltimore and Washington, D.C. metro areas. Demographic and diagnostic characteristics of the study sample are summarized in **Table 1**. Diagnoses were determined with the Structured Clinical Interview for DSM-5 (SCID-5) (52). The majority of clinical participants were prescribed various forms of antipsychotic medication, including atypical antipsychotics (n = 46, 61%), typical antipsychotics (n = 10; 13%), or a combination of atypical and typical antipsychotics (n = 10; 13%). Other prescribed medications for clinical participants included antidepressants (n = 42, 61%), antianxiety (n = 32, 52%), mood stabilizers (n = 30, 40%), and antiparkinsonian medications (n = 21, 28%). We have previously reported on symptom correlates of sleep problems in this sample (53).

Inclusion criteria for clinical participants included (1) aged 18–60, (2) lifetime history of a psychotic disorder, (3) clinical stability (i.e., no inpatient hospitalizations for 3 months before enrollment, no changes in psychoactive medication in the 4 weeks before enrollment) as indicated by approval of clinician and medical record review, and (4) fluent in English. Community participants were recruited *via* online advertisements, and inclusion criteria included (1) aged 18–60, (2) no current clinical disorder or psychiatric medications, (3) no lifetime history of a psychotic or mood disorder, (4) no avoidant, paranoid, schizotypal, or schizoid personality disorder, and (5) fluent in English. Exclusion criteria for all participants included (1) current substance use disorder, (2) neurological conditions (e.g., epilepsy, multiple sclerosis), (3) evidence of intellectual disability as determined by medical history or cognitive testing, (4) any history of serious head injury, (5) any MRI contraindications (e.g., MRI unsafe metal in body, weight that exceeds the limitations of MRI machine), and (6) unwillingness to be videotaped during study participation.

Assessment of Sleep

Sleep assessments utilized the National Institutes of Health Patient-Reported Outcomes Measurement Information System (PROMIS™) Sleep Disturbance and Sleep-Related Impairment short-form scales (54). The Sleep Disturbance scale includes items such as "I had difficulty falling asleep" and "I had trouble staying asleep". The Sleep-Related Impairment scale includes items such as "I had a hard time concentrating because of poor sleep" and "I had a hard time getting things done because I was sleepy". These scales were developed using rigorous item-response theory methods as well as clinical judgement from content experts. The PROMIS™ Sleep Disturbance scale has demonstrated high convergent validity with the Pittsburgh Sleep Quality Index and both the PROMIS™ Sleep Disturbance and Sleep-Related Impairment scales are capable of differentiating healthy individuals from those with clinically diagnosed sleep disorders (54). The PROMIS™ sleep scales have also been shown to be sensitive to treatment effects of positive airway pressure therapy (55). Although not intended to measure symptoms of specific sleep disorders, the PROMIS™ scales do tap sleep quality and sleep dissatisfaction; thus, they are useful in assessing global severity of insomnia (54).

Assessment of Functioning

The Adult Social Relationships Scales (ASRS) (56) consists of six self-report scales assessing for participant appraisals of social relationships over the past month across multiple domains. Domains assessed include perceived social rejection, perceived hostility, loneliness, friendship, instrumental support, and emotional support. The ASRS is part of the NIH Toolbox for the Assessment of Neurological and Behavioral Function and each scale has good internal reliability and concurrent validity with other instruments (56).

The Specific Levels of Functioning Scale (SLOF) (57) is a self-report measure that assesses community functioning. It consists of four subscales related to social and community functioning (Interpersonal Relationships, Social Acceptability, Involvement in Activities and Work Skills). The SLOF has been judged to be the best available measure of real-world functioning (21). Consistent with the procedures used in other samples with psychosis [see (21)], participants completed a 30-item self-report measure of their "*typical* level of functioning" rated on a five-point Likert scale. Higher ratings indicate better functioning.

The Social Network Index (SNI) (58) is a 13-item self-report measure assessing for social network size. Social network size is the total number of individuals whom the respondent has had contact with at least once in the previous two weeks. The SNI has been used to study social relationships in samples at ultra-high risk for psychosis (59) and has been shown to relate to neuromorphology and brain function in neuroimaging studies (60, 61).

The UCSD Performance-Based Skills Assessment Brief Version (UPSA-B) (7) utilizes the Financial and Communications subscales, two out of the five original subscales that make-up the full UPSA. The UPSA-B uses role-playing tasks to assess an individual's capacity to perform everyday tasks as an indicator of their real-world functioning in the community. The financial skills subscale asks participants to count and make change using monetary props (i.e., US dollar bills and coins), and analyze and fill out a check for a utility bill. The Communication skills subscale asks participants to demonstrate their knowledge of using the telephone by rescheduling an appointment, dialing emergency services, and dialing directory assistance to obtain a telephone number. The total score ranges from 0 to 100 and is calculated by summing each of the two subscales with standardized scores ranging on a 0 to 50 scale. Higher scores indicate higher functional capacity. The UPSA-B has been found to be a valid behavioral measure of functional milestones and has good predictive validity for vocational outcomes (7). In a recent review (62), the UPSA was found to have robust relations with social functioning as assessed with the SLOF.

The MATRICS Consensus Cognitive Battery (MCCB) (63) is a cognitive battery designed specifically for people with psychosis. It includes 10 measures assessing for cognitive functioning in seven domains. Domains include speed of processing, attention, working memory, verbal learning, visual learning, reasoning and problem solving, and social cognition. Each of the measures included in the battery has demonstrated acceptable validity and test-retest reliability (63). The MCCB has been shown to be related to functional outcomes in schizophrenia [e.g., (64)].

Assessment of Symptomology

Brief Psychiatric Rating Scale, expanded version (BPRS) (65), is a 24-item clinical interview designed to assess current clinical symptomatology as experienced over the previous week. For the purposes of this study, an overall BPRS score was used to assess total symptom severity. The BPRS has shown acceptable test-rest reliability, internal correlation coefficients, and discriminant validity (66).

Procedures

Data were collected from within a larger fMRI study exploring the links between social affiliation and neurological threat response along with social reward processing. Study procedures were approved by the University of Maryland School of Medicine Institutional Review Board. Participants completed a standardized informed consent process with trained recruiters and signed an informed consent document. A brief questionnaire was administered by trained study staff to verify that participants were competent to provide consent and understood the consent document. After the consent process, participants completed in-person clinical interviews and self-report paper-and-pencil questionnaires related to diagnoses, cognitive functioning, social affiliation, and social functioning. Participants were also compensated for their participation.

Data Analysis

Descriptive statistics for the sleep and social functioning measures are presented in **Table 2**. As reflected in the T-score values, PROMIS™ scales of sleep disturbance (range = 28.90–76.50) and sleep-related impairment (range = 30.00–76.90) represented a wide range, including values that were greater than two standard deviations above the population average (54). There were no significant differences between male and female participants in sleep disturbance ($t = 1.88$, $p = .07$) or sleep impairment ($t = 0.52$, $p = .61$). Age was not correlated with either sleep disturbance ($r = .14$, $p = .20$) or sleep impairment ($r = -.04$, $p = .72$). Given these null results, sex and age were not considered in the analyses. Descriptive statistics for total symptoms and MATRICS cognitive measures are presented in **Table 3**. Correlational analyses were conducted to assess the relation between sleep and social measures with additional partial

TABLE 2 | Descriptive statistics for sleep and social functioning assessments.

	M (SD)
Sleep Disturbance (n = 90)	17.74 (7.73)
T-Score	46.00 (10.58)
Sleep-Related Impairment (n = 90)	17.02 (7.21)
T-Score	49.37 (10.64)
Adult Social Relationship Scales	
Emotional Support (n = 90)	32.28 (7.45)
Instrumental Support (n = 89)	26.42 (8.84)
Friendship (n = 88)	25.41 (7.92)
Loneliness (n = 89)	10.82 (5.64)
Perceived Rejection (n = 89)	15.01 (6.99)
Hostility (n = 88)	14.67 (6.82)
Social Functioning (SLOF)	
Interpersonal (n = 90)	27.78 (6.08)
Social Acceptability (n = 90)	27.58 (2.67)
Social Function (n = 90)	55.36 (7.48)
Activities (n = 89)	52.21 (6.33)
Work Skills (n = 89)	26.54 (3.81)
Comm Living Skills (n = 88)	83.31 (9.19)
Social Network Size (n = 90)	11.16 (7.37)
Social Competence (UPSA)	
Financial (n = 89)	41.09 (8.12)
Communication (n = 90)	37.00 (9.10)

SLOF, Specific Level of Function Scale; UPSA, University of California, San Diego (UCSD) Performance-Based Skills Assessment.

TABLE 3 | Descriptive statistics for symptoms and cognitive functioning.

	M (SD)
BPRS Total Symptom Score (n = 90)	37.24 (9.81)
MATRICS Consensus Cognitive Battery:	
Trail Making Test, Part A (n = 90)	49.69 (29.30)
Symbol Coding (n = 89)	40.46 (14.81)
Category Fluency (n = 88)	18.60 (5.80)
Verbal Learning (n = 90)	19.81 (6.67)
Spatial Span (n = 89)	12.97 (3.66)
Letter-Number Span (n = 89)	10.73 (4.30)
Mazes (n = 87)	9.53 (6.64)
Visuospatial Memory (n = 86)	15.83 (8.76)
Managing Emotions (n = 88)	88.96 (14.70)
Continuous Performance Test (n = 87)	3.40 (16.14)

correlation analyses conducted to control for symptomatology and cognitive impairment.

RESULTS

Correlations between sleep variables and social variables are presented in **Table 4**. Results from the Adult Social Relationship Scale indicated that greater sleep disturbance and sleep-related impairment were related to self-reports of lower perceived emotional support (but not instrumental support), lower ratings of friendship and greater loneliness (range of rs = −.25 to −.28, ps < 05). Greater sleep disturbance and sleep-related impairment were related to greater social distress as reflected by associations with perceived social rejection and hostility from others (range of rs = .36 to .44, ps < .01).

TABLE 4 | Social correlates of sleep disturbance and sleep-related impairment.

	Sleep Disturbance	Sleep-Related Impairment
Adult Social Relationship Scales		
Emotional Support	−.28**	−.25*
Instrumental Support	−.09	−.16
Friendship	−.27*	−.26*
Loneliness	.36**	.36**
Perceived Rejection	.36**	.41***
Hostility	.37***	.44***
Social Functioning (SLOF)		
Interpersonal	−.33***	−.36***
Social Acceptability	−.40***	−.50***
Overall Social Function	−.41***	−.47***
Activities	−.16	−.06
Work Skills	−.41***	−.49***
Community Living Skills	−.30**	−.25*
Social Network	−.22*	−.15
Social Competence (UPSA)		
Financial	−.17	−.12
Communication	−.26*	−.33***

*SLOF, Specific Level of Function Scale; UPSA, University of California, San Diego (UCSD) Performance-Based Skills Assessment. *p < .05; **p < .01; ***p < .005.*

With regard to social functioning, greater sleep disturbance and sleep-related impairment were associated with poorer functioning across all domains with the exception of activities (range of rs = −.25 to −.50, ps < .05). Turning to social network size, greater sleep disturbance (but not sleep-related impairment) was related to smaller social networks (r = −.22, p < .05). Finally, greater sleep disturbance and sleep-related impairment were related to poorer social competence as measured by ratings of communication skills (rs = −.26 and −.33, respectively, ps < .05) but not financial skills on the UPSA.

Given that symptoms and cognitive impairment can contribute to social dysfunction, we sought to determine if sleep disturbance continued to hold a relation with social variables after controlling for total symptoms on the BPRS (due to missing data, partial correlations range of n = 83–87) and after simultaneously controlling for all seven MATRICS subtests (due to missing data, partial correlations range of n = 72–76). Results of partial correlations are presented in **Table 5**. After controlling for the BPRS total symptom score, greater sleep disturbance continued to be related to more social distress as reflected by greater perceived rejection and hostility. Sleep disturbance also remained associated with a range of social functioning measures except activities and community living skills. Finally, greater sleep disturbance remained associated with poorer social competence as assessed by the UPSA communication scale. A similar pattern of results was obtained after controlling for cognitive performance with sleep disturbance retaining associations across perceptions of social relationships, social functioning as well as social competence (communication).

DISCUSSION

This study sought to examine the contribution of sleep disturbance and sleep-related impairment to a variety of social

TABLE 5 | Social correlates of sleep disturbance controlling for symptoms and cognitive impairment.

	Sleep Disturbance	
	Controlling for Symptoms partial-r	**Controlling for Cognitive Impairment partial-r**
Adult Social Relationship Scales		
Emotional Support	−.18	−.19
Instrumental Support	−.08	−.14
Friendship	−.17	−.18
Loneliness	.17	.34**
Perceived Rejection	.27*	.33***
Hostility	.30**	.43***
Social Functioning (SLOF)		
Interpersonal	−.23*	−.28*
Social Acceptability	−.34***	−.46***
Overall Social Function	−.32***	−.41***
Activities	.06	−.04
Work Skills	−.38***	−.39***
Community Living Skills	−.11	−.20
Social Network	−.11	−.04
Social Competence (UPSA)		
Financial	−.07	−.15
Communication	−.22*	−.25*

*SLOF, Specific Level of Function Scale; UPSA, University of California, San Diego (UCSD) Performance-Based Skills Assessment. *p < .05; **p < .01; ***p < .005.*

domains within a transdiagnostic sample including psychotic disorders. Sleep disturbance and sleep-related impairment were assessed with standardized and validated measures. A strength of the study was that social assessments spanned several domains including self-reported perceptions of social relationships, social functioning in the community, social network size, and behavioral assessments of social competence.

Regarding perceptions of social relationships, sleep disturbance and sleep-related impairment were related to reports of lower emotional (but not instrumental) support as well as lower reports of friendship and greater loneliness. The results are consistent with findings from non-clinical samples indicating that lower social support and greater loneliness are related to lower sleep quality (32–35) and greater sleep-related impairment (36) and extend these findings to samples with psychosis. Further, both facets of sleep problems were related to greater perceptions of social rejection and hostility from others. These results are consistent with prior findings that social rejection is related to sleep disturbance in healthy individuals (27). The results for perceptions of social relationships as hostile are potentially consistent with findings that greater paranoid ideation is related to poorer sleep quality in clinical [e.g., (67)] and non-clinical [e.g., (68)] samples. The association between greater emotional support and friendship and lower sleep disturbance found in zero-order correlations were no longer maintained when controlling for symptoms or cognitive functioning. However, greater perceived rejection and hostility remained associated with greater sleep disturbance even after controlling for total symptoms and overall cognitive functioning (and loneliness remained related to sleep disturbance after controlling for cognitive performance). This pattern of results indicates that sleep disturbance may have an especially robust impact on negative perceptions of social relations potentially leading to a sense of rejection and perceptions of being treated in a hostile manner by others.

Greater sleep disturbance and sleep-related impairment were associated with social dysfunction across a variety of domains including poorer overall functioning and poorer work functioning. Notably, these correlates reflected medium to large effect sizes. Importantly, these associations between sleep disturbance and poorer social functioning persisted even after controlling for symptoms or cognitive functioning (factors known to contribute to social impairment). These results suggest that sleep disturbance may have a unique contribution to social impairment in psychosis above and beyond symptomatology and cognitive impairment. Our findings replicate and extend those of Afonso et al. (46) indicating that lower sleep quality was related to poorer personal and social functioning in individuals with schizophrenia.

Findings indicated that sleep disturbance and sleep-related impairment were related to behavioral ratings of social competence in the domain of communication (but not finance). Sleep disturbance remained associated with social competency ratings in communication even after controlling for symptoms and cognitive impairment. This is the first demonstration that we are aware of showing that sleep disturbance manifests in behavior with impaired social skill. Given the contribution of social competence to functional impairment (7, 8, 16), this suggests that sleep disturbance may be a relevant factor to consider in models that seek to understand skills deficits and functional impairment in psychotic disorders.

Overall, our results indicate that sleep problems in psychosis are associated with a variety of social problems involving negative social perceptions, poor functioning in the community, and diminished social skill. These results fit with prior work in non-clinical populations indicating the important connections between sleep and social processes (27, 28). The current findings are cross-sectional; thus, we are not able to disentangle to what extent sleep problems precede and give rise to social problems [e.g., (38, 39)] or whether social difficulties contribute causally to sleep problems [e.g., (27)]. However, current models emphasize a bidirectional relationship between sleep and social behavior (27).

The present findings suggest several paths for future research. An examination of how sleep problems impact social functioning is needed to better understand the mechanisms underlying this association. Prior research suggests that sleep insufficiency may lead to behavioral alterations including a lower ratio of positive to negative affect, lower empathic accuracy, and less conflict resolution (38). Sleep loss may also contribute to feelings of loneliness and self-initiated social withdrawal that adversely impacts observers desire to interact with an individual (39).

Beyond clinical, self-report and behavioral assessments, future research should explore neural mechanisms that might underlie the connection between sleep and social dysfunction in psychosis. Simon and Walker (39) found that sleep deprivation results in social withdrawal based on reduced activity in theory of mind neural networks and increased activity in brain regions involved in perceiving threatening approach. Insomnia has been shown to increase amygdala activation and reduce prefrontal-amygdala connectivity (69–71). Given the role of the amygdala and related structures in negative affect and threat perception [e.g., (72, 73)], amygdala activation associated with sleep insufficiency may in part contribute to perceptions of social rejection and hostility. It is interesting that, paralleling findings of amygdala activation in schizophrenia (74), sleep deprivation has been found to result in elevated amygdala activity to both aversive and neutral stimuli (75). Thus, sleep insufficiency may lead to neural changes that contribute to the misinterpretation of neutral or ambiguous stimuli as threatening. Additional research is required to further examine if sleep insufficiency contributes to social impairment through changes in brain circuitry that are involved in social avoidance, threat perception, and negative affect.

Finally, the current results may have implications for developing interventions to improve social functioning in psychosis. Our findings suggest that sleep disturbance may contribute to social impairment beyond overall symptoms and cognitive impairment. Should this finding be replicated, such an association might indicate that targeting sleep disturbance could enhance functional outcomes in psychotic disorders. Prior research has indicated that sleep interventions can positively impact social functioning in non-psychiatric individuals [e.g., (40–42)]. Given the association between negative symptoms and social impairment in psychosis (12) and the relationship between sleep problems and negative symptoms (53), it is interesting to speculate that adding sleep interventions to treatments for negative symptoms and social impairment could potentiate clinical outcomes to further enhance recovery.

Several limitations constrain interpretation of the present findings. First, as noted previously, this is a cross-sectional study and we are not able to establish if sleep disturbance and related impairment are contributing to social problems or if social difficulties give rise to sleep problems. Second, while we adopted an RDoC approach (49–51) to examine transdiagnostic associations from a dimensional perspective, we were not able to explore the potential differential relations of sleep domains across different diagnoses or differences between clinical and non-clinical participants. Third, the majority of clinical participants were receiving various forms of medication and we are not able to examine how different types or dosages of medication may contribute to sleep problems. Finally, assessment of sleep disturbance and sleep-related impairment were limited to self-reports. We do not have information relevant to the presence of clinically diagnosed sleep disorders nor do we have information based on other methods such as sleep diaries or actigraphy—methods that may provide additional information on sleep parameters not captured in our current assessments.

In summary, consistent with our hypotheses, results indicated that sleep disturbance and sleep-related impairment have widespread deleterious impacts on perceptions of social relationships, social functioning, and social competence or behavioral skill. Sleep disturbance retained its associations with perceptions of social relationships, social functioning, and social competence even after controlling for total symptoms or cognitive functioning. These findings have implications for understanding the profound social impairment that occurs in psychosis and suggest novel approaches to treating social dysfunction in these disorders.

AUTHOR CONTRIBUTIONS

JB and MB developed the study design. RO, AJ, and CS assisted with data collection. JB analyzed the data. All authors contributed to writing the manuscript.

ACKNOWLEDGMENTS

The authors would also like to thank all site staff and research participants in the collection of these data.

REFERENCES

1. Simonsen C, Sundet K, Vaskinn A, Ueland T, Romm KL, Hellvin T, et al. Psychosocial function in schizophrenia and bipolar disorder: relationship to neurocognition and clinical symptoms. *J Int Neuropsychol Soc Soc* (2010) 16:771–83. doi: 10.1017/S1355617710000573
2. van Rheenen TE, Rossell SL. Objective and subjective psychosocial functioning in bipolar disorder: an investigation of the relative importance of neurocognition, social cognition and emotion regulation. *J Affect Disord* (2014) 162:134–41. doi: 10.1016/j.jad.2014.03.043
3. Wiersma D, Wanderling J, Dragomirecka E, Ganev K, Harrison G, an der Heiden WA, et al. Social disability in schizophrenia: its development and prediction over 15 years in incidence cohorts in six European centres. *Psychol Med Med* (2000) 30:1155–67. doi: 10.1017/S0033291799002627
4. Green MF, Horan WP, Lee J, McCleery A, Reddy LF, Wynn JK. Social disconnection in schizophrenia and the general community. *Schizophr Bull* (2018) 44:242–9. doi: 10.1093/schbul/sbx082
5. Gayer-Anderson C, Morgan C. Social networks, support and early psychosis: a systematic review. *Epidemiol Psychiatr Sci* (2013) 22:131–46. doi: 10.1017/S2045796012000406
6. Blanchard JJ, Park SG, Catalano LT, Bennett ME. Social affiliation and negative symptoms in schizophrenia: examining the role of behavioral skills and subjective responding. *Schizophr Res* (2015) 168:491–7. doi: 10.1016/j.schres.2015.07.019
7. Mausbach BT, Harvey PD, Pulver AE, Depp CA, Wolyniec PS, Thornquist MH, et al. Relationship of the Brief UCSD Performance-based Skills Assessment (UPSA-B) to multiple indicators of functioning in people with schizophrenia and bipolar disorder. *Bipolar Disord* (2010) 12:45–55. doi: 10.1111/j.1399-5618.2009.00787.x

8. Mueser KT, Bellack AS, Douglas MS, Morrison RL. Prevalence and stability of social skill deficits in schizophrenia. *Schizophr Res* (1991) 5:167–76. doi: 10.1016/0920-9964(91)90044-R
9. Bellack AS, Schooler NR, Marder SR, Kane JM, Brown CH, Yang Y. Do clozapine and risperidone affect social competence and problem solving? *Am J Psychiatry* (2004) 161:364–7. doi: 10.1176/appi.ajp.161.2.364
10. Huxley N, Baldessarini RJ. Disability and its treatment in bipolar disorder patients. *Bipolar Disord* (2007) 9:183–96. doi: 10.1111/j.1399-5618.2007.00430.x
11. Velthorst E, Fett AKJ, Reichenberg A, Perlman G, van Os J, Bromet EJ, et al. The 20-year longitudinal trajectories of social functioning in individuals with psychotic disorders. *Am J Psychiatry* (2016) 174:1075–85. doi: 10.1176/appi.ajp.2016.15111419
12. Blanchard JJ, Bradshaw KR, Garcia CP, Nasrallah HA, Harvey PD, Casey D, et al. Examining the reliability and validity of the Clinical Assessment Interview for Negative Symptoms within the Management of Schizophrenia in Clinical Practice (MOSAIC) multisite national study. *Schizophr Res* (2017) 185:137–43. doi: 10.1016/j.schres.2017.01.011
13. Cohen A, Forbes CB, Mann MC, Blanchard JJ. Specific cognitive deficits and differential domains of social functioning impairment in schizophrenia. *Schizophr Res* (2006) 81:227–38. doi: 10.1016/j.schres.2005.09.007
14. Jabben N, Arts B, van Os J, Krabbendam L. Neurocognitive functioning as intermediary phenotype and predictor of psychosocial functioning across the psychosis continuum: studies in schizophrenia and bipolar disorder. *J Clin Psychiatry* (2010) 71:764–74. doi: 10.4088/JCP.08m04837yel
15. Fett A-KJ, Viechtbauer W, Dominguez M-G, Penn DL, van Os J, Krabbendam L. The relationship between neurocognition and social cognition with functional outcomes in schizophrenia: a meta-analysis. *Neurosci Biobehav Rev* (2011) 35:573–88. doi: 10.1016/j.neubiorev.2010.07.001
16. Bowie CR, Reichenberg A, Patterson TL, Heaton RK, Harvey PD. Determinants of real-world functional performance in schizophrenia subjects: correlations with cognition, functional capacity, and symptoms. *Am J Psychiatry* (2006) 163:418–25. doi: 10.1176/appi.ajp.163.3.418
17. Bowie CR, Depp C, McGrath JA, Wolyniec P, Mausbach BT, Thornquist MH, et al. Prediction of real-world functional disability in chronic mental disorders: a comparison of schizophrenia and bipolar disorder. *Am J Psychiatry* (2010) 167:1116–24. doi: 10.1176/appi.ajp.2010.09101406
18. Benca RM, Obermeyer WH, Thisted RA, Gillin JC. Sleep and psychiatric disorders: a meta-analysis. *Arch Gen Psychiatry* (1992) 49:651–68. doi: 10.1001/archpsyc.1992.01820080059010
19. Klingaman EA, Brownlow JA, Boland EM, Mosti C, Gehrman PR. Prevalence, predictors and correlates of insomnia in US army soldiers. *J Sleep Res* (2017) 27:1–13. doi: 10.1111/jsr.12612
20. Harvey AG. Sleep and circadian rhythms in bipolar disorder: seeking synchrony, harmony, and regulation. *Am J Psychiatry* (2008) 7:820–9. doi: 10.1176/appi.ajp.2008.08010098
21. Harvey AG, Murray G, Chandler RA, Soehner A. Sleep disturbance as transdiagnostic: consideration of neurobiological mechanisms. *Clin Psychol Rev* (2011) 31:225–35. doi: 10.1016/j.cpr.2010.04.003
22. Kaskie RE, Graziano B, Ferrarelli F. Schizophrenia and sleep disorders: links, risks, and management challenges. *Nat Sci Sleep* (2017) 9:227–39. doi: 10.2147/NSS.S121076
23. Klingaman EA, Palmer-Bacon J, Bennett ME, Rowland LM. Sleep disorders among people with schizophrenia: emerging research. *Curr Psychiatry Rep* (2015) 17:616. doi: 10.1007/s11920-015-06167
24. Wee ZY, Yong SWL, Chew QH, Guan C, Lee TS, Sim K. Actigraphy studies and clinical and biobehavioural correlates in schizophrenia: a systematic review. *J Neural Transm* (2019) 126:531–58. doi: 10.1007/s00702-019-01993-2
25. Davies G, Haddock G, Yung AR, Mulligan LD, Kyle SD. A systematic review of the nature and correlates of sleep disturbance in early psychosis. *Sleep Med Rev* (2017) 31:25–38. doi: 10.1016/j.smrv.2016.01.001
26. Reeve S, Nickless A, Sheaves B, Hodgekins J, Stewart SLK, Gumley A, et al. Sleep duration and psychotic experiences in patients at risk of psychosis: a secondary analysis of the EDIE-2 trial. *Schizophr Res* (2019) 204:326–33. doi: 10.1016/j.schres.2018.08.006
27. Gordon AM, Mendes WB, Prather AA. The social side of sleep: elucidating the links between sleep and social processes. *Curr Dir Psychol Sci* (2017) 26:470–5. doi: 10.1177/0963721417712269
28. Troxel WM, Robles TF, Hall M, Buysse DJ. Marital quality and the marital bed: examining the covariation between relationship quality and sleep. *Sleep Med Rev Rev* (2007) 11:389–404. doi: 10.1016/j.smrv.2007.05.002
29. Lallukka T, Sivertsen B, Kronholm E, Bin YS, Øverland S, Glozier N. Association of sleep duration and sleep quality with the physical, social, and emotional functioning among Australian adults. *Sleep Health* (2018) 4:194–200. doi: 10.1016/j.sleh.2017.11.006
30. Léger D, Scheuermaier K, Philip P, Paillard M, Guilleminault C. SF-36: evaluation of quality of life in severe and mild insomniacs compared with good sleepers. *Psychosom Med* (2001) 63:49–55. doi: 10.1097/00006842-200101000-00006
31. Yao KW, Yu S, Cheng SP, Chen IJ. Relationships between personal, depression and social network factors and sleep quality in community-dwelling older adults. *J Nurs Res* (2008) 16:131–9. doi: 10.1097/01.JNR.0000387298.37419.ff
32. Ailshire JA, Burgard SA. Family relationships and troubled sleep among US adults: examining the influences of contact frequency and relationship quality. *J Health Soc Behav* (2012) 53:248–62. doi: 10.1177/0022146512446642
33. Chung J. Social support, social strain, sleep quality, and actigraphic sleep characteristics: evidence from a national survey of US adults. *Sleep Health* (2017) 3:22–7. doi: 10.1001/jama.1997.03540480040036
34. Kent RG, Uchino BN, Cribbet MR, Bowen K, Smith TW. Social relationships and sleep quality. *Ann Behav Med* (2015) 49:912–7. doi: 10.1007/s12160-015-9711-6
35. Cacioppo JT, Hawkley LC, Berntson GG, Ernst JM, Gibbs AC, Stickgold R, et al. Do lonely days invade the nights? Potential social modulation of sleep efficiency. *Psychol Sci* (2002) 13:384–7. doi: 10.1111/1467-9280.00469
36. Hawkley LC, Preacher KJ, Cacioppo JT. Loneliness impairs daytime functioning but not sleep duration. *Health Psychol* (2010) 29:124–9. doi: 10.1037/a0018646
37. Tavernier R, Willoughby T. A longitudinal examination of the bidirectional association between sleep problems and social ties at university: the mediating role of emotion regulation. *J Youth Adolesc* (2015) 44:317–30. doi: 10.1007/s10964-014-0107-x
38. Gordon AM, Chen S. The role of sleep in interpersonal conflict: do sleepless nights mean worse fights? *Soc Psychol Pers Sci* (2014) 5:168–75. doi: 10.1177/1948550613488952
39. Simon EB, Walker MP. Sleep loss causes social withdrawal and loneliness. *Nat Commun* (2018) 9:3146. doi: 10.1038/s41467-018-05377-0
40. Freeman D, Sheaves B, Goodwin GM, Yu L-M, Nickless A, Harrison PJ, et al. The effects of improving sleep on mental health (OASIS): a randomised controlled trial with mediation analysis. *Lancet Psychiatry* (2017) 4:749–58. doi: 10.1016/S2215-0366(17)30328-0
41. Johal A, Battagel J, Hector M. Controlled, prospective trial of psychosocial function before and after mandibular advancement splint therapy. *Am J Orthod Dentofacial Orthop* (2011) 139:581–7. doi: 10.1016/j.ajodo.2009.06.035
42. McFadyen TA, Espie CA, McArdle N, Douglas NJ, Engleman HM. Controlled, prospective trial of psychosocial function before and after continuous positive airway pressure therapy. *Eur Respir J* (2001) 18:996–1002. doi: 10.1183/09031936.01.00209301
43. Brissos S, Afonso P, Cañas F, Bobes J, Bernardo-Fernandez I, Guzman C. Satisfaction with life of schizophrenia outpatients and their caregivers: differences between patients with and without self-reported sleep complaints. *Schizophr Res Treat* (2013) 2013:502172. doi: 10.1155/2013/502172
44. Hofstetter JR, Lysaker PH, Mayeda AR. Quality of sleep in patients with schizophrenia is associated with quality of life and coping. *BMC Psychiatry* (2005) 5:13. doi: 10.1186/1471-244X-5-13
45. Ritsner M, Kurs R, Ponizovsky A, Hadjez J. Perceived quality of life in schizophrenia: relationships to sleep quality. *Qual Life Res* (2004) 13:783–91. doi: 10.1023/B:QURE.0000021687.18783.d6
46. Afonso P, Brissos S, Bobes J, Cañas F, Bernardo-Fernandez I. Personal and social functioning and satisfaction with life in schizophrenia outpatients with and without sleep disturbances. *Rev Port Psiquiatr Saúde Ment* (2015) 1:33–40.
47. Liu D, Myles H, Foley DL, Watts GF, Morgan VA, Castle D, et al. Risk factors for obstructive sleep apnea are prevalent in people with psychosis and correlate with impaired social functioning and poor physical health. *Front Psychiatry* (2016) 7:139. doi: 10.3389/fpsyt.2016.00139

48. Poe SL, Brucato G, Bruno N, Arndt LY, Ben-David S, Gill KE, et al. Sleep disturbances in individuals at clinical high risk for psychosis. *Psychiatry Res* (2017) 249:240–3. doi: 10.1016/j.psychres.2016.12.029
49. Cuthbert BN. The RDoC framework: facilitating transition from ICD/DSM to dimensional approaches that integrate neuroscience and psychopathology. *World Psychiatry* (2014) 13:28–35. doi: 10.1002/wps.20087
50. Insel TR. The NIMH Research Domain Criteria (RDoC) project: precision medicine for psychiatry. *Am J Psychiatry* (2014) 171:395–7. doi: 10.1176/appi.ajp.2014.14020138
51. Insel T, Cuthbert B, Garvey M, Heinssen R, Pine DS, Quinn K, et al. Research Domain Criteria (RDoC): toward a new classification framework for research on mental disorders. *Am J Psychiatry* (2010) 167:748–51. doi: 10.1176/appi.ajp.2010.09091379
52. First MB, Williams JBW, Karg RS, Spitzer RL. *Structured Clinical Interview for DSM-5—research version (SCID-5 for DSM-5, research version; SCID-5-RV).* Arlington, VA: American Psychiatric Association (2015).
53. Blanchard JJ, Andrea A, Orth RD, Savage C, Bennett ME. Sleep disturbance and sleep-related impairment are related to both positive and negative symptoms. *Psychiatry Res* (2020) 286:112857. doi: 10.1016/j.psychres.2020.112857
54. Yu L, Buysse DJ, Germain A, Moul DE, Stover A, Dodds NE, et al. Development of short forms from the PROMIS™ sleep disturbance and sleep-related impairment item banks. *Behav Sleep Med* (2012) 10:6–24. doi: 10.1080/15402002.2012.636266
55. Donovan LM, Rueschman M, Weng J, Basu N, Dudley KA, Bakker JP, et al. The effectiveness of an obstructive sleep apnea screening and treatment program in patients with type 2 diabetes. *Diabetes Res Clin Pract* (2017) 134:145–52. doi: 10.1016/j.diabres.2017.10.013
56. Cyranowski JM, Zill N, Bode R, Butt Z, Kelly MA, Pilkonis PA, et al. Assessing social support, companionship, and distress: National Institute of Health (NIH) Toolbox Adult Social Relationship Scales. *Health Psychol* (2013) 32:293–301. doi: 10.1037/a0028586
57. Schneider LC, Struening EL. SLOF: a behavioral rating scale for assessing the mentally ill. *Soc Work Res Abstr* (1983) 19:9–21. doi: 10.1093/swra/19.3.9
58. Cohen S, Doyle WJ, Skoner DP, Rabin BS, Gwaltney JM. Social ties and susceptibility to the common cold. *JAMA* (1997) 277:1940–4. doi: 10.1001/jama.1997.03540480040036
59. Robustelli BL, Newberry RE, Whisman MA, Mittal VA. Social relationships in young adults at ultra high risk for psychosis. *Psychiatry Res* (2017) 247:345–51. doi: 10.1016/j.psychres.2016.12.008
60. Bickart KC, Wright CI, Dautoff RJ, Dickerson BC, Barrett LF. Amygdala volume and social network size in humans. *Nat Neurosci* (2011) 14:163–4. doi: 10.1038/nn.2724
61. Bickart KC, Hollenbeck MC, Barrett LF, Dickerson BC. Intrinsic amygdala–cortical functional connectivity predicts social network size in humans. *J Neurosci* (2012) 32:14729–41. doi: 10.1523/JNEUROSCI.1599-12.2012
62. Szabo S, Merikle E, Lozano-Ortega G, Powell L, Macek T, Cline S. Assessing the relationship between performance on the University of California Performance Skills Assessment (UPSA) and outcomes in schizophrenia: a systematic review and evidence synthesis. *Schizophr Res Treat* (2018) 2018:9075174. doi: 10.1155/2018/9075174
63. Nuechterlein KH, Green MF, Kern RS, Baade LE, Barch DM, Cohen JD, et al. The MATRICS Consensus Cognitive Battery, part 1: test selection, reliability, and validity. *Am J Psychiatry* (2008) 165:203–13. doi: 10.1176/appi.ajp.2007.07010042
64. Shamsi S, Lau A, Lencz T, Burdick KE, DeRosse P, Brenner R, et al. Cognitive and symptomatic predictors of functional disability in schizophrenia. *Schizophr Res* (2011) 126:257–64. doi: 10.1016/j.schres.2010.08.007
65. Ventura J, Lukoff D, Nuechterlein K, Liberman RP, Green MF, Shaner A. Brief Psychiatric Rating Scale (BPRS) Expanded version (4.0) scales, anchor points and administration manual. *Int J Methods Psychiatr Res* (1993), 227–44.
66. Kopelowicz A, Ventura J, Liberman RP, Mintz J. Consistency of Brief Psychiatric Rating Scale factor structure across a broad spectrum of schizophrenia patients. *Psychopathology* (2007) 41:77–84. doi: 10.1159/000111551
67. Mulligan LD, Haddock G, Emsley R, Neil ST, Kyle SD. High resolution examination of the role of sleep disturbance in predicting functioning and psychotic symptoms in schizophrenia: A novel experience sampling study. *J Abnorm Psychol* (2016) 125:788–97. doi: 10.1037/abn0000180
68. Freeman D, Stahl D, McManus S, Meltzer H, Brugha T, Wiles N, et al. Insomnia, worry, anxiety and depression as predictors of the occurrence and persistence of paranoid thinking. *Soc Psychiatry Psychiatr Epidemiol* (2012) 47:1195–203. doi: 10.1007/s00127-011-0433-1
69. Krause A, Simon EB, Mander BA, Greer SM, Saletin JM, Goldstein-Piekarski AN, et al. The sleep-deprived human brain. *Nat Rev Neurosci* (2017) 18:404–18. doi: 10.1038/nrn.2017.55
70. Motomura Y, Kitamura S, Oba K, Terasawa Y, Enomoto M, Katayose Y, et al. Sleep debt elicits negative emotional reaction through diminished amygdala anterior cingulate functional connectivity. *PloS One* (2013) 8:e56578. doi: 10.1371/journal.pone.0056578
71. Yoo SS, Gujar J, Hu P, Jolesz FA, Walker MP. The human emotional brain without sleep — a prefrontal amygdala disconnect. *Curr Biol* (2017) 17:R877–R878. doi: 10.1016/j.cub.2007.08.007
72. Fox AS, Shackman AJ. The central extended amygdala in fear and anxiety: closing the gap between mechanistic and neuroimaging research. *Neurosci Lett* (2019) 693:58–67. doi: 10.1016/j.neulet.2017.11.056
73. Shackman AJ, Kaplan CM, Stockbridge MD, Tillman RM, Tromp DPM, Fox AS, et al. The neurobiology of dispositional negativity and attentional biases to threat: implications for understanding anxiety disorders in adults and youth. *J Exp Psychopathol* (2016) 7:311–42. doi: 10.5127/jep.054015
74. Dugre JR, Bitar N, Dumais A, Potvin S. Limbic hyperactivity in response to emotionally neutral stimuli in schizophrenia: a neuroimaging meta-analysis of the hypervigilant mind. *Am J Psychiatry* (2019) 176:1021–9. doi: 10.1176/appi.ajp.2019.19030247
75. Simon EB, Oren N, Sharon H, Kirschner A, Goldway N, Okon-Singer H, et al. Losing neutrality: the neural basis of impaired emotional control without sleep. *J Neurosci* (2015) 35:13194–205. doi: 10.1523/JNEUROSCI.1314-15.2015

3

Social Perception and Interaction Database—A Novel Tool to Study Social Cognitive Processes with Point-Light Displays

Łukasz Okruszek[1]* *and Marta Chrustowicz*[2]

[1] *Social Neuroscience Lab, Institute of Psychology, Polish Academy of Sciences, Warsaw, Poland,* [2] *Faculty of Psychology, University of Warsaw, Warsaw, Poland*

Correspondence:
Łukasz Okruszek
lukasz.okruszek@psych.pan.pl

Introduction: The ability to detect and interpret social interactions (SI) is one of the crucial skills enabling people to operate in the social world. Multiple lines of evidence converge to indicate the preferential processing of SI when compared to the individual actions of multiple agents, even if the actions were visually degraded to minimalistic point-light displays (PLDs). Here, we present a novel PLD dataset (Social Perception and Interaction Database; SoPID) that may be used for studying multiple levels of social information processing.

Methods: During a motion-capture session, two pairs of actors were asked to perform a wide range of 3-second actions, including: (1) neutral, gesture-based communicative interactions (COM); (2) emotional exchanges (Happy/Angry); (3) synchronous interactive physical activity of actors (SYNC); and (4) independent actions of agents, either object-related (ORA) or non-object related (NORA). An interface that allows single/dyadic PLD stimuli to be presented from either the second person (action aimed toward the viewer) or third person (observation of actions presented toward other agents) perspective was implemented on the basis on the recorded actions. Two validation studies (each with 20 healthy individuals) were then performed to establish the recognizability of the SoPID vignettes.

Results: The first study showed a ceiling level accuracy for discrimination of communicative vs. individual actions (93% $\pm$ 5%) and high accuracy for interpreting specific types of actions (85 $\pm$ 4%) from the SoPID. In the second study, a robust effect of scrambling on the recognizability of SoPID stimuli was observed in an independent sample of healthy individuals.

Discussion: These results suggest that the SoPID may be effectively used to examine processes associated with communicative interactions and intentions processing. The database can be accessed via the Open Science Framework (https://osf.io/dcht8/).

Keywords: biological motion, communicative intentions, social perception, individual action, social interaction, point-light animations, emotion recognition

INTRODUCTION

Multiple lines of evidence indicate that encounters between other agents are preferentially processed by healthy individuals. Further, communicative interactions have been shown to be easily discriminated from other types of actions (1–3), gain preferential access to awareness (4), and are encoded as a single unit in working memory (5). Psychophysics experiments have also shown that healthy individuals are able to utilize top-down knowledge about the communicative gesture of one agent to predict both the type (6) and timing (7) of another agent's response. Furthermore, the processing of social interactions elicits widespread activation of the main "social brain" networks, compared to the individual actions of multiple agents (8–11). Importantly, these effects may be observed for both naturalistic full displays of agents (12–15) and minimalistic point-light displays of social interactions (8, 10, 11, 16). Developed by Johansson (17), point-light methodology limits the presentation of agents to a set of light-dots representing the head, limbs, and major joints of the agent's body. Despite the extremely limited amount of visual information presented via point-light displays (PLDs), this type of vignette has been shown to carry enough information to enable the recognition of an agent's action (18, 19), affective state (20), and a wide range of physical characteristics. Furthermore, point-light stimuli have also been used to investigate communicative intentions processing from both single (21) and dyadic displays (3).

Manera et al. (3) presented the Communicative Interaction Database (CID)—a set of 20 stimuli that presents dyadic interactions based on the stereotypical use of communicative gestures with point-light motion. CID stimuli have been used to examine both reflective (2) and reflexive (1) social cognitive processes in healthy individuals. Stimuli from the CID have also been used to create a multilingual task for studying communicative interaction recognition (2), which has been effectively applied to study social cognition across various clinical populations [patients with schizophrenia (22, 23), high functioning individuals with autism spectrum disorders (24), patients with temporal lobe epilepsy (25)]. Furthermore, CID stimuli have been applied to investigate the neural correlates of communicative interactions processing (10, 11). Additionally, as the CID database was created in adherence to the protocols used by Vanrie & Verfaillie (19), who presented a set of 22 non-communicative single-agent point-light actions, stimuli from both databases have previously been combined to obtain a broader spectrum of actions for studying the neural correlates of social interaction processing (11). However, the use of such a combination of stimuli from various datasets may be limited by several methodological factors (e.g., different actors presenting communicative vs. individual actions, varying length of the stimuli).

At the same time, given the widespread nature of social interactions (SI) processing across neural networks, a recent review of neural and behavioral findings in this area concluded that the development of SI localizers, which entail various types of social interaction vignettes, may facilitate research in this area (9). Studies based on static pictures of various types of social interactions have observed differential patterns of brain activity (14) and connectivity (26) in affective vs. cooperative interactions. Yet, due to the limited availability of point-light stimuli, previous studies on SI processing from PLDs either pooled various types of communicative interactions into one category [e.g. (8)] or presented only certain types of interactions (usually encounters based on the typical use of communicative gestures: (10, 11). Furthermore, it has been shown that communicative intentions may be differentially processed from the second person (receiver) and third person (observer) perspective (27). Thus, to address the second *person neuroscience* postulates (28), future studies should compare the processing of communicative intentions from the second person (single figure presenting gesture toward observer) and third person (displays of two agents acting toward each other) perspectives. The aim of the current project was to develop a database of point-light stimuli (Social Perception and Interaction Database; SoPID) that addresses the above listed issues by allowing for the creation of point-light animations with a wide range of communicative and individual actions, while flexibly manipulating the number of agents presented (one vs. two), the viewing perspective, and display options.

DATABASE CREATION

Pre-capturing Session

Two pairs of professional actors took part in the motion capture procedure. One dyad consisted of male actors and one of female actresses. During the pre-capturing session, actors were familiarized with the list of actions that were to be recorded. The list of situations to be recorded consisted of six categories, each with 5–10 situations (see **Data Sheet 1** for a full list of the SoPID stimuli). For the communicative interactions (COM), each of the actors was asked to play both the person initiating the interaction via a communicative gesture (Agent A) and the person responding to the communicative gesture of the other agent (Agent B), thus producing two different takes on each COM situation. A short description of each action was provided to ensure that each dyad was enacting similar communicative intention and a similar behavioral response. To ensure the temporal synchronization of the animations, three sound signals were presented during each recording: first to signal the onset of the recording (played at T = 0 s.), second to signal the half-time of the recording (played at T = 1.5 s.), and third to signal the end of the recording (played at T = 3 s.). For animations that presented the sequential actions of both agents (e.g., Agent A asks Agent B to stand up, Agent B stands up), the actor playing Agent A was asked to start his action at T = 0, while the actor playing Agent B was asked to start responding at T = 1.5 s. The situations were rehearsed until both actors were able to perform them with the required timing. Moreover, to ensure the naturalistic yet expressive movement of the actors during the capturing sessions, a professional choreographer oversaw the actors' rehearsal during the pre-capturing session.

Motion Capture

The motion capture session was performed via a motion-capture studio (*White Kanga* studio; Warsaw) using an OptiTrack

(NaturalPoint, Corvallis, OR, USA) motion tracking system. Twelve OptiTrack Prime 13 cameras were utilized to record the movements of the actors at a 120 Hz rate. The actors wore 41 reflective spherical markers placed according to the OptiTrack Baseline+Hinged Toe system [full list and anatomical locations of the markers available at https://v20.wiki.optitrack.com/index.php?title=Baseline_%2B_Hinged_Toe,_with_Headband_(41)]. The motion capture room was a 7 x 7 meters square with a 3.8 meter high ceiling; a white line was painted on the floor of the motion capture room to mark each actor's subspace (7 x 3.5 meter). With the exception of enactments that included physical contact between the agents, the actors were asked to confine their actions within their subspaces. Similarly, most of the sequences were recorded with actors facing each other at a proximity of around 3 meters. At the beginning and end of each recording, the actors were asked to perform a T-pose (reference pose) at the central position of their subspace. Additional props were used for the sequences that included object-related actions (i.e., shovel, carton box, ax, saw, broom, glass, hammer, toothbrush, football, chair). No markers were used to tag the prop positions during the session, and thus the objects were not displayed in animations. For the stimuli that presented interaction between the agents (communicative interactions, happy/angry and synchronous interactive activity), the actions of both agents were recorded simultaneously to ensure that the response of one agent was congruent with the action of the other agent in terms of position, proxemics, and timing. Actions for object- and non-object related displays were recorded individually to minimize the potential effects of between-agents synchrony while performing the actions. Similarly, as during the pre-capturing session, sound cues were used to inform actors about beginning (T = 0 s.), middle (T = 1.5 s), and end (T = 3 s.) points of each three-second period. Furthermore, the point-light figures were previewed during the session to enable instantaneous re-takes for unsuccessful takes (**Figure 1**, upper).

Data Processing

Data from the motion capture session were further processed using OptiTrack Motive 1.9 beta software. 2-D data from 12 cameras were used to obtain the 3-D coordinates of each marker. Skeleton models consisting of 13 bright dots corresponding to the head, arms, elbows, wrists, hips, knees, and ankles of each actor were animated. Data preprocessing included inspection of each of the recordings, data trimming to the period between the onset (T = 0 s.) and offset (T = 3 s.) of the action, and manual smoothing in case of any vibrating or fluttering movements. The preprocessed data were extracted to FBX files.

Social Perception and Interaction Database

To enable users without programming skills to access and customize the stimuli according to their needs, preprocessed stimuli may be accessed via an interface that is based on the Unity engine (SoPID). The SoPID interface (which is visualized in the **Figure 2**) allows for modification of numerous stimuli characteristics and exports the customized stimuli to movie files (.mp4) using the FFmpeg codec. Overall, 64 different actions of each agent can be accessed via the SoPID and used to create experimental stimuli. Each of the recorded actions may be accessed either separately as a solo action or merged with a second action to produce a stimulus presenting a pair of agents. This way, the SoPID allows for a wide range of animations presenting a single agent's communicative or individual actions to be produced. It also allows for the actions of two agents to be combined into either congruent (by selecting one out of four Agent A's "Communicative Gestures" and any of the corresponding responses of Agent B or by using a combination of either "Happy," "Angry," or "Synchronous Interactive Activity" actions) or incongruent (e.g., by mixing Agent A's communicative action with a non-corresponding action of Agent B) social interactions or parallel individual actions of agents. The whole list of actions available in the SoPID is presented in **Supplementary Table 1**.

The SoPID interface also allows for flexible adjustment of camera position. Four standard camera positions may be selected, with the "Front" position corresponding to a 270 degree display from the CID (Agent A on the left and Agent B on the right) with the camera being placed on the middle line between the agents, at a height of one meter and 15 meters from the agents. Furthermore, by using the "Free" option, both the camera placement (x—left/right; y—up/down; z—closer/further; values in meters) and rotation (x—up/down; y—left/right; z—horizontal/vertical; values in degrees) can be fully customized. Both ortographic (with no depth cues—all points are same size) and perspective (containing depth cues—parts of the actor that are further from the observer are depicted by smaller points) projections may be used to manipulate the availability of depth cues in the animations. Additionally, marker size may be changed ("Marker size," values in centimeters) to modify the agents' appearances and stick figures can be created instead of point-light displays ("Show skeleton"). Finally, two standard modifications that are commonly used in point-light studies can be applied directly via the SoPID. First, by using the "Flicker" option, the visual availability of the stimuli may be limited by selecting the maximal number of simultaneously displayed markers (0–13) and the time range for marker display/disappearance. Markers are flickered by randomly assigning the onset and offset time values separately for each marker with regard to the time range provided by the user. In addition, by using the "Scramble" option, the initial spatial position of each marker can be spatially scrambled. Scrambling is applied by randomly drawing one out of three dimensions for each marker and relocating its initial position by X centimeters from its initial position in the selected direction (e.g., 100% scrambling moves each marker by one meter in either the x, y or z dimension). "Flicker" and "Scramble" can be applied to both agents or selectively to each agent. The database, as well as raw motion capture files, can be accessed via the Open Science Framework (https://osf.io/dcht8/).

METHODS

To examine the recognizability of the presented actions and the effectiveness of the scrambling mechanism, two SoPID validation

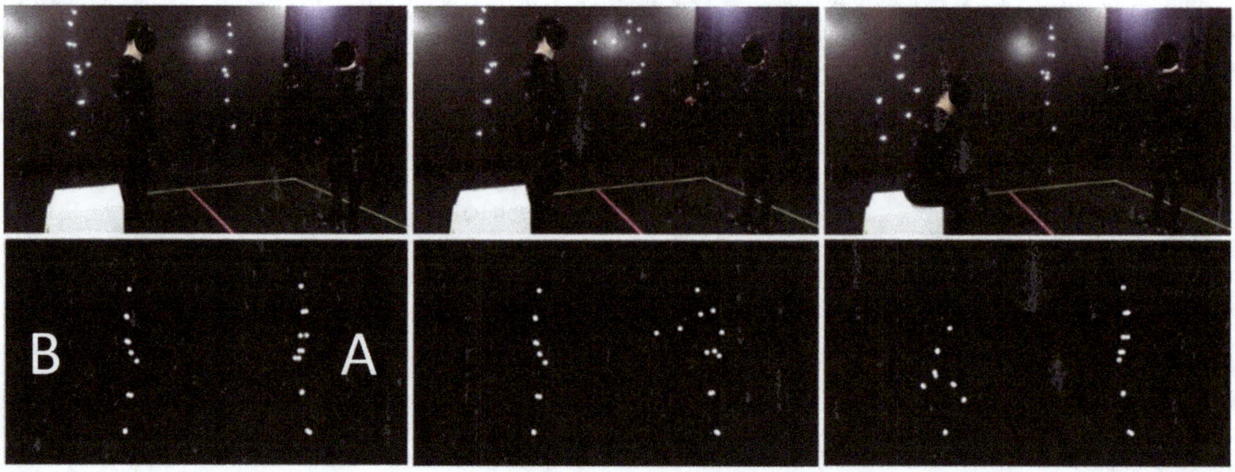

FIGURE 1 | Original (**upper**) and PLD (**lower**) version of the item presenting communicative interaction from SoPID [A (on the right) asks B (on the left) to sit down; B sits down].

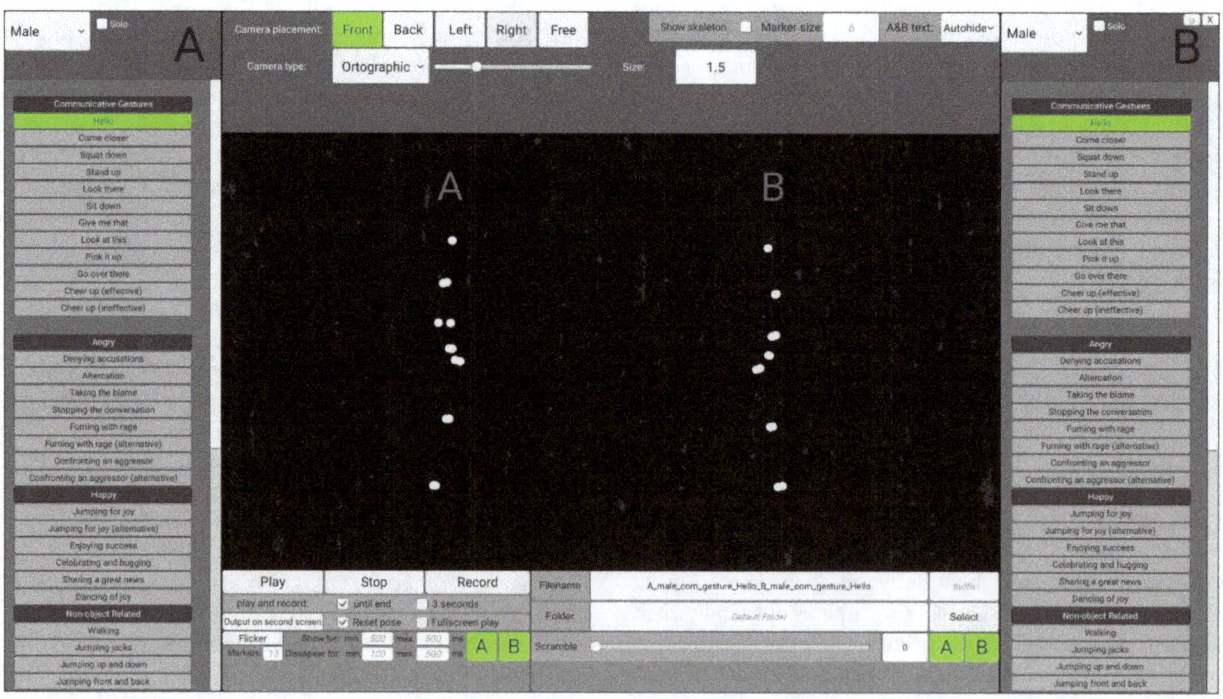

FIGURE 2 | Social Perception and Interaction Database interface.

studies were performed. The aim of Study 1 was to investigate the detection of communicative intentions and the recognition of specific actions of agents across a wide range of social interactions and parallel non-communicative actions included in SoPID. The goal of Study 2 was to examine the effectiveness of the display manipulation procedures (in particular biological motion scrambling procedure) implemented in SoPID, by comparing the recognizability of human motion under various levels of scrambling.

Stimuli

Study 1

Fifty-seven animations presenting the actions of two agents were created using the SoPID (perspective camera with FoV = 10°, camera position = front, and marker size = 6). Six types of stimuli were presented throughout the study: Communicative gestures [COM, 10 animations: "Hello" (Female 2 as Agent A); "Come closer" (Male 1 as Agent A), "Squat down" (F2), "Stand up" (M1), "Look there" (F1), "Sit down" (M2), "Give me that" (F2), "Look at this" (M1), "Pick it up" (F2), "Go over there" (M2)]; Angry exchanges (Angry, 5 animations: "Denying accusations," "Taking the blame," "Stopping the conversation," "Fuming with rage," "Confronting an aggressor (alternative)"); Happy exchanges (Happy: 5 animations: "Jumping for joy," "Enjoying success," "Celebrating and hugging," "Sharing a great news," "Dancing of joy"); Non-object related parallel individual actions (NORA, 10 animations: "Walking," "Jumping jacks," "Jumping up and down," "Jumping front and back," "Arm waving," "Hip swinging," "Torso twist," "A-Skip," "Squat down," "Lateral step," "Lateral kick"); Object related parallel individual actions (ORA, 9 animations: "Shoveling," "Lifting the box," "Chopping wood," "Sawing," "Digging," "Sweeping the floor," "Drinking," "Hammering a nail," "Brushing teeth"); and Synchronous interactive activity of two agents [SYNC, 8 animations: "Dancing" (M/F), "Fencing" (M), "Football" (F), "Throwing the ball" (M), "Boxing" (F), "Kickboxing" (M/F)]. To ensure that a similar number of stimuli were presented for each category and to increase the comparability of recognition accuracy levels across the categories, two stimuli (one with male and one with female actors) were created for each situation from the Angry and Happy categories. ORA and NORA movies were created by merging the displays of two different actions performed by two same-sex actors. Displays of each set of actions with either male or female actors were included, thus producing 11 NORA and 9 ORA movies in total.

Study 2

Twenty movies ["come closer" (F), "squat down" (M), "stand up" (M, F), "go over there" (F), "altercation" (M, F), "jumping for joy" (F), "denying accusations" (M), "jumping for joy (alternative)" (M), "walking" (F), "lateral kick" (F), "hip swinging" (M), "A-skip" (M), "squat down" (M), "lifting the box" (F), "sweeping the floor" (F), "brushing teeth" (F), "chopping wood" (M), "digging" (M)] presenting the action of a single agent (Agent A in case of COM, Angry and Happy) were created from the SoPID (ortographic camera (size = 1.5), camera position = right, and marker size = 6). Each animation was rendered at four scrambling levels: 0, 15, 30, and 100%. Thus, 80 animations were presented during the experimental procedure.

Participants

Participants for each of the studies were recruited from the students of Warsaw-based universities. All of the participants were right-handed. Participants were tested individually, and had not participated in point-light experiments prior to the examination. Twenty participants (9M/11F; 25.9 ± 9.1 yrs. old) completed Study 1, while 20 participants (10M/10F; 24.2 ± 7.7 years old), who did not participate in Study 1, completed Study 2.

Apparatus and Procedures

Study 1

Each stimulus was presented twice, after which participants were asked to: (1) classify whether the presented action was an interaction (behavior of one agent affects the behavior of the other) or not by responding to the response screen with two options (Interaction vs. No interaction), and (2) to provide a verbal description of the actions of the agents (which was written down by the experimenter). The order of stimuli presentation was pseudorandomized to avoid subsequent presentation of more than two stimuli from the same category. The paradigm was programmed using NBS Presentation 20, and the whole procedure took ~1 h. Verbal descriptions provided by the participants were scored by a rater who did not participate in data collection. Spontaneous descriptions for COM, SYNC, Happy, and Angry were scored in a dichotomic manner (2 points for a correct verbal description vs. 0 points for an incorrect description). Accuracy for ORA and NORA stimuli was calculated by scoring one point for each correctly recognized action from male and female presentations (0–2 points). For interaction vs. individual actions classification, COM, Angry, Happy and SYNC were treated as falling into the category "interaction", while ORA and NORA were treated as "individual actions." Two items ("Dancing for joy" and "Fuming with rage") without any explicit communicative cues were discarded from this part of the analysis.

Study 2

Upon presentation of each animation, participants were asked to indicate whether the presented animation resembled human motion. Completion of the whole experimental procedure took approximately 20 min.

Statistical Analysis

Study 1

To examine between-category differences in accuracy levels, one way ANOVAs with Type of animation (six levels) were performed separately for interaction recognition and spontaneous identification of actions.

Study 2

The number of stimuli classified as "human" at each scrambling level was compared to examine the effectiveness of the scrambling procedure. The results were analyzed using rmANOVA with the within-subject factor Scrambling (4 levels: 0, 15, 30, 100%).

RESULTS

Study 1

Behavioral accuracies for each type of the task are presented below in **Table 1**.

Recognition of Communicative Intentions

No between category differences were observed for classifying actions as either communicative or individual [$F_{(5, 15)} = 1.3$; n.s., $\eta_p^2 = 0.07$], with ceiling level recognition for all types of items. As ceiling effects were observed for most of the categories in Study 1, we re-examined the results with a non-parametric Friedman test of differences among repeated measures, which provided a Chi-square value of 8.94 ($p > 0.05$).

Identification of Specific Action

A main effect of category was observed for the accuracy of identification of specific actions [$F_{(5, 15)} = 23.9$, $p < 0.001$, η_p^2

TABLE 1 | Behavioral accuracy for recognition of communicative intentions and identification of specific actions in Study 1 (mean ± standard deviation is given for each category).

	Angry	Happy	COM	SYNC	NORA	ORA
Study 1 results						
Recognition of communicative intentions (%)	95 ± 9	89 ± 13	95 ± 10	91 ± 11	94 ± 10	93 ± 8
Identification of specific action (%)	81 ± 12	92 ± 11	78 ± 12	96 ± 6	95 ± 5	67 ± 13

TABLE 2 | Percentage of stimuli classified as a human motion for various levels of scrambling in Study 2 (mean ± standard deviation is given for each category).

Scrambling level	0%	15%	30%	100%
Study 2 results				
Percentage of stimuli classified as a human motion	98 ± 3	68 ± 18	20 ± 13	3 ± 5

= 0.56]. Further investigation of this effect revealed the highest recognition for SYNC, NORA and Happy, each of which were identified at higher level than Angry and COM. Furthermore, actions from all of the categories were identified more accurately than ORA. As in the case of Study 1, we re-examined these non-normally distributed variables with the Friedman test, which provided a Chi-square value of 49.24 ($p < 0.001$).

Study 2

One participant with results over three standard deviations from the mean value in two conditions (0 and 100%) was excluded from the analysis. A robust effect of scrambling was observed [$F_{(3,16)} = 400.9$; $p < 0.001$, $\eta_p^2 = 0.96$]. Unscrambled stimuli were classified as human motion significantly more often than 15, 30, and 100% scrambled motion. Similarly, 15% stimuli were classified as human motion more often than 30 and 100% scrambled displays, and 30% scrambled stimuli were classified as human more often than 100% scrambled displays. All of the contrasts were significant at $p < 0.001$. Similarly to Study 1, as a non-normal distribution of results was observed for 0 and 100% scrambled motion classification, we re-examined the results with the Friedman test and found a significant ($p < 0.001$) effect with a Chi-square of 55.68. The percentage of the stimuli classified as a human motion at each scrambling level is presented in **Table 2**.

DISCUSSION

The present paper describes the Social Perception and Interaction Database, a novel set of point-light displays that enables study of the processing of a wide range of communicative and individual actions from single-agent and two-agent vignettes. The SoPID includes 32 animations presenting various types of social interactions between two agents, including standard use of communicative gestures (COM), synchronous interactive physical activity (SYNC) and affective exchanges (either Happy or Angry), as well as 20 animations of each actor performing either object- (ORA) or non-object-related (NORA) individual actions. Furthermore, by performing two validation studies, we established that SoPID vignettes elicit similar effects to those previously described in studies on intention and emotion processing from PLDs.

Previous studies that used the CID database showed high accuracy in recognition of communicative vs. individual actions in healthy individuals (2, 29). Similarly, we observed a ceiling level accuracy for classifying stimuli as either communicative or individual across the six categories of stimuli included in the first of the validation studies (ranging from 89% for Happy to 95% for COM). Furthermore, the accuracy of identification of specific communicative actions from the COM category (78% ± 12%) was at a similar level as previously reported for the multilingual CID task [74% ± 18%; (29)]. Interestingly, more accurate identification of specific actions was observed for three other categories of stimuli included in the study (Happy, NORA, SYNC). This result may be linked to the fact that both NORA and SYNC stimuli presented physical activity that is usually associated with whole-body motion (e.g., jumping or kick-boxing), which may have higher salience compared to the more restricted actions (e.g., hand gestures) presented across other categories. Thus, (1) as a salient movement may have been easier to classify and (2) communicative gestures need higher-order processing, and attribution of intent, both of these aspects may have contributed to the better accuracy for NORA and SYNC. Increased recognition of positively-valenced social exchanges (Happy) compared to neutral communicative interactions (COM) and negatively-valenced social exchanges (Angry) is congruent with previous findings showing that the positive emotional valence of stimuli facilitates biological motion processing from single (30) and dyadic (31) point-light displays. Finally, we observed that while object-related individual actions were identified less accurately than any other type of SoPID animations (67% ± 13%), their recognition rate was at a similar level as the recognition rates of individual actions from the well-established stimuli set by Vanrie et al. (19), which reported a mean accuracy rate of 63% for a set of individual point-light actions in 11 observers producing spontaneous descriptions of the animations. In a second validation study, a robust effect of the scrambling mechanism implemented in SoPID was found: unscrambled and 100% scrambled stimuli were almost unanimously categorized as, respectively, human and non-human motion. Furthermore, the more subtle effects of scrambling were also observed: a significant portion of the 15% scrambled stimuli were classified by participants as resembling human motion, while a large majority (80%) of the 30% scrambled stimuli were classified as non-human motion.

These results suggest that the SoPID stimuli may be effectively used in a wide range of experiments examining both basic (e.g., recognition of biological vs. scrambled motion) and higher-order (e.g., recognition of communicative intentions of affective states from PLDs) processing of biological motion. Moreover, a recent review of the findings on emotion and intention processing from biological motion in psychiatric disorders (32), has concluded that disorder-specific social cognitive biases (e.g., negativity bias in depression, abnormal threat perception in anxiety) may be effectively elicited by biological motion vignettes. The use of recorded situations during which two or more actors interact with each other is currently the primary method for social cognitive assessment of communicative interactions processing (33, 34). However, patients with neuropsychiatric disorders have been shown to present decreased ability to process a wide range of social signals (e.g., facial expressions, non-verbal prosody, bodily movements), which need to be successfully integrated to correctly process such complex situations. Thus, between-group differences observed in studies based on paradigms that utilize full-displays of actors to examine communicative interactions processing in neuropsychiatric populations may be affected by other perceptual issues or potentially distracting elements of visual displays. Decreased recognition of affective states and/or communicative intentions from point-light displays have previously been documented in individuals with ASD (35), patients with schizophrenia (36), affective disorders (37), neurodegenerative diseases (38) and temporal lobe epilepsy (25). Furthermore, previous studies that used CID stimuli have provided evidence that a double dissociation between explicit and implicit processes associated with communicative interactions detection may be observed in two neuropsychiatric populations (23, 24). Okruszek et al. (23)observed that patients with schizophrenia, while being less accurate in explicitly interpreting communicative interactions presented with point-light displays, are able to use the communicative action of one agent to predict the response of another agent during an implicit task ("interpersonal predictive coding"). However, the reverse pattern (intact explicit recognition of actions, but no interpersonal predictive coding during an implicit task) was observed in high-functioning individuals with ASD (24). At the same time, the scope of the previous research in this area, due to the limited availability of the stimuli, has been limited to recognition of intentions from standard communicative gestures from either single (38) or dyadic (22, 24, 25) displays. Therefore, use of the SoPID may extend the area of investigation of future studies to neuropsychiatric populations, by enabling the examination of behavioral and neural responses to a wide range of individual actions and communicative actions with or without emotional content.

Investigation of the behavioral and neural correlates of social interactions processing has been the focus of increasing interest in recent years (9). Additionally, a framework integrating current knowledge about the factors shaping the perception of social interactions has recently been proposed [Integrative Model of Relational Impression Formation, IMRIF; (39)]. The IMRIF emphasizes that accuracy of the perception of social interactions is determined by four main types of attributes: (1) content attributes (factors related to the specifics of the interaction which is being perceived), (2) target attributes (characteristics of the interacting agents), (3) perceiver attributes (characteristics of the person perceiving the interaction), and (4) context attributes (specific circumstances under which an interaction is being perceived) (39). By providing a rich source material that can be further customized in multiple ways, the SoPID may be effectively used to examine a wide range of research questions regarding the factors impacting SI processing that have been suggested by IMRIF.

Firstly, by including a wide range of actions from various semantic categories and allowing users to create stimuli by combining the actions of both agents, both within each category and between the categories, a wide range of novel stimuli can be created to study the impact of the content attributes on social interaction processing. In addition, by enabling the congruency of the actions in dyadic displays to be manipulated to create both typical and novel ambiguous or paradoxical situations (e.g., agent B performs an action that is opposite to the request of agent A). Secondly, target attributes can also be changed by either modifying the presentation of the agents (e.g., point-light agents vs. stick figures) or, as the SoPID includes actions produced by four different actors (two male and two female), by presenting the same situations involving different agents. Finally, by enabling one to manipulate the observer's visual perspective and the presence of the second agent's response, contextual factors impacting the SI processing can also be studied. For example, by presenting the same stimuli from a second- and third-person perspective, the impact of the participant vs. observer role for communicative intentions processing can be examined. It has been shown that communicative intentions directed toward the participant (second person perspective) elicit larger activity within the crucial nodes of the mentalizing network (medial prefrontal cortex, mPFC) and mirroring (bilateral premotor cortex) compared to the observation of the same communicative intentions observed from the third person perspective (27). Similarly, the specific impact of the egocentric (second-person) vs. allocentric (third-person) perspective on neural activity elicited by coverbal gestures was observed in the anterior cingulate region (40). These findings, which suggest that neural computations supporting communicative intention processing may be affected by the observer vs. participant point of view, emphasize the importance of further investigating the role of contextual factors in communicative interactions processing.

The necessity of developing new tasks to study the factors impacting third party encounter processing has recently been stressed (9). By introducing a tool that enables manipulation of SI content, target characteristics and contextual factors, the SoPID allows for flexible creation of stimuli to develop novel tasks for behavioral and neuroimaging research and to address novel research hypotheses.

AUTHOR CONTRIBUTIONS

ŁO contributed conception and design of the study, performed the statistical analysis, and wrote the first draft of the manuscript. MC collected the data and wrote a section of the manuscript. All authors contributed to manuscript revision, read, and approved the submitted version.

ACKNOWLEDGMENTS

We would like to thank to the Bartłomiej Leszek, Marcin Kocik, and White Kanga studio personnel, as well as Aleksandra Matlingiewicz, Sonia Jachymiak, Piotr Sedkowski, Piotr Watroba, Artur Marchlewski, and Grzegorz Pochwatko for their help in stimuli creation. This manuscript has been released as a Pre-Print (41).

REFERENCES

1. Manera V, Becchio C, Schouten B, Bara BG, Verfaillie K. Communicative interactions improve visual detection of biological motion. *PLoS ONE.* (2011) 6:e14594. doi: 10.1371/journal.pone.0014594
2. Manera V, Ianì F, Bourgeois J, Haman M, Okruszek ŁP, Rivera SM, et al. The multilingual CID-5: a new tool to study the perception of communicative interactions in different languages. *Front Psychol.* (2015) 6:1724. doi: 10.3389/fpsyg.2015.01724
3. Manera V, Schouten B, Becchio C, Bara BG, Verfaillie K. Inferring intentions from biological motion: a stimulus set of point-light communicative interactions. *Behav Res Methods.* (2010) 42:168–78. doi: 10.3758/BRM.42.1.168
4. Su J, van Boxtel JJA, Lu H. Social interactions receive priority to conscious perception. *PLoS ONE.* (2016) 11:e0160468. doi: 10.1371/journal.pone.0160468
5. Ding X, Gao Z, Shen M. Two equals one: two human actions during social interaction are grouped as one unit in working memory. *Psychol Sci.* (2017) 28:1311–20. doi: 10.1177/0956797617707318
6. Manera V, Del Giudice M, Bara BG, Verfaillie K, Becchio C. The second-agent effect: communicative gestures increase the likelihood of perceiving a second agent. *PLoS ONE.* (2011) 6:e22650. doi: 10.1371/journal.pone.0022650
7. Manera V, Schouten B, Verfaillie K, Becchio C. Time will show: real time predictions during interpersonal action perception. *PLoS ONE.* (2013) 8:e54949. doi: 10.1371/journal.pone.0054949
8. Centelles L, Assaiante C, Nazarian B, Anton J-L, Schmitz C. Recruitment of both the mirror and the mentalizing networks when observing social interactions depicted by point-lights: a neuroimaging study. *PLoS ONE.* (2011) 6:e15749. doi: 10.1371/journal.pone.0015749
9. Quadflieg S, Koldewyn K. The neuroscience of people watching: how the human brain makes sense of other people's encounters. *Ann N Y Acad Sci.* (2017) 1396:166–82. doi: 10.1111/nyas.13331
10. Isik L, Koldewyn K, Beeler D, Kanwisher N. Perceiving social interactions in the posterior superior temporal sulcus. *Proc Natl Acad Sci USA.* (2017) 114:E9145–52. doi: 10.1073/pnas.1714471114
11. Walbrin J, Downing P, Koldewyn K. Neural responses to visually observed social interactions. *Neuropsychologia.* (2018) 112:31–9. doi: 10.1016/j.neuropsychologia.2018.02.023
12. Wang Y, Huang L, Zhang W, Zhang Z, Cacioppo S. Spatio-temporal dynamics of kind versus hostile intentions in the human brain: an electrical neuroimaging study. *Soc Neurosci.* (2015) 10:253–67. doi: 10.1080/17470919.2014.990641
13. Quadflieg S, Gentile F, Rossion B. The neural basis of perceiving person interactions. *Cortex.* (2015) 70:5–20. doi: 10.1016/j.cortex.2014.12.020
14. Canessa N, Alemanno F, Riva F, Zani A, Proverbio AM, Mannara N, et al. The neural bases of social intention understanding: the role of interaction goals. *PLoS ONE.* (2012) 7:e42347. doi: 10.1371/journal.pone.0042347
15. Van den Stock J, Hortensius R, Sinke C, Goebel R, de Gelder B. Personality traits predict brain activation and connectivity when witnessing a violent conflict. *Sci Rep.* (2015) 5:13779. doi: 10.1038/srep13779
16. Petrini K, Piwek L, Crabbe F, Pollick FE, Garrod S. Look at those two!: the precuneus role in unattended third-person perspective of social interactions. *Hum Brain Mapp.* (2014) 35:5190–203. doi: 10.1002/hbm.22543
17. Johansson G. Visual perception of biological motion and a model for its analysis. *Percept Psychophys.* (1973) 14:201–11. doi: 10.3758/BF03212378
18. Dekeyser M, Verfaillie K, Vanrie J. Creating stimuli for the study of biological-motion perception. *Behav Res Methods Instrum Comput.* (2002) 34:375–82. doi: 10.3758/BF03195465
19. Vanrie J, Verfaillie K. Perception of biological motion: a stimulus set of human point-light actions. *Behav Res Methods Instrum Comput.* (2004) 36:625–9. doi: 10.3758/BF03206542
20. Vaskinn A, Sundet K, Østefjells T, Nymo K, Melle I, Ueland T. Reading emotions from body movement: a generalized impairment in schizophrenia. *Front Psychol.* (2015) 6:2058. doi: 10.3389/fpsyg.2015.02058
21. Zaini H, Fawcett JM, White NC, Newman AJ. Communicative and noncommunicative point-light actions featuring high-resolution representation of the hands and fingers. *Behav Res Methods.* (2013) 45:319–28. doi: 10.3758/s13428-012-0273-2
22. Okruszek Ł, Haman M, Kalinowski K, Talarowska M, Becchio C, Manera V. Impaired recognition of communicative interactions from biological motion in schizophrenia. *PLoS ONE.* (2015) 10:e0116793. doi: 10.1371/journal.pone.0116793
23. Okruszek Ł, Piejka A, Wysokinski A, Szczepocka E, Manera V. Biological motion sensitivity, but not interpersonal predictive coding is impaired in schizophrenia. *J Abnorm Psychol.* (2018) 127:305–13. doi: 10.1037/abn0000335
24. von der Lühe T, Manera V, Barisic I, Becchio C, Vogeley K, Schilbach L. Interpersonal predictive coding, not action perception, is impaired in autism. *Philos Trans R Soc Lond B, Biol Sci.* (2016) 371:1–8. doi: 10.1098/rstb.2015.0373
25. Bala A, Okruszek Ł, Piejka A, Głebicka A, Szewczyk E, Bosak K, et al. Social perception in mesial temporal lobe epilepsy: interpreting social information from moving shapes and biological motion. *J Neuropsychiatry Clin Neurosci.* (2018) 30:228–35. doi: 10.1176/appi.neuropsych.17080153
26. Arioli M, Perani D, Cappa S, Proverbio AM, Zani A, Falini A, et al. Affective and cooperative social interactions modulate effective connectivity within and between the mirror and mentalizing systems. *Hum Brain Mapp.* (2018) 39:1412–27. doi: 10.1002/hbm.23930
27. Ciaramidaro A, Becchio C, Colle L, Bara BG, Walter H. Do you mean me? Communicative intentions recruit the mirror and the mentalizing system. *Soc Cogn Affect Neurosci.* (2014) 9:909–16. doi: 10.1093/scan/nst062
28. Schilbach L, Timmermans B, Reddy V, Costall A, Bente G, Schlicht T, et al. Toward a second-person neuroscience. *Behav Brain Sci.* (2013) 36:393–414. doi: 10.1017/S0140525X12000660
29. Manera V, von der Lühe T, Schilbach L, Verfaillie K, Becchio C. Communicative interactions in point-light displays: choosing among multiple response alternatives. *Behav Res Methods.* (2016) 48:1580–90. doi: 10.3758/s13428-015-0669-x
30. Lee H, Kim J. Facilitating effects of emotion on the perception of biological motion: evidence for a happiness superiority effect. *Perception.* (2017) 46:679–97. doi: 10.1177/0301006616681809
31. Piwek L, Pollick F, Petrini K. Audiovisual integration of emotional signals from others' social interactions. *Front Psychol.* (2015) 9:116. doi: 10.3389/fpsyg.2015.00611
32. Okruszek Ł. It is not just in faces! processing of emotion and intention from biological motion in psychiatric disorders. *Front Hum Neurosci.* (2018) 12:48. doi: 10.3389/fnhum.2018.00048
33. Dziobek I, Fleck S, Kalbe E, Rogers K, Hassenstab J, Brand M, et al. Introducing MASC: a movie for the assessment of social cognition. *J Autism Dev Disord.* (2006) 36:623–36. doi: 10.1007/s10803-006-0107-0
34. McDonald S, Flanagan S, Rollins J, Kinch J. TASIT: a new clinical tool for assessing social perception after traumatic brain injury. *J Head Trauma Rehabil.* (2003) 18:219–38. doi: 10.1097/00001199-200305000-00001
35. Couture SM, Penn DL, Losh M, Adolphs R, Hurley R, Piven J. Comparison of social cognitive functioning in schizophrenia and high functioning autism: more convergence than divergence. *Psychol Med.* (2010) 40:569–79. doi: 10.1017/S00332917099 9078X
36. Okruszek Ł, Pilecka I. Biological motion processing in schizophrenia

- systematic review and meta-analysis. *Schizophr Res.* (2017) 190:3–10. doi: 10.1016/j.schres.2017.03.013

37. Kaletsch M, Pilgramm S, Bischoff M, Kindermann S, Sauerbier I, Stark R, et al. Major depressive disorder alters perception of emotional body movements. *Front Psychiatry.* (2014) 5:4. doi: 10.3389/fpsyt.2014.00004
38. Jaywant A, Wasserman V, Kemppainen M, Neargarder S, Cronin-Golomb A. Perception of communicative and non-communicative motion-defined gestures in Parkinson's disease. *J Int Neuropsychol Soc.* (2016) 22:540–50. doi: 10.1017/S1355617716000114
39. Quadflieg S, Westmoreland K. Making sense of other people's encounters: towards an integrative model of relational impression formation. *J Nonverbal Behav.* (2019) 43:1–24. doi: 10.1007/s10919-019-00295-1
40. Nagels A, Kircher T, Steines M, Straube B. Feeling addressed! The role of body orientation and co-speech gesture in social communication. *Hum Brain Mapp.* (2015) 36:1925–36. doi: 10.1002/hbm.22746
41. Okruszek Ł, Chrustowicz M. Social perception and interaction database - a novel tool to study social cognitive processes with point-light displays. *biorxiv. [Preprint].* (2019). doi: 10.1101/729996

4

Sexual Abuse in Adolescents is Associated with Atypically Increased Responsiveness within Regions Implicated in Self-Referential and Emotional Processing to Approaching Animate Threats

Karina S. Blair[1], Johannah Bashford-Largo[1], Niraj Shah[1], Jennie Lukoff[1], Jaimie Elowsky[1], Steven Vogel[1], Amanda Emmert[2], Ru Zhang[1], Matthew Dobbertin[1], Seth Pollak[3†] and James R. Blair[1]*

[1] Center for Neurobehavioral Research, Boys Town National Research Hospital, Boys Town, NE, United States, [2] Department of Psychiatry, Creighton University School of Medicine, Omaha, NE, United States, [3] Department of Psychology, University of Wisconsin, Madison, WI, United States

***Correspondence:**
Karina S. Blair
karina.blair@boystown.org

†ORCID:
Seth Pollak
orcid.org/0000-0001-5184-9846

Childhood sexual abuse is associated with significant subsequent pathology and neurodevelopmental disruption. In particular, childhood sexual abuse has been associated with heightened threat sensitivity. However, little work has directly investigated this issue. In this study, we examine the association of childhood sexual abuse to neural and behavioral responses to looming, threatening face stimuli. The study involved 23 adolescents with significant past sexual abuse and 24 comparison individuals matched on IQ, age, and sex. Participants were scanned during a looming threat task that involved negative and neutral, human faces and animals that appeared to either loom toward or recede from the participant. We found that adolescents who had been previously subjected to sexual abuse, relative to comparison adolescents, showed increased neural responses to *threatening looming stimuli* in regions including rostral and superior frontal gyrus as well as posterior cingulate gyrus. In addition, they were significantly more slowed by looming stimuli, particularly if these were human faces, than adolescents who had not been exposed. These data demonstrate that prior sexual abuse was associated with heightened neural responsiveness to looming threats in a series of regions beyond the amygdala. These data are interpreted within models of rostromedial frontal and posterior cingulate cortices that stress their role in self-referential emotional processing and emotional maintenance.

Keywords: childhood sexual abuse, threat responsiveness, looming threat, adolescents, functional Magnetic Resonance Imaging (fMRI)

INTRODUCTION

Childhood sexual abuse is relatively common and a major risk factor in the development of psychopathology [e.g., (1–3)]. It may have a particularly adverse impact relative to other forms of maltreatment (4, 5) with epidemiological work indicating that it is the most common cause of posttraumatic stress disorder (PTSD) (6). Despite this, studies focusing on the neurodevelopmental impact of sexual abuse are relatively rare [cf. (7, 8)].

Individuals subjected to maltreatment report difficulty regulating emotional responses to adverse events (9, 10). This is associated with increased responses to threat within the amygdala (9, 11–14). However, there has been less attention with respect to maltreatment and regions beyond the amygdala though regions though reports exist of regions such as medial frontal, posterior cingulate (PCC), and superior temporal cortices showing atypical responding to threat following maltreatment (8, 11, 15, 16). While there are no definitive accounts of the roles of these regions in threat processing, cases can be made that ventromedial frontal and PCC cortices are critically involved in the representation of stimulus value [e.g., (17)] while rostromedial frontal cortex may be particularly implicated in the maintenance of emotional responses (18).

Neural responses to threat are not uniform (19). Neural responses to relatively basic threats (e.g., a stimulus looming toward the individual) show overlaps with, but also distinctions from, those to threats that are more visually complex; e.g., facial expressions and threatening animal images (e.g., a snarling wolf); see **Supplemental Figure 1**. Moreover, core neural regions implicated in the response to threats such as the amygdala also respond to other stimulus classes such as human faces (20, 21). Yet again, the differential response to the human faces vs. animal stimulus dimension is rather different from those to the looming or visual threat dimensions properties; see Coker-Appiah et al. (19) and **Supplemental Figure 1**. It is currently unclear the extent to which maltreatment, and particularly sexual abuse, exaggerates responsiveness to particular types of threat stimuli and, perhaps more critically, to social stimuli such as faces that recruit at least partially overlapping neural circuitry (e.g., the amygdala). The level of responsiveness to social stimuli is interesting for two reasons: First, heightened responsiveness to such social stimuli is associated with social anxiety (22–24) that would further detrimentally affect the lives of individuals who had suffered abuse. Second, it allows a determination of the extent to which hyperresponsiveness to threat in specific neural systems (amygdala, vmPFC) is stimulus specific or neural region specific (i.e., to threats only or to all stimuli types that these regions respond to).

The current study aimed to determine the extent to which childhood sexual abuse is associated with increased threat responsiveness to both basic threat properties of a stimulus (e.g., looming relative to receding) as well as more visually complex properties (e.g., angry relative to neutral expressions/ snarling threatening animals relative to neutral animals). In addition, it sought to determine whether increased responsiveness is also seen to human faces relative to animals given the degree of overlap of neural systems engaged by both human faces and threatening stimuli (21). This was investigated with a group of participants previously subjected to sexual abuse and an age, IQ, and sex matched comparison group. Participants performed the Looming task (19). On the basis of the previous literature (9, 11–13), we predicted that participants subjected to prior sexual abuse would show increased responses to both looming relative to receding, and threatening relative to neutral images and potentially particularly strong responses to *looming threatening* images within the amygdala but also associated structures (medial frontal, anterior insula, PCC, and superior temporal gyrus). With respect to human relative to nonhuman faces, we predicted that if sexual abuse has a general impact in increasing responsiveness within regions such as the amygdala and medial frontal cortex, then individuals subjected to sexual abuse will show greater responses within these regions to human faces than comparison individuals. In contrast, if the impact of sexual abuse more selectively impacts the responsiveness of these regions to threat, we anticipated observing group differences only in response to threat variables.

MATERIALS AND METHODS

Participants

Twenty-three adolescents who reported significant past sexual abuse and 24 adolescents who did not report past sexual abuse participated in the study. The two groups were matched on age, sex, and IQ (see **Table 1**). Past sexual abuse was indexed *via* the Childhood Trauma Questionnaire (CTQ). Following validated thresholds [e.g., (25, 26)], individuals were considered to have experienced significant past sexual abuse if they endorsed three or more items pertaining to sexual abuse on the CTQ (see below for details about the CTQ). All sexual abuse reported was officially documented and under care. Psychiatric characterization was done through psychiatric interviews by licensed and board-certified psychiatrists with the participants and their parents, to adhere closely to common clinical practice. Individuals in the healthy comparison (HC) group reported

TABLE 1 | Participant characteristics.

	No past abuse (N = 24)	Past sexual abuse (N = 23)
CTQ Sexual Abuse score^	–	16.5 (SD = 5.32); R: 8–25
Age	15.1 (SD = 1.87)	15.1 (SD = 1.58)
IQ	99.9 (SD = 10.82)	95.3 (SD = 8.57)
% Female[a]	63% (N = 15)	74% (N = 17)
MDD[b]	0% (0)	30.4% (N = 7)
PTSD[b]	0% (0)	43.5% (N = 9)
Stimulants[c]	0% (0)	17.4% (N = 4)
Antidepressants[c]	0% (0)	34.8% (N = 8)
Antipsychotics[c]	0% (0)	34.8% (N = 8)

^Sexual Abuse as indexed by the Childhood Trauma Questionnaire (CTQ) Sexual Abuse subscale; MDD, major depressive disorder; PTSD, posttraumatic stress disorder.
[a]self-identified as female; [b]clinical diagnosis by psychiatrist; [c]medication currently prescribed.

no past sexual abuse and no current/past history of psychiatric illness.

Participants who had experienced sexual abuse were recruited shortly after their arrival at a residential care facility. Comparison adolescents were recruited from the community. Participants were excluded if IQ was below 75 assessed with the Wechsler Abbreviated Scale of Intelligence (WASI two-subtest form) or if they had nonpsychiatric medical illnesses that required the use of medication that may have psychotropic effects, such as beta-blockers or steroids. However, medications provided for psychiatric disorders (specifically antipsychotic, stimulant, or mood stabilizing medications) were not exclusory. Exclusion criteria also included braces, claustrophobia, active substance dependence, pervasive developmental disorder, Tourette's syndrome, lifetime history of psychosis, neurological disorder, head trauma, non-English speaking, and presence of active safety concerns.

Written informed consent and assent was taken. In all cases, youth had the right to decline participation at any time before or during the study. Consent documents were reviewed with the parent/legal guardians and written permission was obtained (1) at the initial visit for community participants or (2) at the time of intake for youth placed in Boys Town programs. Assent was obtained from the Boys Town youth in a separate session. It was made clear to all participants and their parents that their decision with respect to participation had no influence on their clinical care. The Boys Town National Research Hospital institutional review board approved this study.

Measures

History of sexual abuse was assessed using the CTQ, a 28-item self-report measure that indexes childhood/adolescent maltreatment. The CTQ indexes sexual abuse *via* 5 items: (1) Someone tried to touch me in a sexual way/made me touch them; (2) Someone threatened me unless I did something sexual; (3) Someone tried to make me do/watch sexual things; (4) Someone molested me; and (5) I believe that I was sexually abused. In addition to the sexual abuse scale, the CTQ contains four other subscales indexing emotional abuse (EA), physical abuse (PA), emotional neglect (EN), and physical neglect (PN). The CTQ has excellent psychometric properties including internal consistency, test-retest reliability, and convergent and discriminant validity with interviews and clinician reports of maltreatment (27). Individuals respond to each item using a five-point Likers scale: (1) never true, (2) rarely true, (3) sometimes true, (4) often true, and (5) very often true. Thus, individuals can score between 5 (no history of abuse) and 25 (extreme abuse) on the sexual abuse subscale of the CTQ. Psychiatric diagnoses were made according to the Diagnostic and Statistical Manual of Mental Disorders-5 (American Psychiatric Association, 2013) through psychiatric interviews by licensed and board-certified child and adolescent psychiatrists with the participants and their parents, to adhere closely to common clinical practice.

fMRI Task

The participants performed the looming task *(adapted from Coker-Appiah et al., 2013)*. They were presented with an image that appeared to either loom toward or recede away from them. Images were human or animal faces and were either threatening or neutral in valence.

Images were rapidly presented in a series of sixteen 50-ms frames of increasing or decreasing size in the center of the screen to create the effect of either looming (i.e., increasing in size in rapid succession) or receding (i.e., decreasing in size in rapid succession; total stimulus duration: 800 ms); see **Figure 1**. Stimulus presentations were followed by a fixation point, which was on screen for a jittered duration of 1,250–4,250 ms. The task included a single run of 160 stimuli (20 of each of the 8 trial types). Each individual image was presented only twice; once looming toward and once receding from the participant. In order to ensure attention to the task, participants were instructed to press a button with their right index finger as quickly as possible when an image appeared on the screen.

fMRI Parameters

Whole-brain blood oxygen level dependent (BOLD) fMRI data were acquired using a 3.0 Tesla Siemens Skyra Magnetic Resonance Scanner. Functional images were taken with a T2* weighted gradient echo planar imaging (EPI) sequence [repetition time (TR) = 2, 500 ms, echo time (TE) = 27 ms, flip angle = 90° field-of-view (FOV) = 240 mm]. Whole-brain coverage was obtained with 43 axial slices (thickness, 2.5mm; voxel size 2.6 × 2.6 × 2.5 mm^3; distance factor 21%). In the same session, a high-resolution T1-weighed anatomical image was acquired to aid with spatial normalization (MP-RAGE, repetition time = 2,200 ms, echo time = 2.48 ms; 230-mm field of view; 8° flip angle; 256 × 208 matrix) was acquired to register with the EPI dataset. Whole-brain coverage was obtained with 176 axial slices (thickness 1 mm; voxel size 0.9 × 0.9 × 1 mm^3, distance factor 50%).

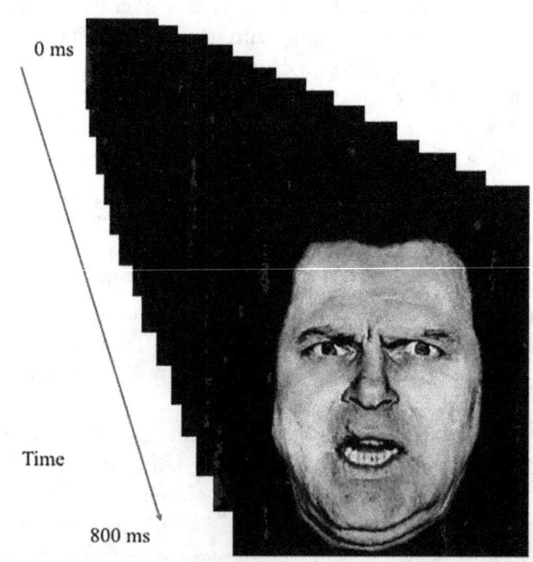

FIGURE 1 | Task illustration. Example of Looming Threatening Human face trial.

fMRI Analysis: Data Preprocessing and Individual Level Analysis

Functional MRI data were preprocessed and analyzed using Analysis of Functional NeuroImages (AFNI) software (28). Data from the first four repetitions were collected prior to magnetization equilibrium and were discarded. The anatomical scan for each participant was registered to the Talairach and Tournoux atlas (29) and each participant's functional EPI data were registered to their Talairach anatomical scan in AFNI. Functional images were motion corrected and spatially smoothed with a 6-mm full width half maximum Gaussian kernel. The data then underwent time series normalization and these results were multiplied by 100 for each voxel. Therefore, the resultant regression coefficients are representative of a percentage of signal change from the mean.

A model was generated using six motion regressors and the following eight regressors: Looming Threatening Human, Looming Neutral Human, Looming Threatening Animal, Looming Neutral Animal, Receding Threatening Human, Receding Neutral Human, Receding Threatening Animal, Receding Neutral Animal. GLM fitting was performed with these eight regressors, six motion regressors, and a regressor modeling baseline drift. All regressors were convolved with a canonical hemodynamic response function (HRF) to account for the slow hemodynamic response (with time point commencing at time of first image onset). This produced a β coefficient and associated *t* statistic for each voxel and regressor. There was no significant regressor collinearity.

Statistical Analyses

Behavioral Data: A 2 (Group: Subjected to sexual abuse, Comparison) by 2 (Direction: Looming, Receding) by 2 (Type: Human, Animal) by 2 (Valence: Threatening, Neutral) ANOVA was conducted on the participant's mean reaction times (RT) for each trial type. Outliers (RTs 3 standard deviations greater or lesser than the participant's mean RT for that trial type) were excluded (approximately 1% of the data).

MRI Data: Our hypotheses were tested by a full 2 (Group: Subjected to sexual abuse, Comparison) by 2 (Direction: Looming, Receding) by 2 (Type: Human, Animal) by 2 (Valence: Threatening, Neutral) ANOVA performed on the BOLD data. Subsequently, we ran a second group-based ANCOVA where total levels of other forms of maltreatment (physical and emotional abuse and physical and emotional neglect) was the covariate. For the follow-up ANCOVAs a Blom Transformation was applied to the participants' CTQ sexual abuse and the CTQ other maltreatment (EA + PA + EN + PN) scores. This is a normalization procedure which rank orders, and then standardizes values within a dataset (30). To facilitate future meta-analytic work, effect sizes [partial eta square (ηp^2)] are reported in the Tables [though note that our relatively small sample size may result in an overestimate of the size of the true population effect; (31)].

Correction for multiple comparisons was performed using a spatial clustering operation in AFNI's 3dClustSim utilizing the autocorrelation function (-acf) with 10,000 Monte Carlo simulations for the whole-brain analysis. Spatial autocorrelation was estimated from residuals from the individual-level GLMs. The initial threshold was set at p =.001. This process yielded an extant threshold of k = 20 voxels for the whole brain (multiple comparison corrected $p < 0.05$). Follow-up testing was conducted within the Statistical Package for the Social Sciences (SPSS) version 22.0.0.2 (IBM Corporation, Armonk, NY).

RESULTS

Behavioral Data

A 2 (Group: Subjected to sexual abuse, Comparison) by 2 (Direction: Looming, Receding) by 2 (Type: Human, Animal) by 2 (Valence: Threatening, Neutral) ANOVA was conducted on the reaction time (RT) data. There was a main effect of Direction [$F(1,45) = 68.92$; $p < 0.001$; $\eta p^2 = 0.616$]; participants were faster to respond to receding than looming stimuli (461.55 vs. 411.26 ms). In addition, there was a significant: (i) main effect of Group [$F(1,45) = 9.05$; $p = 0.004$; $\eta p^2 = 0.174$; participants that had been subjected to sexual abuse were significantly slower to respond than comparison adolescents; M(subjected to sexual abuse) = 481.46 ms; M(Comparison) = 391.35 ms]; (ii) Group-by-Direction interaction [$F(1,45) = 5.02$; $p = 0.030$; $\eta p^2 = 0.104$]. Participants that had been subjected to sexual abuse showed a significantly greater increase in RT for looming relative to receding stimuli relative to comparison adolescents [$F(1,45) = 5.21$; $p = 0.030$; M(subjected to sexual abuse: Looming-Receding) = 63.87ms; M(Comparison: Looming-Receding) = 36.73ms]; and (ii) a significant Group-by-Direction-by-Type interaction [$F(1,45) = 7.08$; $p = 0.010$; $\eta p^2 = 0.14$]. Participants who had been subjected to sexual abuse showed significantly greater increases in RT to looming human faces than receding human faces relative to comparison adolescents {$t[45]=-3.31$; $p=0.002$; M[subjected to sexual abuse: Looming-Receding(human faces)] = 83.09ms; M [Comparison: Receding-Looming(human faces)] = 36.87ms}. However, there were no significant group differences for animal stimuli {$t[45] = -0.566$; $p = 0.574$; M[subjected to sexual abuse: Receding-Looming(animal stimuli)] = 44.64 ms; M[Comparison: Receding-Looming(animal stimuli)] = 36.59 ms}.

Movement Data

Volumes were censored if there was >0.5 mm motion across adjacent volumes. No participant in the final sample for the current study had >5% censored volumes. There were no significant group differences in terms of censored volumes ($F < 1$; ns), average motion per volume ($F < 1$; ns)], or maximum displacement during scanning ($F = 1.73$; $p = 0.195$).

fMRI Data

The analysis of the BOLD response data revealed regions showing significant Group-by-Direction-by-Valence interactions (see **Table 2**). All other significant results are

TABLE 2 | Significant areas of activation from the initial 2 (Group: Subjected to sexual abuse, Comparison) by 2 (Direction: Looming, Receding) by 2 (Type: Human, Animal) by 2 (Valence: Threatening, Neutral) ANOVA.

REGION	BA	Voxels	X	Y	Z	F-value	ηp^2
Group-by-Direction-by-Valence							
L medial frontal gyrus	10	68	−1	59	20	26.32	0.369
L superior frontal gyrus	10	29	−22	53	26	24.22	0.350
L superior frontal gyrus	8	26	−13	44	41	24.82	0.356
L posterior cingulate cortex	31	49	−1	−49	32	21.37	0.322
R superior temporal gyrus	38	31	41	14	−31	28.71	0.389
R inferior temporal gyrus	20	23	50	−7	−19	30.04	0.400

Activations are from whole brain analyses significant at $p < 0.001$, corrected for multiple comparisons significant at $p < 0.05$.

listed in **Supplemental Table 1**. Images of the main effects of Direction, Valence and Type are presented in **Supplemental Figure 1**.

Group-by-Direction-by-Valence Interactions

Regions showing significant Group-by-Direction-by-Valence interaction included rostromedial prefrontal cortex (rmPFC) (BA 10), superior frontal gyrus (BA 8 & BA 10), as well as superior (BA 38) inferior (BA 20) and superior temporal gyrus, and PCC (BA 31); **Table 2**. Within all these regions, participants who had been subjected to sexual abuse, relative to comparison individuals, showed significantly greater BOLD responses to *looming threatening* stimuli relative to both *looming neutral* (F range = 7.35 to 14.20; p < range = 0.01 to 0.001) and *receding threatening* stimuli (F range = 4.35 to 12.93; p < range 0.005 to 0.001); see **Figure 2**. A region of amygdala also showed a Group-by-Direction-by-Valence interaction but at marginal levels ($p < 0.05$, uncorrected).

Follow-Up Analyses

1. ***Excluding Participants With PTSD:*** Given the potential influences of PTSD pathology (nine participants subjected to sexual abuse had diagnoses of PTSD), we reran the initial group-based analysis excluding the participants with PTSD diagnosis. Even when excluding those participants, the Group-by-Direction-by-Valence result pattern reported above and in **Table 2** largely remained; see **Supplemental Table 2**).
2. ***Excluding Participants With MDD:*** Given the potential influences of MDD pathology (seven participants subjected to sexual abuse had diagnoses of MDD), we also reran the initial group-based analysis excluding the participants with MDD diagnosis. The exclusion of those participants did not significantly change the results reported above in the main analysis and in **Table 2**; see **Supplemental Table 3**).
3. ***Excluding Participants on Medication:*** Given the potential influences of mediation use, the group-based ANOVA above was re-run excluding participants on medication (stimulants, antidepressant, and antipsychotics). Again, excluding these participants did not change the Group-by-Direction-by-Valence result pattern reported above and in **Table 2**. See **Supplemental Tables 4–6**.
4. ***Other Maltreatment as an Added Covariate to CTQ Sexual Abuse Scores:*** Given the potential overlap in neural correlates associated with other types of maltreatment, we followed up our initial ANOVA analysis with a group based ANCOVA where Blom transformed total levels of other forms of maltreatment (physical and emotional abuse and physical and emotional neglect) was the covariate. The Group-by-Direction-by-Valence interactions for the left medial, left superior frontal gyrus (BA 8) and the superior temporal gyrus remained; see **Supplemental Table 7**. In contrast, there were no interactions surviving for the Other-Maltreatment-by-Direction-by-Valence interaction.

DISCUSSION

In this study, we investigated the extent to which past sexual abuse is associated with increased responsiveness to threat (looming stimuli and threat images) and social cues (human faces). There were three main findings: First, participants who had been subjected to sexual abuse showed heightened neural responsiveness to looming threats in a series of regions beyond the amygdala (e.g., rmPFC and PCC). Second, participants who had been subjected to sexual abuse did not show heightened responsiveness specifically to social stimuli. Third, looming stimuli were generally associated with slower reaction times and this exaggerated in participants previously subjected to sexual abuse particularly if the looming stimulus was a human face.

Previous work has reported that participants who have experienced maltreatment show heightened responsiveness to threat (8, 11, 13–15). However, much of this work has focused on the amygdala (9, 11–14). There was a Group-by-Direction-by-Valence interaction within the amygdala in the current study. However, this was of marginal significance ($p < 0.05$ uncorrected). Instead, the results of the current study join other work stressing the impact of maltreatment, in this case past sexual abuse, in increasing responsiveness in regions beyond the amygdala [cf. (16, 32)]. This failure to observe more of an increase in amygdala responsiveness in participants who had been subjected to sexual abuse did *not* reflect task or imaging parameters. As reported in **Supplemental Table 1**, and seen in **Supplemental Figure 1**, the amygdala showed strong responses to looming relative to receding stimuli, threat relative to neutral images and human faces relative to animals. However, this amygdala responsiveness was not modulated by previously

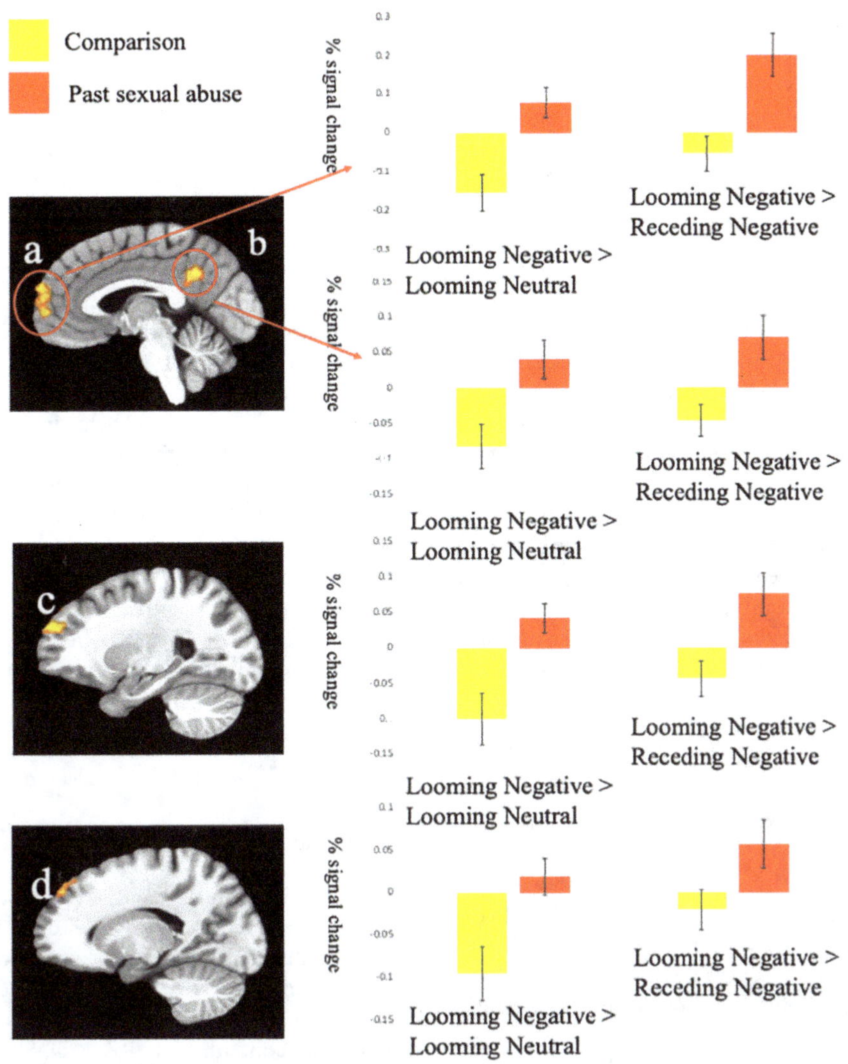

FIGURE 2 | Interactions of Group-by-Direction-by-Valence. Blood oxygen level dependent (BOLD) responses within **(A)** left medial prefrontal gyrus (−1, 59, 20); **(B)** left posterior cingulate cortex (−1, −49, 32); **(C)** left superior frontal gyrus BA 10 (−22, 53, 26); and **(D)** superior frontal gyrus BA 8 (−13, 44, 41) to the Looming Negative trials compared to the Looming Neutral and Receding Neutral trials.

being subjected to sexual abuse. There was no significant Group-by-Direction, Group-by-Valence, or Group-by-Type within the amygdala even at $p < 0.05$. We assume that this reflects a Type II error perhaps as a result of specific features of the task/scanner but future work will investigate this further.

rmPFC, vmPFC, and PCC have been implicated in assessing the salience and relevance of emotional stimuli (17, 18, 33, 34). The suggestion has been made that the intensity of an emotional experience is due in part to the role of these cortical midline structures in affect-based self-referent processing (35, 36). In addition, it has been suggested that rmPFC is particularly implicated in the maintenance of this emotional response (18). As such, it can be speculated on the basis of the current data that being previously subjected to sexual abuse may lead to a heightened emotional response that reflects self-referential emotional processing and emotional maintenance. The amygdala may be implicated but the functioning of other structures, particularly those involved in affect-based self-referent processing and emotional maintenance, may be even more impacted (at least by being previously subjected to sexual abuse). One feature of the current results that is interesting in this regard is that the interactions of group were with Direction-by-Valence, not Direction or Valence alone. This is interesting because in the current results and similar to our previous experience with this task (19), there were no regions showing a significant Direction-by-Valence (i.e., without Group) but instead many regions showing strong (and partly regionally overlapping) main effects for Direction *and* Valence (see **Supplemental Figure 1** and **Supplemental Table 1**). In short, it can be speculated the Group-by-Direction-by-Valence interaction represents a heightened appraisal of a self-referential threat (i.e., a threat moving toward the individual) beyond more stimulus-driven responses to looming and threat information in participants previously subjected to sexual abuse.

The amygdala and rmPFC/vmPFC are not only responsive to emotional stimuli but also to social stimuli, including human faces (20, 21, 37, 38). This was seen in the current study also (see **Supplemental Table 1** and **Supplemental Figure 1**). Moreover, patients with social anxiety disorder show atypically increased activations or connectivity between the amygdala and rmPFC in response to face stimuli (39, 40). However, being previously exposed to sexual abuse was not associated with heightened responsiveness to face stimuli in the current data. These data indicate that while being previously subjected to sexual abuse may increase threat responsiveness and increase propensity for anxiety generally, it does not, at least according to these data, particularly increase responsiveness of neural responses associated with social anxiety.

The behavioral data are worthy of note. Participants were generally faster to respond to receding than looming stimuli. This presumably reflects a freeze response to approaching dangers [cf. (41)]. Interestingly, adolescents previously subjected to sexual abuse showed significantly greater increases in RT to looming relative to receding (looming-receding) stimuli relative to comparison adolescents. Notably, these group differences in increases in RT for looming relative to receding stimuli were most marked for human face stimuli. In short, these data indicate that past sexual abuse may exaggerate the acute threat response. In the context of the current study, with relatively low level threats, this manifested as increased freezing. However, with more intense threats, increased flight or even reactive aggression can be anticipated [cf. (41)]. Moreover, this may be particularly marked for the highly salient threat of approaching humans (even though a greater response to human face stimuli was not seen in the BOLD response data).

There are several caveats that should be noted with respect to the current results. First, consistent with considerable previous work (1–3), past sexual abuse was associated with significant psychiatric psychopathology (see **Table 1**). Accordingly, the current results might reflect psychopathology rather than maltreatment. Ameliorating this concern is the fact that the results of the main analysis largely held even after removal of participants with the most common psychiatric diagnoses in this sample (PTSD, MDD). Second, most adolescents who had experienced sexual abuse had also experienced other forms of maltreatment. As such, the findings might be associated with other forms of maltreatment. This possibility cannot be discounted. The current study was not designed to differentiate associations with sexual abuse relative to other forms of maltreatment. However, it is worth noting that core findings remained even when other forms of maltreatment were included as a covariate (see **Supplemental Table 7**). Third, medication rates were significantly higher for participants who had been subjected to prior sexual abuse relative to those who had not. However, the results of the main analysis held even after excluding participants on medication (stimulants, antidepressant, antipsychotics); see **Supplemental Tables 4–6**. Fourth, the face stimuli used in this study were both male and female. It is possible that face stimuli matching the sex of the perpetrator of the adolescent's sexual abuse might exaggerate responsiveness to looming faces relative to animals.

In conclusion, we found that past sexual abuse was associated with heightened neural responsiveness to looming threats in a series of regions beyond the amygdala such as rmPFC and PCC. At the neural level, there were no group differences with respect to face stimuli or looming faces in particular. Behaviorally, participants were slower to respond to looming than receding stimuli and this effect was exaggerated in participants previously subjected to sexual abuse particularly if the looming stimulus was a human face. As such the behavioral data mirrored the BOLD response data with respect to the interaction of sexual abuse with the looming variable. However, they also suggested that there may be differential sensitization to face stimuli following sexual abuse that did not emerge in the neural data. These data are interpreted within models of rmPFC and PCC cortices that stress their role in self-referential emotional processing and emotional maintenance (18, 35, 36). Sexual abuse may lead to an exaggerated appraisal and maintenance of self-referential threats (i.e., threat, perhaps particularly human threats, moving toward the individual).

AUTHOR CONTRIBUTIONS

Study PI KB conducted and is responsible for the data analysis. She had full access to all the data in the study and takes responsibility for the integrity of the data and the accuracy of the data analysis. NS, JL, JE, AE, and SV contributed to the acquisition and critical revision of the manuscript for important intellectual content. JB-L, RZ, MD, SP, and JB contributed with interpretation of the data and critical revision of the manuscript for important intellectual content.

FUNDING

This research was in part supported by the National Institute of General Medical Sciences of the National Institutes of Health under award number 5P20GM109023-05 (KB) and the National Institute of Mental Health under award number K22-MH109558 (JB). SP was supported by the National Institute of Mental Health [R01MH61285] and the National Institute of Child Health and Human Development [U54 HD090256]. The funders had no role in the design and conduct of the study; collection, management, analysis, and interpretation of the data; preparation, review, or approval of the manuscript; and decision to submit the manuscript for publication.

ACKNOWLEDGMENTS

We would like to thank Ron Copsey, Kim VanHorn, Michael Wright, Mark Timm, and Rhonda Tuel for their contributions to data collection. We would like to thank all participants and their families for their participation. This work was supported by Boys Town National Research Hospital.

REFERENCES

1. Edwards VJ, Holden GW, Felitti VJ, Anda RF. Relationship between multiple forms of childhood maltreatment and adult mental health in community respondents: results from the adverse childhood experiences study. *Am J Psychiatry* (2003) 160:1453–60. doi: 10.1176/appi.ajp.160.8.1453
2. Kendler KS, Kuhn JW, Prescott CA. Childhood sexual abuse, stressful life events and risk for major depression in women. *Psychol Med* (2004) 34:1475–82. doi: 10.1017/s003329170400265x
3. Post RM, Leverich GS, Xing G, Weiss RB. Developmental vulnerabilities to the onset and course of bipolar disorder. *Dev Psychopathol* (2001) 13:581–98. doi: 10.1017/s0954579401003091
4. Heim CM, Mayberg HS, Mletzko T, Nemeroff CB, Pruessner JC. Decreased cortical representation of genital somatosensory field after childhood sexual abuse. *Am J Psychiatry* (2013) 170:616–23. doi: 10.1176/appi.ajp.2013.12070950
5. Cassiers LLM, Sabbe BGC, Schmaal L, Veltman DJ, Penninx B, Van Den Eede F. Structural and Functional Brain Abnormalities Associated With Exposure to Different Childhood Trauma Subtypes: A Systematic Review of Neuroimaging Findings. *Front Psychiatry* (2018) 9:329. doi: 10.3389/fpsyt.2018.00329
6. Kessler RC, Sonnega A, Bromet E, Hughes M, Nelson CB. Posttraumatic stress disorder in the National Comorbidity Survey. *Arch Gen Psychiatry* (1995) 52:1048–60. doi: 10.1001/archpsyc.1995.03950240066012
7. Andersen SL, Tomada A, Vincow ES, Valente E, Polcari A, Teicher MH. Preliminary evidence for sensitive periods in the effect of childhood sexual abuse on regional brain development. *J Neuropsychiat Clin Neurosci* (2008) 20:292–301. doi: 10.1176/jnp.2008.20.3.292
8. Skokauskas N, Carballedo A, Fagan A, Frodl T. The role of sexual abuse on functional neuroimaging markers associated with major depressive disorder. *World J Biol Psychiatry : Off J World Fed Societies Biol Psychiatry* (2015) 16:513–20. doi: 10.3109/15622975.2015.1048723
9. Pechtel P, Pizzagalli DA. Effects of early life stress on cognitive and affective function: an integrated review of human literature. *Psychopharmacol (Berl)* (2011) 214:55–70. doi: 10.1007/s00213-010-2009-2
10. Shackman JE, Pollak SD. Impact of physical maltreatment on the regulation of negative affect and aggression. *Dev Psychopathol* (2014) 26:1021–33. doi: 10.1017/S0954579414000546
11. Hein TC, Monk CS. Research Review: Neural response to threat in children, adolescents, and adults after child maltreatment - a quantitative meta-analysis. *J Child Psychol Psychiatry* (2017) 58:222–30. doi: 10.1111/jcpp.12651
12. Tottenham N, Galvan A. Stress and the adolescent brain: Amygdala-prefrontal cortex circuitry and ventral striatum as developmental targets. *Neurosci Biobehav Rev* (2016) 70:217–27. doi: 10.1016/j.neubiorev.2016.07.030
13. Kaiser RH, Clegg R, Goer F, Pechtel P, Beltzer M, Vitaliano G, et al. Childhood stress, grown-up brain networks: corticolimbic correlates of threat-related early life stress and adult stress response. *Psychol Med* (2018) 48:1157–66. doi: 10.1017/S0033291717002628
14. McCrory EJ, Gerin MI, Viding E. Annual Research Review: Childhood maltreatment, latent vulnerability and the shift to preventative psychiatry - the contribution of functional brain imaging. *J Child Psychol Psychiatry* (2017) 58:338–57. doi: 10.1111/jcpp.12713
15. Elsey J, Coates A, Lacadie CM, McCrory EJ, Sinha R, Mayes LC, et al. Childhood trauma and neural responses to personalized stress, favorite-food and neutral-relaxing cues in adolescents. *Neuropsychopharmacology* (2015) 40:1580–9. doi: 10.1038/npp.2015.6
16. McCrory EJ, De Brito SA, Sebastian CL, Mechelli A, Bird G, Kelly PA, et al. Heightened neural reactivity to threat in child victims of family violence. *Curr Biol* (2011) 21:R947–8. doi: 10.1016/j.cub.2011.10.015
17. Clithero JA, Rangel A. Informatic parcellation of the network involved in the computation of subjective value. *Soc Cognit Affect Neurosci* (2014) 9:1289–302. doi: 10.1093/scan/nst106
18. Waugh CE, Lemus MG, Gotlib IH. The role of the medial frontal cortex in the maintenance of emotional states. *Soc Cognit Affect Neurosci* (2014) 9:2001–9. doi: 10.1093/scan/nsu011
19. Coker-Appiah DS, White SF, Clanton R, Yang J, Martin A, Blair RJ. Looming animate and inanimate threats: The response of the amygdala and periaqueductal gray. *Soc Neurosci* (2013) 8:621–30. doi: 10.1080/17470919.2013.839480
20. Pessoa L, Adolphs R. Emotion processing and the amygdala: from a 'low road' to 'many roads' of evaluating biological significance. *Nat Rev Neurosci* (2010) 11:773–83. doi: 10.1038/nrn2920
21. Yang J, Bellgowan PS, Martin A. Threat, domain-specificity and the human amygdala. *Neuropsychologia* (2012) 50:2566–72. doi: 10.1016/j.neuropsychologia.2012.07.001
22. Fonzo GA, Etkin A. Affective neuroimaging in generalized anxiety disorder: an integrated review. *Dialogues Clin Neurosci* (2017) 19:169–79.
23. Schulz C, Mothes-Lasch M, Straube T. Automatic neural processing of disorder-related stimuli in social anxiety disorder: faces and more. *Front Psychol* (2013) 4:282. doi: 10.3389/fpsyg.2013.00282
24. Blair RJR. Emotion-based learning systems and the development of morality. *Cognition* (2017) 167:38–45. doi: 10.1016/j.cognition.2017.03.013
25. Walker EA, Unutzer J, Rutter C, Gelfand A, Saunders K, VonKorff M, et al. Costs of health care use by women HMO members with a history of childhood abuse and neglect. *Arch Gen Psychiatry* (1999) 56:609–13. doi: 10.1001/archpsyc.56.7.609
26. McLaughlin KA, Peverill M, Gold AL, Alves S, Sheridan MA. Child Maltreatment and Neural Systems Underlying Emotion Regulation. *J Am Acad Child Adolesc Psychiatry* (2015) 54:753–62. doi: 10.1016/j.jaac.2015.06.010
27. Bernstein DP, Ahluvalia T, Pogge D, Handelsman L. Validity of the Childhood Trauma Questionnaire in an adolescent psychiatric population. *J Am Acad Child Adolesc Psychiatry* (1997) 36:340–8. doi: 10.1097/00004583-199703000-00012
28. Cox RW. AFNI: software for analysis and visualization of functional magnetic resonance neuroimages. *Comput Biomed Res* (1996) 29:162–73. doi: 10.1006/cbmr.1996.0014
29. Talairach J, Tournoux P. *Co-planar stereotaxic atlas of the human brain.* New York, NY: Thieme Publishers (1988).
30. Blom G. *Statistical Estimates and Transformed Beta-Variables.* Hoboken, NJ: Wiley and Sons Publishers (1958).
31. Cremers HR, Wager TD, Yarkoni T. The relation between statistical power and inference in fMRI. *PLoS One* (2017) 12(11). doi: 10.1371/journal.pone.0184923
32. Puetz VB, Viding E, Palmer A, Kelly PA, Lickley R, Koutoufa I, et al. Altered neural response to rejection-related words in children exposed to maltreatment. *J Child Psychol Psychiatry* (2016) 57:1165–73. doi: 10.1111/jcpp.12595
33. Wager TD, Waugh CE, Lindquist M, Noll DC, Fredrickson BL, Taylor SF. Brain mediators of cardiovascular responses to social threat: part I: Reciprocal dorsal and ventral sub-regions of the medial prefrontal cortex and heart-rate reactivity. *Neuroimage* (2009) 47:821–35. doi: 10.1016/j.neuroimage.2009.05.043
34. Waugh CE, Hamilton JP, Chen MC, Joormann J, Gotlib IH. Neural temporal dynamics of stress in comorbid major depressive disorder and social anxiety disorder. *Biol Mood Anxiety Disord* (2012) 2:11. doi: 10.1186/2045-5380-2-11
35. Waugh CE, Hamilton JP, Gotlib IH. The neural temporal dynamics of the intensity of emotional experience. *Neuroimage* (2010) 49:1699–707. doi: 10.1016/j.neuroimage.2009.10.006
36. De Pisapia N, Barchiesi G, Jovicich J, Cattaneo L. The role of medial prefrontal cortex in processing emotional self-referential information: a combined TMS/fMRI study. *Brain Imaging Behav* (2018) 13(3):603–14 . doi: 10.1007/s11682-018-9867-3

37. Dang TP, Mattan BD, Kubota JT, Cloutier J. The ventromedial prefrontal cortex is particularly responsive to social evaluations requiring the use of person-knowledge. *Sci Rep* (2019) 9:5054. doi: 10.1038/s41598-019-41544-z
38. Hartwright CE, Apperly IA, Hansen PC. Representation, control, or reasoning? Distinct functions for theory of mind within the medial prefrontal cortex. *J Cognit Neurosci* (2014) 26:683–98. doi: 10.1162/jocn_a_00520
39. Blair KS, Otero M, Teng C, Geraci M, Lewis E, Hollon N, et al. Learning from other people's fear: amygdala-based social reference learning in social anxiety disorder. *Psychol Med* (2016) 46:2943–53. doi: 10.1017/S0033291716001537
40. Robinson OJ, Krimsky M, Lieberman L, Vytal K, Ernst M, Grillon C. Anxiety-potentiated amygdala-medial frontal coupling and attentional control. *Trans Psychiatry* (2016) 6:e833. doi: 10.1038/tp.2016.105
41. Blanchard RJ, Blanchard DC, Takahashi LK. Attack and defensive behaviour in the albino rat. *Anim Behav* (1977) 25:197–224. doi: 10.1016/S0091-6773(77)90308-X

5

Social Media usage and Development of Psychiatric Disorders in Childhood and Adolescence

Ilaria Cataldo [1,2], Bruno Lepri [2], Michelle Jin Yee Neoh [3] and Gianluca Esposito [1,3,4]*

[1] Affiliative Behavior and Physiology Lab, Department of Psychology and Cognitive Science, University of Trento, Trento, Italy, [2] Mobile and Social Computing Lab, Bruno Kessler Foundation, Trento, Italy, [3] Social and Affective Neuroscience Lab, Psychology Program, School of Social Sciences, Nanyang Technological University, Singapore, Singapore, [4] Lee Kong Chian School of Medicine, Nanyang Technological University, Singapore, Singapore

***Correspondence:**
Gianluca Esposito
gianluca.esposito@ntu.edu.sg;
gianluca.esposito@unitn.it

Social media platforms, such as Facebook, Twitter, and Instagram, are now part of almost everyone's social life, especially for the newer generations. Children and teenagers grew up together with these Internet-based services, which have become an integral part of their personal and social life. However, as reported in various studies, psychological and psychiatric problems are sometimes associated with problematic usage of social media. The primary purpose of this review is to provide an overview of the cognitive, psychological, and social outcomes correlated with a problematic use of social media sites during the developmental stages, from age 10 to 19 years. With a specific focus on depression, anxiety, eating, and neurodevelopmental disorders, the review also discusses evidence related to genetic and neurobiological issues, together with the implications in clinical work and future directions under a multidisciplinary perspective. While the scientific community has made significant progress in enhancing our understanding of the impact of social media on teenagers' lives, more research integrating biological and environmental factors is required to fully elucidate the development of these disorders.

Keywords: social media, Facebook, Instagram, Twitter, depression, anxiety, adolescence, psychiatric disorders

1. SOCIAL MEDIA: AN INCREASING PHENOMENON IN HUMAN BEHAVIOR

In our global digital world, social connections are embedded within the external environment we are physically engaged in and the life that we virtually share on social media. Social media is a class of mobile and Internet-based applications that allow people to receive information and to build and share user-generated content. Through the creation of a virtual profile, it is possible to interact with real-life friends, meet new people from all over the world, connect with one's favorite celebrities, and to maintain both online and offline relationships. Since 2004, the use of social media has been increasing rapidly, with the possibility to be connected to the Internet anytime and anywhere. According to the nature of the content, the user can choose, from a wide range of applications, the platform that best suits the purpose of the communication. For example, Facebook is more focused on real-life friends and relatives and encourage interactions through services such as sharing pictures, videos, status updates, and joining groups with specific interests.

Social platforms like Twitter, which are also known as "microblogs," are characterized by brief communication. Other applications, like Instagram or Snapchat, provide photo- and video-sharing services, together with the possibility to like, comment, and re-post preferred content. **Figure 1** shows the popularity of the leading social networks, ranked by the worldwide number of active users (source: ourworldindata.org).

Social media platforms are widely used across different age groups and cultures, but especially for children and teenagers, online communication represents "*a window into the secret world of adolescent peer culture, even as it offers young people a new screen for the projection of adolescent developmental issues*" (1). While social media offers tremendous potential in allowing self-expression of personality and maintaining contact with a network of friends, some studies have also highlighted the risk of negative consequences of excessive online social platforms usage (2, 3). Online social interaction, the blurring of lines between offline and virtual life (4, 5), and the concept of digital identity (6) have become topics of great interest in psychology and mental health fields (7). Researchers in the field are attempting to find a consensual definition of the concept of "problematic social media use," as it is often confused with a description of addictive behavior related to general Internet services, which has been included in the 5th edition of the Diagnostic and Statistical Manual of mental disorders (8). In accordance with a biopsychosocial framework, problematic use of social media involves a set of alterations affecting biological functions (i.e., neurotransmitters regulation and circadian rhythm); cognitive, psychological, and affective mechanisms (i.e., attention, salience, mood fluctuation, and anxiety), and aspects related to the social sphere (i.e., social desirability, popularity, and conflicts), resulting in a decreased perceived quality of life. Feedback from people belonging to the virtual social community can affect individual self-esteem and, generally, well-being (9–13). A problematic use can also affect other aspects of a teenager's daily life, such as academic performance, time management issues, procrastination, distraction (14), and sleep disturbances (15). In severe cases, averse outcomes could arise and, if prolonged, can become highly impactful, with the further risk of developing psychiatric disorders (16). As the Internet and social media are a recent phenomenon, it is more likely that the effect of excessive or problematic usage will affect individuals during more sensitive temporal frames, such as childhood and adolescence. A survey conducted in the United States in 2018 reported that 45% of the teenagers interviewed say they are almost constantly online, without differences among sexes, ethnicities, family incomes, and parental level of education (for the full report, see Teens, Social Media & Technology 2018). Given the continuous exposure to the virtual environment, it is essential to understand the impact that online social relationships have on mental health and interpersonal functioning in developmental stages. The aim of our review, compared to other recent publications [see (17, 18)], is to provide a detailed overview of not only the effect of social media in general but also of the associations between specific platforms and psychopathology. We believe that this point is relevant, as it is important to distinguish among the different social media platforms given that each of them has specific, unique features that drive young users' preferences.

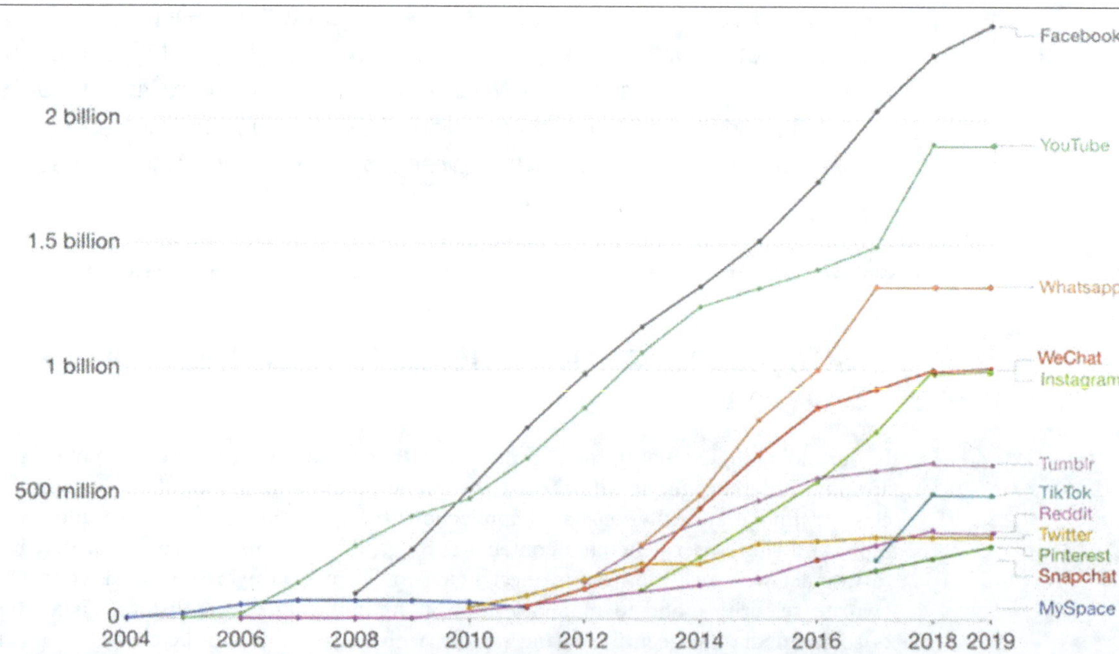

FIGURE 1 | Number of people using social media from 2004 until the end of 2019; estimates correspond to monthly active users, defined as those who logged in during the past 30 days.

Furthermore, social media usage is often included in the broader category of Internet usage, despite the social connotation that primarily describes and defines these kinds of sites. Moreover, the included articles were discussed according to specific disorders that can develop during childhood and adolescence, not merely depression and anxiety that are the most explored disorders but also addictive behaviors toward substances and eating disorders (EDs), as both start to develop during adolescence. In fact, developmental stages are more vulnerable to environmental insults just because of the greater plasticity of the central nervous system, the multiple biological changes, and the formation of psychological mechanisms that drive social behaviors (19, 20). Due to the differences that define each platform, one of the main purposes of the present review is to provide evidence related to targeted social media services, instead of a more general discussion on social media. In fact, we retain that the multifaceted manifestation of diverse psychological issues might be expressed differently through the multiple ways of communication, such as text, video, or picture. As social behavior and the risk for psychiatric disorders is related to the activity of determined brain regions and biological features (21, 22), and since we are addressing the outcomes of problematic social media usage (PSMU) under a biopsychosocial perspective, we will also provide an overview about the neuroscientific and gene-by-environment contribution to the interplay between social media and the development of psychiatric disorders in adolescence.

2. METHODS AND RESULTS

The review adopted the Preferred Reporting Items for Systematic reviews and Meta-Analyses (PRISMA) model in conducting a systematic literature review. A search of four scientific electronic databases yielded 42 papers for qualitative evaluation. We searched PubMed Central, PubMed, PsycInfo, and Scopus databases for articles on psychiatric disorders in youths related to social media. Since this topic embraces multiple fields, such as computer science and information and communication technologies, we also browsed the Association for Computing Machinery Digital Library and the Institute of Electrical and Electronics Engineers Xplore Digital Library to find relevant research articles in the proceedings of conferences focused on the role of social media in explaining psychological issues in the developmental age. We comparatively analyzed the literature from 2006 up to the end of July 2020, combining different keywords and Boolean operators. A database was generated by combining terms and Boolean operators, such as "social media" AND "child*," "social media use" AND "child*," "social media" AND "disorder" AND "youth*". To include more targeted records, we conducted a further search on the same databases using terms describing the specific issues we meant to address in this review: ("YouTube" OR "WeChat" OR "TikTok" OR "Reddit" OR "Pinterest" OR "Facebook" OR "Instagram" OR "Twitter" OR "Tumblr" OR "MySpace" OR "Whatsapp") AND ("psychiatric disorder" OR "mental health" OR "psychological well-being") AND ("adolescent*" OR "youth*" OR "teenager*").

2.1. Eligibility Criteria

From a methodological perspective, studies had to fulfill the following criteria to be included: journals and proceedings of conference papers published up to the end of July 2020, published in English, and meeting the following criteria:

1. participants: children and adolescents until the age of 19 with a profile on at least one of the most popular social media platforms (Facebook, YouTube, WhatsApp, WeChat, Instagram, Twitter, TikTok, Tumblr, Reddit, Pinterest, Snapchat, MySpace, Q-Zone); we opted to consider the age of 19 as the upper limit of adolescence, in accordance with the definition provided by the World Health Organization https://apps.who.int/adolescent/second-decade/section2/page1/recognizing-adolescence.html;
2. interventions: assessment of psychiatric disorders in the developmental ages (depressive symptoms, anxiety and related issues, EDs and body dissatisfaction, neurodevelopmental disorders, substance misuse or abuse);
3. comparison: it is not applicable, as we only included studies based on the sample of social media users;
4. outcomes: we considered the levels of psychological well-being or diagnosis of psychiatric disorders as the outcome;
5. study design: we included studies containing quantitative approaches to produce empirical data and qualitative designs.

2.2. Results

For the selection procedure for the included articles, please refer to **Figure 2**. In the results, we will discuss only the studies resulting from the literature research. In **Table 1**, all the articles included in the review are listed, together with the principal information. Effect size computations for each study have been performed using an effect size calculator (64) or calculated manually. When more variables were analyzed in the study, we reported the range of values for effect sizes (Cohen's *d*). Disorders will be discussed in distinguished macro-categories, divided by diagnostic class, according to the DSM-5(65). Relevant topics such as involvement/changes of neural correlates and genetic contribution will also be discussed. A total of 31,823 papers were screened by title and abstract, 1,394 were considered for further screening, and 511 duplicate papers were removed. Note that 839 papers were removed after assessment for eligibility according to the exclusion criteria, resulting in 44 papers included in the review.

2.3. Depressive Symptoms and Mood Disorders

Depression is a prevalent mood disorder, in which symptoms include persistent sadness and a loss of interest in activities that the person enjoys typically, together with the inability to carry out daily activities (65). With regard to childhood and adolescence, interpersonal models of depression in developmental ages accentuate the cyclical associations between social experiences and depressive symptoms. New schemes in the interpersonal environment, with more articulated, frequent, and unsupervised contacts, may represent a further complication as the influence of peer relationships may affect a person's identity and psychological

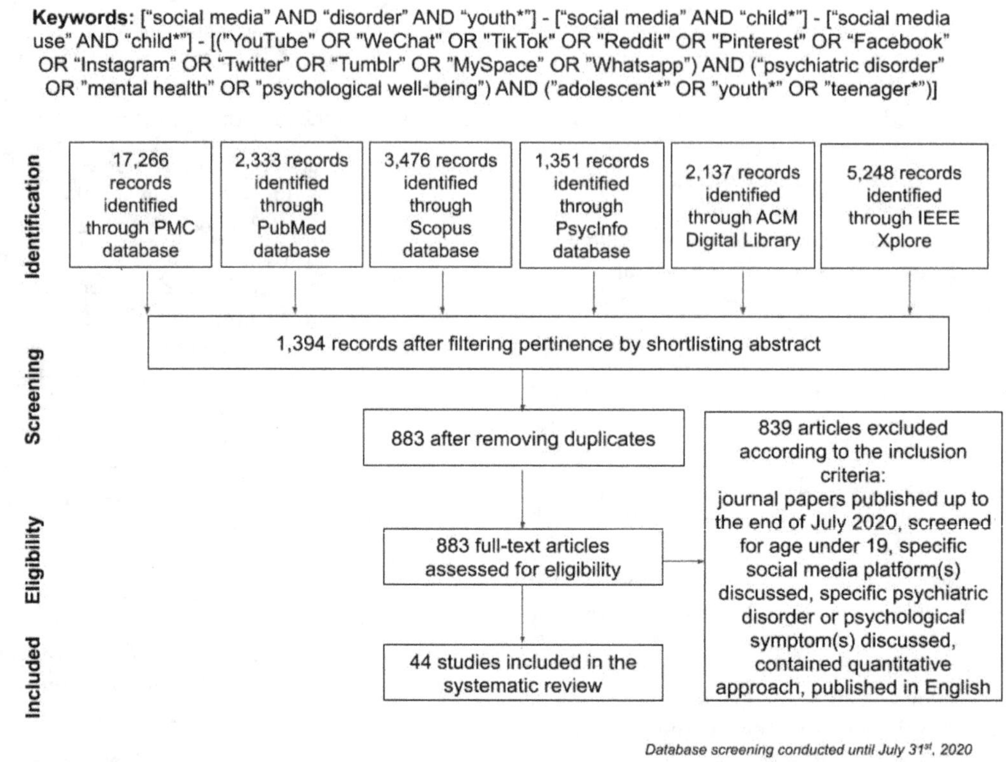

FIGURE 2 | Flow chart of procedural articles shortlisting according to the Preferred Reporting Items for Systematic reviews and Meta-Analyses (PRISMA) guidelines.

well-being (66). As depression and internalizing symptoms have increased among youths in the last decade (67), it is vital to question to what extent social media usage is directly linked to this and to understand how they impact each other.

2.3.1. Effects of Social Media Usage on Depressive Symptoms

Given that social media provide users with a range of possible activities, it is possible to identify specific patterns of usage. For instance, a set of actions such as browsing other users' photos or scrolling through comments or news feeds has been labeled as passive social media use. Recent research indicates that this sort of behavior and depression are linked in both directions. Passive social media usage could directly aggravate depressive symptoms, like loss of interest or blue mood, and thwart personal well-being (16, 32, 68, 69). High social media use appears to be predictive of depressive symptoms and low offline social support from both family and peers (57). It might also act indirectly through mediators such as reduced sense of belonging (70), hence increasing levels of loneliness first (43) and, subsequently, depressive mood and stress (16), which, in turn, reinforce each other (68).

2.3.2. Effects of Depressive Symptoms on Social Media Usage

Passive social media use appears to be increased by depressive symptoms, loneliness, and high levels of stress. In a longitudinal study, Kross and colleagues have demonstrated that a sense of loneliness is a predictor for more intense usage of social media (71), as it might represent a solution to alleviate depressed mood, reinforcing PSMU (68). Specific kinds of actions on social media, related to the peculiarity of the site, were found to be associated with adverse emotional and relational outcomes at different times and vice versa. With regard to Instagram, Frison and Eggermont reported that former browsing behavior was related to a later increase in depressed mood (38). Moreover, levels of depressed mood at Time 1 were associated with increased Instagram posting at Time 2, without differences between boys and girls (38). As for Facebook, levels of depressive symptoms at the first stage can be predictive of a lower number of Facebook friends and fewer ties between friends in the second stage (52). Another study based on Facebook data highlights the relationships between internalizing symptoms and online communication in terms of received comments offering support in response to posts indicating negative or depressive emotional states, with girls receiving more backing compared to boys. Such rumination-like behavior through social media might affect negatively not only the mood of the person who posts but also of those who respond, increasing levels of internalizing symptoms and depression (72). Depressive symptoms, together with sleep problems, can represent a positive predictor for excessive involvement in Facebook-related activities (53). Similarly, emotional dependence on Facebook has been found to be negatively correlated to several aspects of adolescents' psychological well-being, such as autonomy, purpose in life, positive relationships, personal growth, self-acceptance, and ability to manage one's environment

TABLE 1 | List of the studies included in the review.

n	Article	Age	*N*	Social media	Disorder/symptoms	Findings	*ES*
1	Szwedo et al. (23)	13/20	89	f, MS	Depressive symptoms, social anxiety	− (depr); + (s.anx)	0.40–0.60
2	Moreno et al. (24)	18–19	66	f	Alcohol use	+	0.72
3	Pumper and Moreno (25)	12–14	315	f	Alcohol use	+	0.15
4	Tiggemann and Slater (26)	13–15	1,087	f, MS	Body image concerns	+	0.26
5	D'Angelo et al. (27)	18–19	312	f	Alcohol use	+	0.20
6	Huang et al. (28)	14–15	1,563	f, MS	Alcohol and cigarette use	ns	na
7	Birnbaum et al. (29))	12–21	80	f, Instagram, Twitter	Psycotic-spectrum and mood disorder	na	na
8	Nesi and Prinstein (30)	12–16	619	f, Instagram	Depressive symptoms	+	0.53
9	Bert et al. (31)	18	341	Twitter	Pro-anorexia	na	na
10	Ehrenreich and Underwood (2016)	18	125	f	Internalizing symptoms	+	0.58
11	Frison et al. (32)	12–19	1,612	f	Depressive symptoms	ns	0.58
12	Marczinski et al. (33)	19	146	f	Alcohol use	+	0.44
13	Moreno et al. (34)	17–19	94	f, Twitter	Alcohol use	+	0.47–0.92
14	Naeemi and Tamam (35)	13–16	401	f	Psychological well-being	−	0.67
15	Sampasa-Kanyinga and Chaput (36)	11–19	4,468	f, Twitter, Skype, WhatsApp	Body image concerns	+	0.39
16	Abar et al. (37)	19	252	f	Substance use	na	na
17	Frison and Eggermont (38)	12–19	671	Instagram	Depressed mood	+	0.42
18	Gul et al. (39)	13–19	289	f	ADHD	+	0.69
19	Jacob et al. (40)	16–24	21	t	Self-injury	+	na
20	Nesi et al. (30)	15–16	658	f	Alcohol use	+	0.43
21	Nesi et al. (30)	13–16	816	f, Instagram	Depressive symptoms	+	0.85
22	Pontes (41)	10-18	509	f	Depressive symptoms, anxiety	+	0.62–0.68
23	Spilkova et al. (42)	16	4,887	f, Twitter, Skype, WhatsApp	Binge drinking, marjiuana use	+ (drink); ns (marj)	0.88
24	van Rooij et al. (43)	12–15	3,945	Twitter	Depressive symptoms, social anxiety	+	0.45–0.95
25	Weinstein (44)	14–18	507	Instagram	Depressive symptoms	+	0.68
26	Brown et al. (45)	16	52	Instagram	Self-injury, suicidal ideation	na	na
27	Muzaffar et al. (46)	12–20	102	f	Depressive symptoms, social anxiety	ns	na
28	Niu et al. (47)	12–18	764	QZ	Depressive symptoms	+	0.44
29	Settanni et al. (48)	15	283	f	ADHD symptoms	+	0.56
30	Chang et al. (49)	12–16	303	Instagram	Body esteem	−	0.58
31	de Vries et al. (50)	12–19	440	f	Body dissatisfaction	+	0.49
32	Louragli et al. (51)	12–19	541	f	Anxiety, nomophobia	+	0.50–0.98
33	Negriff (52)	13/21	319	f	Depressive symptoms	-	0.58
34	Przepiorka and Blachnio (53)	12–17	426	f	Depressive symptoms	+	0.83
35	Raudsepp and Kais (54)	13	397	f, Instagram, Twitter	Depressive symptoms	+	0.72
36	Savolainen et al. (55)	15–25	4,816	f, Instagram, Twitter, YouTube	Alcohol use	+	0.12–0.43
37	Shakir et al. (2019)	12–18	537	f, Instagram, Twitter, Snapchat, t	Cyberbullying	na	na
38	Steers et al. (56)	17–19	316	f	alcohol use	+	0.69
39	Vannucci and Ohannessian (57)	11-14	1205	f, Instagram, Twitter, Snapchat, t	Depressive symptoms, panic disorder symptoms	+	0.28-.92
40	Yurdagül et al. (58)	14–19	491	Instagram	Depressive symptoms, anxiety, social anxiety, body dissatisfaction	+	0.28–0.50
41	Boursier et al. (59)	13–19	693	f, Instagram, YouTube, WhatsApp	Body image concerns	+	0.36
42	Fardouly et al. (60)	10–12	528	Instagram, Snapchat, YouTube	Depressive symptoms, social anxiety, body satisfaction	+ (depr.); ns (s.anx); − (body)	0.43–0.82
43	Stockdale and Coyne (61)	17/19	385	f, Instagram, Twitter	Depressive symptoms, anxiety	ns (depr.); + (anx)	0.36
44	Brown et al. (62)	16	59	Instagram	Self-injury	na	na

Age, range of age of the participants; N, sample size; ES, effect size; +, directly proportional; −, inversely proportional; ns, non-significant; na, not applicable; f, Facebook; Instagram; Twitter; YouTube; Snapchat; t, Tumblr; Skype; MS, MySpace; QZ, QZone. Icons of social media platforms have been created using the fontawesome package (63).

(35). An addictive attitude toward Facebook was found to be positively correlated with depression, regardless of age (age range 10–18) and gender (41). Longitudinal research on adolescent girls found an association between changes in PSMU and changes in depressive symptoms in both directions, with baseline levels of depressive symptoms being predictive of PSMU (54).

2.3.3. Social Comparison and Negative Affect

Social comparison is a mechanism highly involved in the development of a person's identity starting from childhood, where evaluations are more distorted especially in a positive way, throughout adolescence, when the greater development of cognitive skills permit the generation of more realistic estimates (73). Social comparison, as a consequence, can generate both a positive or a negative self-appraisal, affecting the way people, especially teenagers, perceive themselves and their quality of life. Evidence in literature suggests that PSMU and depressive symptoms might be mediated by social comparisons with others' lives as they appear on their profiles (44, 47, 66), generating a sense of inferiority and feelings of worthlessness (74–78). As a consequence, people showing downward social comparisons are more likely to seek offline feedback for reassurance (66). Social comparison is closely linked to self-esteem, which, in turn, resents of the effect of individual cognitive appraisal, acting as a moderator in the processing of comparison. As a consequence, lower levels of self-esteem can represent a risk factor when making comparisons with others' lives (47). These results appear to be more evident in girls, compared to boys, (44, 66) suggesting that intrinsic features of female identity development can represent a vulnerability for a more negative self-appraisal, especially when comparing or evaluating physical features or attractiveness (49, 54). Moreover, it is possible that online parasocial relationships may amplify distorted perceptions, due to the filtered and selective nature of the information shared, principally when evaluating profiles of users that do not belong to a close or offline network (44).

2.3.4. Controversial Results in the Association Between Depressive Symptoms and Social Media Usage

Amid the research investigating the connection between social media usage and depressive symptoms, a few studies reported no evidence linking social media sites and depression. A recent study investigated the relationships between reasons for Facebook use and psychological and mental health outcomes for a 3-year period in late adolescents, aged from 17 to 19 years. According to their results, none of the possible motivations, which were social connection, boredom, and information seeking, were correlated to depression at any stage of the experimental procedure (61). As for the short-term consequences of negative experiences on Facebook, online peer victimization is not predictive of increased depressive symptoms after 6 months (79). In addition, Fardouly and colleagues did not find differences between users and non-users of the most popular social media platforms (Youtube, Instagram, and Snapchat) among Australian preadolescents in terms of depressive symptoms. Taken together, these results suggest that low mood derived from social media usage might be explained through different factors, such as worry about how youths appear on their preferred social networks sites and their tendency to compare their own image to someone else's image (60). Finally, a longitudinal study by Szwedo and colleagues investigated the preference for Facebook and/or MySpace communication in a cohort of adolescents in relation to depressive symptoms, assessing the sample at the age of 13 (Time 1) and 20 (Time 2). Interestingly, higher depressive symptoms at Time 1 predicted a preference for communication via social media, but at Time 2, higher depressive symptoms were predictive of lesser online disclosure (23). This change in direction might be explained by the different ways, especially social withdrawal, through which depression is manifested in early adolescence and early adulthood. With regard to psychotic and non-psychotic mood disorders, social platforms such as Facebook and Twitter represent an initial avenue to seek help by diagnosed youths (29) and a potential base to examine depressive symptoms and perceived social support from online friends (80).

2.4. Anxiety Disorders

Symptoms relating to anxiety often overlap with depression, especially in youths; just like depression, anxious manifestations may result from a set of internal and external circumstances. In social media, where the relational component is strong, anxiety can derive from a perception of being connected inappropriately, from negative online peer-comparison, or from reduced emotion-regulation abilities, as online interaction can be used as a surrogate for offline physical interaction (81). Targeted Facebook features, such as seeking online approval and support through the number of "likes," or only retaining the visibility of posts and pictures that received lots of positive feedback on one's profile, can promote or elicit non-adaptive behaviors (i.e., excessive social comparison and rumination) and increase anxiety-related traits, such as socially prescribed perfectionism, aggravating pre-existing symptoms in youths diagnosed with an anxiety disorder (82). Facebook can also be used by teenagers as a pastime when feeling bored: a 3-year study found that usage of Facebook in order to alleviate boredom at stage 1 (17 years old) was correlated with increased levels of anxiety at a following stage (19 years old), indicating that the anxiety might be a secondary product of the problematic use of social media developed over the two time-points (61). This could reflect the fact that a 3-year window frame can encompass different stages of a teenager's life, especially when approaching emerging adulthood. As the high school period is over, fewer amounts of structured time, coupled with less monitoring behavior by parents and teachers and greater accessibility to smartphones or other electronic devices, can result in an increase in problematic usage of social media and, as a consequence, underlying anxiety-related mechanisms (61). The type and the reiteration of a set of behaviors that Facebook users could engage in (e.g., posting a photo/comment/status update, "liking" behavior, or using the instant message) can be linked with levels of general anxiety. This might be explained by the need to keep worries related to that driving the person to frequently check a previous posting behavior (46). With regards to Instagram, which is more focused on visual contents, one study reported a direct association between Instagram usage with general anxiety in boys, while in girls this link was mediated by body image dissatisfaction, leading to different adverse outcomes in the two groups (58). This difference between genders suggests that females might be more prone to engage in social comparison, especially when it involves physical appearance. This might be because their perception of their ideal body image as being thin is affected by their excessive exposure to attractive celebrity and peer images on Instagram. Moreover, it underlines once again the importance of considering the possible concurrent mechanisms that contribute to the development of psychological issues.

2.4.1. Online Social Anxiety

Social anxiety is described by the enduring preoccupation of being judged negatively by others during a social performance or social circumstances (65). The worry of receiving unfavorable feedback is even stronger during adolescence, when the identity of the self is developing. Online activity on social media can be very attractive, especially for young people with such fears, as it is possible to share information or content in a more controllable environment. Although this allows people with social anxiety issues to overcome, even partially, the fear of being exposed to public judgment, it can lead to the development of a problematic usage of social media platforms. With regard to Facebook, a longitudinal study by Szwedo and colleagues found that at 13 years of age (Time 1), social anxiety does not explain preference for virtual communications, and at 20 years of age (Time 2), it was positively correlated with a predilection for online relations, especially for those expressing increased levels of maternal behavior undermining autonomy at Time 1 (23). Levels of social anxiety in social media young users have been shown to be positively correlated with online behavioral dimensions such as the attitude of comparing one's appearance with other people's pictures on YouTube, Instagram, and Snapchat (60). As a consequence, the approach toward social media can be conflicting: the person desires at the same time to be recognized as interesting and "liked," but would also like to avoid being judged negatively or ridiculed. The awareness of these mechanisms might intensify pre-existing symptoms of social anxiety, leading to non-adaptive patterns of behavior (82).

2.4.2. Fear of Missing Out and Nomophobia: The Urge to Be Constantly Online

The more people share their lives on their online profiles, the more they are at risk of being afraid of missing updates and feeling the urge to check their profiles for feedback (16, 83). This specific phenomenon has been labeled "fear of missing out" (FoMO), defining the pervasive anxiety experienced by a user when thinking that other people might be enjoying gratifying experiences in their physical absence, pushing him/her to be connected constantly to check upon updates about these experiences, hence fostering the addictive behavior circuit (16, 84–86). FoMO has been shown to be associated with the severity of Facebook usage through a process that is likely to be activated by users as a way to temporarily compensate or regulate negative affect and anxious manifestations (87). Specific social needs may underlie FoMO and reasons for social media usage, like the desire to be popular, or at least not unpopular in the eyes of peers and the need for social affiliation, especially during adolescence when peers acquire greater value compared to the family (88). To this purpose, online interaction can represent a constantly available means of gratification but, at the same time, an attractive risk as it might trigger addictive behaviors and aggravate symptoms of anxiety. This combination of behavioral and cognitive patterns, in the context of social media usage, appears to be mediated by nomophobia, which is described as the fear of not being able to use the mobile phone. Evidence in literature reports a direct association among levels of anxiety, addictive behavior toward social media (41) and nomophobia, with a negative impact on academic performances (51).

2.5. Feeding, Eating Disorders, and Body Dissatisfaction

Adolescence is a temporal frame during which physical changes and identity development occur, and teenagers acquire a greater awareness of the body, both their own and those of their peers (49). Posting pictures on social media is one of the most common practices among young people, especially self-photos (commonly known as "selfies") (89). Exposing and being exposed massively to pictures of body might lead to negative outcomes, such as body image dissatisfaction, defined as "*the discrepancy between identification of one's own figure (actual) and the figure chosen as the desirable self-image*" (90), or alterations in nutrition habits, to the extent of the development of EDs. With regard to Instagram, body image dissatisfaction mediates the relationship between PSMU and internalizing symptoms differently in males and females, with the latter showing a stronger indirect effect (58). Evidence from a study involving Singaporean girls showed that selfie practice on Instagram (browsing and editing) and body esteem are mediated by appearance comparison operated by peers' groups with a negative association, while posting self photos and body esteem are directly correlated (49). With regard to Facebook, Tiggemann and colleagues investigated social media exposure and body image concerns in girls, finding that time spent on the online platform was strongly correlated to body surveillance and the ideal of a thin body shape (26). An analysis of a Canadian sample of teenagers highlights that more frequent and prolonged usage of social media services is associated with body dissatisfaction, with a trend to perceive oneself overweight in both boys and girls (36). Recent findings from a study by Fardouly and colleagues indicate that more frequent appearance comparisons with others on social media and considering them to be more attractive than oneself is negatively correlated with body image satisfaction and positively linked with eating-related disorders in both male and female teenagers (60). Evidence from a sample of Italian adolescents highlights the role played by appearance control beliefs and body image control in photos, as these dimensions could be configured as predictors of problematic usage of social media and negative mental health outcomes (59). Overall, the findings indicate a higher vulnerability for girls to develop a negative image of their own body. This risk can be compounded by misleading and harmful content that can be found on social media.

2.5.1. Presentation of Eating Disorders on Social Media Platforms

In recent years, groups supporting anorexia nervosa in several ways (endorsement and promotion of dysfunctional eating behavior, maintenance of the disorder, and interference with recovery) have been spreading across social media platforms. The dynamics of the Proana Movement, which promotes behaviors relating to anorexia nervosa, have been examined using Twitter, finding that adhering people and/or promoters were almost totally teenage girls (31). In the midst of the factors mediating the risk to develop body dissatisfaction or EDs, one study focused on teenagers' offline social environment, finding that a positive mother-adolescent relationship can exert a protective function against the adverse effects of social media usage on body perception (50). An alarming factor is determined by the support of pro-EDs in online networks. As popular platforms started blocking pro-ED related terms, users supporting dangerous eating habits have begun altering the hashtags, bringing forward their approval toward endangering conducts. On the other hand, it is not unusual that people rehabilitating from an ED seek support during their journey to recovery by sharing their testimony through textual posts or visual media (i.e., pictures, video, and gif). This dual nature of online communication represents a great challenge for research, as the analysis focused uniquely on hashtags may be misleading (91). Moreover, people supporting ED behaviors often alter the terms in hashtags or post them in comments in order to overcome social media censorship policy, with a possible risk to expose more fragile or sensitive people to explicit content.

2.6. Alcohol Use/Abuse and Addiction

Adolescence is the stage of life where people gain more independence and make new experiences in their social environment, where peer influence might encourage and provide opportunities to come into contact with alcohol, potentially leading to the development of an addictive behavior toward the substance. As the social environment is now composed of two realities, online and offline, it is crucial to understand the contribution of social media in fostering, maintaining, or conveying contents related to substances. Studies on drinking behavior among teenagers and social media use highlight that online platforms like Facebook might represent a helpful tool to detect problematic alcohol use (25, 33, 34, 92, 93), or advertise for healthy behavior in settings such as popular alcohol-related events and parties (24). A higher number of alcohol-related posts has been shown to be linked to greater drinking conduct and approval from friends, although heavier consumers seem to tend to post less over time compared to light drinkers (56). A longitudinal study revealed that in the Facebook profiles of individuals identified as dependent alcohol users, alcohol references increased and half of those identified referenced intoxication or problematic drinking after 1 year (25), while another longitudinal study indicated that alcohol references at a first stage can predict binge drinking later in time (27). With regard to alcohol-related attitudes, binge drinkers appear to be more prone to use social media excessively (42). Moreover, posts containing references to alcohol predict the number of weekly substance consumption (93), the risk of developing an addiction, and alcohol cravings (92). In order to predict drinking conduct, Marczinski and colleagues have developed the Alcohol-Related Facebook Activity (ARFA) questionnaire (33) based on a sample of college students. The preference for the virtual environment as a platform to share alcohol-related experiences has been studied by Moreno and colleagues, who report that students owning a profile on both Facebook and Twitter tended to post more alcohol references on Facebook compared to Twitter (34), as they were entertaining more social connections on the former site. Online social networks often include connections with offline friends; therefore, the exposure to a friend's drinking pictures or posts can be associated with higher alcohol consumption (28, 30). Risky alcohol behavior can differ according to the country; a cross-cultural study examined the relationship between daily usage of popular social media platforms and alcohol consumption among youths in the United States, Spain, Finland, and South Korea. In the targeted countries, the different platforms were correlated with greater hazardous alcohol usage as follows: Facebook and Instagram in Spain, Finland, and South Korea, YouTube in South Korea, and Twitter in Spain (55). These results suggest that specific social media sites might play an attractive or inspiring role in risky alcohol consumption but, on the other hand, they could also turn out to contribute greatly to online-based interventions. According to a study on nicotine, alcohol, and marijuana consumption in high school, being friends on Facebook with one's own parents and not hiding contents can represent a protective factor against substance use (37). Parental inclusion on social media interactions, without undermining autonomy and privacy of youths, can depict an important element in substance use prevention targeted toward youths.

2.7. Self-Harm and Suicidal Ideation

Amid the psychological issues potentially occurring in young people, self-harm is a primary concern, with harmful behaviors lying on a continuum between non-suicidal self-injury (NSSI) and suicidal intention (40). Social media can influence self-injury tendencies negatively, through fostering conducts, contagion, or competitions (94), but they can also represent the first foothold when support is needed. A study based on the analysis of MySpace profiles indicates that teenagers utilize personal virtual space to share their suicidal ideation and behaviors directly or by reporting desperation, hopelessness, and despair (95). From the interviews with adolescents recently collected by Jacob and colleagues about self-harm behaviors, it emerges that Tumblr is the preferred platform to share self-injuring content, like pictures, in an anonymous way, with the consequent risk to normalize such harmful behaviors (40). Looking into the motives that push young people to share self-injury related content such as their own wounds on Instagram, there are mostly social purposes, like the need to belong to a group where the person can feel understood (62). Another reason might be the need to self-disclose in an environment that can guarantee anonymity. These reasons are reported to be valid both for the first NSSI post and for the general NSSI ones. Beyond self-oriented motives, another aim is to raise awareness about the topic in order to help other people (62). Although results concerning Instagram do not report any risk for acute suicidality (96), photos of self-injury practices might play a reinforcement role as they are often posted (45) and frequently concealed behind ambiguous hashtags (97). In fact, as users often resort to the use of hashtags to track the shared contents and to find images or discussions related to specific topics, those regarding self-harming behaviors can contain non-related words (i.e., "blithe" for self-cutting pictures) or be constantly changed, in order to make them easily accessible only to a restricted community (98). Social media-related suicidal behavior is a topic of increasing interest and critical importance that has garnered the attention of newspapers and newscasts all over the world, concerning popular and unpopular people (see Channel News Asia for a recent episode). Although researchers attempted to study the extent of social media on suicidal behaviors in-depth, complexities derive from legal and privacy issues, as well as from the indirect association between the usage on web-based platforms and the suicide itself (99).

2.8. Cyberbullying

Suicidal ideation can also derive from the non-adaptive usage of online communication by others, as in the case of cyberbullying. Cyberbullying can be defined as the intentional use of information and communication technologies such as electronic mail, smartphone, short message services, and social media platforms, carried out repeatedly by a group or an individual, to support deliberate, repeated, and hostile behaviors against a victim who cannot easily defend him- or herself (100, 101). Cyberbullying constitutes a possible worrisome phenomenon, given its devastating, occasionally even fatal, consequences on a person's life. Recent statistics point out that cyberbullying is prevalent on platforms based on visual content, such as Instagram (42%), Facebook (37%), and Snapchat (31%) (see the article by Petrov C. on statistics about cyberbullying, February 28, 2019). As the contents are shared and spread quickly online, the victim can experience, besides a lack of control, a series of highly negative psychological consequences, such as social anxiety (102), depression, and suicidal ideation and attempt, especially when bullying behavior perpetuates across time (103, 104). An investigation on social media usage and youths' mental health revealed that cyberbullying appears to mediate this relation occurring in a set of negative outcomes, such as sleep problems and anxiety, more than the frequency of exposure to social media itself, with girls being more exposed to these effects (10). However, social media started adding certain features including the ability to report inappropriate content, comments, and to block users in order to stem violent and inappropriate behaviors.

2.8.1. Safety Measures Adopted by Social Media Sites

Initially, the different platforms did not take responsibility for single users' online behaviors. However, the growing prevalence of cyberbullying in recent years has gained increased relevance, resulting in the implementation of several measures aimed at both children and parents. For instance, in 2013, Facebook launched a safety section on its site, providing information on policies, tools to increase profile protection, and relevant resources and contacts to access in the case of cyber abuse (see Facebook Safety page). Likewise, in 2015, Twitter activated a safety center for parents and teens with guidelines for a more secure navigation and utilization of the site. Furthermore, they founded the Twitter Trust and Safety Council that works in partnership with several institutions and organizations in order to direct users to the appropriate service in case of abuse (see Twitter Safety Partner). With regard to Instagram, which has been owned by Facebook since 2012, the platform presents the community guidelines and another section where parents can find more information about the accessibility and visibility of their children by other users. Moreover, an online form is available for reporting self-injury material, hate comments, abusive or inappropriate content, and profiles belonging to teens younger than 13 years old, which is the requirement to own a profile (see Instagram Privacy and Safety Center page). The same subscription criteria are applied to YouTube, although videos posted by other users are accessible even without owning a profile. Because of this, it is possible for parents to set restrictions in order to avoid potentially dangerous or improper material. In addition, together with the site policies, informative material about harmful behaviors such as self-injury, suicide, harassment, and cyberbullying is provided (see YouTube Community Guidelines). So far, statistics about the efficacy of these safety measures have not being available. Generally, targeted services for prevention have been made known on the most popular online platforms by providing users with links to websites, hotlines, and information about how to detect warning signs of suicide. Web communities focused on suicide prevention have been founded, giving their members the opportunity to share their own direct or indirect experience in an anonymous way and to support each other, without the constraints of physical boundaries (99).

2.9. Neurodevelopmental Disorders

Neurodevelopmental disorders are characterized by altered functioning of the neurological system and brain, affecting cognitive functions and social behavior. Although social media interfere with offline interaction by reducing the investment of time and resources in them while offering a more immediate alternative to satisfy social needs, they can also simplify the engagement in social contacts. This feature might be suitable, for instance, for youths with autism spectrum disorders, as they can have difficulties in decoding complex social information (105, 106). As adolescence is a crucial developmental stage where interactions with peers occur both online and offline, it is of pivotal relevance to understand the impact of social media platforms on teenagers with neurodevelopmental disorders. With regard to ASD, evidence shows a positive association between Facebook usage and friendship quality, moderated by anxiety levels, suggesting that online platforms might act as a means to improve friendship quality (105). For this purpose, Gwynette and colleagues explored Facebook's therapeutic potential as a tool to improve social skills in adolescents with ASD. Their web-based intervention, according to the authors, could have the potential to facilitate interventions, leading to higher engagement with peers through the virtual environment (106). In the context of neurodevelopmental disorders, Asperger syndrome is characterized by significant difficulties in social interaction and non-verbal communication; as a consequence, they could be more vulnerable to cyberbullying victimization on online applications. Findings in the literature suggest that, although adolescents with Asperger syndrome use social media less than their peers, the percentage and frequency of cyberbullying are similar (107). Another neurodevelopmental condition is attention-deficit/hyperactivity disorder (ADHD), which is defined by persistent inattention, hyperactivity, and sometimes impulsivity. These features, combined with online-based platforms, might lead to addictive social media behaviors, with further consequences on mental health, productivity, and academic scores (48). Studies analyzing the correlation between ADHD traits and social media found that a large number of adolescents with ADHD own more than one Facebook account, showed greater overuse compared to their counterparts (39), and ADHD symptoms are positively associated with Facebook addictive use (48). Furthermore, teenagers with more marked ADHD traits were more likely to develop problematic usage of Internet-based services and less likely to remit from problematic Internet usage (108).

3. GENE-BY-ENVIRONMENT CONTRIBUTION TO UNDERSTAND BEHAVIOR ON SOCIAL MEDIA

The hypothesis that genetic features influence behavior and social interactions has been corroborated in several studies [for a review, see (109)], and so is the notion that human behavior and psychological traits are modulated by the interaction between genetic variation and environmental factors (21). Due to the intrinsic interactional nature of social media platforms, it is important to deepen the exploration of concurrent factors that could explain underlying mechanisms related to online interaction adopting integrated methodologies widely used for offline social behavior, that is, the gene-by-environment interaction framework. Few studies report results about genetic contribution in Internet-related usage. Two studies on Turkish twins on communication and social media reported that genetic and environmental effects were equally influential on problematic Internet usage especially in male twin-pairs (110). Another twin study highlighted the impact of genetics on mobile phone use (111). These results have been corroborated by a more recent investigation by York, who focused specifically on social media use (e.g., contact friends and contact family) even after controlling for demographic factors (112). A recent study by Deryakulu and Ursavaş examines the extent to which nomophobia can be explained by genetic and environmental factors, revealing that the dimensions which were more explained by genes were "losing connectedness" and "giving up convenience," while environmental factors were more related to the fear of "not being able to communicate" and "not being able to access" (113). Familiar context represents a factor of great interest in shaping social behavior, especially at the developmental stage, and perception of parental warmth or intrusiveness can influence social media usage in adolescents. With regard to the genetic contribution within the frame of recalled parental bonding, a recent exploration found that people who are genetically more sensitive to environmental factors, represented by oxytocin receptor polymorphisms, with a history of perceived high maternal overprotection tend to show a higher social desirability index on Instagram (114). This index, which describes the ratio between the number of following and followed profiles, could be used for future studies to unveil some tendencies underlying user behavior on Instagram.

4. SOCIAL MEDIA USAGE AND NEURAL MECHANISMS

Evidence deriving from the neuroscientific field reveals a link between online social behaviors and regulation of neural mechanisms. A functional magnetic resonance imaging (fMRI) study conducted by Meshi and colleagues reports that social media engagement is linked to activity in the ventral striatum (vSTR) and adjoining structures of the nucleus accumbens (115). More precisely, the authors found an association between levels of activation of these areas and in response to social feedback identified that were relevant to participants' social reputation (a surrogate for "likes" on Facebook). Another study describes greater recruitment of the vSTR in relation to more popular shared pictures compared to less socially endorsed ones (116). As for structural evidence on gray matter volume and social media habits, the striatal region was found to be linked to daily smartphone checking (117) and heavy social media usage (118). Recent evidence also suggests the involvement of the right lateral orbitofrontal cortex, linking a decreased volume in that area with an excessive usage of social media sites (119). With regard to impulse control, reduced gray matter volume in the anterior cingulate cortex was found in people with high tendencies in developing an addictive attitude toward instant messaging services (120) and "multitasking" users, suggesting that social media usage is highly involved in the control of inhibitory mechanisms (121). Another relevant study by Moisala and colleagues on media multitasking showed increased activity in the right side of the prefrontal cortex while participants were subjected to a cognitive task; this result was explained by the authors as a reflection of mental struggle in recruiting resources in executive control (122). With regard to social cognition in adolescence, fMRI studies found that online rejection by peers or other users elicits an increased activity in the medial prefrontal cortex, which is strongly associated with offline rejection (20), and elicits neural responses in the dorsal anterior cingulate cortex, the subgenual anterior cingulate cortex, and the anterior insula, which are areas generally linked to "social pain" (20, 123) and depression (124). The immediate and long-term effects of frequent and prolonged social media usage on neural structures and activity have yet to be elucidated.

5. CONCLUSION

In just one decade, individuals' lives and their social behavior have been tremendously changed by the phenomenon of social media. Emerging technologies and platforms provide users with a wide range of activities, leisure, and the possibility to interact with friends, families, or strangers. Although different patterns of usage are moderated by a set of individual features concerning genetic, environment, temperament, and personal needs, it is undeniable that online social media have become an integrated part of people's daily lives. This leads to the necessity, in research fields linked to human behavior, to understand if, how, and to what extent these platforms are modifying our brain mechanisms, interactions, and the concept of well-being. During developmental stages, such as adolescence and early adulthood, several changes occur not only with regard to neural functions but also in social patterns, as young people have increasing opportunity to test themselves as individuals in more autonomous social interactions. As for social media, the most popular platforms require users to be at least 13 years old to own a profile and have access to the services. Although this limit is easily bypassed, it is difficult to have a clear overview of the sociodemographic information of young users and of different patterns of usage or effects of social media in early adolescence (10–14), middle adolescence (15–17), and young adulthood (18–21), as the early adolescence population should not be able to access and be engaged in virtual interactions on such platforms. This issue rebounds in a lack of studies considering this distinction, representing a further challenge to future research. Lots of efforts have been invested in creating new tools for assessing people's attitudes toward social media usage, such as the creation and validation of new scales (84, 125–129) and to interpret results within a fitting theoretical frame. Social media provide unprecedented opportunities to trace online activity and to keep track of interaction dynamics at different stages. This allows researchers to overcome issues related to self-report questionnaires and to benefit from leveraging real-time data over time more easily. Specifically, the increasing utilization of hashtags might help in detecting and monitoring targeted topics or risky behaviors, despite the risk of misappropriate use of words (for instance, sometimes people refer to "anxiety" or "depression" when perceiving alterations in preoccupation or mood but with these not being of clinical interest or diagnosed. For sure, the use of hashtags is a powerful tool to build communities and support people's journey to recover, to witness, to join a cause, or to increase awareness around a specific topic related to mental health.

As the number of social media applications increases, with each having its own specific features, there is a need to separate problematic behaviors or effects according to the platforms. In fact, since the advent of social networks sites, multiple platforms have succeeded one another, gaining immediate popularity. Some of them are not used anymore, such as Google+, or had a drastic loss of users, like MySpace. Lately, a new social network site named TikTok, formerly known as Musical.ly, has risen especially among the youth, changing to some extent the way social media are used. From the simple sharing of text, music, or pictures, social media has rapidly evolved, becoming more dynamic and providing the possibility to get immediate and abundant feedback, to join wide online communities based on common interests, and to involve users' talents or attitudes with so-called "challenges." Although TikTok had gained terrific popularity in the course of the last year, no studies regarding the potential outcomes deriving from a problematic usage are available. As social media sites are quickly developing, research appears to struggle in keeping pace with not only the new online functionalities but also with ways of interactions among users that, in turn, might alter parameters in longitudinal studies, like the amount of time spent online. This is partially due to the fact that effects can be explored in terms of both a short and long term, each with different consequences. Moreover, the social media platforms resent of the users' preferences and mass tendencies, and what is new and trendy today might swiftly lose people's interest (130). Since keeping track of how communication technologies evolve across the years can be a precious resource on developmental trajectories, it becomes of great importance for researchers to build and rely on constantly updated evidence. The creation and rise of new technologies has resulted in new behaviors and, consequently, new names for these behaviors. Neologisms like "*nomophobia*," "*selfie*," "*phubbing*," "*FoMO*," and "*vaguebooking*" have appeared for some years, defining specific behaviors or state of minds, that need further analysis, as they represent new, unexplored facets of human behavior. Research in psychological fields would also benefit from the exploration of specific types of interaction, such as the creation of multiple accounts, the fruition of live streaming video services, and behaviors like un-tagging people from posts or pictures or unfollowing/unfriending people in order to better understand the effects of mechanisms related to virtual social inclusion or exclusion. Although social media allows for greater ease of recruitment and testing of a greater number of participants in more efficient ways—sometimes comparable to laboratory testing sessions (131)—a lack of knowledge still persists regarding the involvement of specific brain regions or genetic susceptibility in developing a certain social media-related disorder.

In addition, only a few studies adopted a longitudinal design, while most of the evidence is still based on a cross-sectional methodology that does not fully allow researchers to study in detail the direction of the association between social media usage and psychological well-being. Furthermore, the mental health community should commit to find a solution in considering social media-related issues as being separate from other forms of problematic online behaviors or usage. As there is no separated diagnosis, social media concerns are often included or subsumed within the Internet addiction frame, leading to an incorrect framing of the problem, especially with regard to the social connotation that primarily describes and defines these kinds of services. New evidence in these fields would be of great support for practitioners in a twofold way: on the one hand, information shared on social media sites and patterns of usage of new technologies could be implemented in clinical work for both a more complete assessment, and, on the other hand, it would be possible to profile more user-based interventions merging both online and offline strategies.

AUTHOR CONTRIBUTIONS

IC, GE, and BL conceived the paper. IC performed the search, interpreted the literature, and wrote the paper. GE, MN, and BL reviewed and edited the paper. GE submitted the paper. All the authors reviewed the final version of the paper before submission.

REFERENCES

1. Greenfield P, Yan Z. Children, adolescents, and the Internet: a new field of inquiry in developmental psychology. *Dev Psychol.* (2006) 42:391. doi: 10.1037/0012-1649.42.3.391
2. Lloyd A. Social media, help or hindrance: what role does social media play in young people's mental health. *Psychiatr Danub.* (2014) 26(Suppl. 1):340–6.
3. Radovic A, Gmelin T, Stein BD, Miller E. Depressed adolescents' positive and negative use of social media. *J Adolesc.* (2017) 55:5–15. doi: 10.1016/j.adolescence.2016.12.002
4. Lieberman A, Schroeder J. Two social lives: how differences between online and offline interaction influence social outcomes. *Curr Opin Psychol.* (2020) 31:16–21. doi: 10.1016/j.copsyc.2019.06.022
5. Khan S, Gagné M, Yang L, Shapka J. Exploring the relationship between adolescents' self-concept and their offline and online social worlds. *Comput Hum Behav.* (2016) 55:940–5. doi: 10.1016/j.chb.2015.09.046
6. Warburton S. *Digital identity and social media.* Hershey, PA: IGI Global (2012).
7. Sa'ed HZ, Sweileh WM, Awang R, Al-Jabi SW. Global trends in research related to social media in psychology: mapping and bibliometric analysis. *Int J Ment Health Syst.* (2018) 12:4. doi: 10.1186/s13033-018-0182-6
8. Bányai F, Zsila Á, Király O, Maraz A, Elekes Z, Griffiths MD, et al. Problematic social media use: results from a large-scale nationally representative adolescent sample. *PLoS ONE.* (2017) 12:e0169839. doi: 10.1371/journal.pone.0169839
9. Twenge JM. More time on technology, less happiness? Associations between digital-media use and psychological well-being. *Curr Dir Psychol Sci.* (2019). 28:372–9. doi: 10.1177/0963721419838244
10. Viner RM, Aswathikutty-Gireesh A, Stiglic N, Hudson LD, Goddings AL, Ward JL, et al. Roles of cyberbullying, sleep, and physical activity in mediating the effects of social media use on mental health and wellbeing among young people in England: a secondary analysis of longitudinal data. *Lancet Child Adolesc Health.* (2019) 3:685–96. doi: 10.1016/S2352-4642(19)30186-5
11. Tran BX, Hinh ND, Nguyen LH, Le BN, Nong VM, Thuc VTM, et al. A study on the influence of internet addiction and online interpersonal influences on health-related quality of life in young Vietnamese. *BMC Public Health.* (2017) 17:138. doi: 10.1186/s12889-016-3983-z
12. Kuss DJ, Griffiths MD. Excessive online social networking: can adolescents become addicted to Facebook? *Educ Health.* (2011) 29:63–6.
13. Valkenburg PM, Peter J. Adolescents' identity experiments on the Internet: consequences for social competence and self-concept unity. *Commun Res.* (2008) 35:208–31. doi: 10.1177/0093650207313164
14. Kirschner PA, Karpinski AC. Facebook® and academic performance. *Comput Hum Behav.* (2010) 26:1237–45. doi: 10.1016/j.chb.2010.03.024
15. Reinecke L, Meier A, Beutel ME, Schemer C, Stark B, Wölfling K, et al. The relationship between trait procrastination, internet use, and psychological functioning: results from a community sample of German adolescents. *Front Psychol.* (2018) 9:913. doi: 10.3389/fpsyg.2018.00913
16. Hussain Z, Griffiths MD. Problematic social networking site use and comorbid psychiatric disorders: a systematic review of recent large-scale studies. *Front Psychiatry.* (2018) 9:686. doi: 10.3389/fpsyt.2018.00686
17. Keles B, McCrae N, Grealish A. A systematic review: the influence of social media on depression, anxiety and psychological distress in adolescents. *Int J Adolesc Youth.* (2020) 25:79–93. doi: 10.1080/02673843.2019.1590851
18. Abi-Jaoude E, Naylor KT, Pignatiello A. Smartphones, social media use and youth mental health. *CMAJ.* (2020) 192:E136–41. doi: 10.1503/cmaj.190434
19. Paulus MP, Squeglia LM, Bagot K, Jacobus J, Kuplicki R, Breslin FJ, et al. Screen media activity and brain structure in youth: evidence for diverse structural correlation networks from the ABCD study. *Neuroimage.* (2019) 185:140–53. doi: 10.1016/j.neuroimage.2018.10.040
20. Crone EA, Konijn EA. Media use and brain development during adolescence. *Nat Commun.* (2018) 9:588. doi: 10.1530/ey.15.7.4
21. Cataldo I, Azhari A, Lepri B, Esposito G. Oxytocin receptors (OXTR) and early parental care: an interaction that modulates psychiatric disorders. *Res Dev Disabil.* (2018) 82:27–38. doi: 10.1016/j.ridd.2017.10.007
22. Feldman R, Monakhov M, Pratt M, Ebstein RP. Oxytocin pathway genes: evolutionary ancient system impacting on human affiliation, sociality, and psychopathology. *Biol Psychiatry.* (2016) 79:174–84. doi: 10.1016/j.biopsych.2015.08.008
23. Szwedo DE, Mikami AY, Allen JP. Qualities of peer relations on social networking websites: predictions from negative mother–teen interactions. *J Res Adolesc.* (2011) 21:595–607. doi: 10.1111/j.1532-7795.2010.00692.x
24. Moreno MA, Kacvinsky L, Pumper M, Wachowski L, Whitehill JM. Associations between social media displays and event-specific alcohol consumption by college students. *WMJ.* (2013) 112:251.
25. Pumper MA, Moreno MA. Identifying high-risk alcohol users in first-year college students: attitude, intention, and Facebook. *J Alcohol Drug Depend.* (2013) 1:1000128. doi: 10.4172/2329-6488.1000128
26. Tiggemann M, Slater A. NetGirls: the Internet, Facebook, and body image concern in adolescent girls. *Int J Eat Disord.* (2013) 46:630–3. doi: 10.1002/eat.22141
27. D'Angelo J, Kerr B, Moreno MA. Facebook displays as predictors of binge drinking: from the virtual to the visceral. *Bull Sci Technol Soc.* (2014) 34:159–69. doi: 10.1177/0270467615584044
28. Huang GC, Unger JB, Soto D, Fujimoto K, Pentz MA, Jordan-Marsh M, et al. Peer influences: the impact of online and offline friendship networks on adolescent smoking and alcohol use. *J Adolesc Health.* (2014) 54:508–14. doi: 10.1016/j.jadohealth.2013.07.001
29. Birnbaum ML, Rizvi AF, Correll CU, Kane JM, Confino J. Role of social media and the I nternet in pathways to care for adolescents and young adults with psychotic disorders and non-psychotic mood disorders. *Early Interv Psychiatry.* (2017) 11:290–5. doi: 10.1111/eip.12237
30. Nesi J, Rothenberg WA, Hussong AM, Jackson KM. Friends' alcohol-related social networking site activity predicts escalations in adolescent drinking: mediation by peer norms. *J Adolesc Health.* (2017) 60:641–7. doi: 10.1016/j.jadohealth.2017.01.009
31. Bert F, Gualano MR, Camussi E, Siliquini R. Risks and threats of social media websites: twitter and the Proana movement. *Cyberpsychol Behav Soc Netw.* (2016) 19:233–8. doi: 10.1089/cyber.2015.0553
32. Frison E, Eggermont S. Exploring the relationships between different types of Facebook use, perceived online social support, and adolescents' depressed mood. *Soc Sci Comput Rev.* (2016) 34:153–71. doi: 10.1177/0894439314567449
33. Marczinski CA, Hertzenberg H, Goddard P, Maloney SF, Stamates AL, O'Connor K. Alcohol-related Facebook activity predicts alcohol use patterns in college students. *Addict Res Theor.* (2016) 24:398–405. doi: 10.3109/16066359.2016.1146709
34. Moreno MA, Arseniev-Koehler A, Litt D, Christakis D. Evaluating college students' displayed alcohol references on facebook and twitter. *J Adolesc Health.* (2016) 58:527–32. doi: 10.1016/j.jadohealth.2016.01.005
35. Naeemi S, Tamam E. The relationship between emotional dependence on facebook and psychological well-being in adolescents aged 13–16. *Child Indic Res.* (2017) 10:1095–106. doi: 10.1007/s12187-016-9438-3

36. Sampasa-Kanyinga H, Chaput JP. Use of social networking sites and alcohol consumption among adolescents. *Public Health.* (2016) 139:88–95. doi: 10.1016/j.puhe.2016.05.005
37. Abar CC, Farnett S, Mendola K, Koban K, Sarra S. Relationships between parent–child social media interactions and health behaviors. *J Subst Use.* (2018) 23:335–7. doi: 10.1080/14659891.2017.1410586
38. Frison E, Eggermont S. Browsing, posting, and liking on Instagram: the reciprocal relationships between different types of Instagram use and adolescents' depressed mood. *Cyberpsychol Behav Soc Netw.* (2017) 20:603–9. doi: 10.1089/cyber.2017.0156
39. Gul H, Yurumez Solmaz E, Gul A, Oner O. Facebook overuse and addiction among Turkish adolescents: are ADHD and ADHD-related problems risk factors? *Psychiatry Clin Psychopharmacol.* (2018) 28:80–90. doi: 10.1080/24750573.2017.1383706
40. Jacob N, Evans R, Scourfield J. The influence of online images on self-harm: a qualitative study of young people aged 16–24. *J Adolesc.* (2017) 60:140–7. doi: 10.1016/j.adolescence.2017.08.001
41. Pontes HM. Investigating the differential effects of social networking site addiction and Internet gaming disorder on psychological health. *J Behav Addict.* (2017) 6:601–10. doi: 10.1556/2006.6.2017.075
42. Spilkova J, Chomynova P, Csemy L. Predictors of excessive use of social media and excessive online gaming in Czech teenagers. *J Behav Addict.* (2017) 6:611–9. doi: 10.1556/2006.6.2017.064
43. Van Rooij AJ, Ferguson CJ, Van de Mheen D, Schoenmakers TM. Time to abandon Internet Addiction? Predicting problematic Internet, game, and social media use from psychosocial well-being and application use. *Clin Neuropsychiatry.* (2017) 14:113–21.
44. Weinstein E. Adolescents' differential responses to social media browsing: exploring causes and consequences for intervention. *Comput Hum Behav.* (2017) 76:396–405. doi: 10.1016/j.chb.2017.07.038
45. Brown RC, Fischer T, Goldwich AD, Keller F, Young R, Plener PL. # cutting: non-suicidal self-injury (NSSI) on Instagram. *Psychol Med.* (2018) 48:337–46. doi: 10.1017/S0033291717001751
46. Muzaffar N, Brito EB, Fogel J, Fagan D, Kumar K, Verma R. The association of adolescent Facebook behaviours with symptoms of social anxiety, generalized anxiety, and depression. *J Can Acad Child Adolesc Psychiatry.* (2018) 27:252.
47. Niu GF, Luo YJ, Sun XJ, Zhou ZK, Yu F, Yang SL, et al. Qzone use and depression among Chinese adolescents: a moderated mediation model. *J Affect Disord.* (2018) 231:58–62. doi: 10.1016/j.jad.2018.01.013
48. Settanni M, Marengo D, Fabris MA, Longobardi C. The interplay between ADHD symptoms and time perspective in addictive social media use: a study on adolescent Facebook users. *Child Youth Serv Rev.* (2018) 89:165–70. doi: 10.1016/j.childyouth.2018.04.031
49. Chang L, Li P, Loh RSM, Chua THH. A study of Singapore adolescent girls' selfie practices, peer appearance comparisons, and body esteem on Instagram. *Body Image.* (2019) 29:90–9. doi: 10.1016/j.bodyim.2019.03.005
50. de Vries DA, Vossen HGM, van der Kolk-van der Boom P. Social media and body dissatisfaction: investigating the attenuating role of positive parent–Adolescent relationships. *J Youth Adolesc.* (2019) 48:527–36. doi: 10.1007/s10964-018-0956-9
51. Louragli I, Ahami A, Khadmaoui A, Aboussaleh Y, Lamrani AC. Behavioral analysis of adolescent's students addicted to facebook and its impact on performance and mental health. *Acta Neuropsychol.* (2019) 17:427–39. doi: 10.5604/01.3001.0013.6550
52. Negriff S. Depressive symptoms predict characteristics of online social networks. *J Adolesc Health.* (2019) 65:101–6. doi: 10.1016/j.jadohealth.2019.01.026
53. Przepiorka A, Blachnio A. The role of Facebook intrusion, depression, and future time perspective in sleep problems among adolescents. *J Res Adolesc.* (2019) 30:559–69. doi: 10.1111/jora.12543
54. Raudsepp L, Kais K. Longitudinal associations between problematic social media use and depressive symptoms in adolescent girls. *Prev Med Rep.* (2019) 15:100925. doi: 10.1016/j.pmedr.2019.100925
55. Savolainen I, Oksanen A, Kaakinen M, Sirola A, Miller BL, Paek HJ, et al. The Association between social media use and hazardous alcohol use among youths: a four-country study. *Alcohol Alcohol.* (2020) 55:86–95. doi: 10.1093/alcalc/agz088
56. Steers MLN, Neighbors C, Wickham RE, Petit WE, Kerr B, Moreno MA. My friends, I'm# SOTALLYTOBER: A longitudinal examination of college students' drinking, friends' approval of drinking, and Facebook alcohol-related posts. *Digit Health.* (2019) 5:2055207619845449. doi: 10.1177/2055207619845449
57. Vannucci A, Ohannessian CM. Social media use subgroups differentially predict psychosocial well-being during early adolescence. *J Youth Adolesc.* (2019) 48:1469–93. doi: 10.1007/s10964-019-01060-9
58. Yurdagül C, Kircaburun K, Emirtekin E, Wang P, Griffiths MD. Psychopathological consequences related to problematic instagram use among adolescents: the mediating role of body image dissatisfaction and moderating role of gender. *Int J Ment Health Addict.* (2019) 1–13. doi: 10.1007/s11469-019-00071-8
59. Boursier V, Gioia F, Griffiths MD. Objectified body consciousness, body image control in photos, and problematic social networking: the role of appearance control beliefs. *Front Psychol.* (2020) 11:147. doi: 10.3389/fpsyg.2020.00147
60. Fardouly J, Magson NR, Rapee RM, Johnco CJ, Oar EL. The use of social media by Australian preadolescents and its links with mental health. *J Clin Psychol.* (2020) 76:1304–26. doi: 10.1002/jclp.22936
61. Stockdale LA, Coyne SM. Bored and online: reasons for using social media, problematic social networking site use, and behavioral outcomes across the transition from adolescence to emerging adulthood. *J Adolesc.* (2020) 79:173–83. doi: 10.1016/j.adolescence.2020.01.010
62. Brown RC, Fischer T, Goldwich DA, Plener PL. "I just finally wanted to belong somewhere"--Qualitative analysis of experiences with posting pictures of self-injury on instagram. *Front Psychiatry.* (2020) 11:274. doi: 10.3389/fpsyt.2020.00274
63. Danaux X, Gandy D. *FontAwesome.* (2016). Available online at: http://mirror.kumi.systems/ctan/fonts/fontawesome/doc/fontawesome.pdf
64. Lenhard W, Lenhard A. *Calculation of Effect Sizes.* Dettelbach (2016).
65. American Psychiatric Pub. *Diagnostic and Statistical Manual of Mental Disorders (DSM-5®).* Washington, DC: American Psychiatric Pub (2013).
66. Nesi J, Prinstein MJ. Using social media for social comparison and feedback-seeking: gender and popularity moderate associations with depressive symptoms. *J Abnorm Child Psychol.* (2015) 43:1427–38. doi: 10.1007/s10802-015-0020-0
67. Twenge JM, Cooper AB, Joiner TE, Duffy ME, Binau SG. Age, period, and cohort trends in mood disorder indicators and suicide-related outcomes in a nationally representative dataset, 2005–2017. *J Abnorm Psychol.* (2019) 128:185–99. doi: 10.1037/abn0000410
68. Aalbers G, McNally RJ, Heeren A, Wit SD, Fried EI. Social media and depression symptoms: a network perspective. *J Exp Psychol Gen.* (2018) 148:1454–62. doi: 10.1037/xge0000528
69. Brooks S, Longstreet P. Social networking's peril: cognitive absorption, social networking usage, and depression. *Cyberpsychology.* (2015) 9:21–39. doi: 10.5817/CP2015-4-5
70. Tobin SJ, Vanman EJ, Verreynne M, Saeri AK. Threats to belonging on Facebook: lurking and ostracism. *Soc Influence.* (2015) 10:31–42. doi: 10.1080/15534510.2014.893924
71. Kross E, Verduyn P, Demiralp E, Park J, Lee DS, Lin N, et al. Facebook use predicts declines in subjective well-being in young adults. *PLoS ONE.* (2013) 8:e69841. doi: 10.1371/journal.pone.0069841
72. Ehrenreich SE, Underwood MK. Adolescents' internalizing symptoms as predictors of the content of their Facebook communication and responses received from peers. *Transl Issues Psychol Sci.* (2016) 2:227. doi: 10.1037/tps0000077
73. Harter S. *The Construction of the Self: Developmental and Sociocultural Foundations.* New York, NY: Guilford Publications (2015).
74. Chou HTG, Edge N. "They are happier and having better lives than I am" : the impact of using Facebook on perceptions of others' lives. *Cyberpsychol Behav Soc Netw.* (2012) 15:117–21. doi: 10.1089/cyber.2011.0324
75. Davila J, Hershenberg R, Feinstein BA, Gorman K, Bhatia V, Starr LR. Frequency and quality of social networking among young adults: associations with depressive symptoms, rumination, and corumination. *Psychol Popul Media Cult.* (2012) 1:72. doi: 10.1037/a0027512
76. Steers MLN, Wickham RE, Acitelli LK. Seeing everyone else's highlight reels: how Facebook usage is linked to depressive symptoms.

J Soc Clin Psychol. (2014) 33:701–31. doi: 10.1521/jscp.2014.33.8.701

77. Appel H, Gerlach AL, Crusius J. The interplay between Facebook use, social comparison, envy, and depression. *Curr Opin Psychol.* (2016) 9:44–9. doi: 10.1016/j.copsyc.2015.10.006
78. Bollen J, Gonçalves B, van de Leemput I, Ruan G. The happiness paradox: your friends are happier than you. *EPJ Data Sci.* (2017) 6:4. doi: 10.1140/epjds/s13688-017-0100-1
79. Frison E, Subrahmanyam K, Eggermont S. The short-term longitudinal and reciprocal relations between peer victimization on Facebook and adolescents' well-being. *J Youth Adolesc.* (2016) 45:1755–71. doi: 10.1007/s10964-016-0436-z
80. McCloskey W, Iwanicki S, Lauterbach D, Giammittorio DM, Maxwell K. Are Facebook "friends" helpful? Development of a Facebook-based measure of social support and examination of relationships among depression, quality of life, and social support. *Cyberpsychol Behav Soc Netw.* (2015) 18:499–505. doi: 10.1089/cyber.2014.0538
81. Hoge E, Bickham D, Cantor J. Digital media, anxiety, and depression in children. *Pediatrics.* (2017) 140(Suppl. 2):S76–80. doi: 10.1542/peds.2016-1758G
82. Calancie O, Ewing L, Narducci LD, Horgan S, Khalid-Khan S. Exploring how social networking sites impact youth with anxiety: a qualitative study of Facebook stressors among adolescents with an anxiety disorder diagnosis. *Cyberpsychology.* (2017) 11. doi: 10.5817/CP2017-4-2
83. Oberst U, Wegmann E, Stodt B, Brand M, Chamarro A. Negative consequences from heavy social networking in adolescents: the mediating role of fear of missing out. *J Adolesc.* (2017) 55:51–60. doi: 10.1016/j.adolescence.2016.12.008
84. Przybylski AK, Murayama K, DeHaan CR, Gladwell V. Motivational, emotional, and behavioral correlates of fear of missing out. *Comput Hum Behav.* (2013) 29:1841–8. doi: 10.1016/j.chb.2013.02.014
85. Andreassen CS. Online social network site addiction: a comprehensive review. *Curr Addict Rep.* (2015) 2:175–84. doi: 10.1007/s40429-015-0056-9
86. Dhir A, Yossatorn Y, Kaur P, Chen S. Online social media fatigue and psychological wellbeing—A study of compulsive use, fear of missing out, fatigue, anxiety and depression. *Int J Inform Manage.* (2018) 40:141–52. doi: 10.1016/j.ijinfomgt.2018.01.012
87. Dempsey AE, O'Brien KD, Tiamiyu MF, Elhai JD. Fear of missing out (FoMO) and rumination mediate relations between social anxiety and problematic Facebook use. *Addict Behav Rep.* (2019) 9:100150. doi: 10.1016/j.abrep.2018.100150
88. Beyens I, Frison E, Eggermont S. "I don't want to miss a thing": Adolescents' fear of missing out and its relationship to adolescents' social needs, Facebook use, and Facebook related stress. *Comput Hum Behav.* (2016) 64:1–8. doi: 10.1016/j.chb.2016.05.083
89. McLean SA, Jarman HK, Rodgers RF. How do "selfies" impact adolescents' well-being and body confidence? A narrative review. *Psychol Res Behav Manage.* (2019) 12:513. doi: 10.2147/PRBM.S177834
90. Forrest KY, Stuhldreher WL. Patterns and correlates of body image dissatisfaction and distortion among college students. *Am J Health Stud.* (2007) 22:18–25.
91. Pater JA, Haimson OL, Andalibi N, Mynatt ED. "Hunger Hurts but Starving Works" Characterizing the Presentation of Eating Disorders Online. In: *Proceedings of the 19th ACM Conference on Computer-Supported Cooperative Work & Social Computing.* San Francisco, CA (2016). p. 1185–200.
92. Curtis BL, Lookatch SJ, Ramo DE, McKay JR, Feinn RS, Kranzler HR. Meta-analysis of the association of alcohol-related social media use with alcohol consumption and alcohol-related problems in adolescents and young adults. *Alcohol Clin Exp Res.* (2018) 42:978–86. doi: 10.1111/acer.13642
93. Westgate EC, Neighbors C, Heppner H, Jahn S, Lindgren KP. "I will take a shot for every 'like'I get on this status": posting alcohol-related Facebook content is linked to drinking outcomes. *J Stud Alcohol Drugs.* (2014) 75:390–8. doi: 10.15288/jsad.2014.75.390
94. Marchant A, Hawton K, Stewart A, Montgomery P, Singaravelu V, Lloyd K, et al. A systematic review of the relationship between internet use, self-harm and suicidal behaviour in young people: the good, the bad and the unknown. *PLoS ONE.* (2017) 12:e0181722. doi: 10.1371/journal.pone.0181722
95. Cash SJ, Thelwall M, Peck SN, Ferrell JZ, Bridge JA. Adolescent suicide statements on MySpace. *Cyberpsychol Behav Soc Netw.* (2013) 16:166–74. doi: 10.1089/cyber.2012.0098
96. Brown RC, Bendig E, Fischer T, Goldwich AD, Baumeister H, Plener PL. Can acute suicidality be predicted by Instagram data? Results from qualitative and quantitative language analyses. *PLoS ONE.* (2019) 14:e0220623. doi: 10.1371/journal.pone.0220623
97. Miguel EM, Chou T, Golik A, Cornacchio D, Sanchez AL, DeSerisy M, et al. Examining the scope and patterns of deliberate self-injurious cutting content in popular social media. *Depress Anxiety.* (2017) 34:786–93. doi: 10.1002/da.22668
98. Moreno MA, Ton A, Selkie E, Evans Y. Secret society 123: understanding the language of self-harm on Instagram. *J Adolesc Health.* (2016) 58:78–84. doi: 10.1016/j.jadohealth.2015.09.015
99. Luxton DD, June JD, Fairall JM. Social media and suicide: a public health perspective. *Am J Public Health.* (2012) 102:195–200. doi: 10.2105/AJPH.2011.300608
100. Pettalia JL, Levin E, Dickinson J. Cyberbullying: eliciting harm without consequence. *Comput Hum. Behav.* (2013) 29:2758–65. doi: 10.1016/j.chb.2013.07.020
101. Barlett CP, Gentile DA, Chng G, Li D, Chamberlin K. Social media use and cyberbullying perpetration: a longitudinal analysis. *Violence Gender.* (2018) 5:191–7. doi: 10.1089/vio.2017.0047
102. Shakir, T., Bhandari, N., Andrews, A., Zmitrovich, A., McCracken, C., Gadomski, J., et al. (2019). Do our adolescents know they are cyberbullying victims? *J. Infant Child Adolesc. Psychother.* 18, 93–101. doi: 10.1080/15289168.2018.1565004
103. Chatzakou D, Leontiadis I, Blackburn J, De Cristofaro E, Stringhini G, Vakali A, et al. Detecting cyberbullying and cyberaggression in social media. *arXiv preprint* arXiv:190708873 (2019). doi: 10.1145/3343484
104. Plemmons G, Hall M, Doupnik S, Gay J, Brown C, Browning W, et al. Hospitalization for suicide ideation or attempt: 2008–2015. *Pediatrics.* (2018) 141:e20172426. doi: 10.1542/peds.2017-2426
105. van Schalkwyk GI, Marin CE, Ortiz M, Rolison M, Qayyum Z, McPartland JC, et al. Social media use, friendship quality, and the moderating role of anxiety in adolescents with autism spectrum disorder. *J Autism Dev Disord.* (2017) 47:2805–13. doi: 10.1007/s10803-017-3201-6
106. Gwynette MF, Morriss D, Warren N, Truelove J, Warthen J, Ross CP, et al. Social skills training for adolescents with autism spectrum disorder using facebook (project rex connect): a survey study. *JMIR Ment Health.* (2017) 4:e4. doi: 10.2196/mental.6605
107. Iglesias OB, Sanchez LEG, Rodríguez MÁA. Do young people with Asperger syndrome or intellectual disability use social media and are they cyberbullied or cyberbullies in the same way as their peers? *Psicothema.* (2019) 31:30–7.
108. Choi BY, Huh S, Kim DJ, Suh SW, Lee SK, Potenza MN. Transitions in problematic internet use: a one-year longitudinal study of boys. *Psychiatry Invest.* (2019) 16:433–42. doi: 10.30773/pi.2019.04.02.1
109. Ebstein RP, Israel S, Chew SH, Zhong S, Knafo A. Genetics of human social behavior. *Neuron.* (2010) 65:831–44. doi: 10.1016/j.neuron.2010.02.020
110. Deryakulu D, Ursavaş ÖF. Genetic and environmental influences on problematic Internet use: a twin study. *Comput Hum Behav.* (2014) 39:331–8. doi: 10.1016/j.chb.2014.07.038
111. Miller G, Zhu G, Wright MJ, Hansell NK, Martin NG. The heritability and genetic correlates of mobile phone use: a twin study of consumer behavior. *Twin Res Hum Genet.* (2012) 15:97–106. doi: 10.1375/twin.15.1.97
112. York C. A regression approach to testing genetic influence on communication behavior: social media use as an example. *Comput Hum Behav.* (2017) 73:100–9. doi: 10.1016/j.chb.2017.03.029
113. Deryakulu D, Ursavaş ÖF. Genetic and environmental sources of nomophobia: a small-scale Turkish Twin study. *Addicta.* (2019) 6:147–62. doi: 10.15805/addicta.2019.6.1.0028
114. Bonassi A, Cataldo I, Gabrieli G, Foo JN, Lepri B, Esposito G. Oxytocin Receptor Gene polymorphism and early parental bonding interact in shaping Instagram social behaviour. *PsyArXiv.* (2019). Available online at: psyarxiv.com/n6mgv.

115. Meshi D, Morawetz C, Heekeren HR. Nucleus accumbens response to gains in reputation for the self relative to gains for others predicts social media use. *Front Hum Neurosci.* (2013) 7:439. doi: 10.3389/fnhum.2013.00439
116. Sherman LE, Payton AA, Hernandez LM, Greenfield PM, Dapretto M. The power of the like in adolescence: effects of peer influence on neural and behavioral responses to social media. *Psychol Sci.* (2016) 27:1027–35. doi: 10.1177/0956797616645673
117. Montag C, Markowetz A, Blaszkiewicz K, Andone I, Lachmann B, Sariyska R, et al. Facebook usage on smartphones and gray matter volume of the nucleus accumbens. *Behav Brain Res.* (2017) 329:221–8. doi: 10.1016/j.bbr.2017.04.035
118. He Q, Turel O, Brevers D, Bechara A. Excess social media use in normal populations is associated with amygdala-striatal but not with prefrontal morphology. *Psychiatry Res Neuroimaging.* (2017) 269:31–5. doi: 10.1016/j.pscychresns.2017.09.003
119. Lee D, Namkoong K, Lee J, Lee BO, Jung YC. Lateral orbitofrontal gray matter abnormalities in subjects with problematic smartphone use. *J Behav Addict.* (2019) 8:404–11. doi: 10.1556/2006.8.2019.50
120. Montag C, Zhao Z, Sindermann C, Xu L, Fu M, Li J, et al. Internet Communication Disorder and the structure of the human brain: initial insights on WeChat addiction. *Sci Rep.* (2018) 8:2155. doi: 10.1038/s41598-018-19904-y
121. Loh KK, Kanai R. Higher media multi-tasking activity is associated with smaller gray-matter density in the anterior cingulate cortex. *PLoS ONE.* (2014) 9:e106698. doi: 10.1371/journal.pone.0106698
122. Moisala M, Salmela V, Hietajärvi L, Salo E, Carlson S, Salonen O, et al. Media multitasking is associated with distractibility and increased prefrontal activity in adolescents and young adults. *Neuroimage.* (2016) 134:113–21. doi: 10.1016/j.neuroimage.2016.04.011
123. Bayer JB, O'Donnell MB, Cascio CN, Falk EB. Brain sensitivity to exclusion is associated with core network closure. *Sci Rep.* (2018) 8:16037. doi: 10.1038/s41598-018-33624-3
124. Pandya M, Altinay M, Malone DA, Anand A. Where in the brain is depression? *Curr Psychiatry Rep.* (2012) 14:634–42. doi: 10.1007/s11920-012-0322-7
125. Andreassen CS, Torsheim T, Brunborg GS, Pallesen S. Development of a Facebook addiction scale. *Psychol Rep.* (2012) 110:501–17. doi: 10.2466/02.09.18.PR0.110.2.501-517
126. Van den Eijnden R, Lemmens J, Valkenburg P. The social media disorder scale: validity and psychometric properties. *J Behav Addict.* (2016) 5:13. doi: 10.1037/t53816-000
127. Nick EA, Cole DA, Cho SJ, Smith DK, Carter TG, Zelkowitz RL. The Online Social Support Scale: measure development and validation. *Psychol Assess.* (2018) 30:1127. doi: 10.1037/pas0000558
128. Kwon M, Kim DJ, Cho H, Yang S. The smartphone addiction scale: development and validation of a short version for adolescents. *PLoS ONE.* (2013) 8:e83558. doi: 10.1371/journal.pone.0083558
129. Landoll RR, La Greca AM, Lai BS. Aversive Peer Experiences on Social Networking Sites: development of the Social Networking-Peer Experiences Questionnaire (SN-PEQ). *J Res Adolesc.* (2013) 23:695–705. doi: 10.1111/jora.12022
130. Anderson KE. Getting acquainted with social networks and apps: it is time to talk about TikTok. *Library Hi Tech News.* (2020).
131. Casler K, Bickel L, Hackett E. Separate but equal? A comparison of participants and data gathered via Amazon's MTurk, social media, and face-to-face behavioral testing. *Comput Hum Behav.* (2013) 29:2156–60. doi: 10.1016/j.chb.2013.05.009

6

The Presence of Another Person Influences Oscillatory Cortical Dynamics During Dual Brain EEG Recording

*Max J. Rolison, Adam J. Naples, Helena J. V. Rutherford and James C. McPartland**

Child Study Center, Yale School of Medicine, New Haven, CT, United States

***Correspondence:**
James C. McPartland
james.mcpartland@yale.edu

Humans are innately social creatures and the social environment strongly influences brain development. As such, the human brain is primed for and sensitive to social information even in the absence of explicit task or instruction. In this study, we examined the influence of different levels of interpersonal proximity on resting state brain activity and its association with social cognition. We measured EEG in pairs of 13 typically developing (TD) adults seated in separate rooms, in the same room back-to-back, and in the same room facing each other. Interpersonal proximity modulated broadband EEG power from 4–55 Hz and individual differences in self-reported social cognition modulated these effects in the beta and gamma frequency bands. These findings provide novel insight into the influence of social environment on brain activity and its association with social cognition through dual-brain EEG recording and demonstrate the importance of using interactive methods to study the human brain.

Keywords: EEG, resting state, dual brain, social cognition, interactive social neuroscience, autism spectrum disorder

INTRODUCTION

Social interaction is central to human experience and necessary for normative brain development. The presence of another person is environmentally salient, drawing attention and neural resources (1). During development, such social interactions provide required information to experience-expectant brain systems supporting specialization of a network of brain regions for processing social information (2, 3), and it is hypothesized that primate brains evolved to support complex social cognition (4, 5). Thus, in addition to actively supporting social performance, this network remains engaged even when a person is "at rest" rather than engaged in an explicitly social activity (6).

The association between resting state brain activity and social cognition is incompletely understood. Neuroimaging studies consistently implicate atypical resting activity across multiple modalities in clinical populations with impaired social cognition (7–10). Even in nonclinically ascertained populations, EEG studies have identified alterations in power in the alpha frequency range (8–13 Hz) associated with social cognition (11). Despite strong evidence for an association between at-rest brain activity and social function, the majority of research has measured brain activity when participants are in isolation in an EEG recording chamber, MRI, or MEG; we know little about brain activity during *in vivo* social interactions. Interactive social neuroscience (12), or second person neuroscience (13), the study of brain function during live social interaction, seeks to measure brain activity in a more ecologically valid manner.

Increasing efforts have focused on using EEG hyperscanning to understand the neural basis of social interactions, with protocols being developed to allow this approach to be more widely implemented across research groups (14). EEG hyperscanning during cooperative games reveals variability in the activity of different frequency bands in prefrontal areas (15), with activity in prefrontal and anterior cingulate regions differentiating player order during card games (16). EEG hyperscanning has also evidenced value during cooperative (17–19) and competitive social interactions (20, 21). Additionally, EEG hyperscanning has demonstrated interpersonal synchrony when people are performing coordinated movements (22–26). Importantly, correlations between participants' EEG activity may be shaped by a host of individual differences, including empathy, social closeness, and autistic traits (27, 28). Clinically, hyperscanning approaches may also be especially relevant to our understanding of the neural basis of autism (12). Using fNIRS, children with ASD evidenced variability in neural synchronization in frontal areas when interacting with their parents compared to when they were completing the task alone under parental observation or during a no interaction comparison condition (29).

Using these methods, researchers have identified task-related differences (28) and differences in the alpha, beta, and theta frequency bands when participants were together versus alone, which were modulated by anxious attachment style (30), but relationships with resting brain activity and social performance remain unexplored.

In this study, we examined how the presence of another person modulated resting state brain activity. We recorded EEG simultaneously from pairs of participants during three social contexts: in separate rooms, together seated back-to-back, and together facing each other. EEG data was recorded when participants had their eyes open and their eyes closed across the three social contexts. We predicted that variation in social context would alter resting-state oscillatory brain activity. Specifically, we expected that alpha would be sensitive to changing social dynamics based on the well-established evidence that alpha indexes vigilance and arousal, as well as prior work demonstrating an association between alpha activity and autistic traits (11). Additionally, we expected that variation in oscillatory activity between contexts, as a marker of sensitivity to social context, would be associated with social cognition, as measured through self-report of social ability.

METHODS

Participants

Twenty college-aged participants from the New Haven community (M=21.7 years, SD=0.45, 6 male) participated in 10 same-sex dyads (recruited independently and paired arbitrarily). Exclusionary criteria included prescription medications affecting cognitive processes (including benzodiazepines, barbiturates, antiepileptics, carbamazepine, and valproic acid), history of head trauma or serious brain or psychiatric illness, or history of learning or intellectual disability. All procedures were conducted with the understanding and written consent of participants and with approval of the Human Investigations Committee at the Yale School of Medicine. Participants were compensated for their participation in the study.

Behavioral Measures

Participants completed a series of self-report questionnaires designed to measure variation across subclinical to clinical levels of social and communicative performance and impairment: the Social Responsiveness Scale 2nd Edition (31) and the Broad Autism Phenotype Questionnaire (32).

EEG Procedures

Task

Following separate consenting procedures, participants were introduced to one another and seated in the same room for EEG application. During EEG recording, participants sat quietly for two minutes in two eye orientations (eyes opened (EO) or eyes closed (EC)) across three conditions: (1) "separate" rooms, (2) the same room "back-to-back", and (3) the same room "facing" each other (**Figure 1A**). During EC across all three social contexts, participants were instructed to remain still with their eyes closed. During EO, when participants were in separate rooms and back-to-back, they were instructed to remain still and pick a point straight ahead and fixate on the point. When participants were facing, they were instructed to remain still while looking into each other's eyes. Therefore, the facing EO condition demonstrated joint-gaze. While a fixed order precludes estimation of order effects, a full counterbalancing of experimental conditions was not possible with the planned sample size. Moreover, in order to draw comparisons between the current study and prior studies of resting-state EEG recorded in isolation, we similarly began by recording in separate rooms. Additionally, we speculated that the novelty of the face-to-face condition would limit the interpretation of subsequent conditions. For these reasons, we adopted this fixed order of social context administration.

EEG was recorded using the B-Alert X-24 20 channel wireless EEG sensor net (Advanced Brain Monitoring Inc., Carlsbad CA). Continuous EEG data was recorded at 256 Hz using B-Alert acquisition software [Version 2.05.05; (33)] with joint mastoid reference. Electrode impedance was kept under 10 kOhms with Synapse Conductive Electrode Cream. Continuous EEG data across systems was synchronized using a pair of ABM External Sync Units (ESU) connected to the stimulus presentation computer *via* a split cable TTL pulse. An audio tone signaling the start and end of each condition was presented using E-Prime 2.0 (34). EEG was marked every 1000 milliseconds during each condition.

EEG Processing

EEG was filtered from 0.5 to 100 Hz and preprocessed using EEGLAB (35). Data was selected from frontal electrodes due to

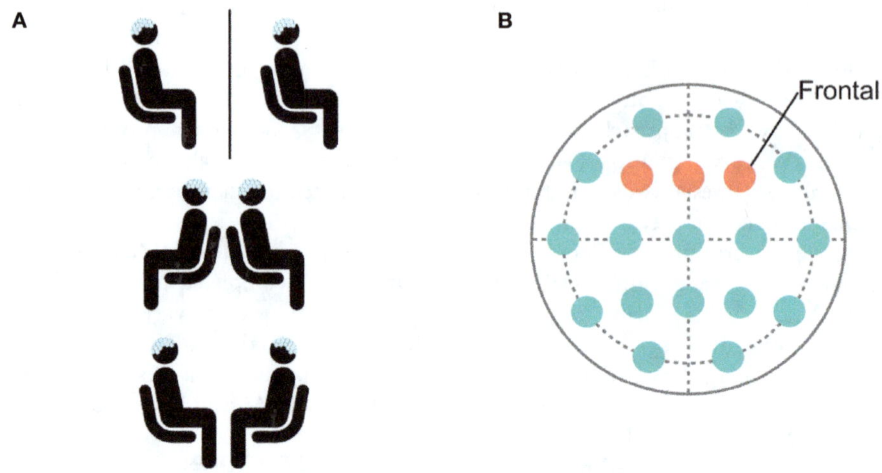

FIGURE 1 | (A) Participants were seated in separate rooms, back-to-back, and facing each other. **(B)** Data was selected and analyzed from frontal electrodes F3, Fz, and F4.

the importance of the frontal cortex in modulating attention (**Figure 1B**). PREP pipeline (36) was used to remove line-noise, detect, and interpolate bad channels. Next, independent component analysis (ICA) was performed and eye-blink components were manually identified based on scalp topography and removed. Data was epoched into 1,000-ms segments. Artifact detection was performed with a 40-μV threshold using a 50-ms moving window in 25-ms steps, and epochs containing artifact were rejected. Participants with more than 50% rejected epochs per category were excluded from analyses. Included participants had an average of 7.2% rejected epochs.

Frequency decomposition was performed using the Fieldtrip Toolbox (37). Theta (4–7 Hz), alpha (8–12 Hz), beta (12–24 Hz), and gamma (30–40 Hz) frequency bands were defined based on prior studies (30). Epochs were zero padded to contain 25,600 samples, mean detrended, windowed with a Hann window, and power was calculated using a multitaper fast Fourier transform (FFT) with four tapers.

Analyses

Data from 13 participants was included in analyses following artifact detection. Parametric data was analyzed using repeated measures analysis of variance (ANOVA), and data not meeting criteria for normality as indicated by Shapiro-Wilk's test was analyzed using Friedman's 2-way ANOVA by Rank. EEG power in the theta and gamma frequency ranges was analyzed separately using 3 (separate/back-to-back/facing) × 2 (EO/EC) repeated measures ANOVA. EEG power in the alpha and beta frequency ranges was analyzed separately using Friedman's two-way ANOVA by rank for eye orientation and condition. Planned comparisons were performed to investigate directionality of observed effects, utilizing paired samples *t* tests for parametric data and Wilcoxon Signed Rank test for nonparametric data. Spearman's rank correlations were used for assessing the relationship between changes in EEG power and social function. Difference scores were calculated by subtracting the absolute power between different conditions (SEP-BACK, BACK-FACE) For all analyses, the statistical significance level was set at $\alpha < 0.05$, and Bonferroni correction was applied to correct for multiple comparisons. Effect size estimates for analyses of variance, t-tests, and behavioral correlations were calculated with partial eta-squared ($\eta^2_{partial}$), Cohen's d (d), and Spearman's rank correlation coefficient (ρ, rho), respectively. Confidence intervals (CI) for Spearman's rank correlations were calculated based on the Fisher r-to-z transformation.

RESULTS

Theta Power

Spectral plots are shown in **Figure 2**. Results revealed a main effect of eye orientation on theta power, $F(1,12)=6.6$, $p=0.03$, $\eta^2_{partial}=0.35$, with participants demonstrating greater theta-band activity during EO relative to EC. Furthermore, there was a main effect of condition, $F(2,24)=4.2$, $p=0.03$, $\eta^2_{partial}=0.26$, indicating that theta activity was greater when separate compared to back-to-back, $p=0.01$, or facing, $p=0.04$ (**Figures 3A, B**). There was no interaction between eye orientation and condition, $p=0.48$.

Alpha Power

Results revealed greater alpha activity during EC than EO when resting separately $Z=-2.7$, $p < 0.01$, back-to-back, $Z=-2.2$, $p=0.03$, and facing, $Z=-3.2$, $p < 0.01$. Additionally, there was an effect of condition during EC, $\chi^2(2)=11.2$, $p < 0.01$, such that alpha activity was greater when back-to-back compared to when resting separately, $Z=1.3$, $p < 0.01$. There was no effect of condition during EO, $\chi^2(2)=3.2$, $p=0.20$ (**Figures 3C, D**).

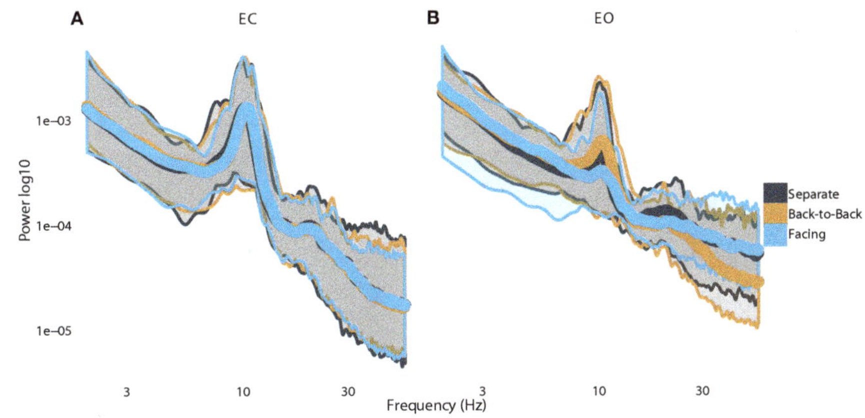

FIGURE 2 | Plots of power spectra with standard error while resting with **(A)** eyes closed and **(B)** eyes open.

Beta Power

Results revealed greater beta activity during EC than EO when resting separately, Z=−3.0, $p < 0.01$, back-to-back, Z=−3.0, $p < 0.01$, and facing, Z=−3.1, $p < 0.01$. There was no effect of condition during EC, $\chi^2(2)=1.1$, p=0.58. However, there was an effect of condition during EO, $\chi^2(2)=12.2$, $p < 0.01$, such that beta activity was greater during joint-gaze while facing compared to resting separately, Z=1.3, $p < 0.01$, or resting back-to-back, Z=1.0, p=0.03 (**Figures 3E, F**).

Gamma Power

A significant interaction between eyes and condition, F(2,24)= 5.9, $p < 0.01$, $\eta^2_{partial}=0.33$, revealed that gamma activity was greater during EO than EC when separate, t(12)=4.7, $p < 0.01$, d=1.25, and when facing, t(12)=3.3, $p < 0.01$, d=0.84, but was not different when back-to-back, t(12)=1.6, p=0.13. During EO, gamma activity was greater when resting separately than resting back-to-back, t(12)=4.2, $p < 0.01$, d=1.23, or facing with joint-gaze, t(12)=2.4, p=0.03, d=0.73. However, there was no difference between resting back-to-back or facing with joint-gaze during EO, t(12) =−2.0, p=0.08. During EC, gamma activity was greater when resting separately than resting back-to-back, t(12) =2.5, p=0.03, d=0.51. Gamma activity was not different when resting separately versus resting while facing, t(12)=2.1, p=0.06, or back-to-back versus facing, t(12) =−1.3, p=0.21 (**Figures 3G, H**).

Behavioral Correlations

Greater difference in EC beta power when back-to-back versus facing was associated with lower scores on the BAPQ, *r*=0.60, *p*=0.03, 95% CI [0.074, 0.865] (**Figure 4A**).

Higher total score on the BAPQ was associated with greater difference in EC gamma activity between separate and back-to-back, ρ=0.61, p=0.03, 95% CI [0.089, 0.868] (**Figure 4B**). Additionally, this difference score between separate and back-to-back was associated with higher total score on the SRS, ρ=0.70, $p < 0.01$, 95% CI [0.243, 0.902] (**Figure 4C**).

DISCUSSION

The current study recorded resting-state EEG simultaneously from two adults while social context was manipulated–with participants separated, in the same room but back-to-back, or in the same room and facing one another. Differential oscillatory power in the theta, alpha, and gamma bands was observed when participants were isolated; when in the presence of another person, facing towards one another or away from one another did not influence resting neural activity. These results suggest that the social presence of another human, regardless of interpersonal orientation, modulates brain activity. We interpret these findings as suggestive of the adoption of an "interpersonally-oriented stance" when in proximity to a potential social partner. The activity was not modulated by facing towards or away from the potential partner which suggests that without an explicit social task, default mode activity is tuned to the presence of another person rather than more granular levels of information, such as face-to-face orientation. Specifically, theta, alpha, and gamma activity attenuation in the presence of another person suggest that activity in these frequency bands may be suppressed in preparation for social interaction.

Additionally, theta and gamma activity was greater when resting with eyes open, while alpha and beta power was greater while resting with eyes closed. These results are consistent with prior studies demonstrating a balance of excitatory and inhibitory activity with a U-shaped profile (38).

Greater difference in beta activity between being back-to-back and facing another person with eyes closed was associated with better self-reported social function. These findings suggest that greater sensitivity to differences in the social environment may contribute to better social cognition. Within the gamma band, differential neural response to isolation versus presence of another person was associated with self-reported social function. Specifically, a greater difference in gamma activity between separate and back-to-back was associated with more

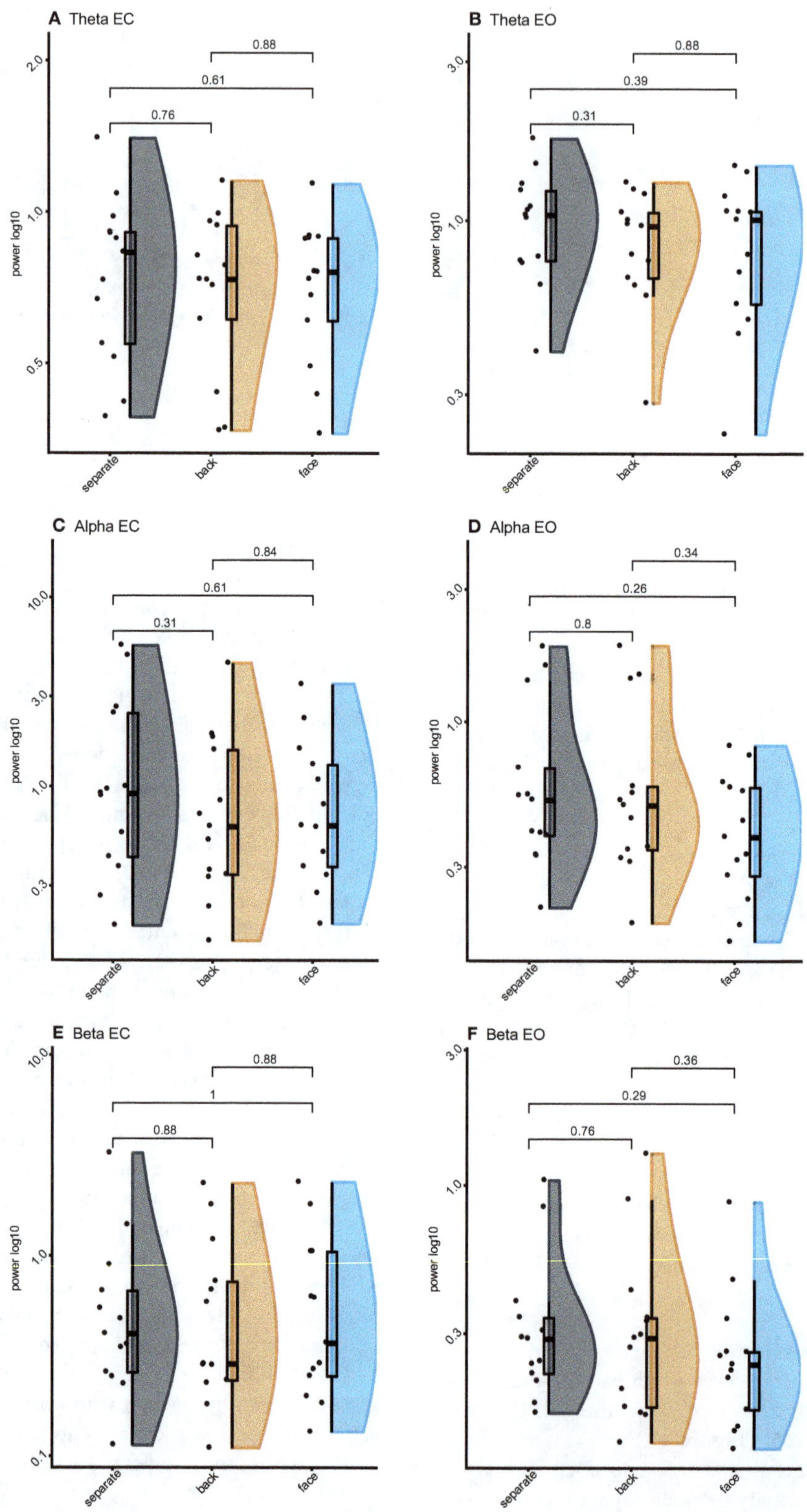

FIGURE 3 | Continued

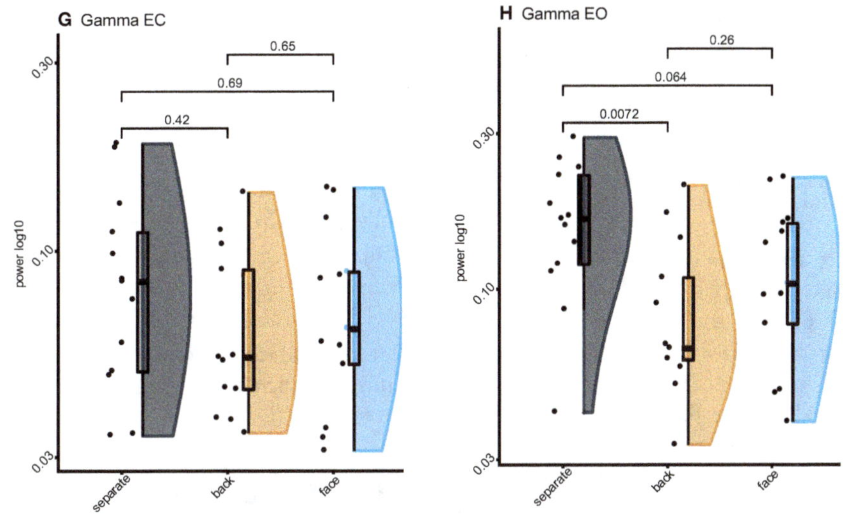

FIGURE 3 | Raincloud plots of spectral power for varying levels of interpersonal proximity: **(A)** Eyes closed (EC) theta power; **(B)** Eyes opened (EO) theta power; **(C)** EC alpha power; **(D)** EO alpha power; **(E)** EC beta power; **(F)** EO beta power; **(G)** EC gamma power; **(H)** EO gamma power.

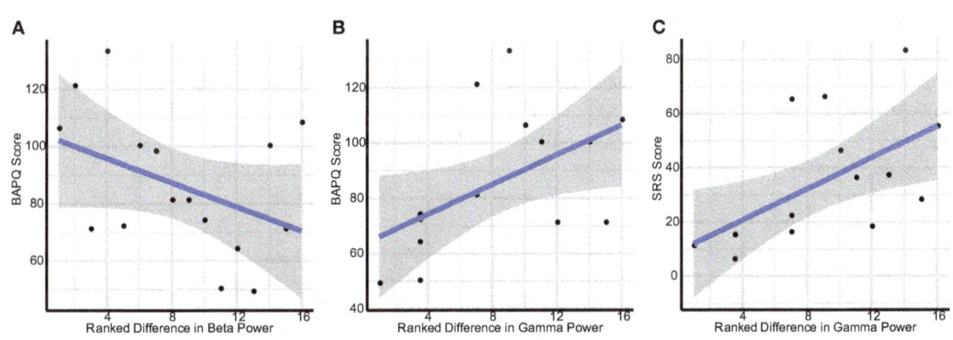

FIGURE 4 | Scatterplots depicting association of self-reported social cognition and variation in interpersonal proximity: **(A)** Ranked difference in eyes closed (EC) beta power between facing versus back-to-back and BAPQ score; **(B)** Ranked difference in EC gamma power between separate and back-to-back and BAPQ score; **(C)** Ranked difference in EC gamma power between separate and back-to-back and SRS score.

impaired self-reported social function. Gamma activity has been associated with social cognition and mentalizing (39), suggesting a relationship between neural attunement to conspecifics and social performance. Specifically, it has been hypothesized that gamma activity is associated with the integration of sensory with socially and emotionally salient information (39, 40), as well as with emotional regulation (41). Additionally, gamma activity has been associated with brain-to-brain synchronization during social interactions (42). Our finding of a relationship between gamma activity and social function aligns with prior research demonstrating correlated resting gamma activity in familiar, but not unfamiliar, dyads (42). These results add to a nascent literature showing relationships among psychological attributes and modulation of resting brain activity by the presence of another person; for example, other studies have shown this modulation to be related to attachment status (30). Given the relevance of social interaction to many clinical conditions, such as autism spectrum disorder, this study reveals a novel avenue for investigating social brain function dissociated from active social tasks.

These findings indicate the overarching influence of interpersonal proximity on resting brain activity. The observation of neural modulation based on mere presence of another person has significant implications for electrophysiological brain research on resting neural activity. Many investigations presume that resting state brain activity represents a task-free "absolute" baseline. Our findings demonstrate that the social environment influences baseline brain activity, suggesting that methodological variation, such as the presence of an examiner in the room, may exert significant influence on results. These findings add to a growing literature demonstrating the importance of studying the brain during social interaction across a variety of contexts. In particular, EEG hyperscanning offers promise for the investigation of these questions because EEG is relatively scalable, cost-effective, and produces a robust signal (12, 14, 43).

Several limitations of the present study should be addressed in future research. Our sample size was limited and precluded more complex and exploratory analytic approaches, such as whole scalp analyses, functional connectivity, and interbrain synchrony. Replication and a more comprehensive analytic approach will be required in future studies with larger samples. Although our analyses do not examine interbrain synchronization between dyads, we consider the simultaneous recording an important part of the experimental procedure in that both participants were in comparable circumstances (e.g., both observed), which would not be the case with only one recording device (e.g., observer and observed). We felt that this arrangement was necessary to be consistent with a naturalistic social interaction. Because we utilized a fixed order for conditions, we were not able to fully explore the effects of a changing social context. Since we utilized only same-sex dyads we could not examine the influence of sex on interpersonal modulation of brain activity. We could not monitor eye gaze during our face-to-face condition; given the importance of eye contact, use of eye-tracking would enable more nuanced investigation of the influence of eye contact during face-to-face interactions. Additionally, gamma activity has been associated with a multitude of cognitive processes, as well as eye movements, thus unexplored factors may contribute to the observed effects.

CONCLUSIONS

The current study recorded resting-state EEG simultaneously from two adults in varying social contexts to investigate the influence of the social environment on baseline brain activity. Results reveal modulation of brain activity based on varying levels of interpersonal proximity, specifically in the theta, alpha, and gamma frequency bands. This study adds to a growing body of evidence suggesting that resting state brain activity is strongly subject to the influence of social context and that these differences in resting state brain activity are associated with social cognition. Our findings provide new insight into resting state neural dynamics and further emphasize the utility of interactive social neuroscience approaches for the study of varying brain states.

AUTHOR CONTRIBUTION

MR, AN, and JM conceived of and designed the experiment. MR performed data collection. MR, AN, and HR analyzed the data. MR, AN, HR, and JM wrote the manuscript.

ACKNOWLEDGMENTS

We thank Advanced Brain Monitoring, Inc. for loaning the EEG equipment and Katherine Stavropoulos and Jennifer Foss-Feig for theoretical contributions.

REFERENCES

1. Klin A, Jones W, Schultz R, Volkmar F. the Enactive Mind, or From Actions to Cognition: Lessons From Autism. *Philos Trans R Soc Lond B Biol Sci* (2003) 358(1430):345–60. doi: 10.1098/rstb.2002.1202
2. Hari R, Henriksson L, Malinen S, Parkkonen L. Centrality of Social Interaction in Human Brain Function. *Neuron* (2015) 88(1):181–93. doi: 10.1016/j.neuron.2015.09.022
3. Leppänen JM, Nelson CA. Tuning the Developing Brain to Social Signals of Emotions. *Nat Rev Neurosci* (2008) 10:37. doi: 10.1038/nrn2554
4. Dunbar RIM. The Social Brain Hypothesis. Evolutionary Anthropology: Issues. *News Rev* (1998) 6(5):178–90. doi: 10.1002/(SICI)1520-6505(1998)6:5<178::AID-EVAN5>3.0.CO;2-8
5. Dunbar RIM, Shultz S. Understanding Primate Brain Evolution. Philosophical. *Trans R Soc B: Biol Sci* (2007) 362(1480):649–58. doi: 10.1098/rstb.2006.2001
6. Schilbach L, Eickhoff SB, Rotarska-Jagiela A, Fink GR, Vogeley K. Minds At Rest? Social Cognition as the Default Mode of Cognizing and Its Putative Relationship to the "Default System" of the Brain. *Conscious Cognit* (2008) 17 (2):457–67. doi: 10.1016/j.concog.2008.03.013
7. Hull JV, Dokovna LB, Jacokes ZJ, Torgerson CM, Irimia A, Horn JDV. Resting-State Functional Connectivity in Autism Spectrum Disorders: a Review. *Front Psychiatry* (2017) 7:205. doi: 10.3389/fpsyt.2016.00205
8. Von Dem Hagen EA, Stoyanova RS, Baron-Cohen S, Calder AJ. Reduced Functional Connectivity Within and Between 'Social' Resting State Networks in Autism Spectrum Conditions. *Soc Cognit Affect Neurosci* (2013) 8(6):694–701. doi: 10.1093/scan/nss053
9. Murias M, Webb SJ, Greenson J, Dawson G. Resting State Cortical Connectivity Reflected in EEG Coherence in Individuals With Autism. *Biol Psychiatry* (2007) 62(3):270–3. doi: 10.1016/j.biopsych.2006.11.012
10. Mcvoy M, Lytle S, Fulchiero E, Aebi ME, Adeleye O, Sajatovic M. a Systematic Review of Quantitative EEG as a Possible Biomarker in Child Psychiatric Disorders. *Psychiatry Res* (2019) 279:331–44. doi: 10.1016/j.psychres.2019.07.004
11. Leno V, Tomlinson SB, Chang S-AA, Naples AJ, Mcpartland JC. Resting-State Alpha Power Is Selectively Associated With Autistic Traits Reflecting Behavioral Rigidity. *Sci Rep* (2018) 8(1):11982. doi: 10.1038/s41598-018-30445-2
12. Rolison MJ, Naples AJ, Mcpartland JC. Interactive Social Neuroscience to Study Autism Spectrum Disorder. *Yale J Biol Med* (2015) 88(1):17–24.
13. Schilbach L, Timmermans B, Reddy V, Costall A, Bente G, Schlicht T, et al. Toward a Second-Person Neuroscience. *Behav Brain Sci* (2013) 36(4):393–414. doi: 10.1017/S0140525X12000660
14. Liu D, Liu S, Liu X, Zhang C, Li A, Jin C, et al. Interactive Brain Activity: Review and Progress on EEG-Based Hyperscanning in Social Interactions. *Front Psychol* (2018) 9:1862. doi: 10.3389/fpsyg.2018.01862
15. Babiloni F, Cincotti F, Mattia D, Mattiocco M, De Vico Fallani F, Tocci A, et al. "Hypermethods for EEG Hyperscanning," in *Conf Proc IEEE Eng Med Biol Soc*, (2006) p. 3666–9. doi: 10.1109/IEMBS.2006.260754
16. Babiloni F, Cincotti F, Mattia D, Fallani FDV, Tocci A, Bianchi L, et al. "High resolution eeg hyperscanning during a card game.," in *2007 29th Annual International Conference of the IEEE Engineering in Medicine and Biology Society* (2007).
17. Babiloni F, Astolfi L, Cincotti F, Mattia D, Tocci A, Tarantino A, et al. "Cortical activity and connectivity of human brain during the prisoner's dilemma: an EEG Hyperscanning Study," in *Conf Proc IEEE Eng Med Biol Soc*, 2007. (2007). p. 4953–6. doi: 10.1109/IEMBS.2007.4353452
18. Astolfi L, Cincotti F, Mattia D, De Vico Fallani F, Salinari S, Vecchiato G, et al. "Imaging the social brain: multi-subjects EEG recordings during the "Chicken's game"," in *2010 Annual International Conference of the IEEE Engineering in Medicine and Biology*, Buenos Aires. (2010). p. 1734–7.
19. De Vico Fallani F, Nicosia V, Sinatra R, Astolfi L, Cincotti F, Mattia D, et al. Defecting or Not Defecting: How to "Read" Human Behavior During

Cooperative Games by EEG Measurements. *PloS One* (2010) 5(12):E14187. doi: 10.1371/journal.pone.0014187
20. Balconi M, Vanutelli ME. Functional EEG Connectivity During Competition. *BMC Neurosci* (2018) 19(1):63. doi: 10.1186/s12868-018-0464-6
21. Spape MM, Kivikangas JM, Jarvela S, Kosunen I, Jacucci G, Ravaja N. Keep Your Opponents Close: Social Context Affects EEG and Femg Linkage in a Turn-Based Computer Game. *PloS One* (2013) 8(11):E78795. doi: 10.1371/journal.pone.0078795
22. Tognoli E, Lagarde J, Deguzman GC, Kelso JA. the Phi Complex as a Neuromarker of Human Social Coordination. *Proc Natl Acad Sci U S A* (2007) 104(19):8190–5. doi: 10.1073/pnas.0611453104
23. Naeem M, Prasad G, Watson DR, Kelso JA. Functional Dissociation of Brain Rhythms in Social Coordination. *Clin Neurophysiol* (2012) 123(9):1789–97. doi: 10.1016/j.clinph.2012.02.065
24. Konvalinka I, Bauer M, Stahlhut C, Hansen LK, Roepstorff A, Frith CD. Frontal Alpha Oscillations Distinguish Leaders From Followers: Multivariate Decoding of Mutually Interacting Brains. *Neuroimage* (2014) 94:79–88. doi: 10.1016/j.neuroimage.2014.03.003
25. Dumas G, Nadel J, Soussignan R, Martinerie J, Garnero L. Inter-Brain Synchronization During Social Interaction. *PloS One* (2010) 5(8):E12166. doi: 10.1371/journal.pone.0012166
26. Menoret M, Varnet L, Fargier R, Cheylus A, Curie A, Des Portes V, et al. Neural Correlates of Non-Verbal Social Interactions: a Dual-EEG Study. *Neuropsychologia* (2014) 55:85–97. doi: 10.1016/j.neuropsychologia.2013.10.001
27. Dikker S, Michalareas G, Oostrik M, Serafimaki A, Kahraman HM, Struiksma ME, et al. Crowdsourcing Neuroscience: Inter-Brain Coupling During Face-To-Face Interactions Outside the Laboratory. *Biorxiv* (2019), 822320. doi: 10.1101/822320
28. Rolison MJ, Naples AJ, Rutherford HJV, Mcpartland JC. Modulation of Reward in a Live Social Context as Revealed Through Interactive Social Neuroscience. *Soc Neurosci* (2018) 13(4):416–28. doi: 10.1080/17470919.2017.1339635
29. Wang Q, Han Z, Hu X, Feng S, Wang H, Liu T, et al. Autism Symptoms Modulate Interpersonal Neural Synchronization in Children With Autism Spectrum Disorder in Cooperative Interactions. *Brain Topogr* (2020) 33(1) doi: 10.1007/s10548-019-00731-x
30. Verbeke WJ, Pozharliev R, Van Strien JW, Belschak F, Bagozzi RP. "I Am Resting But Rest Less Well With You." the Moderating Effect of Anxious Attachment Style on Alpha Power During EEG Resting State in a Social Context. *Front Hum Neurosci* (2014) 8:486. doi: 10.3389/fnhum.2014.00486
31. Constantino JN, Gruber CP. *the Social Responsiveness Scale.* Los Angeles: Western Psychological Services (2012).
32. Hurley RS, Losh M, Parlier M, Reznick JS, Piven J. the Broad Autism Phenotype Questionnaire. *J Autism Dev Disord* (2007) 37(9):1679–90. doi: 10.1007/s10803-006-0299-3
33. Advanced Brain Monitoring. *B-Alert Control GUI.* Carlsbad, California: Advanced Brain Monitoring (2013).
34. Schneider W, Eschman A, Zuccolotto A. *E-Prime: User's Guide.* Pittsburgh, PA: Psychology Software Incorporated (2002).
35. Delorme A, Makeig S. EEGLAB: an Open Source Toolbox for Analysis of Single-Trial EEG Dynamics Including Independent Component Analysis. *J Neurosci Methods* (2004) 134(1):9–21. doi: 10.1016/j.jneumeth.2003.10.009
36. Bigdely-Shamlo N, Mullen T, Kothe C, Su KM, Robbins KA. the PREP Pipeline: Standardized Preprocessing for Large-Scale EEG Analysis. *Front Neuroinf* (2015) 9:16. doi: 10.3389/fninf.2015.00016
37. Oostenveld R, Fries P, Maris E, Schoffelen JM. Fieldtrip: Open Source Software for Advanced Analysis of MEG, EEG, and Invasive Electrophysiological Data. *Comput Intell Neurosci* (2011) 2011:156869. doi: 10.1155/2011/156869
38. Wang J, Barstein J, Ethridge LE, Mosconi MW, Takarae Y, Sweeney JA. Resting State EEG Abnormalities in Autism Spectrum Disorders. *J Neurodev Disord* (2013) 5(1):24. doi: 10.1186/1866-1955-5-24
39. Cohen MX, David N, Vogeley K, Elger CE. Gamma-Band Activity in the Human Superior Temporal Sulcus During Mentalizing From Nonverbal Social Cues. *Psychophysiology* (2009) 46(1):43–51. doi: 10.1111/j.1469-8986.2008.00724.x
40. Symons AE, El-Deredy W, Schwartze M, Kotz SA. the Functional Role of Neural Oscillations in Non-Verbal Emotional Communication. *Front Hum Neurosci* (2016) 10:239. doi: 10.3389/fnhum.2016.00239
41. Kang JH, Ahn HM, Jeong JW, Hwang I, Kim HT, Kim SH, et al. the Modulation of Parietal Gamma Oscillations in the Human Electroencephalogram With Cognitive Reappraisal. *Neuroreport* (2012) 23 (17):995–9. doi: 10.1097/WNR.0b013e32835a6475
42. Kinreich S, Djalovski A, Kraus L, Louzoun Y, Feldman R. Brain-To-Brain Synchrony During Naturalistic Social Interactions. *Sci Rep* (2017) 7(1):17060. doi: 10.1038/s41598-017-17339-5
43. Mcpartland JC. Considerations in Biomarker Development for Neurodevelopmental Disorders. *Curr Opin Neurol* (2016) 29(2):118–22. doi: 10.1097/WCO.0000000000000300

7

Empathic Accuracy in Clinical Populations

Yonat Rum and Anat Perry*

Psychology Department, The Hebrew University of Jerusalem, Jerusalem, Israel

***Correspondence:**
Anat Perry
anat.perry@mail.huji.ac.il

Empathy, broadly defined as the ability to understand the other and to share others' emotions, motivates prosocial behavior and underlies successful interpersonal relations. Dysfunctions in this ability may cause fundamental difficulties in social communication. Empathy has been measured in various ways, from self-report questionnaires to laboratory objective performance tests. Empathic accuracy (EA), i.e., the ability to accurately empathize, is measured using more complex and ecological paradigms, such as asking participants to infer filmed interactions, or having people narrate personal emotional stories then assessing the correspondence between the perceiver and the target of empathy as the criteria for empathic ability. This measure is particularly useful in the study of clinical populations, where deconstructing the multifaceted concept of empathy may contribute to a more complete understanding of specific clinical profiles. This paper presents a scoping review of the literature on EA in clinical populations, and on EA and clinical traits and states in nonclinical or high-risk populations. Following an exhaustive literature search, 34 studies were found eligible to be included in this review. The largest category was studies focused on EA in people with schizophrenia (31%; 11 papers), followed by studies focused on EA in autism spectrum disorders (ASD) and autistic traits in a nonclinical population (22%; 8 papers). Studies were also found on EA and depression tendencies, psychopathy, social anxiety, behavior disorders, and personality disorders, and a few other clinical conditions. The included studies varied on research aims, designs, sample sizes, and male:female ratios. The overall synthesized results suggest that EA is reduced in schizophrenia and ASD. In other clinical populations, the number of studies was very limited. We urge researchers to further examine EA in these less-studied populations. The review reveals a general underrepresentation of female participants in studies on EA in clinical populations. We suggest that future research address understudied clinical populations, such as those diagnosed with psychopathy. Subject, target, and situational variables should also be considered, with special attention to gender differences (and similarities), the association between EA abilities and adaptive functioning, and the study of individuals with clinical conditions as targets, not just observers, in EA tasks.

Keywords: empathic accuracy, autism, schizophrenia, psychopathy, depression, anxiety, behavior disorders, personality disorders

INTRODUCTION

Every well-adjusted social interaction—for example, between parents and children, between peers or between partners—requires recognition, understanding and sometimes sharing each other's thoughts, feelings, and emotions. Applying these complex skills, while maintaining a self/other distinction, is termed *empathy* (1–3). An evolutionary perspective suggests that the basic need to care for offspring explains why human beings developed empathy (4). Empathy motivates prosocial behavior and interpersonal relations (2). On the other hand, dysfunction or lack of empathic abilities may cause not only misunderstandings and unpleasantness but also fundamental difficulties living in society. The multifaceted concept of empathy can be divided into *cognitive empathy* (or *mentalizing*)—the recognition and understanding of others' mental states—and *emotional empathy* (or *experience sharing*)—in which the affective experience is similar to that of the other, or there is an emotional response to the mental state of the other [(5–7); for a review see: (2, 8)].

As a sophisticated yet fundamental ability that plays a central role in human relationships, empathy has been extensively researched for decades, and it has been examined specifically in clinical populations in which social dysfunctions are key. For example, autism spectrum disorder (ASD), psychopathy and schizophrenia are clinical conditions that according to several theories are associated with pronounced empathic dysfunction (9–15). In both ASD and psychopathy, a social deficit is not only a characteristic, it is a diagnostic criterion (16, 17). While some have suggested that both cognitive and emotional domains of empathy are impaired in schizophrenia (18), others claim that schizophrenia and psychopathy are characterized by deficits in emotional empathy but not cognitive empathy (11, 19, 20). Aberrant empathic functioning, specifically impairments in cognitive empathy, was also found in borderline personality disorder [BPD; (21)] and bipolar disorder (22), two conditions associated with interpersonal deficits. However, other findings support a hypothesis according to which individuals with BPD are uncommonly sensitive or "over empathic" to the internal experience of others (23–25). Findings from clinical populations are of great value for understanding the multifaceted concept of empathy on the one hand, and specific clinical profiles on the other hand, but these are not always consistent. One possible explanation for the inconsistencies may be the varied operationalizations of empathy in research.

Researchers in the fields of developmental, social, cognitive, educational, and clinical psychology, as well as cognitive neuroscience, use different methods and instruments to measure empathy in the general population, and in clinical or high-risk populations. In early childhood, empathy is often measured through observations, as a behavioral response to a simulation of others' distress (26–28) or by caregivers' reports [e.g., (29)]. In older children, empathy is measured using different tasks, including the evoked emotional response in the child (30, 31). In schoolchildren, adolescents, and adults, empathy can be measured using either self-report questionnaires [e.g., IRI, (32); EQ, (33); CEAQ, (34)] or objective performance tests, which compare participants' output to predefined "correct" responses. These kinds of tasks include emotion recognition tasks in still pictures, and reading a vignette describing a mental state or a social situation. Theory of Mind (ToM) and traditional false beliefs and "Faux-Pas" tasks are also related to some extent to the cognitive component of empathy (35–40). Generally, some tasks or questionnaires primarily measure the cognitive empathic component, while others capture more of the emotional output. Objective performance tests offer some integration between the individual's perspective and the observed behavioral output, but such laboratory tasks usually fail to capture the dynamic nature and complexities involved in social communication, including rapid and nuanced changes in facial expression, intonation and other pragmatic characteristics of the speech, posture and gestures of the target social partner (41). Other limitations in some of the methods mentioned above include the fact that reading and comprehension abilities and executive functions (e.g., in questionnaires, vignettes) may present a potential confound, and the fact that some measures refer to a very narrow aspect of empathy (e.g., emotion recognition from facial expressions). In studying empathy in clinical populations, these limitations need to be considered.

Empathic accuracy (EA) tasks have tried to offer a more ecological setting to measure empathic abilities. EA is the ability to accurately judge the cognitive and affective mental states of others (42, 43). Accordingly, in the original lab procedure developed by Ickes and his colleagues, a dyad is videotaped while interacting. Then each member of the dyad views the videotape separately and reports his or her own thoughts and feelings during the interaction, as well as inferences regarding the partner's thoughts and feelings during the interaction. EA is measured by the similarity between the explicit reported mental states of the target and those reported by the perceiver (42, 43). In the current review we refer to this prototype paradigm (and later adaptations and variations of it) as a dyadic interaction paradigm.

A more recent EA paradigm developed by Zaki and colleagues is based on the perceiver's interpretation of a target's videotaped autobiographical emotional story as the stimulus (instead of a dyadic interaction), and the correspondence between the perceiver's and the target's ratings of *valence* (i.e., how positive or negative the target felt while telling the story) instead of the exact mental content. In this paradigm, both the target and the perceiver use a rating dial to continuously rate the valence of the videotaped story, and the perceiver's EA score results from the correlation between the two continuous ratings (41, 44, 45). This method comes from an earlier attempt by Levenson and Ruef (46) to create a measure of behavioral empathy that relies on rating dials to provide continuous responses to a given videotaped stimulus. Here, we refer to this method as an emotional story inferring paradigm.

Another EA paradigm, which has been utilized mostly in research on romantic partners, uses experience-sampling diaries [e.g., (47, 48)]. In this approach, participants provide daily reports of their own mental states and their inferences regarding their partner's perceived mental states over a period of time. Then reports of each participant on his/her partner's (the target's) thoughts and feelings are compared to the target's own reports to arrive at an EA score. In this review, this is referred to as a daily diary paradigm.

All three prototypes of EA paradigms yielded various studies, and some of them applied specific variations and adaptations to the original developed tests. Common to all is the reliance on the concordance between the perceiver's (the subject of the EA measure) view of the target and the target's (the object of the EA measure) own report on their internal states to generate the EA measure. As such, EA measures provide more ecologically valid data on interpersonal perception in comparison to other experimental techniques. Moreover, an fMRI study by Zaki and colleagues suggests that both cognitive and emotional mechanisms contribute to the ability of the perceiver to accurately match her state with the emotions or thoughts experienced by a social target (49). Thus, measuring EA seems to capture a more nuanced measure of empathy and reflect its complexity.

The main objective of this review is to provide an overview of the existing literature on EA in clinical populations or high-risk subclinical populations, and on clinical states and traits measured in nonclinical samples. To this end, we aim to (1) conduct a systematic search of the published peer-reviewed papers on EA in clinical populations; (2) map the characteristics and range of findings and conclusions in the identified papers; (3) examine reported challenges and limitations of measuring EA in clinical populations; and (4) propose recommendations for future research directions. Within the scope of this review are studies measuring EA conducted on clinical populations, as well as studies focusing on clinical traits in a high-risk or nonclinical population. We considered studies measuring valence (negative-positive) or content (thoughts, feelings), and measuring EA as a primary or secondary aim of the study (for example, studies measuring EA in a clinical sample as part of a battery of tests assessing social cognition). We also considered a variety of paradigms used to assess EA, including the dyadic interaction paradigm, the emotional story inferring paradigm and the daily diary paradigm. Common to all studies was the aim to assess the perceivers' ability to accurately understand and report on the targets' affective or mental state when the criteria are the target's own representations of his or her mental state.

METHODS

The methodology was based on the framework outlined by Arksey and O'Malley's (50) review and recommendations made by Levac et al. (51). It consisted of five key phases: (1) identifying the research question; (2) identifying potentially relevant studies; (3) selection of studies; (4) charting the data; and (5) organizing, summarizing, and reporting the findings. The Preferred Reporting Items for Systematic Reviews and Meta-Analyses (52) were used in the current review as a guide, where applicable.

Research Question

This review was guided by the following two questions: (1) What are the characteristics of studies measuring EA in clinical populations? and (2) What are the main findings and conclusions in the literature regarding EA in clinical populations? For the purposes of this review, all papers that used the term "empathic accuracy" and referred to a concordance or correlation between two partners (i.e., a target and a perceiver) were included.

Data Sources and Search Strategy

The initial search was implemented in July 2019, using PsycNET and PubMed. The search query included the term "empathic accuracy" AND (permutations of) the terms: "autism"; "psychopathy"; "schizophrenia"; "depression"; "dyslexia"; "attention deficit"; "anxiety"; "OCD"; "behavior disorders"; "personality disorders"; "mood disorders"; "affective disorders"; "neurodegenerative disease"; "mental disability"; "learning disability"; "neurodevelopmental disorder"; "clinical population"; "mental disorders." The reference lists of all potentially relevant papers were screened in a two-phase process: (a) title and abstract screening; and (b) full-text screening. Empathy measures were examined in the selected studies with respect to the extent to which they tapped into EA. A "snowball" technique was also utilized in which citations within papers were searched to look for potentially relevant studies. A follow-up search was conducted on September 24, 2019, to identify any additional relevant papers published after the initial search, resulting in the final list of papers for the review (see **Table 1**).

Eligibility Criteria

Peer-reviewed papers written in English were eligible for inclusion if they explicitly aimed to measure *"empathic accuracy"* (EA) in a clinical population. Studies published in any year were considered. Papers that referred to *empathy* in clinical populations without measuring EA and review papers were excluded from the analysis, but their reference list was reviewed to identify additional relevant papers. Papers aiming to measure the relation between EA and *clinical traits* in nonclinical populations were also included in the current review. Exclusion criteria included: papers in languages other than English; nonpeer-reviewed papers (such as theses or dissertations); and papers aiming to measure EA in the general/nonclinical/typically developing population.

Data Characterization and Analysis

All papers deemed relevant after the title and abstract screening were procured for subsequent review of the full text. Studies were excluded at this phase if they were found not to meet the eligibility criteria. The following characteristics of each full-text article were then extracted: objectives; participants (clinical population, N, age, gender); definition of EA; EA paradigm used; main findings and main conclusions regarding EA. All references, abstracts and data characteristics were imported into Microsoft Excel. Descriptive statistics were calculated to

TABLE 1 | Summary of studies' characteristics.

Study	Objective/Research Question	Design and Participants	EA paradigm	Main conclusions regarding EA
Schizophrenia Spectrum and Psychotic Disorders				
van Donkersgoed et al. (53)	To assess the moderating role of the target's gender and expressivity and the valence of the story on EA performance; the correlation between EA and other commonly used empathy measures.	Schizophrenia group (n=92, 67 males) Nonclinical control group (n=42, 32 males) matched for age, gender, and education	Emotional story	Schizophrenia group performed worse than controls in EA. Individuals with schizophrenia benefit less from the emotional expressivity of targets. No correlations were found between EA and questionnaire scores, suggesting a distinction between self-report empathy and actual empathy performance.
de Jong et al. (54)	To investigate which measures of social cognition and metacognition are related to violent history in patients with psychotic disorder; which domains of metacognition were indicative of a violent history in psychosis.	Violent psychotic disorder in care at a forensic clinic for a violent crime (n=23) Clinical group 2: nonviolent psychotic disorder (n=27, all males) Nonclinical control group (n=33, all males)	Emotional story	EA differentiated between the violent and nonviolent psychotic patients, while scores on social cognition (such as ToM) and a metacognition scale did not. EA may offer an important contribution to statistical models of violence risk in psychotic disorder.
Harenski et al. (55)	To explore the hypothesis that lower EA and smaller brain volumes in regions implicated in social cognition are related to past suicide attempts in offenders with a psychotic disorder.	Criminals with a psychotic disorder and a history of suicide attempts (n=18, all males) Criminals with a psychotic disorder and no past suicide attempts (n=25, all males) Nonclinical group: criminals with no history of a psychotic disorder (n=59, all males) Nonclinical control group (n=26; all males)	Emotional story	Criminal offenders with psychotic disorders and suicide attempts had lower EA and smaller temporal pole volumes compared to the other groups. EA and temporal pole volumes were significantly associated with past suicide attempts independent of other risk factors.
Horan et al. (56)	To evaluate correlations of the Questionnaire of Cognitive and Affective Empathy (QCAE) in schizophrenia with EA (and other empathy measures).	Schizophrenia group (n=145, 108 males) Nonclinical control group (n=45, 32 males)	Emotional story	No significant association was found between the QCAE and EA performance in either group, indicating that self-reported beliefs about empathic characteristics are not necessarily correlated with an actual understanding of others' affective states.
Davis et al. (57)	To assess whether oxytocin (OT) enhances the effectiveness of a social cognitive training. The final four sessions of training focused on improving EA.	Individuals with schizophrenia (n=27, all males) were randomly assigned to an OT condition (n=13) or to a placebo condition (n=14). (Double-blind drug administration with before and after treatment comparison)	Emotional story	Administration of OT before a psychosocial intervention targeting social cognition improved EA and not other measures of social cognition, in individuals with schizophrenia.
Ripoll et al. (58)	To test schizotypal personality disorder (SPD) participants and healthy controls on the EA paradigm and the Reading of the Mind in the Eyes Test (RMET).	SPD group (n=19, 13 males, 6 females) Nonclinical control group (n=19, 6 males, 13 females)	Emotional story	SPD individuals demonstrated lower EA than controls during negative-valence videos, associated with lower social support. RMET did not differ between groups, suggesting that EA paradigms may be more effective at capturing interpersonal dysfunction than static image tasks. Schizotypal severity, trait empathy and cognitive dysfunction did not account for the empathic dysfunction.
Olbert et al. (59)	To examine the relationship between EA (and three other social cognitive paradigms adapted from social neuroscience) and functionally meaningful outcomes in schizophrenia (incremental, external validity).	Within-subject design on participants with schizophrenia (n=173, 124 males)	Emotional story	The EA paradigm was found to have the broadest external validity, and it is the most recommended measure from the four paradigms that were evaluated. EA had a significant association with functional outcome measures: Higher EA was associated with greater nonsocial cognitive ability, functional capacity, social skills and community functioning.
Kern et al. (60)	To evaluate psychometric properties of EA (and three other social cognitive paradigms adapted from social neuroscience) to inform	Schizophrenia group (n=173, 124 males) Nonclinical control group (n=88,	Emotional story	The EA task had the best psychometric properties of the four paradigms checked: The largest between-group difference was seen

(Continued)

TABLE 1 | Continued

Study	Objective/Research Question	Design and Participants	EA paradigm	Main conclusions regarding EA
	possible use in clinical trials that assess treatment-related changes in social cognition in schizophrenia.	57 males) within subject (test-retest) in the schizophrenia group		on EA; of all measures, only a long version of the EA task met acceptable test-retest reliability standards; EA task was the strongest measure in regard to practice effects.
Harvey et al. (61)	To examine the neural correlates of EA and targets' expressivity in schizophrenia.	Schizophrenia group (n=15, 13 males) Nonclinical control group (n=15, 13 males)	Emotional story	Schizophrenia patients demonstrated impaired EA, failed to benefit from targets' emotional expressivity (wherein controls did benefit from targets' expressivity), and demonstrated reduced neural sensitivity to targets' affective cues.
Lee et al. (62)	To determine the relative extent of impairment in social and nonsocial cognitive domains in schizophrenia and bipolar disorder patients compared with healthy controls.	Schizophrenia group (n=38, 21 males) Bipolar disorder group (68, 38 males) Nonclinical control group (n=36, 20 males)	Emotional story	Schizophrenia patients performed significantly worse on EA than bipolar patients and controls, who did not differ from each other. *see findings regarding bipolar patients under Bipolar Disorder*
Lee et al. (63)	To examine whether schizophrenia patients showed lower EA compared with controls; whether emotional expressivity of a target moderated group differences; whether EA is associated with self-reported trait empathy or clinical characteristics in the schizophrenia sample.	Schizophrenia group (n=30, 25 males) Nonclinical control group (n=22, 17 males)	Emotional story	Schizophrenia patients were impaired in EA relative to controls. Both groups showed better accuracy for positive- vs. negative-valence videos. Both groups showed greater EA for highly expressive targets, but this effect was significantly smaller in schizophrenia patients. EA was not related to the participants' self-reports or clinical symptoms.
ASD and Autistic Traits				
Adler et al. (64)	To compare levels of empathic embarrassment accuracy among individuals with ASD with those of matched controls.	ASD group (n=17, 16 males, high functioning/Asperger's syndrome) Nonclinical control group matched for age and IQ (n=24, 21 males)	A paradigm designed to measure empathic *embarrassment* accuracy[1]	The ASD group displayed less empathic embarrassment accuracy compared with the control group. Higher AQ scores predicted low EA in the ASD group (a marginal correlation).
aan het Rot and Hogenelst (65)	To investigate the influence of autistic traits and trait affective empathy on EA.	Nonclinical sample (n=100, 50 male and 50 female)	Emotional story	Perceivers with more autistic traits demonstrated worse EA, particularly when their trait affective empathy was relatively low. Higher perceiver EA was predicted by a higher perceiver affective empathy and the target being female (rather than male), but there was no significant interaction between these two predictors.
Demurie et al. (66)	To investigate and compare the mind-reading abilities of adolescents with ASD, adolescents with ADHD and typically developed (TD) adolescents.	ASD group (n=13, 12 males) ADHD group (n=13, 12 males) Nonclinical control group (n=18, 14 males) adolescents	Dyadic interaction In each dyad one of two targets was TD, and the other was ASD or ADHD	Adolescents with ASD demonstrated impairment on both EA and a static task. *see findings regarding ADHD under ADHD*
Bartz et al. (67)	To test whether normal variance in social proficiency moderates the effects of oxytocin (OT) on social-cognitive performance.	Nonclinical sample (n=27, all males). Participants were randomly assigned to either an OT condition or a placebo condition, followed by an EA task. Participants returned 3 to 5 weeks later, received the alternate compound, and completed the EA task again.	Emotional story	Oxytocin selectively improved EA for people with higher (but not lower) autistic traits.
Ponnet et al. (68)	To investigate EA of participants with ASD asked to infer the mental states of targets in a highly structured conversation vs. a less structured/more naturalistic conversation.	ASD group (n=22, all males) Nonclinical control group (n=22, all males) matched for chronological age and IQ	Dyadic interaction One interaction was more structured than the other.	Differences between ASD and control groups in EA were more pronounced when participants had to infer the thoughts and feelings of other persons in a less structured conversation.

(Continued)

TABLE 1 | Continued

Study	Objective/Research Question	Design and Participants	EA paradigm	Main conclusions regarding EA
Ponnet et al. (69)	To measure the social functioning of adults with pervasive developmental disorder (PDD) during a conversation with a TD stranger and to explore whether EA of both groups was affected by behavioral characteristics and by the content of the interaction.	Part 1: Eleven dyads, each composed of a partner with ASD (n=11, 9 males; PDD) and a TD partner (n=11, 9 males), interacted in a lab task, then performed the EA task on each other within each dyad. PDD participants with the highest scores in the EA task of Roeyers et al. (70) were invited to participate in this study. TD participants were matched based on sex, age, education and main interests. Part 2: TD participants (n=13, 8 males), with the filmed interactions from part 1 as the stimuli for EA measure.	Dyadic interaction ASD participants take part in the interaction	No significant difference was found between controls and PDD participants in EA. No significant associations were found between EA and IQ scores, age or the time needed to complete the task. EA scores of the 11 participants with PDD correlated significantly with their EA scores on the previous study (Roeyers et al., (70); on a video of structured interaction). No significant difference was found among participants in part 2 in EA towards TD or PDD individuals as targets. Being in the interaction yields higher EA scores than just perceiving the interaction: participants in part 1 (PDD and TD) scored higher in EA than participants in part 2 (TD), who inferred EA from an interaction in which they did not previously take part.
Ponnet et al. (71)	To compare individuals with Asperger syndrome and controls' performance in two static mind-reading tasks and the EA task.	ASD group (n=19, 14 males; Asperger's syndrome) Nonclinical control group (n=19, 14 males)	Dyadic interaction	The EA task indicated significant between-group differences, whereas no such differences were found on the static mind-reading tasks. EA in both groups depended on the focus of the target's thoughts and feelings. Participants with ASD needed more time than the controls to complete the EA task.
Roeyers et al. (70)	To compare individuals with PDD with controls on twopreviously used static empathy tests and onan EA task.	ASD group (n=24, 22 males; PDD/high-functioning) Nonclinical control group (n=24, 22 males) matched for sex, education, profession or interests	Dyadic interaction	Participants with PDD demonstrated worse EA in a video presenting a less structured conversation between two stranger targets, whereas no between-group differences were found in a video presenting a more structured conversation. Participants with PDD did not use more time than controls to complete the EA task. EA measure was proven to be a valid alternative to the previously used static tests.
Depression Measured in a Nonclinical or High-Risk Population				
aan het Rot et al. (72)	To examine the impact of light therapy on mood and on cognitive empathy in premenstrual women with complaints indicating a premenstrual disorder.	A nonclinical sample (n=48, all females) divided into two treatment groups (light therapy/sham session; participant-blind between-groups design)	Emotional story	There were no significant effects of light therapy on EA. Participants obtained higher EA scores when watching positive clips compared to negative clips.
Hogenelst et al. (73)	To investigate the effect of acute tryptophan depletion (ATD), which reduces brain serotonin, on social functioning, EA, and oxytocin levels.	High risk for MDD group (n=20, 10 males) Nonclinical matched control group A randomized, double-blind, crossover design (2 treatment conditions) with between-group comparison	Emotional story	EA remains unaffected by acute reductions in brain serotonin, even though brain oxytocin levels may be reduced.
Gadassi et al. (74)	To examine associations between EA and depression as a possible mechanism underlying gender differences in the association between interpersonal difficulties and depression in an intimate relationship.	Nonclinical sample of romantic couples (51 dyads; measurement of subclinical depression traits in couples)	Dyadic interaction and Diary	Depressive symptoms were associated with lower EA among females and may have a stronger impact on interpersonal perception in intimate relationships among females than among males. When a female is depressed, both her own and her partner's EA levels are lower. When males are depressed, neither their own nor their partner's levels of EA are lower. Depressive symptoms predicted lower EA regarding negative moods and feelings, but not regarding positive ones.

(Continued)

TABLE 1 | Continued

Study	Objective/Research Question	Design and Participants	EA paradigm	Main conclusions regarding EA
Papp et al. (75)	To examine affectivity in marital interaction: to test partners' EA and assumed similarity in marital conflict interactions and whether they are moderated by spouses' levels of depressive symptoms; to examine whether spouses' ratings of their partner's specific emotions depend on how they felt themselves in the same conflict interaction.	Nonclinical sample of romantic couples (267 dyads; measurement of subclinical depression traits in couples)	Dyadic interaction The interaction was focused on a topic of conflict	Females with higher levels of depressive symptoms demonstrated higher EA (and lower assumed similarity) compared to females with lower levels of symptoms. In rating negative emotions, spousal depressive symptoms weakened females' abilities to rate their partners' emotions; in rating positivity, higher females' depressive symptoms strengthened their ratings of their partner's emotions. Females' depressive symptoms were associated with lower EA ratings *by their partners* (for anger, but not for sadness); males' depressive symptoms were associated with lower EA in rating their partner's anger. Males' EA in rating their partner's sadness was higher when their partner had a higher level of depressive symptoms. Partners of spouses with elevated depressive symptoms demonstrated particular difficulty in assessing partner anger in marital conflict.
Thomas et al. (76)	To examine the correlates of online EA in a sample of married couples in the context of problem-solving discussions, considering depression, relationship length and educational attainment.	Nonclinical sample of romantic couples (74 dyads; measurement of subclinical depression traits in married couples)	Dyadic interaction The interaction was focused on a topic of conflict	EA was not significantly correlated with depression in either males or females.
SAD and Trait/State Social Anxiety				
Morrison et al. (77)	To compare cognitive empathy and affective empathy in individuals with SAD to that of matched controls; to assess empathy with an adapted version of the EA task, with an additional behavioral index of *affective empathy*—by examining the degree of congruency between the target's self-rating of emotion and the participant's self-rating of his/her own emotions.	SAD group (n=32, 18 males) Nonclinical matched control group (n=32, 18 males)	Emotional story	No between-group differences were found in EA, indicating intact cognitive empathy in SAD. For positively valenced (but not for negatively valenced) clips, individuals with SAD exhibited significantly lower empathic congruence (affective empathy) than controls, indicating that affective empathy may be impaired in SAD.
Auyeung and Alden (78)	To examine whether individual differences in social anxiety moderate EA.	A nonclinical sample (n=121, 95 females) measured to assess social interaction anxiety in to conditions: experimental condition (a manipulation designed to increase state anxiety) and a control condition	Emotional story Specifically, targets narrated experiences when they felt: (1) socially excluded (2) socially included	Social anxiety was associated with greater EA for others' social pain, but only when participants experienced social threat: Individuals with lower levels of social anxiety were less accurate in judging others' negative emotions following a social threat.
Simpson et al. (79)	To test how people with more anxious-ambivalent attachment orientations react when their relationships are threatened by alternative dating partners.	Nonclinical sample of romantic couples (82 dyads; measurement of subclinical anxiety traits)	Dyadic interaction	Highly anxious-ambivalent individuals demonstrated higher EA (than those rated lower on anxiety) in a relationship-threatening situation (watching their partners rating opposite-sex optional dating partners), greater distress, and less confidence in their partners and relationships. The more anxious-ambivalent females reported a slight decrease in the perceived closeness of their relationships. More anxious-ambivalent males' relationships were more likely to have ended by follow-up.
Borderline Personality Disorder (BPD)				
Miano et al. (80)	To investigate whether BPD patients show motivated inaccuracy by measuring their EA during a relationship-threatening	Dyadic analysis of BPD couples (30 couples; the female partner diagnosed with BPD) vs. a	Dyadic interaction Specifically focused on: (1)	Reduced EA when facing a relationship-threatening situation was found in couples in the nonclinical control group, while females with BPD did not show this pattern of

(Continued)

TABLE 1 | Continued

Study	Objective/Research Question	Design and Participants	EA paradigm	Main conclusions regarding EA
	conversation with their own romantic partner.	nonclinical control group of couples (34 couples)	a personally threatening topic (2) a relationship-threatening topic	motivated inaccuracy and instead increased their EA, a finding that supports the concept of borderline empathy. Male partners of BPD females did not have a different EA pattern than control males. Neutral and personally threatening contexts did not significantly affect EA between BPD and control females.
Flury et al. (81)	To explore the phenomenon of borderline empathy (elevated empathy among individuals with BPD) with the use of EA.	A nonclinical sample (n=76, 46 females), composed of high vs. low risk for BPD, assigned to dyads each composed of a high-risk for BPD partner and low-risk for BPD partner.	Dyadic interaction In each dyad one "borderline" (high-risk) and one "nonborderline" (low-risk)	The empathic advantage displayed by high BPD individuals may not reflect greater ability, but result from the comparison to the ratings of their partner, who had difficulty inferring emotions of the BPD partners.
Conduct Disorder and Callous-Unemotional Traits				
Martin-Key et al. (82)	To assess EA, emotion recognition and affective empathy in male adolescents with Conduct Disorder (CD) and higher versus lower levels of callous-unemotional (CU) traits.	Clinical group: CD (n=37, all males) Nonclinical control group (n=40, all males) adolescents	Emotional story	Adolescents with CD did not differ in EA from TD adolescents but displayed significant impairments in emotion recognition and affective empathy (measured by asking participants to report whether they experienced the same emotion as the target). No difference in EA was found between high and low CU traits subgroups.
De Ridder et al. (83)	To assess everyday EA in institutionalized adolescents with high and low CU traits, and how EA is related to adolescents' own behavior, and own affective and relational experience.	A sample of institutionalized adolescents (n=71, 45 males) divided into high CU traits vs. low CU traits *adolescents	A procedure similar to the diary paradigm[2]	High CU adolescents unexpectedly did not differ from low CU adolescents in EA (specifically inferring anger and distress in staff members) and notably overestimated the general intensity of both anger and distress, and in particular, inferred more anger when they (the adolescent themselves) were misbehaving.
Psychopathy				
Brook and Kosson (84)	To examine relationships between psychopathy and cognitive empathy. To design an improved EA task, with multiple targets, and a standardized forced-choice response format.	A sample of incarcerated offenders (n=103, all males)	Emotional story	Inverse association between psychopathy and EA was found, as well as robust group differences between psychopathic and nonpsychopathic inmates, findings that corroborate the deficient empathy hypothesis.
Bipolar Disorder				
Lee et al. (62)	See the same study in the category: Schizophrenia spectrum and Psychotic disorders.			Bipolar groups did not differ from the control group on EA but outperformed the schizophrenia group. Bipolar patients performed significantly better on social relative to nonsocial cognitive domains, whereas schizophrenia patients showed the opposite pattern.
Risk for Hypomania				
Devlin et al. (85)	To utilize a naturalistic, dynamic social stimulus (EA paradigm) in order to investigate the relationship between hypomania risk and empathy.	Nonclinical sample (n=121, 69 females), divided into high vs. low risk for hypomania	Emotional story	Risk for hypomania was associated with elevated EA of increases in positive emotion for targets describing positive events; however, it was also associated with overestimating global positive emotion for targets describing negative events.
ADHD				
Demurie et al. (66)	See the same study in the category: ASD and autistic traits in a subclinical population.			ADHD did not significantly differ in EA from either the control group or ASD group; thus, it was determined to be an intermediate group between the clinical and nonclinical groups. Thoughts and feelings of target persons with

(Continued)

TABLE 1 | Continued

Study	Objective/Research Question	Design and Participants	EA paradigm	Main conclusions regarding EA
				ADHD seemed to be less easy to read than the thoughts and feelings of TD targets.
Neurodegenerative Disease				
Brown et al. (86)	To investigate whether deficits in EA in patients with neurodegenerative disease are associated with greater depression in their caregivers.	Two independent cross-sectional samples (n=172, n=63) of patients with a variety of neurodegenerative diseases and their caregivers (usually spouses) vs. a nonclinical control group of healthy couples.	Dyadic interaction	Lower EA in patients was associated with higher depression in their caregivers. In study 1, this relationship was found using EA (after controlling for patient cognitive and functional symptoms) and was not found when using other more traditional tasks. In study 2, the relationship was found after accounting for caregiver characteristics that have previously been associated with caregiver depression.

[1] *Participants watch films in which protagonists performed embarrassing actions and are asked to rate how embarrassed they feel (empathic embarrassment-EE) and how embarrassed they think the protagonist feels. The participant's ratings are compared with the protagonist's own ratings to produce a measure of empathic embarrassment accuracy.*
[2] *Adolescents reported the intensity of anger and distress they perceived in staff members; staff members reported their own levels of anger and distress after each period of at least 1 hour spent with the adolescent.*

summarize data characteristics when applicable. The main findings and conclusions of all reviewed papers were discussed in light of the known data characteristics, limitations, and strengths of the included studies.

RESULTS

Search and Selection of Papers

The original search conducted in July 2019 yielded 17 potentially relevant citations for EA and *"autism"* (using "ASD" as a search word instead of "autism" yielded no additional papers). For EA and *"schizophrenia,"* 24 potentially relevant citations were found (using "schizophrenic" as a search word instead of schizophrenia yielded no additional papers). For EA and *"psychopathy,"* four potentially relevant citations were found. For EA and *"depression,"* 26 potentially relevant citations were found (using "depressive" as a search word instead of "depression" yielded one additional potentially relevant paper). For EA and *"attention deficit,"* five potentially relevant citations were found (using "ADHD" as a search word instead of "attention deficit" yielded no additional papers). For EA and *"anxiety,"* 22 potentially relevant citations were found. For EA and *"behavior disorders,"* 16 potentially relevant citations were found (using "conduct disorder" or "disruptive behavior disorders" as a search word instead of "behavior disorders" yielded one additional potentially relevant paper). For EA and *"personality disorders,"* five potentially relevant citations were found (using "borderline disorder" as a search word instead of "personality disorders" yielded no additional papers). For EA and *"neurodegenerative,"* one potentially relevant citation was found (using "degenerative" or "Alzheimer's disease" or "Alzheimer" or "dementia" as a search word instead of "neurodegenerative" yielded no additional papers). One potentially relevant paper was found for EA and *"learning disabilities"* (using "learning disability" as a search word instead of "learning disabilities" yielded no additional papers). No potentially relevant papers were found for EA and *"dyslexia"* or "dyslexic", for EA and *"OCD,"* for EA and *"mood disorders,"* or for EA and *"epilepsy."* No potentially relevant papers were found for EA and *"mental disabilities"* or *"mental disability,"* or for EA and *"clinical populations."* For EA and *"mental disorders,"* five potentially relevant citations were found in the search.

Thus, the initial list consisted of 128 references. After the first phase of relevance screening, 70 citations were considered to potentially meet the eligibility criteria based on title and abstract, and the full-text articles were reviewed. In the second phase of reviewing full texts, 34 papers were excluded. Among the excluded papers, two mentioned measuring EA, but no results regarding EA were reported, and two papers were not available. During the full-text screening, the "snowball" search technique resulted in two additional eligible papers. The updated search in September 2019 produced two more potentially relevant citations, one of which was found to be eligible and was included. During the full-text screening phase, two studies were excluded, as the current inclusion criteria referred to EA as a measure comparing the subject's perception to the target's own perceptions: one study (87) that used the term "empathic accuracy" to refer to the "Reading the Mind in the Eyes" test [RMET; (36)], and one (88) that referred to EA as the correlation between a perceiver's rating and a panel of judges' ratings of the emotions of the same target (and not the concordance between the perceiver's and the target's rating). Thus, the final list of papers selected for inclusion in the current review consists of 34 peer-reviewed papers. **Figure 1** presents the search flow diagram.

Characteristics of Included Papers

EA Definition

An explicit definition or description of what the authors mean by *"empathic accuracy"* was reported in all but four of the papers. Most definitions/paradigms centered on *the ability to accurately judge the valence and/or content of emotions or thoughts experienced by another person*, mostly citing Ickes et al. (43), Ickes (42), and Zaki et al. (44). However, there was some

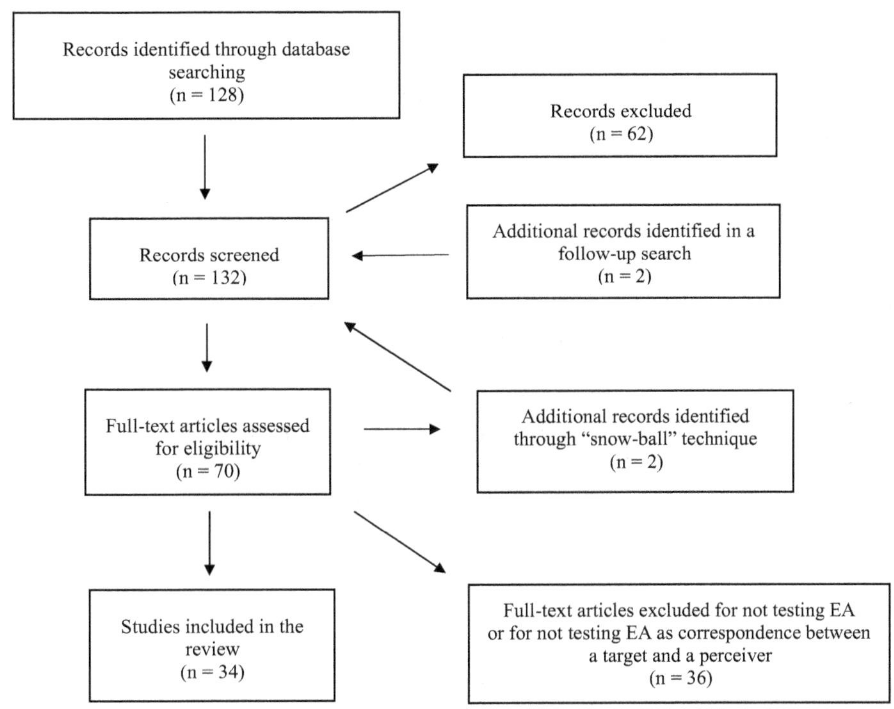

FIGURE 1 | Studies search flow diagram.

divergence in how authors characterized EA. Some studies referred to EA as a measure of cognitive empathy (53, 65, 73, 77, 83, 84). In contrast, some other authors mentioned that because EA is the ability to correctly infer the *emotional* state of a target, it has a relatively affective character (54, 75). Harvey et al. (61) claim that EA is not solely a measure of mental-state attribution (associated with cognitive empathy) or of experience sharing (associated with affective empathy), but that it is *the product of these two processes* [this definition was also used by Martin-Key et al. (82)].

Clinical Populations

Included papers referred to EA in the following categories of clinical populations and traits in high-risk, subclinical or nonclinical populations: schizophrenia spectrum and psychotic disorders (31%; 11 papers); ASD and autistic traits in a nonclinical population (22%; eight papers); depression measured in a nonclinical or high-risk population (14%; five papers); social anxiety disorder (SAD), social anxiety, and trait/state anxiety in a nonclinical population (8%; three papers); BPD (5%; two papers); conduct disorder and callous-unemotional traits (5%; two papers); and one paper in each of the following categories: psychopathy; hypomania; attention deficit and hyperactivity disorder (ADHD); bipolar disorder and neurodegenerative disease. Two papers were assigned to two categories, as they compared two clinical samples in the study [an ASD group was compared to an ADHD group in Demurie et al. (66); a bipolar disorder group was compared to a schizophrenia group in Lee et al. (62)]. In most of the papers, learning about the nature of EA in a clinical population was the primary aim; thus, a between-group design was assigned, comparing the clinical group to a matched control group. In some of the studies, this was a secondary aim, as when EA was part of a battery of tests to assess social cognition (62), or when the primary aim was evaluating interventions (57, 67, 72, 73) or evaluating the psychometric properties of an EA paradigm (59, 60).

Clinical Sample Sizes

Of the final list of eligible papers, 23 (67%) reported studies done directly on participants from a clinical population (i.e., participants have a diagnosis of one of the above-mentioned conditions), while the rest referred to clinical traits in healthy, nonclinical or high-risk populations. Of the 23 studies that included participants with a clinical diagnosis, the largest sample size was n = 173 [(59, 60)]; schizophrenia spectrum and psychotic disorders category), and the smallest sample size was n = 11 [(69)]; ASD category), with 48% (11/23) of the studies based on n < 30. In the studies with nonclinical or high-risk populations, samples were usually larger, with all studies but one ((67); n = 27) based on n > 30, and 6 of them with sample size of n > 100 (see **Table 1**).

Male : Female Ratio

In six studies where EA was measured on clinical samples, there was no representation of females (0 female participants; see **Table 1**). In one study (BPD category), there was no male representation. In the rest of the reviewed studies on clinical populations, the male to female ratio was in favor of male participants and ranged from 1.2:1 to 16:1. Aggregating the number of all participants diagnosed with a disorder from one of the above categories across studies reveals a male-to-female ratio of 2.9:1, with 887 male and 306 female participants. In the studies on nonclinical or high-risk populations, in one study [(67); ASD and autistic traits category] all participants were males; in one study [(72)]; Depression measured in a nonclinical or high-risk population category) all participant were females; in six studies the number of male and female participants was even; and in the remaining two studies more females than males participated. When aggregating numbers of all participants in the 10 nonclinical studies, the male:female ratio was 1.16:1. The male:female ratio also differed among categories of clinical condition. As can be seen in **Figure 2**, while studies on psychopathy, ADHD, conduct disorder and callous-unemotional traits, schizophrenia spectrum and psychotic disorders, and ASD and autistic traits relied more on male participants, studies in the categories of depression (depressive traits in a nonclinical or high-risk population), SAD, social anxiety and trait/state anxiety, BPD and risk for Hypomania relied more on female participants.

EA Paradigm Used

Most of the studies (22 papers) were based on the emotional story inferring paradigm (or similar); about a third (10 papers) were based on the dyadic interaction paradigm; one study relied on the diary procedure; and one study utilized a similar procedure to that of the daily diary, though slightly modified.

Limitations mentioned by researchers were mainly a small sample size, underrepresentation of females in the sample, comorbidity with other conditions, use of medications, and a lack of ethnic diversity among targets.

Publishing Year

Although we did not limit the search years, all included papers were published between 1997 and September 2019, with 82% (28/34) published after 2010.

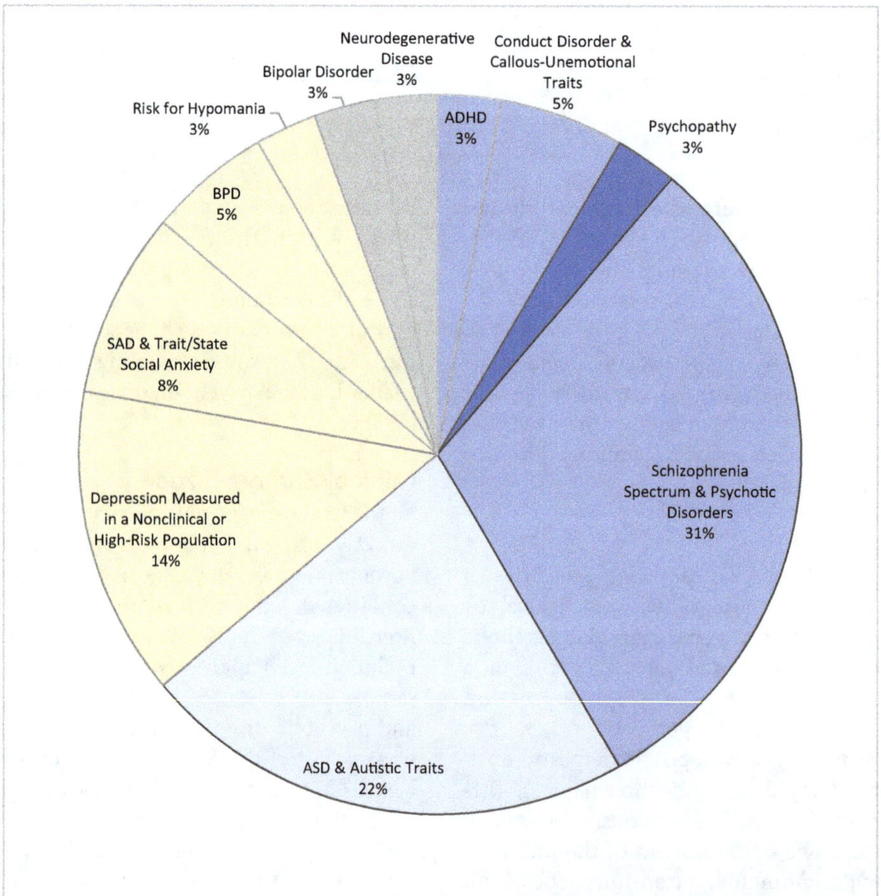

FIGURE 2 | Distribution of studies by clinical population category. Percentages refer to the percentage of papers on that population out of all papers in the current review, and colors refer to the male:female ratio. In blue, categories with overall more males than females among all participants (in all studies together). In yellow, categories with overall more females than males among all participants. The darker the color, the more pronounced the underrepresentation for females, with darker blue = 0 females, lighter blue = a ratio of more than 3:1, lightest blue = a ratio of more than 2:1, and gray = a ratio of less than 2:1. Specific male:female ratios for each category are reported under "Specific Results per Clinical Population".

Specific Results per Clinical Population

Table 1 presents the characteristics, main objective, findings, and conclusion of each of the studies included in this review.

In the following section, we review the main findings from the papers included, organized by clinical populations or clinical traits. Categories of clinical populations/traits are presented according to the number of relevant studies found, from the categories with a larger number of studies to those with the fewest. Two exceptions are categories that include papers referring to two different clinical conditions in the same comparative study. In these cases, the category of the clinical condition with the smaller number of studies will follow the category with the larger number. These cases will be explicitly noted when presenting the new category.

Schizophrenia Spectrum and Psychotic Disorders

Thirty-one percent (eleven papers) of the studies included in the current search focused on EA in the context of schizophrenia and psychotic disorders. In five studies (53, 56, 58, 61, 63), a group of participants with schizophrenia was compared with a nonclinical control group. In Lee et al.'s study (62), a schizophrenia group was compared to both a nonclinical control group and a group of participants diagnosed with bipolar disorder (see below). In de Jong et al.'s study (54), a group of violent participants with a psychotic disorder (a primary diagnosis of schizophrenia or schizoaffective disorder) was compared to a nonviolent psychotic disorder group and to a nonclinical control group. One study (60), which aimed to evaluate psychometric properties of EA and other paradigms to inform possible use in clinical trials, used both a between-group design (schizophrenia group in comparison to nonclinical control group) and a within-subject (test-retest) design in the schizophrenia group. Olbert et al. (59) applied a within-subject design in order to examine the relationship between EA (and other social-cognitive paradigms adapted from social neuroscience) and functionally meaningful outcomes in schizophrenia. Davis et al. (57) assessed whether oxytocin would enhance the effectiveness of a psychosocial intervention—applied both before and after treatment with a double-blind drug administration design. Harenski et al. (55) compared criminal offenders with psychotic disorders to criminal offenders with no history of psychotic disorders and to a nonclinical nonoffenders control group. Within the first group, psychotic offenders with a history of suicide attempts were compared to psychotic offenders without such a history. In all studies but one, the EA tests were based on Zaki et al. (44), where EA assessment is based on the *valence* rating of a target's emotional states while s/he tells an autobiographical *emotional story*. In Harenski et al. (55), participants watched video clips in which people described autobiographical events, and participants indicated the *content* of emotions the people most likely experienced during the event, and additionally *ranked* the emotions (84).

The number of participants with schizophrenia ranged from 15 (61) to 173 [(59, 60)]—two studies based on the same sample), with the control groups usually similar to or smaller than the schizophrenia group. In three studies (54, 55, 57) all participants were males. In all the other studies there were more male participants than female participants, with a male:female ratio ranging from 1.2:1 (62) to 6.5:1 (61).

A synthesis of findings and conclusions from all studies together indicates *reduced overall EA abilities in people with schizophrenia spectrum disorders in comparison to nonclinical controls*. This is a robust finding that holds cross-culturally (53, 54, 56, 61–63). The EA impairment in schizophrenia is not easily explained by attention or motor deficits (61), and no correlation was found between EA performance and schizophrenia symptoms (63). Also, no significant effects of gender or gender by diagnosis were found on EA (58). However, the valence of the content that targets convey and participants need to infer may be an important variable that moderates results: In one study (58) it was found that the EA impairment in schizophrenia is specific to negative content, while in positive content participants with schizophrenia scored similarly to controls. Interestingly, this difficulty understanding others' negative affect was associated with lower indices of social support. Harvey et al. (61) found that participants with schizophrenia were more impaired than controls in EA in the context of negative videos compared with positive videos. In Lee et al. (63), both groups showed better accuracy for positive valence; however, participants in the schizophrenia group demonstrated impairment in the positive as well as in the negative valence stimuli.

Findings also indicate that EA is a sensitive measure that captured a group difference between individuals with schizophrenia and controls, even where other tasks (e.g. RMET) did not (58). EA differentiated not only between people with schizophrenia and healthy individuals, but also within a group of patients with a psychotic disorder, EA differentiated between those with and without a violent history (54), and between psychotic offenders with and without past suicide attempts, and nonpsychotic offenders and nonclinical controls (55), where lower EA was associated with a greater likelihood of a past suicide attempt, beyond other risk factors such as depression and substance use. EA was found to be a sensitive differentiating measure in such cases even when other measures (such as ToM, "understanding the other's mind") were not (54). In a research project evaluating the psychometric properties of four different social-cognitive paradigms adapted from social neuroscience (basic biological motion, emotion in biological motion, self-referential memory and EA) that were administered to participants with schizophrenia, EA had the broadest external validity (59). The other examined paradigms all had limitations for use in clinical trials, at least without further adaptation (60).

Similar to findings from the general population, associations between EA measures and self-report empathy measures from questionnaires in participants with schizophrenia were found to be weak (53, 56, 63). This might suggest a discrepancy between subjectively experienced empathy and actual empathy performance in a dynamic, interpersonal task. Another possible explanation is that the EA measure captures a certain aspect of empathy, while questionnaires [in these cases: IRI; (32);

QCAE, (89)] capture a different aspect. This lack of a significant correlation between EA tasks and empathy self-report questionnaires, alongside the fact that other tasks designed to measure empathy did not always differentiate between participants with schizophrenia and controls (54, 58) may also indicate that at least some aspects of empathy are intact in schizophrenia. It seems that people with schizophrenia do not respond to others' greater emotional expressivity as much as healthy individuals do (53, 61, 63). Level of expressivity of the targets in all these studies was based on their score on the Berkeley Expressivity Questionnaire [BEQ; (90)], a self-report questionnaire that assesses tendencies to experience and express strong emotions in general (example items: "Whenever I feel positive emotions, people can easily see exactly what I am feeling"; "I sometimes cry during sad movies"; "I've learned it is better to suppress my anger than to show it"; "I am an emotionally expressive person". Van Donkersgoed et al. (53) found that with less expressive targets, participants with schizophrenia and controls had similarly low EA scores, but with more expressive targets, the control group performed better on EA than the patients with schizophrenia. On the neural level, it was found that expressivity elicited activity in specific regions more powerfully in controls than in participants with schizophrenia (61). Lee et al. (63) found that although both schizophrenia and control groups showed greater EA for more expressive targets, this effect was significantly smaller in schizophrenia participants. What seems to improve EA performance in schizophrenia is oxytocin: Participants assigned to oxytocin demonstrated significantly greater improvements than placebo on the measure of EA [but not on other social-cognitive measures; (57)].

Lastly, two studies utilized fMRI (61) and structural MRI (55) scans. Supporting the idea that both mental-state attribution and experience-sharing processes contribute to EA, Harvey et al. (55) found that in healthy controls, EA was associated with increased activity in brain regions typically linked to cognitive effort (i.e., lateral PFC), visual attention (i.e., parietal and occipital cortices), socioemotional processes, including mental-state attribution (i.e., mPFC, precuneus, posterior cingulate), experience sharing (i.e., inferior frontal, inferior parietal), and social context processing (i.e., parahippocampal gyrus). However, in participants with schizophrenia, the pattern of accuracy-related brain activity was relatively sparse (61). Harenski et al. (55) found that offenders with psychotic disorders and suicide attempts demonstrated lower EA and had smaller temporal pole volumes relative to controls, to nonpsychotic offenders and to psychotic offenders without past suicide attempts (this association was significant independent of other risk variables).

Bipolar Disorder

One of the studies described in the schizophrenia category (62) was a comparative study aiming to determine the relative extent of impairment in social (and nonsocial) cognitive domains in individuals with bipolar disorder compared with schizophrenia patients. EA was thus a part of a battery measuring social cognition within these two groups and in a nonclinical control group. Participants in the bipolar group did not differ from comparison participants on EA, nor in each of the other social-cognitive tasks, whereas schizophrenia patients showed impaired social-cognitive performance compared with both bipolar patients and the control group. Bipolar disorder was found in this study to be associated with less impairment on social relative to nonsocial-cognitive performance, whereas schizophrenia was associated with more impairment on social relative to nonsocial-cognitive performance.

ASD and Autistic Traits

Twenty-two percent (eight papers) of the studies that were found in the current search focused on EA in the context of ASD or autistic traits. In five of them (64, 68–71), a group of participants with ASD was compared with a nonclinical control group. In one study (66), a group of participants with ASD was compared to both a nonclinical control group and a group of participants diagnosed with ADHD. In two studies (65, 67), autistic traits were assessed in nonclinical samples. In five studies (66, 68–71), participants were mostly high-functioning individuals (sometimes defined as Asperger's syndrome, or PDD). EA measurement was based on a *dyadic interaction* paradigm, with perceivers asked to infer the *content* of the targets' mental states (43, 91). In Demurie et al. (66), one of the targets featured in each filmed interaction was diagnosed with ADHD while the other was a typically developed participant. In Ponnet et al. (69), all members of dyads who participated as targets also participated later as participants for measuring EA; each dyad included a participant with ASD and a typically developed participant. Two studies (65, 67) relied on Zaki et al. (44), where EA assessment is based on the *valence* rating of a target's emotional states while s/he tells an autobiographical *emotional story*. One study focused on empathic *embarrassment* accuracy among individuals with ASD in comparison to the control group, using a similar paradigm (64). One study (67) aimed to test whether variance in social proficiency moderates the effects of *oxytocin* on social-cognitive performance, applying a randomized, double-blind, placebo-controlled design: Participants completed a questionnaire measuring autistic traits [AQ; (92)] and then self-administered intranasal oxytocin or a matching placebo before completing an EA task. EA scores were then compared between the experimental and the control (placebo) group.

The number of participants with ASD ranged from 11 participants (69) to 24 participants (70), with the control groups usually the same size, or slightly larger. Females were generally underrepresented in all six studies with participants with ASD: The number of female participants with ASD ranged from 0 (68) to 5 (71), resulting in an overall male-to-female ratio of around 10:1. In the two studies that were based on a nonclinical sample (65, 67), sample sizes were larger (n = 100; n = 27). In aan het Rot and Hogenelst's study (65), the male-to-female ratio was 1:1, and in the Bartz et al. study (67), all participants were males.

The synthesis of the findings and conclusions from all the studies together shows that individuals with ASD exhibit a deficit in EA abilities (64, 66, 68–71). More pronounced autistic traits in typically developed individuals were also associated with poorer

EA abilities (65, 67). However, this may be true only for individuals who have more autistic traits as well as less trait affective empathy (5). Additionally, this association was found to be moderated by the hormone oxytocin: Bartz et al. (67) showed that oxytocin selectively improved EA for people with more pronounced autistic traits. In this study, participants with less pronounced autistic traits performed better on the EA task in the placebo condition and maintained this performance level in the oxytocin condition, whereas participants with more pronounced autistic traits performed worse in the placebo condition but significantly better in the oxytocin condition, such that in the oxytocin condition, the performance of participants with more and less pronounced autistic traits did not differ. Roeyers et al. (70) found that participants with ASD did not use more time than the control group to complete the EA assessment, while in Ponnet et al. (71), participants with ASD needed more time than the controls to carry out the EA task.

Importantly, the measurement of EA in a naturalistic, ecological paradigm captured the difference between the ASD group and a control group when static mind-reading tasks did not (71). Ponnet et al. (68) found that when participants were presented with two filmed interactions, one more structured than the other, participants with ASD demonstrated better EA abilities on the more structured video than on the less structured one, while no such difference was found in the control group. Thus, the findings from both studies (68, 71) emphasize the role of *structure* in bringing out empathic abilities of individuals with ASD, indicating that they perform better in more structured settings, tasks or situations. Ponnet et al. (69) found that when participants with ASD who had to infer the thoughts and feelings of a target in a videotaped interaction also took part in these prerecorded interactions, they did not differ from a nonclinical control group in their EA scores. The researchers concluded that being in the interaction yields higher EA scores than perceiving a social interaction without participating in it (69). In terms of people with ASD, this may be a result of the opportunity to review a social situation that was previously experienced, hence reflecting practice and learning. It is also possible that the interactive experience itself enhanced EA due to attention, motivation or even bio-behavioral factors, such as oxytocinergic influences. Roeyers et al. (70) noted that although impairments in EA were observed among people with ASD, the underlying *mechanisms* accounting for this remain unexplained. They added that as the advanced EA measure proved to be a valid alternative for the static tests, they believe that future work incorporating the EA paradigm could expand the research on deficient mind reading in ASD.

Attention Deficit and Hyperactivity Disorder

In one of the studies reviewed above (66), adolescents with ASD (n = 13) were compared to adolescents with ADHD (n = 13) and to a nonclinical control group (n = 18) on EA performance, in a dyadic interaction paradigm. In each dyad, one of two interacting targets was a typically developing adolescent, and the other was diagnosed with ADHD. Thus, participants with ADHD were examined in this study not only as subjects but also as the targets for EA (participants with ASD were examined only as subjects/perceivers). The study results demonstrate the impairment in EA abilities of adolescents with ASD. Participants with ADHD performed as an intermediate category between the ASD and the control group in EA abilities: Their scores did not differ significantly from those of the control group nor from those of the ASD individuals. As targets, participants with ADHD were less accurately understood than the typically developing participants, and their thoughts and feelings seemed to be less easy to read.

Depression Measured in a Nonclinical or High-Risk Population

In 14% of the papers (five papers), the relationship between EA and depressive traits or states in a nonclinical or high-risk population was examined. Two studies (72, 73) used an EA test based on the valence rating of targets narrating autobiographical stories (44, 65). One of them (73) aimed to examine the effects of reduced brain serotonin on EA, oxytocin and mood in never-depressed individuals with low vs. high risk for major depressive disorder. This study utilized a double-blind cross-over design, with an order of treatment randomized by gender and group (high vs. low risk, 10 males and 10 females in each group, and two treatment conditions). The other study (72) aimed to examine the impact of light therapy on mood and on cognitive empathy in premenstrual women with symptoms indicating a premenstrual disorder (PMS). The sample was characterized by mild depression [assessed using the Quick Inventory of Depressive Symptoms; (93)]. This study utilized a participant-blind between-groups (two treatment groups) design and included 48 females. In both studies, participants' EA performance was not affected by intervention. aan het Rot et al. (72) found that the therapy improved mood (only in women not using hormonal contraceptives), but found no differential effects of light therapy on EA, even when potential moderators such as valence (positive or negative) of the stimuli, the target's emotional expressivity, PMS severity, participants' depression and contraceptive use were taken into account. Similarly, Hogenelst et al. (73) found that the procedure used to model reduced serotonin (acute tryptophan depletion; ATD) did not significantly alter EA in the high-risk group, nor in the control group. In both studies, participants obtained higher EA scores when watching positive stimuli compared to negative stimuli, but without moderating the overall results. To sum, in both studies EA and depression were measured in the context of an intervention aimed to target depression (light therapy, ATD), and in both EA was not affected by the intervention.

The other three studies all used samples of romantic couples [51 couples in Gadassi et al. (74)]; 267 couples in Papp et al. (75); 74 couples in Thomas et al. (76)). These studies measured both EA and depressive symptoms and utilized a dyadic interaction paradigm (Actor–Partner Interdependence Model). All three studies measured EA using a lab procedure where couples are videotaped while interacting (discussing a given topic or an issue of conflict); then they separately review the recording, write the content of their own experienced mental states during the interaction and infer their partner's mental states. One study (74) additionally utilized the daily diary procedure, measuring both content and valence of the partner's thoughts and feelings. Thomas et al. (76) examined the predictors of EA and assumed similarity (judgments of how closely linked partner emotions are) in a sample of married couples, in the context of problem-solving discussions, considering depression. They found no association between depression and EA. It is interesting to note, however, that lower levels of depression tended to produce higher levels of assumed similarity. Based on the procedure applied by Thomas et al. (74), Papp et al. (75) tested partners' EA and assumed similarity in marital conflict interactions, and whether they are moderated by spouses' levels of depressive symptoms. They found that higher levels of depressive symptoms were associated with reduced EA for negative emotions (among both males and females) and, surprisingly, with increased EA for positive emotions among females. Gadassi et al. (74) aimed to examine gender differences in the association between depressive symptoms and interpersonal perception. In the lab measures, they found that females' (but not males') higher levels of depressive symptoms were associated with lower EA. In the daily diary procedure, females' depressive symptoms were specifically associated with lower levels of EA for negative (but not for positive) feelings, and with lower levels of their partner's EA for the females' negative feelings. Males' depressive symptoms were again unrelated to levels of EA. They concluded that when a woman is depressed, first her own EA is lowered, and second, her partner's EA when trying to infer her emotional state is also lowered. This pattern was valence-specific and gender-specific. Taken together, findings from these three studies present some inconsistencies regarding the association between EA and depressive symptoms and indicate that the mechanism underlying this potential association may be modified both by valence and by gender.

SAD and Trait/State Social Anxiety

Three studies examined associations between EA and social anxiety. One study (77) compared 32 participants with a SAD to a nonclinical matched control group. These researchers aimed to compare cognitive empathy and affective empathy in individuals with SAD to that of nonanxious controls. They used an adapted version of an emotional story inferring paradigm (44), adding to the procedure a measure of "empathic congruence." According to Morrison et al. (77), while perceiver inference of the target's emotional valence provides a measure of *cognitive empathy*, a measure of *emotional empathy* can be gained by examining the degree of congruence between the target's self-rating of emotion and the participant's self-rating of emotion. They found that individuals with SAD did not differ from controls in continuously rating how negative or positive they thought the targets felt (i.e., in EA, cognitive empathy). However, they did differ from controls in their empathic congruence (rating how they themselves felt): For positively valenced (but not for negatively valenced) clips, individuals with SAD exhibited significantly lower empathic congruence.

In the remaining two studies (78, 79), social anxiety was measured in a nonclinical population. Auyeung and Alden (78) examined whether individual differences in social anxiety moderated EA. They randomly assigned 121 participants to an experimental condition designed to increase state anxiety *via* social threat or to a control condition; they then asked the participants to observe videos of target individuals discussing either a socially painful or a nonpainful event. Both targets and participants rated the negative emotions that the targets were feeling while discussing the event. The researchers found that social anxiety was associated with higher EA for others' negative social emotions (social pain), but only when participants experienced social threat (under the social-threat condition). Simpson et al. (79) tested how people with more anxious-ambivalent attachment orientations [a measure of anxiety in the context of relationships; (94, 95)] react when potential alternative dating partners threaten their relationship. Eighty-two dating couples inferred their partner's mental states from a videotaped interaction in which they each rated pictures of opposite-sex individuals for attractiveness. EA was operationalized in this study as the degree to which one participant's inference about the content of each of his or her partner's thoughts and feelings matched the partner's actual thoughts and feelings (by independent coders). Highly anxious participants demonstrated higher EA in this relationship-threatening situation. These more anxious participants also showed greater relational instability when they more accurately read their partners' thoughts and feelings, and their relationships were more likely to have ended 4 months later, measured in a follow-up screening. According to Simpson et al. (79), their findings demonstrate that in relationship-threatening situations, anxious-ambivalent individuals appear to be particularly vulnerable to the negative implications of their partner's thoughts and feelings.

Borderline Personality Disorder

Two studies (80, 81) measured EA in the context of BPD. Both utilized a dyadic interaction paradigm. Miano et al. (80) measured EA in 30 romantic couples, with a female partner diagnosed with BPD, in comparison to a control nonclinical group of 37 couples. They aimed to investigate whether females with BPD show *inaccuracy* during a relationship-threatening conversation with their partner (the authors note that motivated inaccuracy is a protective mechanism for couples in healthy relationships during some relationship-threatening situations). Their findings indicate that when facing a relationship-threatening situation, couples in the control group demonstrated inaccuracy, i.e., reduced EA. In contrast, females with BPD tended to increase their EA compared with females in the control group, in a relationship-threatening context. Male partners of BPD females did not differ from males in the control group in the EA pattern.

Flury et al. (81) aimed to explore the "borderline empathy phenomenon," i.e., the claim, suggested by clinical psychologists, that patients with BPD are unusually accurate at "reading" other people (23–25, 96, 97). The authors used an assessment of EA.

They recruited 30 males and 46 females from a larger sample of participants who completed the Borderline Syndrome Index [BSI; (98)], and scored in the upper and lower quartiles, to create a group of individuals at high risk for BPD and a low-risk group. Participants were then assigned to same-sex dyads, each composed of one "borderline" (high-risk) and one "nonborderline" (low-risk) participant, and EA was measured within this dyadic interaction paradigm. Researchers found that the high-risk BPD dyad members displayed better EA than the low-risk BPD dyad members, which seemed to support the borderline empathy phenomenon. However, further analyses [with the Actor–Partner Interdependence Model, APIM; (99–101)] revealed that between those at high risk versus those at low risk, these effects were not a consequence of greater abilities on the part of the BPD participants, but poorer abilities on the part of their partners, meaning that for high-BPD members, EA was harder to predict and more difficult to infer by their partners. The authors emphasize the importance of considering the fact that "high BPD individuals do not have greater empathic ability; they are simply harder to 'read'." [(81), p.326]

Conduct Disorder and Callous-Unemotional Traits

Two studies evaluated EA abilities in the context of conduct disorder in adolescents. In one study, Martin-Key et al. (82) compared male adolescents with Conduct Disorder (CD) and higher versus lower levels of callous-unemotional (CU) traits (n = 37) and a nonclinical control group of male adolescents (n = 40), using an emotional story inferring paradigm. This study employed a modified version of the EA task developed by Zaki et al. (49) in order to draw three measures: the participants' ability to track changes in the intensity of the target's emotion, i.e., EA; their ability to recognize the specific emotion displayed by the target after watching the full video clip, i.e., emotion recognition; and the participants' reported experience of the same emotion as the target, i.e., emotional empathy. They found that relative to controls, participants with CD showed deficits in emotion recognition and emotional empathy (deficits were particularly evident for sadness, fear and disgust), but not in EA. Comparison between the subgroups of high versus low CU traits did not yield any significant differences in EA either.

In the second study, De Ridder et al. (83) assessed EA of male institutionalized adolescents toward staff members, over eight days, in 71 participants with high and low CU traits. Their findings indicate that adolescents with high CU traits perform in the normal range for anger recognition, and they are as accurate as low CU in inferring distress among staff members. The adolescents with high CU traits overestimated the intensity of both anger and distress, in particular during their own misbehavior. The authors suggest that this may reflect overrelying on cognitive empathy ability, instead of their impaired emotional empathy abilities. Thus, the two studies, conducted using two different methods, in two different settings, imply that in the context of conduct disorder, EA as a measure of cognitive EA is intact (when the participant is asked to track the intensity of the target's emotion). However, accuracy in emotion recognition is impaired, as is the ability to accurately share the affective experience of the target, as a measure of emotional empathy.

Psychopathy

Surprisingly, only one paper (84) was found in the search to study EA in psychopathy. This study aimed to examine the relationship between psychopathy and cognitive empathy, with a procedure similar to that of the emotional story inferring, using standardized forced-choice response format for both the videotaped targets and the perceivers (and not a continuous rating scale). Findings revealed an inverse association between psychopathy and EA scores, as well as robust group differences between psychopathic and nonpsychopathic male inmates.

Risk for Hypomania

One study (85) measured the association between EA and high risk for hypomania. The study included 121 participants (57% females) and utilized an emotional story inferring paradigm. The researchers examined how the risk for hypomania contributes to the emotional experiences upon encountering another person's emotions and EA of that target's emotions. The risk for hypomania [assessed by The Hypomanic Personality Scale; (102)] was found to be associated with heightened moment-by-moment detection of positive emotions for targets describing positive events, and with overestimating global positive emotion for targets describing negative events. Hypomania risk was also significantly associated with a higher positive emotional experience after viewing a high-intensity negative emotional story video, but not after viewing a low-intensity negative video or high/low-intensity positive video.

Neurodegenerative Disease

Lastly, one paper (86) investigated the association between EA in patients with neurodegenerative disease and their caregivers' depressive symptoms. Across two independent studies (n = 172, n = 63), lower EA in neurodegenerative patients was found to be associated with greater depressive symptoms in their caregivers (who were mainly partners). This association was found when accuracy was measured *via* caregiver report or with a dynamic tracking task. Patients' ability to recognize specific emotions portrayed in photographs or films was not found to be associated with caregivers' depressive symptoms.

DISCUSSION

The current review aimed to scope the existing literature on EA in clinical populations. An exhaustive systematic search yielded 34 peer-reviewed papers aiming to measure EA in a clinical population or to assess links between EA and clinical trait or state in a nonclinical or a high-risk population. Overall, the review indicates a growing interest in the EA measure, a dynamic ecological measure that enables greater sensitivity in detecting between-group differences, and more nuanced characterization of empathic functioning.

An Overview and a Different View of the Main Findings

While ASD and psychopathy are considered to be the two main conditions traditionally associated with empathic dysfunction (11), surprisingly, only one study was found to focus on EA in psychopathy, and two more on conduct disorder in adolescents. The category with the most studies found is schizophrenia (with 31% of the studies). Some of the studies assessed EA in people with a diagnosed clinical condition, while others assessed clinical states or traits in nonclinical or high-risk populations. EA was measured in individuals from clinical groups for various purposes: looking for between-group differences, evaluating interventions and assessing measurements or tools. Accordingly, various designs were used: clinical condition group versus nonclinical control group, randomized or test-retest designs and dyadic designs. Studies also varied in sample sizes and male:female ratios, which will be further discussed.

Almost all studies utilized the emotional story inferring paradigm (or similar), or a dyadic interaction paradigm. These are difficult to compare as they were never used in the same study and were usually used in different contexts or with different populations. For example, the category with the largest number of studies, schizophrenia and psychotic disorders, consists only of studies based on the emotional story inferring paradigm, while all studies focusing on romantic partners used dyadic interactions. This may reflect the tendency of different research groups to use different research paradigms. While there does not seem to be an advantage of one EA paradigm over the other, each has its advantages and limitations. The dyadic paradigm better simulates real-life face-to-face interactions, and it can be used with actual partners expressing emotions from their actual lives together; however, each interaction will end up very different and thus can be difficult to compare. Moreover, this paradigm requires a more demanding coding and scoring process, and it relies on the judgment of raters in assessing the similarity between the target and the perceiver. The emotional story inferring paradigm, on the other hand, is simpler and easier to facilitate as a lab procedure, with the main advantage being the use of the same stimuli for all participants. This can enable a clear separation between the effects of target and perceiver characteristics (as all perceivers see the exact same targets), but it is by nature less ecological. The diary procedure is the most ecological in the sense of having a longer temporal window in which one can examine EA; however, it is suitable mainly for couples, it is the hardest to manipulate and control, and it relies heavily on the participants' cooperation in their natural environment. Thus, the review does not provide general support for the use of a specific paradigm over the others, but it suggests that scholars should consider the characteristics of each paradigm in light of the research question, the clinical population and the available resources.

Importantly, EA served as a sensitive measure that detected between-group differences even when other paradigms such as emotion detection from still pictures or ToM measures did not (71) in ASD; [(54, 58) in schizophrenia], suggesting that EA, as a complex ecological paradigm, better captures nuanced deficits. However, it is also possible that EA traces a more specific aspect of empathy impairment in these populations that is not captured by the other tasks. A third potential explanation might be that EA tasks are more difficult for these populations due to attention, executive functions, or motor requirements. These observations should be taken into account when planning future studies with clinical populations, and tasks should be made simpler when possible.

An interesting modification was added to some of the reviewed studies, namely, asking participants to report not only on the target's assumed experience, but also on their own. The authors could then assess not only how accurate participants were in identifying the emotional state of the target, but also how much they themselves shared the target's affective experience. This addition to the EA paradigm seems to be especially valuable in clinical populations, where deconstructing the multifaceted concept of empathy could contribute to a better understanding of unique clinical profiles. For example, Martin-Key et al. (82) found no impairment in the classic EA measure in study participants with conduct disorder, but found a difference in levels of shared experience, which they referred to as emotional empathy. Similarly, Morrison et al. (77), who studied individuals with SAD, measured both EA and *empathic congruence*, comparing the subjects' continuous rating of their own emotion to the targets' ratings. They, too, found no impairment in EA but did find significantly lower empathic congruence in a group of individuals with SAD compared to a nonclinical control group.

Overall, reduced EA was found in schizophrenia, ASD, and psychopathy when compared with nonclinical control groups, and also when compared to individuals with bipolar disorder (in schizophrenia) or ADHD (in ASD). In the context of depression, lower EA was found in the context of negative emotional content (for both males and females), and in higher levels of depressive symptoms in females, but not in males (74). However, other findings indicated no correlation between depression and EA (76)—and even, in certain contexts, an association between higher depressive symptoms and higher EA (75). Negative emotional content conveyed by the target was also associated with lower EA in schizophrenia (58, 61), and this pattern may be true for healthy individuals as well (63). Thus, it may be concluded that negative emotional content is harder to infer accurately, and that gender and clinical condition are among the variables that moderate this specific difficulty. Other variables found to be associated with lower EA were reduced social support (58), the subjects' history of violence (54), smaller temporal pole volumes and past suicide attempts (55). Note, however, that all the above were inferred from the schizophrenia cohorts and may not apply to the general population. Importantly, reduced EA was also evident when participants were asked to infer the thoughts and feelings of targets with ADHD (66) or with BPD (81), meaning that individuals with these clinical conditions were "harder to read." This pattern is demonstrated specifically for depressive tendencies of females within marital relationships, where depression in females was found to be associated with reduced EA in both the females and their partners (74). Interestingly, this was not the case for targets with ASD, who did not differ from TD targets in their "readability" [i.e., did not yield lower EA scores in perceivers; (69)].

A clinical condition that has been hypothesized to be associated with enhanced EA is BPD (23–25, 96, 97). Miano et al. (80) found support for this hypothesis only in females in a romantic relationship setting, and specifically in a relationship-threatening situation. However, Flury et al. (81) remind us that when comparing between a clinical and a nonclinical group within a dyadic setting, EA scores are relative and are not independent. If one group gets a higher score than the other, it may imply better EA, or it may hint at more difficulty inferring from the clinical group as targets. Indeed, after utilizing an Actor–Partner Interdependence Model, that was the authors' conclusion.

A clinical population that does seem to exhibit enhanced EA is SAD, specifically under the experience of social threat (78) or when in a relationship-threatening situation (79). These findings imply better performance under social threat, which may be explained by higher arousal, greater attention or higher motivation in such situations. It is important to note that higher EA may not always be an advantage. For example, Miano et al. (80) claim that the pattern of empathic *inaccuracy* that they found among participants with a low risk for BPD is an adaptive skill in a relationship-threatening situation.

EA performance was improved by oxytocin in schizophrenia (57) and in people with more pronounced autistic traits (67). Feldman et al. (103) found that face-to-face synchronized parent-child interaction had the effect of normalizing oxytocin level in children with ASD, and keeping it high during social contact. This role of social interaction in elevating oxytocin levels in individuals with ASD, alongside the findings on the association between oxytocin and improved EA performance, may relate to the next variable that was found to be associated with better EA functioning in ASD: participation.

In ASD, it was found that participating in the same dyadic interaction that they later had to rate contributed to better EA, compared to inferring from passive observation (69). This could indicate an advantage for the participation itself (over observation), an advantage for learning and rehearsing, or both. Higher arousal, immediate feedback, attention and motivation may also explain this effect. Another variable that was found to be associated with improvement in EA abilities among participants with ASD was the extent to which the situation was more or less structured, i.e., how clear and predictable the social interaction was. ASD participants specifically benefited from a structured versus unstructured situation (68). Thus, in order to better characterize EA in ASD, it is desirable to simulate the complex, dynamic and unstructured daily social interactions, while in planning intervention programs it may be of great value to take into account the potential importance of participation and the role of a structured social situation in encouraging the EA abilities of people with ASD.

Given the dyadic nature of empathy, both the target and the perceiver contribute to EA. The perceiver's ability to accurately infer the target's thoughts and feelings depends not only on his/her states and traits but also on the various characteristics of the target, such as expressivity and motivation. Though some studies referred to such "target effects" on EA [e.g., (53, 63, 66, 75)], much of the reviewed literature emphasized the perceiver's side. Specifically, many studies were designed to investigate whether a clinical condition affects the perceiver's EA performance [e.g., (54–56, 58, 64, 65)]. Another interesting question that is highly relevant on both a social and a clinical level is how a clinical condition of a target affects the way perceivers understand the target's emotional state. Moreover, a target–perceiver interaction effect must also be considered. Such questions relate to the growing literature on "the double empathy problem," which stresses that it's not only autistic people who struggle with empathy—neuro-typical people also struggle to understand the minds of autistic individuals and empathize with them (104, 105). Such ideas challenge the traditional framing of autism as entailing empathic dysfunction. EA measures can be helpful in investigating this dyadic nature of empathy, as they rely on both the target and the perceiver's reports. Such directions are suggested by the findings of Flury et al. (81) on BPD patients' "readability," and of Demurie et in the context of ADHD, and may be of great value in the study of other clinical conditions as well.

We suggest that these variables, discussed in the context of either impairing or enhancing EA, can be further classified as *subject variables* (e.g., the clinical condition, clinical profile, biological characteristics, previous experiences, participation, social support), *target variables* (such as expressivity, content conveyed, clinical condition and specific profile), and *situational variables* (e.g., structured vs. unstructured, threatening, familiar). Within this framework, wherein the subject, the target or the situation can influence EA results, it may be valuable to consider additional variables in future research on empathy in clinical populations. One such variable that was barely directly addressed in the reviewed papers, yet was very pronounced in the process of synthesizing the findings, is gender.

The current review reveals a general underrepresentation of female participants in studies on clinical populations, and a slight underrepresentation for males in studies aiming to evaluate clinical traits or states in nonclinical or high-risk samples. This finding may reflect either a trend in research questions and aims, recruitment challenges (sometimes due to male:female ratio in a specific condition) or both. One consequence of this trend is that while in nonclinical studies gender differences can be (and sometimes are) examined, in studies based on clinical samples, the associations between EA, gender and clinical condition are hardly addressed. For example, without considering the male: female ratio of participants in each study, one might conclude that EA is impaired in ASD, schizophrenia, psychopathy and conduct disorder, and that EA is intact in bipolar disorder, enhanced to some extent in borderline disorder, and that in SAD the dysfunction is due to a lack of protective inaccuracy. But a closer look at the gender of participants in each category reveals that while studies in ASD, schizophrenia, psychopathy and conduct disorder were done mostly on male participants, research on BPD and SAD relied more on female participants. To date, in most studies on clinical populations, the sample size is not large enough to address this question, with the recruitment of clinical participants and specifically females constituting one of the main challenges limiting the studies, as researchers themselves often note (57, 61, 64, 67).

We believe that findings regarding gender, clinical phenotype and EA interactions may have important clinical implications. For example, Gadassi et al. (74) state that according to their findings, when females are depressed, their romantic relationship suffers doubly: first, because their own EA is lower, and second, because their partner's EA is also lower. In contrast, when males are depressed, neither their own nor their partner's levels of EA change. In the field of autism research, for example, there is a growing understanding that the male:female ratio might be different than previously assumed (106–108). New research indicates that females with autism are underdiagnosed and understudied, due to lack of knowledge on the ASD female phenotype, and perhaps to the "camouflage effect" [an hypothesis that females with ASD are better at camouflaging their social deficits; (109)]. Along these lines, we encourage future studies to take gender into account, and call for a deeper investigation of a potential clinical profile, EA and gender interaction.

Lastly, we want to draw attention to a group of studies focusing on EA in the context of violent or aggressive behavior in intimate relationships. These studies did not appear in our systematic search based on the chosen search-words but were brought to our attention by a reviewer, and we agree that they are of clear relevance to this review, as aggressive behavior may relate to various clinical conditions (16). For example, Schweinle et al. (110) investigated whether husbands' wife-directed aggression is related to unusual accuracy (hypersensitivity), or to a bias to infer criticism or rejection inappropriately when they infer women's thoughts and feelings. They used a procedure similar to the dyadic interaction paradigm to assess EA: videotapes depicting female clients participating in a simulated individual psychotherapy session with the same male therapist, focusing on intimate relationships. Each client watched her filmed therapy session and wrote down her thoughts and feelings through the session [originally developed by Marangoni et al. (91)]. The study's participants (all males) were asked to infer the client's thoughts and feelings while watching the videos. Then independent raters rated the similarity between the client's self-report and the participant's inferences of her thoughts and feelings. The results revealed that the greater the husbands' bias to overattribute criticism and rejection to the thoughts and feelings of women they had never met, the more they reported behaving in a verbally aggressive way toward their own wives. The men's overattribution bias, i.e., inaccurately inferring that women's thoughts and feelings are critical or rejecting of their male partners, was related not only to aggression against their wives but to the men's insecure attachment style [see also Clements et al. (111)]. An interesting future research direction may be to study both the violent individuals' EA *and* their clinical profiles. Such an investigation can also examine whether the association between the aggression and the EA profile is unique to the intimate relationship context, or if it reflects a more pervasive personality characteristic.

Strengths and Limitations of the Current Review, and Suggestions for Future Research

To ensure a broad search of the literature, the search strategy included PsycNET and PubMed, as well as the snowball technique (also using Google Scholar search engine), and an updated search was performed in September 2019. This review may not have identified all published papers on EA in clinical populations despite attempts to be as comprehensive as possible. Thus, the main limitation of this study is the possibility that the review may have missed some relevant papers, as the search included many words and terms, and it was spread over many clinical populations and research fields. We did not review unpublished studies such as dissertations, which may have contributed additional knowledge. Exclusion of the gray literature from the search and exclusion of studies published in a language other than English has probably left some valuable information outside the scope of this review.

As our aim was to present an overview of the existing literature on EA in clinical populations, we included all eligible peer-reviewed studies, regardless of methodological quality. Future research should address the methodological issues and aim for a meta-analysis of suitable and well-designed studies. This may be of great value in light of the small sample sizes typical of studies on clinical populations.

It seems that the study of EA in clinical populations could benefit from a modified measure that can capture both EA and empathic congruence (77), or accuracy in sharing the affective experience (82). On the other hand, it is reasonable to assume that clinical populations are even more susceptible than nonclinical populations to the length of a task/fatigue effects, and both those considerations must be taken into account when planning a study evaluating EA in a clinical sample.

Research on EA in clinical populations has added to the accumulating knowledge on the price one pays for not accurately understanding others' affective and mental states. Another interesting and potentially important question refers to the experience of the targets when they are not being understood. We have learned that low EA is associated with depression in the *partners* of the clinical patients with low EA (74, 75, 102). Thus, people who are not accurately understood on a daily basis suffer from the other, less-studied side of the EA model. Therefore, future studies could benefit from not only examining EA in a relevant clinical population, but exploring the effects of EA difficulties on spouses, family members and other social partners as well. It would also be relevant to examine individuals with clinical conditions not just as subjects or perceivers but also as *targets* of EA, i.e., to study not only how accurate individuals with social deficits are at understanding the other and sharing their emotions, but how accurately they are being understood by others, and possible associations with well-being.

To the best of our knowledge, this is the first review of the existing literature on EA in clinical conditions, states and traits. It reveals a growing interest in using these measures to deepen our understanding of clinical profiles, and it indicates that EA assessments have the potential to capture unique and subtle characteristics of empathic function and dysfunction. It also points to the paucity of existing studies on EA in the context of most clinical conditions. Due to the variance between and within clinical populations, and the variety of research aims, designs and methods across existing studies, it is difficult to draw robust meta-analytic conclusions regarding the nature of EA in clinical populations. A promising future research direction would be to integrate the cumulative knowledge on EA in the general (nonclinical) population with emerging data from clinical populations. For example, in the studies reviewed here, anxiety was found to be associated with enhanced EA in a relationship-threatening situation ((79); see also 93 for similar results with BPD). Ickes & Simpson (112) refer to motivational inaccuracy as protective in intimate relationship under certain circumstances of threat to the relationship, and it seems that anxiety and BPD are associated (perhaps only in females) with not applying this protective behavior. An alternative explanation is that enhanced EA is associated with enhanced alertness, sensitivity or arousal, which may characterize BPD patients as well as anxious individuals and individuals under threat [support for such an interpretation also can be found in Auyeung and Alden (78), and Devlin et al. (85)]. This interpretation may account for Ponnet et al.'s finding in which participants with ASD did not differ from a control group in their EA scores after participating in an interaction with the target (69). It may be that real face-to-face interactions cause increased alertness and arousal, and these facilitated EA. More research is needed in order to disentangle the role of personality traits and emotional states in EA in both clinical and nonclinical populations.

In summary, EA is an important measure, paradigm and concept in empathy research in the context of clinical populations. Though some limitations to the use of specific tools for measuring EA in clinical populations need to be considered, it seems that EA paradigms are promising for measuring outcomes and discriminating clinical from nonclinical populations, and subgroups within clinical conditions, even when other paradigms fail to do so. It may be that with further advances in research, EA paradigms could be used as a screening tool, and maybe even in training and practicing empathic abilities. In future research on EA in clinical populations, we suggest addressing understudied populations, such as psychopathy. Subject, target and situational variables should be considered, with special attention to gender differences (and similarities), the association between EA abilities and adaptive functioning, and the study of individuals with clinical conditions as targets of EA. These avenues of investigation may promote a better understanding of the nature of EA, of specific clinical profiles and of social attitudes toward people with clinical conditions.

AUTHOR CONTRIBUTIONS

Both YR and AP equally contributed to the review.

REFERENCES

1. Decety J, Bartal IB, Uzefovsky F, Knafo-Noam A. Empathy as a driver of prosocial behaviour: highly conserved neurobehavioural mechanisms across species. *Philos Trans R Soc B: Biol Sci* (2016) 371(1686):20150077. doi: 10.1098/rstb.2015.0077
2. Uzefovsky F, Knafo-Noam A. Empathy development throughout the life span. In: *Social Cognition*. New York: Routledge (2016). p. 89–115.
3. Walter H. Social cognitive neuroscience of empathy: concepts, circuits, and genes. *Emotion Rev* (2012) 4(1):9–17. doi: 10.1177/1754073911421379
4. Decety J, Norman GJ, Berntson GG, Cacioppo JT. A neurobehavioral evolutionary perspective on the mechanisms underlying empathy. *Prog Neurobiol* (2012) 98(1):38–48. doi: 10.1016/j.pneurobio.2012.05.001
5. Davis MH, Luce C, Kraus SJ. The heritability of characteristics associated with dispositional empathy. *J Personal* (1994) 62(3):369–91. doi: 10.1111/j.1467-6494.1994.tb00302.x
6. Decety J. The neuroevolution of empathy. *Ann New York Acad Sci* (2011) 1231(1):35–45. doi: 10.1111/j.1749-6632.2011.06027.x
7. Eisenberg N, Fabes RA, Carlo G, Speer AL, Switzer G, Karbon M, et al. The relations of empathy-related emotions and maternal practices to children' s comforting behavior. *J Exp Child Psychol* (1993) 55(2):131–50. doi: 10.1006/jecp.1993.1007
8. Abramson L, Uzefovsky F, Toccaceli V, Knafo-Noam A. The genetic and environmental origins of emotional and cognitive empathy: Review and meta-analyses of twin studies. *Neurosci Biobehav Rev* (2020). doi: 10.1016/j.neubiorev.2020.03.023
9. Baron-Cohen S. Empathizing, systemizing, and the extreme male brain theory of autism. In: *Progress in brain research* vol. 186. Oxford, UK: Elsevier (2010) p. 167–75. doi: 10.1016/B978-0-444-53630-3.00011-7
10. Bird G, Viding E. The self to other model of empathy: providing a new framework for understanding empathy impairments in psychopathy, autism, and alexithymia. *Neurosci Biobehav Rev* (2014) 47:520–32. doi: 10.1016/j.neubiorev.2014.09.021
11. Blair RJ. Responding to the emotions of others: Dissociating forms of empathy through the study of typical and psychiatric populations. *Consciousness Cogn* (2005) 14(4):698–718. doi: 10.1016/j.concog.2005.06.004
12. Blair RJ. Neuroimaging of psychopathy and antisocial behavior: a targeted review. *Curr Psychiatry Rep* (2010) 12(1):76–82. doi: 10.1007/s11920-009-0086-x
13. Brüne M. Emotion recognition,'theory of mind,'and social behavior in schizophrenia. *Psychiatry Res* (2005) 133(2-3):135–47. doi: 10.1016/j.psychres.2004.10.007
14. Horan WP, Green MF. Treatment of social cognition in schizophrenia: Current status and future directions. *Schizophr Res* (2019) 203:3–11. doi: 10.1016/j.schres.2017.07.013
15. Tandon R, Gaebel W, Barch DM, Bustillo J, Gur RE, Heckers S, et al. Definition and description of schizophrenia in the DSM-5. *Schizophr Res* (2013) 150(1):3–10. doi: 10.1016/j.schres.2013.05.028
16. DSM-5 American Psychiatric Association. *Diagnostic and statistical manual of mental disorders*. Arlington: American Psychiatric Publishing (2013).
17. Hare RD. *The Hare Psychopathy Checklist-Revised (PCL-R)*. Toronto: Multi-Health Systems (2003).
18. Derntl B, Finkelmeyer A, Toygar TK, Hülsmann A, Schneider F, Falkenberg

DI, et al. Generalized deficit in all core components of empathy in schizophrenia. *Schizophr Res* (2009) 108(1-3):197–206. doi: 10.1016/j.schres.2008.11.009

19. Jones AP, Happé FG, Gilbert F, Burnett S, Viding E. Feeling, caring, knowing: different types of empathy deficit in boys with psychopathic tendencies and autism spectrum disorder. *J Child Psychol Psychiatry* (2010) 51(11):1188–97. doi: 10.1111/j.1469-7610.2010.02280.x
20. Shamay-Tsoory SG, Shur S, Barcai-Goodman L, Medlovich S, Harari H, Levkovitz Y. Dissociation of cognitive from affective components of theory of mind in schizophrenia. *Psychiatry Res* (2007) 149(1-3):11–23. doi: 10.1016/j.psychres.2005.10.018
21. Harari H, Shamay-Tsoory SG, Ravid M, Levkovitz Y. Double dissociation between cognitive and affective empathy in borderline personality disorder. *Psychiatry Res* (2010) 175(3):277–9. doi: 10.1016/j.psychres.2009.03.002
22. Shamay-Tsoory S, Harari H, Szepsenwol O, Levkovitz Y. Neuropsychological evidence of impaired cognitive empathy in euthymic bipolar disorder. *J. Neuropsychiatry Clin Neurosci* (2009) 21(1):59–67. doi: 10.1176/jnp.2009.21.1.59
23. Frank H, Hoffman N. Borderline empathy: An empirical investigation. *Compr Psychiatry* (1986) 27(4):387–95. doi: 10.1016/0010-440X(86)90015-5
24. Guttman HA, Laporte L. Empathy in families of women with borderline personality disorder, anorexia nervosa, and a control group. *Family Process* (2000) 39(3):345–58. doi: 10.1111/j.1545-5300.2000.39306.x
25. Ladisich W, Feil WB. Empathy in psychiatric patients. *Br J Med Psychol* (1988) 61(2):155–62. doi: 10.1111/j.2044-8341.1988.tb02774.x
26. Knafo A, Zahn-Waxler C, Davidov M, Van Hulle C, Robinson JL, Rhee SH. Empathy in early childhood: genetic, environmental, and affective contributions. *Ann New York Acad Sci* (2009) 1167(1):103–14. doi: 10.1111/j.1749-6632.2009.04540.x
27. Van Hulle C, Zahn-Waxler C, Robinson JL, Rhee SH, Hastings PD, Knafo A. Autonomic correlates of children's concern and disregard for others. *Soc Neurosci* (2013) 8(4):275–90. doi: 10.1080/17470919.2013.791342
28. Zahn-Waxler C, Robinson JL, Emde RN. The development of empathy in twins. *Dev Psychol* (1992) 28(6):1038. doi: 10.1037/0012-1649.28.6.1038
29. Mikolajewski AJ, Chavarria J, Moltisanti A, Hart SA, Taylor J. Examining the factor structure and etiology of prosociality. *psychol Assessment* (2014) 26 (4):1259. doi: 10.1037/a0037132
30. Knafo A, Steinberg T, Goldner I. Children's low affective perspective-taking ability is associated with low self-initiated pro-sociality. *Emotion* (2011) 11 (1):194. doi: 10.1037/a0021240
31. Nowicki S, Duke MP. Individual differences in the nonverbal communication of affect: The Diagnostic Analysis of Nonverbal Accuracy Scale. *J Nonverbal Behav* (1994) 18(1):9–35. doi: 10.1007/BF02169077
32. Davis MH. Measuring individual differences in empathy: Evidence for a multidimensional approach. *J Pers Soc Psychol* (1983) 44(1):113. doi: 10.1037/0022-3514.44.1.113
33. Lawrence EJ, Shaw P, Baker D, Baron-Cohen S, David AS. Measuring empathy: reliability and validity of the Empathy Quotient. *psychol Med* (2004) 34(5):911–20. doi: 10.1017/S0033291703001624
34. Funk J, Fox C, Chan M, Curtiss K. The development of the Children's Empathic Attitudes Questionnaire using classical and Rasch analyses. *J Appl Dev Psychol* (2008) 29(3):187–96. doi: 10.1016/j.appdev.2008.02.005
35. Baron-Cohen S, O'riordan M, Stone V, Jones R, Plaisted K. Recognition of faux pas by normally developing children and children with Asperger syndrome or high-functioning autism. *J Autism Dev Disord* (1999) 29 (5):407–18. doi: 10.1023/A:1023035012436
36. Baron-Cohen S, Wheelwright S, Hill J, Raste Y, Plumb I. The "Reading the Mind in the Eyes" Test revised version: a study with normal adults, and adults with Asperger syndrome or high-functioning autism. *J Child Psychol Psychiatry Allied Discipl* (2001) 42(2):241–51. doi: 10.1111/1469-7610.00715
37. Corcoran R, Cahill C, Frith CD. The appreciation of visual jokes in people with schizophrenia: a study of 'mentalizing'ability. *Schizophr Res* (1997) 24 (3):319–27. doi: 10.1016/S0920-9964(96)00117-X
38. Happé FG. Communicative competence and theory of mind in autism: A test of relevance theory. *Cognition* (1993) 48(2):101–19. doi: 10.1016/0010-0277(93)90026-R
39. Mo S, Su Y, Chan RC, Liu J. Comprehension of metaphor and irony in schizophrenia during remission: the role of theory of mind and IQ. *Psychiatry Res* (2008) 157(1-3):21–9. doi: 10.1016/j.psychres.2006.04.002
40. Wimmer H, Perner J. Beliefs about beliefs: Representation and constraining function of wrong beliefs in young children's understanding of deception. *Cognition* (1983) 13(1):103–28. doi: 10.1016/0010-0277(83)90004-5
41. Zaki J, Ochsner K. The need for a cognitive neuroscience of naturalistic social cognition. *Ann New York Acad Sci* (2009) 1167:16. doi: 10.1111/j.1749-6632.2009.04601.x
42. Ickes W. Empathic accuracy. *J Personal* (1993) 61(4):587–610. doi: 10.1111/j.1467-6494.1993.tb00783.x
43. Ickes W, Stinson L, Bissonnette V, Garcia S. Naturalistic social cognition: Empathic accuracy in mixed-sex dyads. *J Pers Soc Psychol* (1990) 59(4):730. doi: 10.1037/0022-3514.59.4.730
44. Zaki J, Bolger N, Ochsner K. It takes two: The interpersonal nature of empathic accuracy. *psychol Sci* (2008) 19(4):399–404. doi: 10.1111/j.1467-9280.2008.02099.x
45. Zaki J, Ochsner KN. The neuroscience of empathy: progress, pitfalls and promise. *Nat Neurosci* (2012) 15(5):675–80. doi: 10.1038/nn.3085
46. Levenson RW, Ruef AM. Empathy: A physiological substrate. *J Pers Soc Psychol* (1992) 63(2):234–46. doi: 10.1037/0022-3514.63.2.234
47. Howland M, Rafaeli E. Bringing everyday mind reading into everyday life: Assessing empathic accuracy with daily diary data. *J Personality* (2010) 78 (5):1437–68. doi: 10.1111/j.1467-6494.2010.00657.x
48. Sened H, Yovel I, Bar-Kalifa E, Gadassi R, Rafaeli E. Now you have my attention: Empathic accuracy pathways in couples and the role of conflict. *Emotion* (2017) 17(1):155. doi: 10.1037/emo0000220
49. Zaki J, Weber J, Bolger N, Ochsner K. The neural bases of empathic accuracy. *Proc Natl Acad Sci* (2009) 106(27):11382–7. doi: 10.1073/pnas.0902666106
50. Arksey H, O'Malley L. Scoping studies: towards a methodological framework. *Int J Soc Res Methodol* (2005) 8(1):19–32. doi: 10.1080/1364557032000119616
51. Levac D, Colquhoun H, O'Brien KK. Scoping studies: advancing the methodology. *Implementation Sci* (2010) 5(1):69. doi: 10.1186/1748-5908-5-69
52. Liberati A, Altman DG, Tetzlaff J, Mulrow C, Gøtzsche PC, Ioannidis JP, et al. The PRISMA statement for reporting systematic reviews and meta-analyses of studies that evaluate health care interventions: explanation and elaboration. *Ann Internal Med* (2009) 151(4):W–65. doi: 10.1016/j.jclinepi.2009.06.006
53. Van Donkersgoed RJ, De Jong S, Aan het Rot M, Wunderink L, Lysaker PH, Hasson-Ohayon I, et al. Measuring empathy in schizophrenia: The Empathic Accuracy Task and its correlation with other empathy measures. *Schizophr Res* (2019) 208:153–9. doi: 10.1016/j.schres.2019.03.024
54. de Jong S, van Donkersgoed R, Renard S, Carter S, Bokern H, Lysaker P, et al. Social-cognitive risk factors for violence in psychosis: A discriminant function analysis. *Psychiatry Res* (2018) 265:93–9. doi: 10.1016/j.psychres.2018.04.048
55. Harenski CL, Brook M, Kosson DS, Bustillo JR, Harenski KA, Caldwell MF, et al. Socio-neuro risk factors for suicidal behavior in criminal offenders with psychotic disorders. *Soc Cogn Affect Neurosci* (2017) 12(1):70–80. doi: 10.1093/scan/nsw164
56. Horan WP, Reise SP, Kern RS, Lee J, Penn DL, Green MF. Structure and correlates of self-reported empathy in schizophrenia. *J Psychiatr Res* (2015) 66:60–6. doi: 10.1016/j.jpsychires.2015.04.016
57. Davis MC, Green MF, Lee J, Horan WP, Senturk D, Clarke AD, et al. Oxytocin-augmented social cognitive skills training in schizophrenia. *Neuropsychopharmacology* (2014) 39(9):2070–7. doi: 10.1038/npp.2014.68
58. Ripoll LH, Zaki J, Perez-Rodriguez MM, Snyder R, Strike KS, Boussi A, et al. Empathic accuracy and cognition in schizotypal personality disorder. *Psychiatry Res* (2013) 210(1):232–41. doi: 10.1016/j.psychres.2013.05.025
59. Olbert CM, Penn DL, Kern RS, Lee J, Horan WP, Reise SP, et al. Adapting social neuroscience measures for schizophrenia clinical trials, part 3: fathoming external validity. *Schizophr Bull* (2013) 39(6):1211–8. doi: 10.1093/schbul/sbt130
60. Kern RS, Penn DL, Lee J, Horan WP, Reise SP, Ochsner KN, et al. Adapting social neuroscience measures for schizophrenia clinical trials, Part 2: trolling the depths of psychometric properties. *Schizophr Bull* (2013) 39(6):1201–10. doi: 10.1093/schbul/sbt127
61. Harvey PO, Zaki J, Lee J, Ochsner K, Green MF. Neural substrates of

empathic accuracy in people with schizophrenia. *Schizophr Bull* (2013) 39 (3):617–28. doi: 10.1093/schbul/sbs042

62. Lee J, Altshuler L, Glahn DC, Miklowitz DJ, Ochsner K, Green MF. Social and nonsocial cognition in bipolar disorder and schizophrenia: relative levels of impairment. *Am J Psychiatry* (2013) 170(3):334–41. doi: 10.1176/appi.ajp.2012.12040490
63. Lee J, Zaki J, Harvey PO, Ochsner K, Green MF. Schizophrenia patients are impaired in empathic accuracy. *psychol Med* (2011) 41(11):2297–304. doi: 10.1017/S0033291711000614
64. Adler N, Dvash J, Shamay-Tsoory SG. Empathic embarrassment accuracy in autism spectrum disorder. *Autism Res* (2015) 8(3):241–9. doi: 10.1002/aur.1439
65. aan het Rot M, Hogenelst K. The influence of affective empathy and autism spectrum traits on empathic accuracy. *PloS One* (2014) 9(6):e98436. doi: 10.1371/journal.pone.0098436
66. Demurie E, De Corel M, Roeyers H. Empathic accuracy in adolescents with autism spectrum disorders and adolescents with attention-deficit/hyperactivity disorder. *Res Autism Spectr Disord* (2011) 5(1):126–34. doi: 10.1016/j.rasd.2010.03.002
67. Bartz JA, Zaki J, Bolger N, Hollander E, Ludwig NN, Kolevzon A, et al. Oxytocin selectively improves empathic accuracy. *psychol Sci* (2010) 21 (10):1426–8. doi: 10.1177/0956797610383439
68. Ponnet K, Buysse A, Roeyers H, De Clercq A. Mind-reading in young adults with ASD: Does structure matter? *J Autism Dev Disord* (2008) 38(5):905–18. doi: 10.1007/s10803-007-0462-5
69. Ponnet K, Buysse A, Roeyers H, De Corte K. Empathic accuracy in adults with a pervasive developmental disorder during an unstructured conversation with a typically developing stranger. *J Autism Dev Disord* (2005) 35(5):585–600. doi: 10.1007/s10803-005-0003-z
70. Roeyers H, Buysse A, Ponnet K, Pichal B. Advancing advanced mind-reading tests: Empathic accuracy in adults with a pervasive developmental disorder. *J Child Psychol Psychiatry Allied Discipl* (2001) 42(2):271–8. doi: 10.1111/1469-7610.00718
71. Ponnet KS, Roeyers H, Buysse A, De Clercq A, Van Der Heyden E. Advanced mind-reading in adults with Asperger syndrome. *Autism* (2004) 8(3):249–66. doi: 10.1177/1362361304045214
72. aan het Rot M, Miloserdov K, Buijze AL, Meesters Y, Gordijn MC. Premenstrual mood and empathy after a single light therapy session. *Psychiatry Res* (2017) 256:212–8. doi: 10.1016/j.psychres.2017.06.052
73. Hogenelst K, Schoevers RA, Kema IP, Sweep FC, aan het Rot M. Empathic accuracy and oxytocin after tryptophan depletion in adults at risk for depression. *Psychopharmacology* (2016) 233(1):111–20. doi: 10.1007/s00213-015-4093-9
74. Gadassi R, Mor N, Rafaeli E. Depression and empathic accuracy in couples: An interpersonal model of gender differences in depression. *psychol Sci* (2011) 22(8):1033–41. doi: 10.1177/0956797611414728
75. Papp LM, Kouros CD, Cummings EM. Emotions in marital conflict interactions: Empathic accuracy, assumed similarity, and the moderating context of depressive symptoms. *J Soc Pers Relationships* (2010) 27(3):367–87. doi: 10.1177/0265407509348810
76. Thomas G, Fletcher GJ, Lange C. On-line empathic accuracy in marital interaction. *J Pers Soc Psychol* (1997) 72(4):839. doi: 10.1037/0022-3514.72.4.839
77. Morrison AS, Mateen MA, Brozovich FA, Zaki J, Goldin PR, Heimberg RG, et al. Empathy for positive and negative emotions in social anxiety disorder. *Behav Res Ther* (2016) 87:232–42. doi: 10.1016/j.brat.2016.10.005
78. Auyeung KW, Alden LE. Social anxiety and empathy for social pain. *Cogn Ther Res* (2016) 40(1):38–45. doi: 10.1007/s10608-015-9718-0
79. Simpson JA, Ickes W, Grich J. When accuracy hurts: Reactions of anxious-ambivalent dating partners to a relationship-threatening situation. *J Pers Soc Psychol* (1999) 76(5):754. doi: 10.1037/0022-3514.76.5.754
80. Miano A, Dziobek I, Roepke S. Understanding interpersonal dysfunction in borderline personality disorder: A naturalistic dyadic study reveals absence of relationship-protective empathic inaccuracy. *Clin psychol Sci* (2017) 5 (2):355–66. doi: 10.1177/2167702616683505
81. Flury JM, Ickes W, Schweinle W. The borderline empathy effect: Do high BPD individuals have greater empathic ability? Or are they just more difficult to "read"? *J Res Personality* (2008) 42(2):312–32. doi: 10.1016/j.jrp.2007.05.008
82. Martin-Key N, Brown T, Fairchild G. Empathic accuracy in male adolescents with conduct disorder and higher versus lower levels of callous-unemotional traits. *J Abnormal Child Psychol* (2017) 45(7):1385–97. doi: 10.1007/s10802-016-0243-8
83. De Ridder J, Pihet S, Suter M, Caldara R. Empathy in institutionalized adolescents with callous-unemotional traits: An ecological momentary assessment study of emotion recognition. *Crim Justice Behav* (2016) 43 (5):653–69. doi: 10.1177/0093854815618431
84. Brook M, Kosson DS. Impaired cognitive empathy in criminal psychopathy: Evidence from a laboratory measure of empathic accuracy. *J Abnormal Psychol* (2013) 122(1):156. doi: 10.1037/a0030261
85. Devlin HC, Zaki J, Ong DC, Gruber J. Tracking the emotional highs but missing the lows: Hypomania risk is associated with positively biased empathic inference. *Cogn Ther Res* (2016) 40(1):72–9. doi: 10.1007/s10608-015-9720-6
86. Brown CL, Lwi SJ, Goodkind MS, Rankin KP, Merrilees J, Miller BL, et al. Empathic accuracy deficits in patients with neurodegenerative disease: association with caregiver depression. *Am J Geriatr Psychiatry* (2018) 26 (4):484–93. doi: 10.1016/j.jagp.2017.10.012
87. Doyle-Thomas KA, Lee W, Foster NE, Tryfon A, Ouimet T, Hyde KL, et al. Atypical functional brain connectivity during rest in autism spectrum disorders. *Ann Neurol* (2015) 77(5):866–76. doi: 10.1002/ana.24391
88. Wells JL, Brown CL, Hua AY, Soyster PD, Chen KH, Dokuru DR, et al. Neurodegenerative Disease Caregivers'5-HTTLPR Genotype Moderates the Effect of Patients' Empathic Accuracy Deficits on Caregivers' Well-Being. *Am J Geriatr Psychiatry* (2019) 27(10):1046–56. doi: 10.1016/j.jagp.2019.04.009
89. Reniers RL, Corcoran R, Drake R, Shryane NM, Völlm BA. The QCAE: A questionnaire of cognitive and affective empathy. *J Pers Assessment* (2011) 93 (1):84–95. doi: 10.1080/00223891.2010.528484
90. Gross JJ, John OP, Richards J. *Berkeley expressivity questionnaire*. Lewiston, NY: Edwin Mellen Press (1995).
91. Marangoni C, Garcia S, Ickes W, Teng G. Empathic accuracy in a clinically relevant setting. *J Pers Soc Psychol* (1995) 68(5):854. doi: 10.1037/0022-3514.68.5.854
92. Baron-Cohen S, Wheelwright S, Skinner R, Martin J, Clubley E. The autism-spectrum quotient (AQ): Evidence from asperger syndrome/high-functioning autism, malesand females, scientists and mathematicians. *J Autism Dev Disord* (2001) 31(1):5–17. doi: 10.1023/A:1005653411471
93. Rush AJ, Trivedi MH, Ibrahim HM, Carmody TJ, Arnow B, Klein DN, et al. The 16-Item Quick Inventory of Depressive Symptomatology (QIDS), clinician rating (QIDS-C), and self-report (QIDS-SR): a psychometric evaluation in patients with chronic major depression. *Biol Psychiatry* (2003) 54(5):573–83. doi: 10.1016/S0006-3223(02)01866-8
94. Brennan KA, Clark CL, Shaver PR. Self-report measurement of adult attachment: An integrative overview. In: Simpson JA, Rholes WS, editors. *Attachment theory and close relationships*. New York: Guilford Press (1998).
95. Griffin DW, Bartholomew K. Models of the self and other: Fundamental dimensions underlying measures of adult attachment. *J Pers Soc Psychol* (1994) 67(3):430. doi: 10.1037/0022-3514.67.3.430
96. Carter L, Rinsley DB. Vicissitudes of' empathy'in a borderline adolescent. *Int Rev Psycho-Analysis* (1977) 4:317–26.
97. Krohn A. Borderline "empathy" and differentiation of object representations: a contribution to the psychology of object relations. *Int J Psychoanal Psychother* (1974) 3(2):142.
98. Conte HR, Plutchik R, Karasu TB, Jerrett I. A self-report borderline scale: Discriminative validity and preliminary norms. *J Nervous Ment Dis* (1980) 168(7):428–35. doi: 10.1097/00005053-198007000-00007
99. Campbell L, Kashy DA. Estimating actor, partner, and interaction effects for dyadic data using PROC MIXED and HLM: A user-friendly guide. *Pers Relationships* (2002) 9(3):327–42. doi: 10.1111/1475-6811.00023
100. Kashy DA, Kenny DA. The analysis of data from dyads and groups. In: Reis HT, Judd CM, editors. *Handbook of research methods in social and personality psychology*. New York: Cambridge University Press (2000) p. 451–77.
101. Kenny DA. Models of non-independence in dyadic research. *J Soc Pers Relationships* (1996) 13(2):279–94. doi: 10.1177/0265407596132007
102. Eckblad M, Chapman LJ. Development and validation of a scale for hypomanic personality. *J Abnormal Psychol* (1986) 95(3):214. doi: 10.1037/0021-843X.95.3.214

103. Feldman R, Golan O, Hirschler-Guttenberg Y, Ostfeld-Etzion S, Zagoory-Sharon O. Parent–child interaction and oxytocin production in pre-schoolers with autism spectrum disorder. *Br J Psychiatry* (2014) 205 (2):107–12. doi: 10.1192/bjp.bp.113.137513
104. Milton DE. On the ontological status of autism: the 'double empathy problem'. *Disability Soc* (2012) 27(6):883–7. doi: 10.1080/09687599.2012.710008
105. Milton DEM, Heasman B, Sheppard E. Double Empathy. In: Volkmar F, editors *Encyclopedia of Autism Spectrum Disorders*. New York, NY: Springer (2018). doi: 10.1007/978-1-4614-6435-8_102273-1
106. Gould J, Ashton-Smith J. Missed diagnosis or misdiagnosis? Girls and women on the autism spectrum. *Good Autism Pract (GAP)* (2011) 12 (1):34–41.
107. Kirkovski M, Enticott PG, Fitzgerald PB. A review of the role of female gender in autism spectrum disorders. *J Autism Dev Disord* (2013) 43 (11):2584–603. doi: 10.1007/s10803-013-1811-1
108. Van Wijngaarden-Cremers PJ, van Eeten E, Groen WB, Van Deurzen PA, Oosterling IJ, Van der Gaag RJ. Gender and age differences in the core triad of impairments in autism spectrum disorders: a systematic review and meta-analysis. *J Autism Dev Disord* Abingdon, Oxon: Routledge (2014) 44(3):627–35. doi: 10.1007/s10803-013-1913-9
109. Carpenter B, Happé F, Egerton J eds. *Girls and autism: educational, family and personal perspectives*. Abingdon, Oxon: Routledge. (2019). Feb 7.
110. Schweinle WE, Ickes W, Bernstein IH. Emphatic inaccuracy in husband to wife aggression: The overattribution bias. *Pers Relationships* (2002) 9(2):141–58. doi: 10.1111/1475-6811.00009
111. Clements K, Holtzworth-Munroe A, Schweinle W, Ickes W. Empathic accuracy of intimate partners in violent versus nonviolent relationships. *Pers Relationships* (2007) 14(3):369–88. doi: 10.1111/j.1475-6811.2007.00161.x
112. Ickes W, Simpson JA. Motivational aspects of empathic accuracy. In: Fletcher GJO, Clark MS, editors, *Blackwell handbook of social psychology: Interpersonal processes*. Malden, MA: Blackwell (2003) pp. 229–49. doi: 10.1002/9780470998557.ch9

8

Speech Prosody as a Bridge between Psychopathology and Linguistics: The Case of the Schizophrenia Spectrum

Valeria Lucarini[1], Martine Grice[2], Francesco Cangemi[2], Juliane T. Zimmermann[3], Carlo Marchesi[1], Kai Vogeley[3,4] and Matteo Tonna[5]*

[1] Psychiatry Unit, Department of Medicine and Surgery, Medical Faculty, University of Parma, Parma, Italy, [2] IfL-Phonetics, University of Cologne, Cologne, Germany, [3] Department of Psychiatry and Psychotherapy, Medical Faculty, University of Cologne, Cologne, Germany, [4] Cognitive Neuroscience (INM-3), Institute of Neuroscience and Medicine, Research Center Jülich, Jülich, Germany, [5] Department of Mental Health, Azienda Unità Sanitaria Locale di Parma, Parma, Italy

***Correspondence:**
Valeria Lucarini
valeria.lucarini@studenti.unipr.it

Patients with schizophrenia spectrum disorders experience severe difficulties in interpersonal communication, as described by traditional psychopathology and current research on social cognition. From a linguistic perspective, pragmatic abilities are crucial for successful communication. Empirical studies have shown that these abilities are significantly impaired in this group of patients. Prosody, the tone of voice with which words and sentences are pronounced, is one of the most important carriers of pragmatic meaning and can serve a range of functions from linguistic to emotional ones. Most of the existing literature on prosody of patients with schizophrenia spectrum disorders focuses on the expression of emotion, generally showing significant impairments. By contrast, the use of non-emotional prosody in these patients is scarcely investigated. In this paper, we first present a linguistic model to classify prosodic functions. Second, we discuss existing studies on the use of non-emotional prosody in these patients, providing an overview of the state of the art. Third, we delineate possible future lines of research in this field, also taking into account some classical psychopathological assumptions, for both diagnostic and therapeutic purposes.

Keywords: communication, non-emotional, prosody, pragmatics, psychopathology, linguistics, schizophrenia spectrum

INTRODUCTION

Schizophrenia Spectrum and Communication: Disorders of Pragmatic Abilities

Patients with schizophrenia spectrum disorders typically present with significant difficulties in social functioning that can occur in various areas, including in interpersonal communication (1). Schizophrenia has traditionally been described primarily as a communication disorder (2–6). There is currently a great interest in this topic in social cognition research (7).

Successful interpersonal communication relies on conversation partners being able to express and perceive different content *via* their verbal or nonverbal messages. Pragmatics, the branch of linguistics that takes into account the relationship between language and its context, including the correct interpretation of non-literal contents, plays a major role (8). Empirical studies focusing on language have shown a severe impairment of pragmatic abilities (like the capacity to comprehend humor, irony and metaphors) (9, 10) in patients with schizophrenia (11). Moreover, pragmatic deficits negatively correlate with global social functioning (8), significantly contributing, therefore, to the difficulties in social interaction displayed by these patients (12).

Impairments in the comprehension of non-literal meanings, referred to as "concretism" (13), have always been considered distinctive traits of the schizophrenia spectrum by psychopathology. In addition, there is a strong connection between these communication difficulties and one of the core features of the disorders (14, 15), the so-called "hypoattunement" (16, 17) with others, i.e., the incapacity to intuitively grasp unwritten rules of social interactions.

Prosody as a Fundamental Pragmatic Tool

One of the most important carriers of pragmatic meaning is prosody, the tone of voice with which words and sentences are pronounced (18–20). Thus, pragmatic abilities are strongly dependent on prosodic encoding and decoding, achieved mostly through the modulation of fundamental frequency, duration and intensity (18). Prosody is used to divide utterances into chunks, or prosodic phrases, involving the insertion of boundary tones marking the edges of these phrases (18). It also has the role of highlighting certain elements within these phrases by means of accentuation (18). It is important to explore the range of meanings prosody can convey which are often difficult to tease apart and frequently expressed simultaneously. Prosody can have grammatical, pragmatic or emotional functions (21), also referred to as linguistic (grammatical and pragmatic) and paralinguistic (emotional) (22), constituting a continuum (22), as proposed by Grice and Baumann in their model (22) (see **Figure 1**).

At a grammatical level, prosody can provide lexical and syntactic information. For example, in some cases prosody indicates a change in grammatical class (e.g., the word "permit" in English with stress on the first syllable is a noun, while with stress on the second syllable, it is a verb) (18). Prosody can also be used to resolve ambiguities in syntactic structure, such as the attachment of modifiers or relative clauses (e.g., "Jane looked at the man with the binoculars", in which the binoculars are either used as a viewing device by Jane, or being held by the man being looked at). Prosody can be used to discriminate between questions and statements (18), a function at the interface of grammar and pragmatics. The pragmatic role of prosody can be crucial. In fact, prosody is often the most important means to transmit and

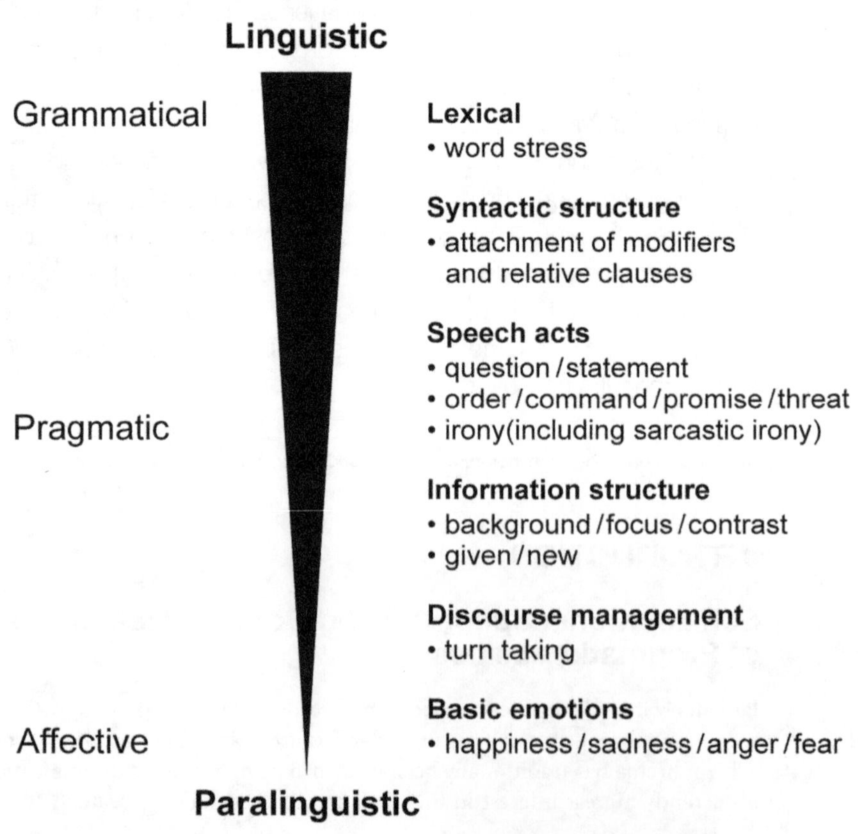

FIGURE 1 | Categorization of prosodic functions [adapted by the authors from Grice and Baumann, (22) and Krüger (18)].

understand the communicative purpose of the speaker, helping to distinguish whether a certain phrase is an order, a desire, a promise or a threat. Another important pragmatic role of prosody is the structuring of the elements of a statement in terms of their "givenness", i.e., whether the element is new or was mentioned before, and therefore given. For example, "I bought a $car_{[NEW]}$" refers to the car for the first time (new). A follow-up utterance "Do you want to *see* the $car_{[GIVEN]}$?" refers to the car for a second time and it is therefore given. Referents can also be in focus or in the background (18). For example, in a context such as "What did you buy?" "I bought *a* $car_{[FOCUS]}$", the car is in focus, whereas in the context "Did you buy a new car?" "No, I *borrowed* [FOCUS] a car[BACKGROUND]" the car is in the background. Moreover, prosody plays a role in controlling turn-taking, e.g., rising pitch indicating the speaker has not yet finished. Finally, prosody can express the emotional state of the speaker (18). Note that such functions (listed in **Figure 1**) are not always clearly distinct and the use of emotional prosody greatly contributes to promoting contextualization in communicative interactions. In recent years, there has been considerable development of technological tools for experimental linguistics, which has permitted the study of these aspects of language in greater depth.

Research on Prosody in Schizophrenia Spectrum Disorders: State of the Art and Purpose of This Review

Most of the literature on prosody in patients with schizophrenia spectrum disorders has focused on recognition of emotional functions. There is a general consensus on significant impairments in this capacity, despite the heterogeneity of the tasks used (23, 24). However, these deficits only partially explain the difficulties in communicative situations displayed by these patients. Some of the communicative impairments could be further accounted for by difficulties with non-emotional prosody which have scarcely been investigated in patients with schizophrenia spectrum disorders.

The present paper summarizes the main existing studies on the topic. It provides an overview of the state of the art, with papers selected from a search on PubMed and Google Scholar of those published in the period between 1990 and November 2019 (search strategies: schizo* AND prosod*; psychosis AND prosod*; schizophrenia AND prosody NOT emotion NOT affect; psychosis AND prosody NOT emotion NOT affect). From the initial 217 papers, we finally selected 11 studies reporting on patients with any of the following diagnoses: schizophrenia, schizoaffective disorder, first episode psychosis, persons at risk of psychosis, schizotypal personality disorder. We considered all the articles referring to schizophrenia spectrum, together with first episode psychosis and conditions at risk of psychosis, in order to include the whole continuum of different stages of schizophrenia psychopathology (from vulnerability and trait conditions to full-blown disorder). Therefore, the diagnoses of affective psychosis or other psychotic, non-schizophrenia disorders were excluded. We only selected studies in which these groups were compared with healthy controls in their ability to perceive and/or produce non-emotional prosody. Finally, studies had to be written in English. In addition, we manually searched for papers from reference lists of the main articles and reviews, finding one additional study. While focusing mainly on findings regarding pragmatic prosody, we also included results on grammatical prosody, as these are not always clearly distinguishable. Building on this review, the aim of the paper is to identify controversies and limitations of this important, though relatively thin, strand of literature and to delineate possible future lines of research in this field, guided by classical psychopathological notions.

PERCEPTION OF NON-EMOTIONAL PROSODY IN PATIENTS WITH SCHIZOPHRENIA SPECTRUM DISORDERS

Although some studies found an intact performance, there is evidence of a deficit in the perception of non-emotional prosody in patients with schizophrenia spectrum disorders. Below we present the empirical evidence following the continuum of prosodic functions (see **Figure 1**). **Table 1** provides an overview of all studies mentioned in this section.

To our knowledge, no study has assessed the role of prosody to provide lexical information in patients with schizophrenia spectrum disorders so far. The perception of prosody to resolve syntactic ambiguity has been tested by Rabagliati and colleagues (30). In their

TABLE 1 | Perception of non-emotional prosody by patients with schizophrenia spectrum disorders.

	Grammatical	**Pragmatic**			
Functions	***Syntactic structure***	***Speech acts***			***Information structure***
Details	**Prosodic phrases**	**Question/Statement**	**Order/Command**	**Irony (including sarcastic irony)**	**Background/Focus/ Contrast**
Diff. bt. Groups	Matsumoto et al. (25) (not sign.)	Pawełczyk et al. (26) Caletti et al. (27)	Pawełczyk et al. (26)	Leitman et al. (28), Kantrowitz et al. (29)	Matsumoto et al. (25)
No diff. bt. Groups	Rabagliati et al. (30)	Matsumoto et al. (25) Edwards et al. (31) Castagna et al. (32) Pawełczyk et al. (26, 33) (FEP, UHR, relatives)	Pawełczyk et al. (26, 33) (FEP, UHR, relatives) Caletti et al. (27)		Murphy and Cutting (34)

study, participants with schizophrenia were instructed to manipulate a set of objects on the basis of sentences with variations in the phrasing, determining a bias toward or against a target instrument [e.g., "You can poke the frog ... with the feather" vs "You can poke ... the frog with the feather" (30)]. The use of the linguistic cues was investigated by tracking eye movements. Results showed that patients and healthy controls did not differ in task performance. This prosodic function was also evaluated by Matsumoto and colleagues (25), who tested patients with schizophrenia and healthy controls in the discrimination of pairs of sentences that differed only in phrasing (like in "Francis, the doctor is ready to begin" and "Francis, the doctor, is ready to begin") (35, 36). Although patients showed a reduced capacity to recognize these changes, the difference did not reach significance. The same study investigated another prosodic function, namely the discrimination between questions and statements. Sentences (e.g., "She plays the flute") (35, 36) were pronounced with an intonation indicating either a question or a statement. Patients had to detect and point out the difference. The authors did not find an impairment regarding this ability. These findings were replicated in studies with a similar design, where sentences spoken with statement or question intonation were to be correctly identified. These studies also enrolled patients with first episode schizophrenia (31, 32). Contrary to these findings, Pawełczyk and colleagues (26, 33, 37) recently reported a significant difference between patients with schizophrenia and healthy controls in the use of prosody to decode the communicative purpose of the speaker. They tested patients with schizophrenia, patients with first episode schizophrenia, participants at ultra-high risk of psychosis and first-degree relatives of patients with schizophrenia by means of the "Right Hemisphere Language Battery". This comprises tasks assessing several pragmatic capacities, including abilities in prosodic processing. Participants listened to sentences read with a statement, question, or command intonation, and indicated for each of them their respective communicative purpose. Apart from the difference between patients with schizophrenia and healthy controls, the authors did not find a difference among subjects at high risk of psychosis, patients with first episode schizophrenia and healthy controls. The ability to detect the same intonation patterns was tested by another recent study (27), which included patients with first episode psychosis (affective and non-affective) and healthy control subjects. Semantically neutral sentences were pronounced with the same three intonation patterns (question/statement/command) and participants had to choose the correct one. The results showed lower scores in both patient groups as compared to controls only regarding the capacity to correctly map question intonation, while no impairment was found for statement and command patterns. Likewise, Leitman and colleagues and Kantrowitz and colleagues (28, 29) investigated the use of prosody to identify speech acts, this time sarcastic irony. They found a deficit in patients with schizophrenia in comparison to healthy controls in the capacity to correctly interpret sentences read in a sincere or sarcastic manner.

Finally, we turn to information structure. Items that are new or in focus are often prosodically highlighted. Murphy and Cutting (34) compared patients with schizophrenia, bipolar disorder in a manic phase, major depression and a group of healthy controls in their ability to recognize the highlighted word in a set of sentences. The authors did not find impairments in patients with schizophrenia. These results conflict with those of Matsumoto and colleagues (25), who also tested patients' ability to discriminate highlighted words. They used sentence pairs (like "The orange *flowers* smell very sweet" vs "The *orange* flowers smell very sweet") (35, 36) and found a significant impairment in patients with schizophrenia as compared to controls.

PRODUCTION OF NON-EMOTIONAL PROSODY IN PATIENTS WITH SCHIZOPHRENIA SPECTRUM DISORDERS

The production of non-emotional prosody in patients with schizophrenia spectrum disorders has been investigated mainly in terms of acoustic parameters of patients' speech. Generally, the experiments used to analyze participants' discourse consisted of clinical interviews (38), free speech tasks (39–43), descriptions of images (44–46) or reading tasks (39, 41, 47). Compared to that of healthy control subjects, the speech of patients on the schizophrenia spectrum appears less fluent (40), contains more and longer pauses (44, 47) as well as less pitch variability (measured as the variance of fundamental frequency for each syllable) (40, 43). Although prosodic parameters were associated neither with antipsychotic dosage (38, 47) nor with positive symptoms (46, 47), an association with negative symptoms was found (38, 40, 46, 48). Moreover, illness-duration had an effect on the performance of patients in prosodic tasks (47). Subjects with schizotypal personality disorder were shown to exhibit a slower speech, with more pauses and less variability in pitch, as compared to healthy controls (41), whereas Cohen and colleagues (45) found differences in prosodic traits only for subjects with negative schizotypal traits.

For the productive use of linguistic prosody, the previously reported study by Murphy and Cutting (34) also tested patients' ability to highlight a specific word (and thus to indicate its information status). The sentences read aloud by participants were recorded and rated by four raters according to the question which word sounded highlighted to them. The authors did not find a difference between the groups in this task. To our knowledge, only one study, conducted by Michelas and colleagues (49), specifically focused on the production of pragmatic prosody. The authors tested a group of patients with schizophrenia and healthy controls regarding their capacity to signal the focus or background status of an element in a sentence. Participants had to explain to a confederate a designated route on a map, with pairs of landmarks, each composed of two noun-adjective fragments. The pairs could contain the same noun and a different adjective, e.g., bonbons marrons ("brown candies") vs. bonbons violets ("purple candies"), (49) or a different noun and the same adjective, e.g., bougies violettes ("purple candles") vs. bonbons violets ("purple candies") (49). Participants had to use prosodic phrasing to encode the contrastive status of the referent. Even though patients had the ability to produce the same types of phrasing as control participants, they did not appropriately adjust their use of phrasing to the context.

DISCUSSION

The Role of Non-Emotional Prosody in Schizophrenia Spectrum: The Evidence So Far

Altogether, there is evidence that in patients with schizophrenia spectrum disorders the capacity for processing grammatical prosody is intact, both with respect to the ability to use phrasing to resolve syntactic ambiguities (30) and with respect to the identification of a question or statement intonation (25, 31, 32), although for the latter there is no general consensus (26, 27). It should be noted that a possible limitation of these studies might be the high simplicity of the tasks, e.g., in (25) patients were required simply to signal if two intonations (question/ statement) were different, without having to identify them. When assessing more specifically the prosodic expression of pragmatic functions, these patients show specific impairments as compared to controls (26, 28, 29). In terms of the identification of the speaker's communicative purpose, the literature focuses on the detection of sarcasm (28, 29) and commands (26). Moreover, patients seem to be impaired in their capacity to use prosody to decode and encode the structural information of a sentence with regard to given/new and focus/background elements (25), although other results conflict with this finding (34). Again, the simplicity of the task of the study of Murphy and Cutting (34) might partially explain the inconsistency of these results.

The use of non-emotional prosody in patients with schizophrenia spectrum disorders has seldom been compared with other clinical groups. Edwards and colleagues (31) did not find significant differences in performance among patients with first episode schizophrenia, first episode affective psychosis or the first episode of other psychotic disorders in their ability to distinguish between a statement and question intonation, similar to the findings of Caletti and colleagues (27). Likewise, in the study of Murphy and Cutting (34), patients diagnosed with schizophrenia, mania, and depression did not differ from the healthy controls regarding their use of pragmatic prosody when recognizing and encoding a highlighted word in a sentence. Few studies investigated a possible association of the perception and production of prosody with clinical measures. Schizophrenia illness duration and antipsychotic treatment dosage have not been shown to correlate with the ability to use prosody to encode the contrastive status of a referent (49) nor with sarcasm detection (29). Results on the relationship with the principal symptom dimensions are controversial. The accuracy to discriminate background/focus information by means of prosodic cues appears negatively correlated with positive symptoms (25), while Michelas and colleagues (49) did not find a relationship between clinical symptomatology and the ability to use prosody to encode the contrastive status of a referent. The ability to detect sarcasm was not associated with positive symptoms, but it correlated with avolition (28). The capacity to correctly map question, statement or command intonation patterns was associated neither with positive symptoms, nor with negative ones (27) in people with first episode psychosis. Altogether, the evidence so far is too scant to draw firm conclusions about these correlations.

Finally, the capacity to use pragmatic prosody was associated with Theory of Mind scores (49) and a significant positive correlation was found between the ability to detect sarcasm and general functioning (29).

In sum, results about the relationship between the use of non-emotional prosody and vulnerability to psychosis (27, 33, 37) are inconclusive. Evidence for impairment in non-emotional prosody processing in first-episode schizophrenia, in ultra-high risk- or in first-degree relative groups was not found, but this last result (33) was not confirmed in larger samples of patients with first episode schizophrenia (27, 37). Interestingly, the Right Hemisphere Language Battery was not originally conceived for patients with schizophrenia. Some tasks may be too simple for less chronically affected patients or unaffected subjects.

The main limitation of the present review is that it is not a systematic one. Nevertheless, to our knowledge this is the first attempt to date to sum up the existing literature about the use of non-emotional prosodic cues by patients with schizophrenia spectrum disorders.

Perspective on Future Research

The existing literature focusing on the use of non-emotional prosody in patients with schizophrenia spectrum disorders is still very limited. Further research is needed to shed light on the existing results. We suggest that these lines of research should be extended, for a deeper understanding of the specific communicative impairments underlying the disorders. This in turn could contribute to a better diagnosis and possibly help discriminating between schizophrenia and other psychiatric conditions in the future. Moreover, there is evidence of the efficacy of training targeting both pragmatic skills and the use of prosody (50, 51). This could help to design specific and more sophisticated tools, paving the way towards new promising therapeutic approaches.

We have identified some possible points to be addressed by the future research agenda regarding the use of non-emotional prosody by patients with schizophrenia spectrum disorders. The following require investigation:

1. *A number of prosodic functions that have not been investigated so far.* These include (a) The capacity to understand other speakers' communicative purposes conveyed through prosody, beyond those already tested (sarcasm and commands), especially the ability to correctly detect a threatening disposition. As previously mentioned, the core feature of schizophrenia spectrum is an impairment in the tacit understanding of social situations (17). This can also affect the ability to capture the communicative purpose of the speaker and may elicit compensatory mechanisms (17), contributing to further misinterpretations of social signals,

for example leading to persecutory ideas. This is in line with the hypothesis of schizophrenic delusions as due to a "disturbance or breakdown of communication" (52). Another prosodic function is (b) the management of turn-taking. There is evidence of a specific impairment of this function in schizophrenia (53), but the role played by prosody has not been explored so far. A fluid transition in turn-taking implies a high level of rhythmicity between partners (54). A disruption in the shared rhythm between the individual and the environment is traditionally considered a central feature in schizophrenia spectrum (55) and there is empirical evidence for impaired interpersonal synchronization in these patients (56). Prosody, which naturally and implicitly reflects interpersonal synchronization, may represent a key feature of intersubjective "desynchronization" (57) in schizophrenia spectrum disorders. A further prosodic function is (c) the structuring of the elements of a sentence into given/new or focus/background partitions. This has only been scarcely assessed in these patients and a specific investigation of this ability should most definitely be a topic of future research.

2. *Further investigation of the link between prosody deficits and social cognition capacities, such as Theory of Mind.* Schizophrenia has been described as a disorder of social cognition (7) and prosody as a tool playing a crucial role in social interaction (18). A deeper understanding of the use of prosody by patients with schizophrenia spectrum disorders could also shed light on its role in social cognition in general.
3. *The comparison of different clinical groups in their use of non-emotional prosody.* This could help to identify specific profiles of capacities and disorders and to understand if linguistic difficulties (in particular prosodic) are to be considered specific to schizophrenia spectrum disorders. Interestingly, schizophrenia has also been described primarily as a linguistic disorder, ("the price that Homo sapiens paid for language" (Crow, 4). From this perspective, the study of prosody in this clinical population warrants even more interest.
4. *A deeper understanding of possible links between the use of non-emotional prosody and clinical variables, in line with the Research Domain Criteria (RDoC) strategy.* This approach aims at combining several data types, e.g., neurobiological or clinical data, to investigate basic domains of functioning underlying human behavior (like cognition and social processes) for the study of psychiatric conditions (58). For example, investigating if prosodic abilities are linked to negative or positive dimensions could help to understand if linguistic capacities are related to the core symptoms of the disorder.
5. *Further studies assessing the use of non-emotional prosody in people with a vulnerability to schizophrenia.* This would enable us to understand if the impairments are to be considered trait or state conditions. Giving the importance of an early diagnosis in these conditions, it is crucial to find signs that can aid the identification of subjects at risk of schizophrenia prior to the full expression of the disorder.
6. *The examination of the interaction between prosody and other non-verbal cues, like gaze behavior or gestures, on the basis of real-life communicative situations.* To investigate this interaction, it is particularly important to pay attention to the ecological validity of experimental tasks.

A deeper knowledge of the use of non-emotional prosody in patients with schizophrenia spectrum disorders could be helpful also for the study of other communication disorders. Further research should extend this approach to other psychiatric conditions that entail impairments regarding the use of prosody, such as autism spectrum disorders (18, 59, 60).

AUTHOR CONTRIBUTIONS

VL wrote the first manuscript version in accordance with theoretical discussions with MG, KV and MT. CM, FC, and JZ contributed with literature and theoretical ideas. All authors read and modified the manuscript several times. All authors contributed to the article and approved the submitted version.

REFERENCES

1. Couture SM, Penn DL, Roberts DL. The functional significance of social cognition in schizophrenia: a review. *Schizophr Bull* (2006) 32(1):44–63. doi: 10.1093/schbul/sbl029
2. Bleuler E. *Dementia praecox oder Gruppe der Schizophrenien*. Neuausgabe, Psychosozialverlag: Gießen (2014). p. 445.
3. Kraepelin E. *Psychiatrie. Ein Lehrbuch für Studierende und Ärzte (6. Auflage)*. Johann Ambrosius Barth: Leipzig (1899). p. 364.
4. Crow TJ. Schizophrenia as the price that Homo sapiens pays for language: a resolution of the central paradox in the origin of the species. *Brain Res Brain Res Rev* (2000) 31:118–29. doi: 10.1016/s0165-0173(99)00029-6
5. Dörr-Zegers O. The group of schizophrenias as logopathies. *J Psychopathol* (2016) 22:55–61.
6. Ruesch J. *Disturbed communication: the clinical assessment of normal and pathological communicative behaviour*. Norton & Company: New York (1957). p. 337.
7. Green MF, Leitman DI. Social cognition in schizophrenia. *Schizophr Bull* (2008) 34(4):670–2. doi: 10.1093/schbul/sbn045
8. Bambini V, Arcara G, Bechi M, Buonocore M, Cavallaro R, Bosia M. The communicative impairment as a core feature of schizophrenia: frequency of pragmatic deficit, cognitive substrates and relation with quality of life. *Compr Psychiatry* (2016) 71:106–20. doi: 10.1016/j.comppsych.2016.08.012
9. Kuperberg GR. Language and schizophrenia. Part 1: an introduction. *Lang Linguist Compass* (2010a) 4:576–89. doi: 10.1111/j.1749-818X.2010.00216.x
10. Kuperberg GR. Language and schizophrenia. Part 2: what can psycholinguistic bring to the study of schizophrenia ... and vice versa? *Lang Linguist Compass* (2010b) 4:590–604. doi: 10.1111/j.1749-818X.2010.00217.x
11. Covington M, He C, Brown C, Naçi L, McClain JT, Fjordbak BS, et al. Schizophrenia and the structure of language: the linguist's view. *Schizophr Res* (2005) 77:85–98-. doi: 10.1016/J.schres.2005.01.016
12. Champagne-Lavau M, Stip E. Pragmatic and executive dysfunction in schizophrenia. *J Neuroling* (2010) 23:285–96. doi: 10.1016/j.ijneuroling.2009.08.009
13. Goldstein K. Concerning the concreteness in schizophrenia. *J Abnorm Psychol* (1959) 59(1):146–8. doi: 10.1037/h0045400

14. Sass L, Pienkos E, Skodlar B, Stanghellini G, Fuchs T, Parnas J, et al. EAWE: Examination of Anomalous World Experience. *Psychopathology* (2017) 50:10–54. doi: 10.1159/000454928
15. Pienkos E, Sass L. Language: On the Phenomenology of Linguistic Experience in Schizophrenia (Ancillary Article to EAWE Domain 4). *Psychopathology* (2017) 50:83–9. doi: 10.1159/000455195
16. Stanghellini G. Vulnerability to schizophrenia and lack of common sense. *Schizophr Bull* (2000) 26(4):775–87. doi: 10.1093/oxfordjournals.schbul.a033493
17. Stanghellini G, Ballerini M, Mancini M. Other Persons: On the Phenomenology of Interpersonal Experience in Schizophrenia (Ancillary Article to EAWE Domain 3). *Psychopathology* (2017) 50:75–82. doi: 10.1159/000456037
18. Krüger M. *Prosodic decoding and encoding of referential givenness in adults with autism spectrum disorders.* [Cologne(IL)]: University of Cologne (2018). [dissertation/doctoral thesis].
19. Lehiste I. *Suprasegmentals.* MIT Press: Cambridge, MA (1970). p. 194.
20. Lehiste I. Suprasegmental features of speech. In: Lass NJ, editor. *Contemporary issues in experimental phonetics.* New York: Academic Press (1976). p. 256–39.
21. Shriberg LD, Paul R, Mc Sweeny JL, Klin AM, Cohen DJ, Volkmar FR. Speech and prosody characteristics of adolescents and adults with high-functioning autism and Asperger syndrome. *J Speech Lang Hear Res* (2001) 44:1097–115. doi: 10.1044/1092-4388(2001/087)
22. Grice M, Baumann S. An introduction to intonation – functions and models. In: Trouvain J, Gut U, editors. *Non-Native Prosody. Phonetic Description and Teaching Practice. Trends in Linguistics. Studies and Monographs [TiLSM].* Berlin & New York: De Gruyter (2007). p. 25–51.
23. Hoekert M, Kahn RS, Pijnenborg M, Aleman A. Impaired recognition and expression of emotional prosody in schizophrenia: review and meta-analysis. *Schizophr Res* (2007) 96:135–45. doi: 10.1016/j.schres.2007.07.023
24. Lin Y, Ding H, Zhang Y. Emotional prosody processing in schizophrenic patients: a selective review and meta-analysis. *J Clin Med* (2018) 7(10):363. doi: 10.3390/jcm7100363
25. Matsumoto K, Samson GT, O'Daly OD, Tracy DK, Patel AD, Shergill SS. Prosodic discrimination in patients with schizophrenia. *Br J Psychiatry* (2006) 189:180–1. doi: 10.1192/bjp.bp.105.009332
26. Pawełczyk A, Kotlicka-Antczak M, Łojek E, Ruszpel A, Pawełczyk T. Schizophrenia patients have higher-order language and extralinguistic impairments. *Schizophr Res* (2018) 192:274–80. doi: 10.1016/j.schres.2017.04.030
27. Caletti E, Delvecchio G, Andreella A, Finos L, Perlini C, Tavano A, et al. Prosody abilities in a large sample of affective and non-affective first episode psychosis patients. *Compr Psychiatry* (2018) 86:31–8. doi: 10.1016/j.comppsych.2018.07.004
28. Leitman DI, Ziwich R, Pasternak R, Javitt DC. Theory of Mind (ToM) and counterfactuality deficits in schizophrenia: misperception or misinterpretation? *Psychol Med* (2006) 36:1075–83. doi: 10.1017/S0033291706007653
29. Kantrowitz JT, Hoptman MJ, Leitman DI, Silipo G, Javitt DC. The 5% difference: early sensory processing predicts sarcasm perception in schizophrenia and schizoaffective disorder. *Psychol Med* (2014) 44(1):25–36. doi: 10.1017/S0033291713000834
30. Rabagliati H, Delaney-Busch N, Snedeker J, Kuperberg G. Spared bottom-up but impaired top-down interactive effect during naturalistic language processing in schizophrenia: evidence from the visual-world paradigm. *Psychol Med* (2019) 49(8):1335–45. doi: 10.1017/S0033291718001952
31. Edwards J, Pattison PE, Jackson HJ, Wales RJ. Facial affect and affective prosody recognition in first-episode schizophrenia. *Schizophr Res* (2001) 48:235–53. doi: 10.1016/s0920-9964(00)00099-2
32. Castagna F, Montemagni C, Milani AM, Rocca G, Rocca P, Casacchia M, et al. Prosody recognition and audiovisual emotion matching in schizophrenia: the contribution of cognition and psychopathology. *Psychiatry Res* (2013) 205:192–8. doi: 10.1016/j.psychres.2012.08.038
33. Pawełczyk A, Kotlicka-Antczak M, Łojek E, Pawełczyk T. Preliminary study of higher-order language and extralinguistic impairments in individuals with high clinical risk of psychosis and first episode of schizophrenia. *Early Interv Psychiatry* (2019) 13:369–78. doi: 10.1111/eip.12482
34. Murphy D, Cutting J. Prosodic comprehension and expression in schizophrenia. *J Neurol Neurosurg Psychiatry* (1990) 53:727–30. doi: 10.1136/jnnp.53.9.727
35. Patel AD, Peretz I, Tramo M, Labreque R. Processing prosodic and musical patterns: a neuropsychological investigation. *Brain Lang* (1998) 61:123–44. doi: 10.1006/brln.1997.1862
36. Nicholson KG, Baum S, Kilgour A, Koh CK, Munhall KG, Cuddy LL. Impaired processing of prosodic and musical patterns after right hemisphere damage. *Brain Cogn* (2003) 52:382–9. doi: 10.1016/S0278-2626(03)00182-9
37. Pawełczyk A, Łojek E, Żurner N, Gawłowska-Sawosz M, Pawełczyk T. Higher-order language dysfunctions as a possible neurolinguistic endophenotype for schizophrenia: evidence from patients and their unaffected first degree relatives. *Psychiatry Res* (2018) 267:63–72. doi: 10.1016/j.psychres.2018.05.070
38. Covington MA, Lunden SL, Cristofaro SL, Wan CR, Bailey CT, Broussard B, et al. Phonetic measures of reduced tongue movement correlate with negative symptom severity in hospitalized patients with first-episode schizophrenia-spectrum disorders. *Schizophr Res* (2012) 142(1–3):93–5. doi: 10.1016/j.schres.2012.10.005
39. Leentjens AF, Wielaert SM, van Harskamp F, Wilmink FW. Disturbances of affective prosody in patients with schizophrenia; a cross sectional study. *J Neurol Neurosurg Psychiatry* (1998) 64:375–8. doi: 10.1136/jnnp.64.3.375
40. Alpert M, Rosenberg SD, Pouget ER, Shaw RJ. Prosody and lexical accuracy in flat affect schizophrenia. *Psychiatry Res* (2000) 97(2–3):107–18. doi: 10.1016/s0165-1781(00)00231-6
41. Dickey CC, Vu M-AT, Voglmaier MM, Niznikiewicz MA, McCarley RW, Panych LP. Prosodic Abnormalities in Schizotypal Personality Disorder. *Schizophr Res* (2012) 142(1–3):20–30. doi: 10.1016/j.schres.2012.09.006
42. Bedwell JS, Cohen AS, Trachik BJ, Deptula AE, Mitchell JC. Speech prosody abnormalities and specific dimensional schizotypy features: are relationships limited to male participants? *J Nerv Ment Dis* (2014) 202(10):745–51. doi: 10.1097/NMD.0000000000000184
43. Compton MT, Lunden A, Cleary SD, Pauselli L, Alolayan Y, Halpern B, et al. The aprosody of schizophrenia: computationally derived acoustic phonetic underpinnings of monotone speech. *Schizophr Res* (2018) 197:392–9. doi: 10.1016/j.schres.2018.01.007
44. Cannizzaro MS, Cohen H, Rappard F, Snyder PJ. Bradyphrenia and bradykinesia both contribute to altered speech in schizophrenia: a quantitative acoustic study. *Cog Behav Neurol* (2005) 18(4):206–10. doi: 10.1097/01.wnn.0000185278.21352.e5
45. Cohen AS, Hong SL. Understanding constricted affect in schizotypy through computerized prosodic analysis. *J Pers Disord* (2011) 25(4):478–91. doi: 10.1521/pedi.2011.25.4.478
46. Cohen AS, Kim Y, Najolia G. Psychiatric symptom versus neurocognitive correlates of diminished expressivity in schizophrenia and mood disorders. *Schizophr Res* (2018) 146(1–3):249–53. doi: 10.1016/j.schres.2013.02.002
47. Martínez-Sánchez F, Muela- Martínez JA, Cortés-Soto P, García-Meilán JJ, Vera Ferr ándiz JA, Caparrós AE, et al. Can the acoustic analysis of expressive prosody discriminate schizophrenia? *Span J Psychol* (2015) 18(e86):1–9. doi: 10.1017/sjp.2015.85
48. Bernardini F, Lunden A, Covington M, Broussard B, Halpern B, Alolayan Y, et al. Association of acoustically measured tongue/jaw movements and portion of time speaking with negative symptom severity in patients with schizophrenia in Italy and the United States. *Psychiatry Res* (2016) 239:253–8. doi: 10.1016/j.psychres.2016.03.037
49. Michelas A, Faget C, Portes C, Lienhart AS, Boyer L, Lançon C, et al. Do patients with schizophrenia use prosody to encode contrastive discourse status? *Front Psychol* (2014) 5:755. doi: 10.3389/fpsyg.2014.00755
50. Joyal M, Bonneau A, Fecteau S. Speech and language therapies to improve pragmatics and discourse skills in patients with schizophrenia. *Psychiatry Res* (2016) 240:88–95. doi: 10.1016/j.psyres.2016.04.010
51. Lado-Codesido M, Méndez Pérez C, Mateos R, Olivares JM, García Caballero A. Improving emotion recognition in schizophrenia with "VOICES": an on-line prosodic self-training. *PLoS One* (2019) 14(1):1–19. doi: 10.1371/journal.pone.0210816
52. Fuchs T. The intersubjectivity of delusions. *World Psychiatry* (2015) 14 (2):178–9. doi: 10.1002/wps.20209
53. Colle L, Angeleri R, Vallana M, Sacco K, Bara BG, Bosco FM.

Understanding the communicative impairments in schizophrenia: a preliminary study. *J Commun Disord* (2013) 46:294–308. doi: 10.1016/j.comdis.2013.01.003

54. Wehrle S, Cangemi F, Vogeley K, Grice M. (2018). The timing of turn-taking in high-functioning autism, in: *Proc. Phonetik und Phonologie im deutschsprachigen Raum (P&P) 2018*, Vienna, Austria, 2018 Sep 14. pp. 136–7.
55. Minkowski E. *Le temps vécu: études phénoménologiques et psychopathologiques.* Payot: Paris (1933). p. 432.
56. Kupper Z, Ramseyer F, Hoffmann H, Tschacher W. Nonverbal Synchrony in Social Interactions of Patients with Schizophrenia Indicates Socio-Communicative Deficits. *PLoS One* (2015) 10(12):e0145882. doi: 10.1371/journal.pone.0145882
57. Vogeley K, Kupke C. Disturbances of time consciousness from a phenomenological and a neuroscientific perspective. *Schizophr Bull* (2007) 33(1):157–65. doi: 10.1093/schbul/sbl056
58. Insel T, Cuthbert B, Garvey M, Heinssen R, Pine DS, Quinn K, et al. Research Domain Criteria (RDoC): toward a new classification framework for research on mental disorders. *Am J Psychiatry* (2010) 167:748–51. doi: 10.1176/appi.ajp.2010.09091379
59. Grice M, Krüger M, Vogeley K. Adults with Asperger syndrome are less sensitive to intonation than control persons when listening to speech. *Culture Brain* (2016) 4(1):38–50. doi: 10.1007/s40167-016-0035-6
60. Krüger M, Cangemi F, Vogeley K, Grice M. (2018). Prosodic Marking of Information Status in Adults with Autism Spectrum Disorders, in: *Proc. 9th International Conference on Speech Prosody 2018*, Poznań, Poland, 2018 Jun 13-16. pp. 182–6. doi: 10.21437/SpeechProsody.2018-37

9

Two-Person Approaches to Studying Social Interaction in Psychiatry: Uses and Clinical Relevance

Yafeng Pan [1,2] *and Xiaojun Cheng* [1*]

[1] *School of Psychology, Shenzhen University, Shenzhen, China,* [2] *Department of Clinical Neuroscience, Karolinska Institutet, Stockholm, Sweden*

Correspondence:
Xiaojun Cheng
chengxiaojun@szu.edu.cn

Social interaction is ubiquitous in human society. The two-person approach—a new, powerful tool to study information exchange and social behaviors—aims to characterize the behavioral dynamics and neural mechanisms of real-time social interactions. In this review, we discuss the benefits of two-person approaches compared to those for conventional, single-person approaches. We describe measures and paradigms that model social interaction in three dimensions (3-D), including eye-to-eye, body-to-body, and brain-to-brain relationships. We then discuss how these two-person measures and paradigms are used in psychiatric conditions (e.g., autism, mood disorders, schizophrenia, borderline personality disorder, and psychotherapy). Furthermore, the advantages of a two-person approach (e.g., dual brain stimulation, multi-person neurofeedback) in clinical interventions are described. Finally, we discuss the methodological and translational challenges surrounding the application of two-person approaches in psychiatry, as well as prospects for future two-/multi-person studies. We conclude that two-person approaches serve as useful additions to the range of behavioral and neuroscientific methods available to assess social interaction in psychiatric settings, for both diagnostic techniques and complementary interventions.

Keywords: two-person approach, social interaction, psychiatry, application, intervention

INTRODUCTION

The scientific study of the neurophysiological mechanisms that underlie social processes is undergoing a major paradigm shift: moving from the examination of single brains to the simultaneous acquisition of data from multiple brains and their interaction [see, e.g., our recent contributions: (1–6); see also (7–9) for reviews]. Within this fast-emerging area of research, we focused on recent advances that examined the relationship between eye gaze/body movement/brain activity recorded from interacting dyads under psychiatric settings. Thus, we attempted to characterize *social interaction in psychiatry* within a two-person framework (9–11).

In the present review, we will first briefly introduce the two-person approach and its benefits compared to those of a single-person approach, as well as potential interpersonal paradigms/markers derived from this approach. We will then focus on two-person studies in two aspects: first, the applications of the two-person approach in multiple cases of psychiatric conditions (e.g., autism, mood disorders, schizophrenia, borderline personality disorder, and psychotherapy), and second, the potential benefits of the two-person approach in psychiatric interventions (e.g., behavioral intervention, dual brain stimulation, multi-person neurofeedback). Finally, we will discuss challenges and future prospects of the applications of the two-person approach.

What Is the Two-Person Approach?

Human society is organized socially. Despite the interactive nature of human social behaviors, conventional neuroscientific studies investigating social cognitive processes have typically been restricted to isolated individual behaviors, leaving the dynamic (neural) interactions between individuals incompletely understood. Methodological advances allow researchers to address this issue by developing a novel technique termed "hyperscanning" or "hypermethod" [e.g., using electroencephalography (EEG) (12), functional near-infrared spectroscopy (fNIRS) (13), or functional magnetic resonance imaging (fMRI) (14)]. This technique first highlights the simultaneous consideration of two individuals in an interacting dyad.

In 2013, Schilbach and colleagues further advanced this field and formally proposed the theoretical framework of "second-person neuroscience" (11) or "two-person neuroscience" (15). Accordingly, recent years have seen fruitful empirical evidence of this two-person approach [for a review, see (9)]. The two-person approach has a basic assumption: behavioral and neural mechanisms supporting social cognition within the context of a real-time reciprocal social interaction are distinguishable from those within the context of social observation (without interaction). To further define two-person studies properly, two criteria were proposed: (*i*) social interactions should occur in real time and be reciprocal, and (*ii*) social interactions elicit psychological engagement (feeling of involvement with one another) between interacting partners. Studies having one of the two criteria could be seen as two-person studies.

Note that *two*-person approaches do not necessarily mean that investigations should be conducted only with *two* interacting individuals; one can also develop variants by monitoring *multiple* persons because social interaction could also take place in multi-person situations (16).

Is "Two" Indeed Better Than "One"?

As described in the previous section, human social behaviors have an interactive nature. To characterize the dynamic social interaction between individuals, it is imperative to adopt the two-person approach. However, one important question should be addressed first:*is "two" indeed better than "one"*? Several neuroimaging studies have attempted to address this issue (6, 17–19). Using fNIRS-based hyperscanning and machine learning approaches, Pan et al. found that two-brain measures served as a better neural-classification feature than single-brain measures (6). Specifically, machine learning techniques were reported to be more successful when decoding instructional approaches from instructor-learner brain coupling data than when using a single-brain method. Supporting these findings, previous fMRI studies reported that two-brain measures, such as brain-to-brain similarities, are more sensitive and better suited to track inter-personal influences, such as social network proximity (17); friends showed more similar neural responses to naturalistic movies, and such similar neural responses decreased with increasing social distance between friends. Monitoring and measuring two individuals simultaneously uncovered additional information beyond conventional single-brain approaches (18, 19). For example, compared to the single-brain method, which reflects a mixture of both neuronal components (i.e., stimulus-induced neural processes) and non-neuronal components (e.g., intrinsic neural processes and non-neuronal noise), two-brain measures using fMRI isolated stimulus-related inter-brain correlations (18). We believe that these prior studies are sufficient to imply that "two" performs better than "one" in several aspects during real-time social interaction; however, more research is needed to clarify the assets of the two-person approach compared to those of the single-person approach.

It is important to note that we do not claim that adopting the single-person approach to investigate the social cognitive process is useless – this contention would discredit various classic and ongoing investigations in this field [e.g., (20–22)]. Instead, we propose that using the two-person approach would add additional value to the exploration of dynamic and truly social interaction, thus advancing our understanding of both behavioral and neural mechanisms underlying human social behaviors.

Modeling Social Interaction in 3-D

To take advantage of the two-person approach, the field calls for interactive paradigms and interpersonal markers of real-time social interaction (23, 24). Here, we highlight three dimensions (3-D) that characterize the behavioral and neural mechanisms of social interaction. These paradigms/markers allow us to model real-time social interaction in 3-D: eye-to-eye, body-to-body, and brain-to-brain.

Eye-to-Eye

Gaze behavior is critical in social interaction and in communication in particular. While many studies have investigated the role of gaze behavior in social observation, research about a person's interactive gaze allowing eye-to-eye contact and face-to-face interaction is still lacking. Pfeiffer et al. reviewed novel approaches to investigate the neural systems that support social gaze behavior, thus requiring active social engagement (25); these novel approaches include interactions with virtual agents (26), live interactions *via* videos (27), and dual eye-tracking setups (28).

Regarding dual-eye-tracking setups, in the last decade, we have seen fruitful applications of the eye-to-eye paradigm in investigating neural mechanisms of social interaction. For example, Saito and colleagues initiated a combination of fMRI hyperscanning and dual eye-tracking. With this novel setup, they found that paired subjects showed higher inter-individual neural synchronization in the right inferior frontal gyrus *during* mutual gaze and joint attention activities than non-paired subjects (28). Using EEG hyperscanning in an eye-to-eye (face-to-face) situation, Lachat et al. found that the joint attention condition

—compared to the no-joint attention condition—induced an 11-13 Hz power decrease over left centro-parieto-occipital regions (29). As Lachat et al. suggested, the power decrease might reflect attention mirroring, social coordination, and mutual attentiveness associated with joint attention. Hirsch et al. combined a two-person eye-tracking system and fNIRS recordings. The results revealed that fronto-temporo-parietal neural systems synchronize within and across brains during live eye-to-eye contact, in contrast with the results for an eye-to-picture gaze (30).

Body-to-Body

Body movement is an important nonverbal cue and signal for social interaction. The coupling between hand/body movements acts as an index for implicit social interaction (31). For example, Yun et al. found that synchrony of both fingertip movement and neural activity between two individuals in a dyad increased after a cooperation interaction. In more complex social interactions, nonverbal interpersonal coordination (body sway) among people was indicative of leadership in joint music making (32).

Furthermore, recent advances also reported that body-to-body coupling was associated with many positive outcomes, including prosociality (2), therapeutic alliances (33), mentalizing (34), and closeness (35). Using a combination of a two-person paradigm and fNIRS recordings, Hu and colleagues found that the manipulation of body-to-body synchrony predicted subsequent prosocial behaviors. Brain-to-brain synchronization between the two participants during ongoing movements might be a potential underlying mechanism. At the behavioral level, Ramseyer et al. (33) quantified nonverbal synchrony between the patient's and therapist's movements. They found that nonverbal synchrony reflected the relationship quality; synchrony was associated with symptom reduction. Baimel et al. found that behavioral synchrony between partners fostered mentalizing capacities. Synchrony increased the mental state attribution to interacting participant dyads (34). Another behavioral study explored the influence of motor synchrony on the experience of intimacy (35). Specifically, the authors examined whether body-to-body synchrony between partners instilled a sense of intimacy. The results suggested that synchrony was strongly associated with intimacy and possibly promoted closeness in intimate situations.

Another subdomain of the body-to-body relationship concerns peripheral physiological signals, including the heart rate, electrodermal activity, and respiration. The relationship between the physiological activity of two or more people is referred to as "interpersonal autonomic physiology" or "physiological synchrony" (36). The concept of physiological synchrony has been incorporated into a wide range of contexts to investigate its relation with a number of social behaviors, including cooperation (37), singing (38), and romantic interaction (39). Specifically, in the field of psychiatry, physiological synchrony serves as a useful tool to track psychotherapy processes (40–42). In 2016, Koole and Tschacher reviewed clinical studies on therapeutic alliances and interpersonal synchrony and then integrated both concepts into the interpersonal synchrony model of psychotherapy. In a later empirical study, Tschacher and Meier explored physiological synchrony in naturalistic psychotherapy sessions and found that synchrony correlated with the therapeutic alliance and psychotherapy session reports.

Brain-to-Brain

The most recent neuroimaging work in this field shifted the focus on single-brain functioning toward two-brain communication during real-time social interaction. As mentioned above, this shift is boosted by a fast-developing technique: "hyperscanning". The concept of hyperscanning was first proposed by Montague et al. (14). In their commentary paper, the authors described simultaneous neuroimaging during linked social interactions; specifically, participants could interact with each other while their brain activity was simultaneously recorded. Regarding data analysis, hyperscanning setups enable us to effectively quantify the relationship between two brain activities. A common finding derived from previous hyperscanning studies is that brain activity from two interacting participants in a dyad tends to be "coupled together", creating a joint networked state. This phenomenon is usually called "brain-to-brain synchrony/ synchronization" (16) or "interpersonal brain/neural synchronization" (4, 5, 43–45).

The mechanisms of brain-to-brain synchrony are still debated. Although some researchers see brain-to-brain synchrony, *per se*, as a mechanism for social behaviors [e.g., (8)], others claim that synchrony is not a mechanism in itself but a measurable reflection of the underlying neural computations that support some psychological processes [e.g., (16)]. Dikker and colleagues proposed "shared attention" as a possible source of brain-to-brain synchrony by successfully demonstrating a positive relationship between alpha band power (a well-characterized index of attention) and synchrony measures. This account is also in line with a series of past studies using mutual gaze tasks (28, 46–48). Apart from this account of shared attention, other studies also posited that social signals (such as gaze, gestures, or vocalizations) could promote mutual temporal alignment of the brains involved, leading to a joint networked state to facilitate information transfer (5, 49).

Note that this review is not intended to be a comprehensive review of two-person approaches, given the excellent reviews previously published on this topic (9, 11, 50). For this reason, we did not go into depth about any techniques but instead refer readers to **Table 1** that briefly describes the commonly used measures and other empirical work [e.g., (58–60)]. Additionally, compared to emerging two-person neuroscience endeavors (i.e., brain-to-brain), two-person behaviors (i.e., eye-to-eye and body-to-body) have long been monitored to investigate social interaction. With this in mind, we mainly discussed behavioral paradigms that were (potentially) related to two-person neuroscience, as that is where our novelty lies.

Readers should keep in mind that the three aforementioned dimensions (eye-to-eye, body-to-body, and brain-to-brain) are not isolated but are strongly associated with each other. For instance, eye contact synchronization might occur in parallel with brain activity synchronization (28, 30), and body-to-body coupling could be associated with brain-to-brain coupling (2,

TABLE 1 | Several commonly used measures in two- or multi-person studies.

Measure	Description	Example References
Motion energy analysis	Computing pixel changes across video frames and generate motion energy time series for both participants during interaction	(33, 51)
Windowed cross-correlation	Tracking the movements of two variables or sets of data relative to each other	(33, 51, 52)
Phase locking value	Measuring the consistency of the phase-difference	(3, 53, 54)
Circular correlation coefficient	Measuring the circular covariance of differences between the observed phase and the expected phase	(55–57)
Wavelet transform coherence	Measuring local correlation between two signals as a function of both frequency and time	(1, 4–6)
Granger causality analysis	Estimating the directional coupling	(1, 4, 5, 45)

31). These novel approaches facilitate the investigation of behavioral dynamics and neural mechanisms of social behaviors (50) and thus yield new insights into the field of *social interaction in psychiatry*.

RECENT APPLICATIONS OF THE TWO-PERSON APPROACH IN SOCIAL INTERACTIONS UNDER PSYCHIATRIC SETTINGS

Autism

Autism spectrum disorder (ASD) is a neurodevelopmental disorder characterized by social deficits in communication and inter-personal interactions, as well as non-social deficits in repetitive behavior (61). Social deficits in communication in individuals with ASD are reflected in various aspects, such as joint attention (62–64), motor imitation (65), and interpersonal coordination (66, 67).

Joint attention is a set of nonverbal behaviors, including eye gaze, pointing, and showing, which are used to reference outside objects during a communicative exchange (62). Generally, joint attention occurs within the context of a social interaction, when one person directs another person's attention to an object (*initiating joint attention*), and the second person's attention follows (*responding to joint attention*). Previous studies have established impaired joint attention in children with ASD (62) and that the early development of joint attention predicts future language and social cognitive skills in children with ASD (68, 69); therefore, joint attention skills are critical targets of intervention for this population.

Atypical joint attention behaviors and brain activation patterns have been observed in individuals with ASD when they were required to view images or movies of real or virtual people (63, 70). However, these traditional experimental setups (i.e., viewing images or movies) might not be a promising method to disclose the neural basis of *initiating joint attention* in individuals with ASD. Concerning this issue, Redcay et al. adopted a dual-video setup that allowed for a face-to-face interaction between the subject and experimenter *via* video during fMRI data collection. By using the two-person approach, they depicted activation patterns related to *initiating joint attention* and *responding to joint attention* in both the ASD group and the normal control group (27). Compared with the normal group, the ASD group showed a reduced brain activation difference between joint attention conditions (including *initiating joint attention* and *responding to joint attention*) and solo attention conditions in the dorsal medial prefrontal cortex and right posterior superior temporal sulcus. Distinct regions included the ventromedial prefrontal cortex for *responding to joint attention* and the intraparietal sulcus and middle frontal gyrus for *initiating joint attention* (27). The lack of differentiation was further characterized by reduced activation during joint attention conditions and relative hyperactivation during solo attention conditions (71).

Although Redcay and colleagues applied the two-person approach and adopted a live face-to-face communication task in their study, they used a single fMRI setting and measured a single brain in an isolated manner. To elucidate the neural substrates of direct, real-time interactions between ASD patients and normal subjects, Tanabe et al. (72) conducted the first fMRI-based hyperscanning study in ASD individuals by using the mutual gaze paradigm developed by Saito et al.. They found that compared to the normal–normal pairs, ASD–normal pairs exhibited less accurate gaze direction detection and less prominent inter-brain coherence in the right inferior frontal gyrus during eye contact (72). The findings suggest that the impairment of joint attention in ASD could be related to the difficulty in understanding shared intention through eye contact, which is represented by reduced inter-subject synchronization of cortical regions including the right inferior frontal gyrus.

Apart from impaired joint attention, most individuals with ASD have deficits in interpersonal motor imitation and coordination (65–67). A related study has shown that in individuals with ASD, a higher degree of autistic traits (i.e., higher Autism Spectrum Quotient score) could predict a lower ability to modulate movements to coordinate with normal individuals (i.e., social interactive tasks) but not differences in movement preparation and planning with a non-biological stimulus (i.e., non-social tasks) (66). This finding suggests that the failure of individuals with ASD to coordinate with others was not due to basic motor or executive function difficulties. Furthermore, the performance of individuals with ASD regarding interpersonal motor coordination could possibly depend on the social skill ability of the individuals with whom they are paired (73). Pairs of participants with widely differing Autism Spectrum Quotient scores performed better than pairs with similar Autism Spectrum Quotient scores in the inter-personal rhythmic movement task. Specifically, participants with relatively higher Autism Spectrum Quotient scores tended to precede their partners in the task.

Recently, Wang and colleagues conducted fNIRS-based hyperscanning studies to further explore brain-to-brain coupling during interpersonal coordination tasks between children with ASD and normal partners (i.e., parents in the study). The results showed that compared to solo and non-interactive behaviors, coordinating interactions with their parents could elicit increased inter-personal neural synchronization in the frontal cortex of children with ASD (67). Neural synchronization was further found to be modulated by the children's autism symptoms and covaried with their cooperation task performance. That is, children with severe autism symptoms showed worse behavioral performance and less neural synchronization with their parents during coordination than children with less severe symptoms.

Mood Disorders

Patients suffering from mood disorders, e.g., major depressive disorder and bipolar disorder, showed atypical interpersonal communication according to their mood state (61). Previous studies have employed fMRI to explore cognitive and emotional dysfunctions and found altered activation of the amygdala, as well as the frontal, cingulate, and temporal cortices, in patients with major depressive disorder and bipolar disorder during various cognitive tasks (74). However, brain activation during conversation has not yet been investigated in patients with mood disorders due to methodological difficulties.

In 2014, Takei and colleagues conducted a fNIRS study in which major depressive disorder and bipolar disorder patients performed a face-to-face conversation with an interviewer who was selected from the hospital staff and had not been previously acquainted with the participants (i.e., a two-person situation with a focus on the patient's brain). In their study, patients' frontal and temporal lobe activation levels were measured during the conversation condition (including speech and listening phases) and control condition (including syllables and silent phases). The results showed less activation in the left dorsolateral prefrontal and left frontopolar cortices in major depressive disorder and bipolar disorder patients than in normal individuals, as well as a rapid decrease in bilateral frontopolar activation in major depressive disorder and bipolar disorder patients. Particularly, in patients with major depressive disorder, the average amount of signal change over time in the frontopolar cortex was positively correlated with their Global Assessment of Functioning scores; in patients with bipolar disorder, the average brain activation during conversation was negatively correlated with the age of onset in the right dorsolateral prefrontal cortex and both middle temporal lobes (75). These findings suggest that both continuous activation and rapid change may reflect the pathophysiological characteristics of major depressive disorder and bipolar disorder.

Schizophrenia

Schizophrenia is marked by poor social-role performance and social-functioning deficits that are well reflected in interpersonal communication (61). Such social deficits could be captured by body-to-body dynamics. For example, Kupper and colleagues found that a low level of nonverbal synchrony was associated with negative symptoms, low social competence, impaired social functioning, and low self-reported competence. Negative symptoms were more prominent when patients reduced their imitation of the movements of the interactant; in turn, positive symptoms were more prominent when interactants reduced their imitation of patients' movements (51).

The social deficits shown by patients with schizophrenia could be associated with reduced volume and/or reduced gray matter activation in specific brain regions, such as the temporal lobe, ventromedial prefrontal cortex, and cingulate cortex (76, 77). Takei et al. used fNIRS to investigate frontal and temporal lobe activation in patients with schizophrenia during the conversation (i.e., a two-person situation with a focus on the patient's brain). The results showed that patients with schizophrenia, compared to normal controls, were characterized by decreased activation in the bilateral temporal lobes and right inferior frontal gyrus during the conversation task (78). The decreased activation in the related brain regions negatively correlated with disorganization and negative symptoms suggested that the disorganization and negative symptoms observed in patients with schizophrenia in clinical situations are related to dysfunction of the left temporal lobe and right inferior frontal gyrus. In addition, frontal lobe dysfunction was also reported to be linked to difficulties in gesture planning and execution (79), which might explain the poor social functioning in schizophrenia patients.

Borderline Personality Disorder

Borderline personality disorder is characterized by repeated interpersonal conflict and unstable relationships (61). Bilek and colleagues recently explored the neurobiological mechanism of social interactive deficits in borderline personality disorder. In their study, current borderline personality disorder patients and remitted borderline personality disorder patients were recruited to perform a joint attention task with normal participants. Compared with the normal-normal pairs, normal-current borderline personality disorder pairs showed reduced interpersonal brain connectivity. Remarkably, for remitted patients, interpersonal brain connectivity was restored. These findings emerged only in the study of information flow between dyads and were not associated with any between-group differences in individual brain structure or function, indicating the necessity of two-person approaches. Cross-brain measurements, therefore, deliver state-associated biomarkers that may help to guide diagnostic and therapeutic procedures in the future (80).

Psychotherapy

As described above, individuals with psychiatric disorders have social deficits that reflect verbal or nonverbal coordination with others to some extent. It is worth noting that the synchrony, especially nonverbal synchrony, between patients and therapists is also highlighted during psychotherapy.

Ramseyer et al. (33) found higher nonverbal coordination in genuine interactions (i.e., real pairs of patients and therapists) in contrast with pseudo-interactions (i.e., random pairs of patients and therapists). More importantly, nonverbal coordination was associated with patients experiencing high quality relationships and high self-efficacy (33). Other studies showed that nonverbal synchrony between patients and therapists could be modulated by therapeutic approaches (81) and varied by disorder (82).

Recently, researchers attempted to disclose the neural mechanisms underlying behavioral synchrony during psychotherapy. In a preliminary study, typical students were recruited as clients, and they were required to have interactions with professional counsellors. By using the fNIRS-based hyperscanning technique, researchers recorded the brain activation of both clients and counsellors in the frontal cortex and right temporoparietal junction during the psychological counselling phase and the chatting phase (83). Better working alliances and increased interpersonal brain synchrony in the right temporoparietal junction between clients and counselors were observed during psychological counseling (versus chatting). Such inter-personal brain synchrony was correlated with the bond of the working alliance. This study refines the neural explanation of behavioral synchrony during psychotherapy.

Briefly, interpersonal body and brain synchrony could play important roles in the processes of psychotherapy. The lack of coordination during psychotherapy may be a risk factor for the condition's recurrence (84). The findings provide insights for psychological interventions for psychiatric disorders.

INTERPERSONAL BODY AND BRAIN COUPLING OFFER INSIGHTS FOR PSYCHOLOGICAL INTERVENTIONS FOR PSYCHIATRIC DISORDERS

Manipulation of Inter-personal Body Synchrony

Given that synchrony has also been associated with the outcome of psychotherapy, "moving together" could possibly be an efficient means to improve psychiatric patients' social dysfunction. Notably, the idea of using imitation and synchronization in clinical interventions to target social functions has a long tradition in dance/movement therapy in general and in working with children with ASD in particular (85–87). Some studies have provided empirical evidence for this notion. For example, a seven-week intervention study focusing on movement mirroring showed that young adults with ASD reported improved well-being, body awareness, self–other distinction, and social skills after the intervention (88). Moreover, patients treated with an interpersonal movement imitation and synchronization intervention showed a significantly larger improvement in emotional inference than those treated with a control movement intervention that focused on individual motor coordination (89).

Interventions targeting social synchronous behavior on social functions can even positively affect two-year-old toddlers with ASD (90). In the study by Landa et al., toddlers with ASD were randomized to either a classroom-based inter-personal synchrony intervention (including imitation, joint attention, and affect sharing) or a non-inter-personal synchrony intervention. It was found that after approximately 200 hours of interpersonal synchrony interventions (versus non-interpersonal synchrony interventions), toddlers showed enhanced socially engaged imitations paired with eye contact with the examiner and demonstrated a trend toward higher levels of nonverbal cognition during posttest assessments (90). The study provided evidence for plasticity in these developmental systems in toddlers with ASD.

Notably, the interventions could initially be conducted *via* a computer-mediated interference. It was reported that individuals with high-functioning autism showed a reduced sensitivity to the other person's responsiveness to one's own behavior when they were required to have real-time sensorimotor interaction with normal individuals; however, they performed equally well as controls under the highly simplified, computer-mediated, embodied form of social interaction. This finding supports the increasing use of virtual reality interfaces to help people with ASD better compensate for their social disabilities (91).

Manipulation of Inter-personal Brain Synchrony

Related studies have revealed that interpersonal brain synchrony reflects social dysfunctions and intervention effects to some extent (80, 83). Thus, it could be possible to improve the social communication and interpersonal relationships of patients with psychiatric disorders by manipulating interpersonal brain synchrony.

To date, some studies have applied transcranial alternating current stimulation (tACS) to specific brain regions of interacting persons to directly examine the relationship between interpersonal brain synchrony and behavioral synchrony (92, 93). For example, Novembre and colleagues induced beta band (20 Hz) oscillations over the left motor cortex in pairs of individuals who both performed a finger-tapping task with the right hand and found that in-phase 20 Hz stimulation enhanced inter-personal movement synchrony compared with anti-phase or sham stimulation, particularly for the initial taps following the preparatory period. However, in the study of Szymanski et al., both the same-phase-same-frequency and the different-phase-different-frequency conditions were associated with greater dyadic drumming asynchrony relative to the sham condition. The inconsistent findings might be related to the different stimulation protocols and experimental paradigms, which need to be verified.

Apart from dual-brain stimulation, neurofeedback is also a promising approach to manipulating brain activity. There is growing evidence to support the idea that a single participant's brain activity can be self-regulated with neurofeedback, yielding specific behavioral effects [see (94, 95) for a review]. During the past several decades, the technique of neurofeedback has been applied to patients with psychiatric disorders (e.g., major depressive disorder, personality disorder, and schizophrenia) to relieve psychiatric symptoms [see (96) for a review]. Previous studies have revealed that a neurofeedback tool that tracks human interaction at the neural level has potential clinical applications for the diagnosis and treatment of social cognition disorders. For example, persons with autism may respond better to explicit cues *via* technological interfaces than to human cues (91).

CHALLENGES

Artifacts and Sample Size

To study the behavioral and neurophysiological mechanisms underlying social interactions, two-person approaches call for highly ecologically valid experimental paradigms. At the methodological level, compared to fMRI and EEG data, fNIRS data offer the advantage of capturing brain activity in realistic social situations while being less affected by motor artifacts (97). Some video-based techniques or peripheral devices restrain participants even less (e.g., motion energy analysis, actigraphy).

However, high ecological validity comes at the cost of having unavoidable artifacts. The (neural) signal is potentially contaminated by at least two factors. First, motion artifacts are likely to be generated in unconstrained environments (98, 99), affecting the reliability of data. Second, spontaneous systemic effects from neural activity or peripheral physiological fluctuations may affect signal quality (100). These artifacts could be mitigated by several artifact correction methods. However, good *post hoc* data processing is never better than good data collection. Future studies should simultaneously consider the ecological validity and motion/systemic artifacts when applying two-person approaches.

A common issue in two-person neuroscientific research relates to the sample size. "Two-person" is a fancy technique, but it also means that a larger sample size would be required. For example, 60 participants indicate a sample size of 60 for single-person studies but only half for two-person studies in many cases (i.e., 60 participants would lead to a sample size of 30 for two-person studies; and an even smaller sample size for multi-person studies). One is encouraged to define the sample size prior to formal experiments by conducting statistical power analyses, e.g., using the G*power toolbox (101). Future studies are needed to consolidate the previous findings from two-person studies by enlarging the sample size to increase statistical power.

Statistical Methods of Assessing Synchrony

There are several techniques that estimate the covariance or directional coupling of time series generated from two interacting partners in previous studies. These include the phase locking value [(53); see also (3, 54)], wavelet transform coherence [(102); see also (4, 13)], windowed cross-correlation [(52); see also (33, 51)], and Granger causality analysis [(103); see also (5, 32, 45)].

However, when evaluating data analyses for two-person data, there is currently no uniform analytical pipeline (i.e., statistical methods for assessing synchrony). Different two-person studies adopt distinct analysis strategies (e.g., with vs. without filtering), making the findings less congruent. In an endeavor to achieve transparency, consistency, and repeatability, future research should reach a consensus on common analysis guidelines. This practice will largely facilitate the replication of findings and their interpretations. Recent advances have seen some efforts in this direction [e.g., (104)].

Indeed, different methods aim at addressing distinctive research questions. For example, interpersonal *phase* synchronization between two participants in a dyad could be addressed using phase locking value or wavelet transform coherence methods, whereas the former was commonly used in behavioral and EEG studies and the latter was widely used in fNIRS research. Windowed cross-correlation not only provides information regarding simultaneous synchrony but can also reveal lagged information (i.e., which time series is leading the other). Granger causality also provides suggestions for coupling directionality, in case one is interested in exploring the direction of information flow between individuals. Researchers should utilize suitable statistical methods for assessing synchrony, targeting specific research aims.

Clinical Translation Application

Current two-person studies are still facing technical and methodological challenges, making the findings difficult to interpret and controversial for direct clinical translation. In addition, considering the limited sample size in previous two-person studies, it is rather inappropriate to generalize the laboratory findings to real-life psychiatric applications. Notwithstanding, previous studies pave the way for the use of two-person approaches in practical psychiatric settings. For example, it was reported that body-to-body synchrony reflected relationship quality and outcomes in psychotherapy (33). This implies that interpersonal markers could be potential tools to aid diagnostic procedures. Additionally, dual brain stimulation was reported to foster behavioral coordination and improve social interactions (92, 93). This is relevant for complementary treatments for social disorders, such as autism.

CONCLUSIONS AND FUTURE PERSPECTIVES

In sum, two-person approaches are promising tools for studying social interaction, particularly in the field of psychiatry. Although still facing several methodological and translational challenges, the two-person approach has its benefits compared to the conventional single-person approach when studying dynamic social interactions. The use of two-person approaches in psychiatry facilitates advancements in our understanding of the mechanism of atypical social interaction in the fields of autism, mood disorders, schizophrenia, borderline personality disorder, and psychotherapy. Two-person approaches also show promise in clinical interventions when combined with brain stimulation and neurofeedback techniques.

A future direction is to integrate the two-person approaches with computational modeling techniques (105), which may help further empower a better understanding of the computational mechanism of social interaction in psychiatry. Another direction is to manipulate the situations during social interaction using virtual reality (106) and test the effects of social factors, such as interpersonal distances and angles on eye-to-eye, body-to-body, and brain-to-brain communications. Eventually, as psychiatric disorders are strongly influenced by genetic factors (107), future studies are also encouraged to combine two-person approaches and multivariate genetic models.

AUTHOR CONTRIBUTIONS

YP and XC wrote the manuscript.

REFERENCES

1. Cheng X, Pan Y, Hu Y, Hu Y. Coordination Elicits Synchronous Brain Activity Between Co-actors: Frequency Ratio Matters. *Front Neurosci* (2019) 13:1–10. doi: 10.3389/fnins.2019.01071
2. Hu Y, Hu Y, Li X, Pan Y, Cheng X. Brain-to-brain synchronization across two persons predicts mutual prosociality. *Soc Cognit Affect Neurosci* (2017) 12:1835–44. doi: 10.1093/scan/nsx118
3. Hu Y, Pan Y, Shi X, Cai Q, Li X, Cheng X. Inter-brain synchrony and cooperation context in interactive decision making. *Biol Psychol* (2018) 133:54–62. doi: 10.1016/j.biopsycho.2017.12.005
4. Pan Y, Cheng X, Zhang Z, Li X, Hu Y. Cooperation in lovers: An fNIRS-based hyperscanning study. *Hum Brain Mapp* (2017) 38:831–41. doi: 10.1002/hbm.23421
5. Pan Y, Novembre G, Song B, Li X, Hu Y. Interpersonal synchronization of inferior frontal cortices tracks social interactive learning of a song. *Neuroimage* (2018) 183:280–90. doi: 10.1016/j.neuroimage.2018.08.005
6. Pan Y, Dikker S, Goldstein P, Zhu Y, Yang C, Hu Y. Instructor-learner brain coupling discriminates between instructional approaches and predicts learning. *Neuroimage* (2020) 211:116657. doi: 10.1016/j.neuroimage.2020.116657
7. Babiloni F, Astolfi L. Social neuroscience and hyperscanning techniques: Past, present and future. *Neurosci Biobehav Rev* (2014) 44:76–93. doi: 10.1016/j.neubiorev.2012.07.006
8. Hasson U, Ghazanfar AA, Galantucci B, Garrod S, Keysers C. Brain-to-brain coupling: A mechanism for creating and sharing a social world. *Trends Cognit Sci* (2012) 16:114–21. doi: 10.1016/j.tics.2011.12.007
9. Redcay E, Schilbach L. Using second-person neuroscience to elucidate the mechanisms of social interaction. *Nat Rev Neurosci* (2019) 20:495–505. doi: 10.1038/s41583-019-0179-4
10. Schilbach L. Eye to eye, face to face and brain to brain: Novel approaches to study the behavioral dynamics and neural mechanisms of social interactions. *Curr Opin Behav Sci* (2015) 3:130–5. doi: 10.1016/j.cobeha.2015.03.006
11. Schilbach L, Timmermans B, Reddy V, Costall A, Bente G, Schlicht T, et al. Toward a second-person neuroscience. *Behav Brain Sci* (2013) 36:393–414. doi: 10.1017/S0140525X12000660
12. Babiloni F, Cincotti F, Mattia D, Mattiocco M, De Fallani FV, Tocci A, et al. Hypermethods for EEG hyperscanning. *Annu Int Conf IEEE Eng Med Biol - Proc* (2006) 1:3666–9. doi: 10.1109/IEMBS.2006.260754
13. Cui X, Bryant DM, Reiss AL. NIRS-based hyperscanning reveals increased interpersonal coherence in superior frontal cortex during cooperation. *Neuroimage* (2012) 59:2430–7. doi: 10.1016/j.neuroimage.2011.09.003
14. Montague PR, Berns GS, Cohen JD, McClure SM, Pagnoni G, Dhamala M, et al. Hyperscanning: Simultaneous fMRI during linked social interactions. *Neuroimage* (2002) 16:1159–64. doi: 10.1006/nimg.2002.1150
15. Leong V, Schilbach L. The promise of two-person neuroscience for developmental psychiatry: Using interaction-based sociometrics to identify disorders of social interaction. *Br J Psychiatry* (2019) 215:636–8. doi: 10.1192/bjp.2019.73
16. Dikker S, Wan L, Davidesco I, Kaggen L, Oostrik M, McClintock J, et al. Brain-to-Brain Synchrony Tracks Real-World Dynamic Group Interactions in the Classroom. *Curr Biol* (2017) 27:1375–80. doi: 10.1016/j.cub.2017.04.002
17. Parkinson C, Kleinbaum AM, Wheatley T. Similar neural responses predict friendship. *Nat Commun* (2018) 9:322. doi: 10.1038/s41467-017-02722-7
18. Simony E, Honey CJ, Chen J, Lositsky O, Yeshurun Y, Wiesel A, et al. Dynamic reconfiguration of the default mode network during narrative comprehension. *Nat Commun* (2016) 7:12141. doi: 10.1038/ncomms12141
19. Balconi M, Pezard L, Nandrino JL, Vanutelli ME. Two is better than one: The effects of strategic cooperation on intra- and inter-brain connectivity by fNIRS. *PloS One* (2017) 12:e0187652. doi: 10.1371/journal.pone.0187652
20. Frith CD. The social brain? *Philos Trans R Soc B Biol Sci* (2007) 362:671–8. doi: 10.1098/rstb.2006.2003
21. Lieberman MD. Social Cognitive Neuroscience: A Review of Core Processes. *Annu Rev Psychol* (2007) 58:259–89. doi: 10.1146/annurev.psych.58.110405.085654
22. Lindström B, Golkar A, Jangard S, Tobler PN, Olsson A. Social threat learning transfers to decision making in humans. *Proc Natl Acad Sci U S A* (2019) 116:4732–7. doi: 10.1073/pnas.1810180116
23. De Jaegher H, Di Paolo E, Gallagher S. Can social interaction constitute social cognition? *Trends Cognit Sci* (2010) 14:441–7. doi: 10.1016/j.tics.2010.06.009
24. Konvalinka I, Roepstorff A. The two-brain approach: How can mutually interacting brains teach us something about social interaction? *Front Hum Neurosci* (2012) 6:1–10. doi: 10.3389/fnhum.2012.00215
25. Pfeiffer UJ, Vogeley K, Schilbach L. From gaze cueing to dual eye-tracking: Novel approaches to investigate the neural correlates of gaze in social interaction. *Neurosci Biobehav Rev* (2013) 37:2516–28. doi: 10.1016/j.neubiorev.2013.07.017
26. Wilms M, Schilbach L, Pfeiffer U, Bente G, Fink GR, Vogeley K. It's in your eyes-using gaze-contingent stimuli to create truly interactive paradigms for social cognitive and affective neuroscience. *Soc Cognit Affect Neurosci* (2010) 5:98–107. doi: 10.1093/scan/nsq024
27. Redcay E, Kleiner M, Saxe R. Look at this: The neural correlates of initiating and responding to bids for joint attention. *Front Hum Neurosci* (2012) 6:1–14. doi: 10.3389/fnhum.2012.00169
28. Saito DN, Tanabe HC, Izuma K, Hayashi MJ, Morito Y, Komeda H, et al. Stay tuned: Inter-individual neural synchronization during mutual gaze and joint attention. *Front Integr Neurosci* (2010) 4:1–12. doi: 10.3389/fnint.2010.00127
29. Lachat F, Hugueville L, Lemaréchal JD, Conty L, George N. Oscillatory brain correlates of live joint attention: A dual-EEG study. *Front Hum Neurosci* (2012) 6:1–12. doi: 10.3389/fnhum.2012.00156
30. Hirsch J, Zhang X, Noah JA, Ono Y. Frontal temporal and parietal systems synchronize within and across brains during live eye-to-eye contact. *Neuroimage* (2017) 157:314–30. doi: 10.1016/j.neuroimage.2017.06.018
31. Yun K, Watanabe K, Shimojo S. Interpersonal body and neural synchronization as a marker of implicit social interaction. *Sci Rep* (2012) 2:1–8. doi: 10.1038/srep00959
32. Chang A, Livingstone SR, Bosnyak DJ, Trainor LJ. Body sway reflects leadership in joint music performance. *Proc Natl Acad Sci* (2017) 114: E4134–41. doi: 10.1073/pnas.1617657114
33. Ramseyer F, Tschacher W. Nonverbal synchrony in psychotherapy: Coordinated body movement reflects relationship quality and outcome. *J Consult Clin Psychol* (2011) 79:284–95. doi: 10.1037/a0023419
34. Baimel A, Birch SAJ, Norenzayan A. Coordinating bodies and minds: Behavioral synchrony fosters mentalizing. *J Exp Soc Psychol* (2018) 74:281–90. doi: 10.1016/j.jesp.2017.10.008
35. Sharon-David H, Mizrahi M, Rinott M, Golland Y, Birnbaum GE. Being on the same wavelength: Behavioral synchrony between partners and its influence on the experience of intimacy. *J Soc Pers Relat* (2019) 36:2983–3008. doi: 10.1177/0265407518809478
36. Palumbo RV, Marraccini ME, Weyandt LL, Wilder-Smith O, McGee HA, Liu S, et al. Interpersonal Autonomic Physiology: A Systematic Review of the Literature. *Pers Soc Psychol Rev* (2017) 21:99–141. doi: 10.1177/1088868316628405
37. Vanutelli ME, Gatti L, Angioletti L, Balconi M. Affective Synchrony and Autonomic Coupling during Cooperation: A Hyperscanning Study. *BioMed Res Int* (2017) 2017:3104564. doi: 10.1155/2017/3104564
38. Müller V, Delius JAM, Lindenberger U. Complex networks emerging during choir singing. *Ann N Y Acad Sci* (2018) 1431:85–101. doi: 10.1111/nyas.13940
39. Chatel-Goldman J, Congedo M, Jutten C, Schwartz J-L. Touch increases autonomic coupling between romantic partners. *Front Behav Neurosci* (2014) 8:95. doi: 10.3389/fnbeh.2014.00095
40. Kleinbub JR. State of the Art of Interpersonal Physiology in Psychotherapy: A Systematic Review. *Front Psychol* (2017) 8:2053. doi: 10.3389/fpsyg.2017.02053
41. Koole SL, Tschacher W. Synchrony in Psychotherapy: A Review and an Integrative Framework for the Therapeutic Alliance. *Front Psychol* (2016) 7:862. doi: 10.3389/fpsyg.2016.00862

42. Tschacher W, Meier D. Physiological synchrony in psychotherapy sessions. *Psychother Res* (2019) 6:1–16. doi: 10.1080/10503307.2019.1612114
43. Dai B, Chen C, Long Y, Zheng L, Zhao H, Bai X, et al. Neural mechanisms for selectively tuning in to the target speaker in a naturalistic noisy situation. *Nat Commun* (2018) 9:2405. doi: 10.1038/s41467-018-04819-z
44. Jiang J, Dai B, Peng D, Zhu C, Liu L, Lu C. Neural synchronization during face-to-face communication. *J Neurosci* (2012) 32:16064–9. doi: 10.1523/JNEUROSCI.2926-12.2012
45. Jiang J, Chen C, Dai B, Shi G, Ding G, Liu L, et al. Leader emergence through interpersonal neural synchronization. *Proc Natl Acad Sci U S A* (2015) 112:4274–9. doi: 10.1073/pnas.1422930112
46. Bilek E, Ruf M, Schäfer A, Akdeniz C, Calhoun VD, Schmahl C, et al. Information flow between interacting human brains: Identification, validation, and relationship to social expertise. *Proc Natl Acad Sci U S A* (2015) 112:5207–12. doi: 10.1073/pnas.1421831112
47. Goelman G, Dan R, Stößel G, Tost H, Meyer-Lindenberg A, Bilek E. Bidirectional signal exchanges and their mechanisms during joint attention interaction – A hyperscanning fMRI study. *Neuroimage* (2019) 198:242–54. doi: 10.1016/j.neuroimage.2019.05.028
48. Oberwelland E, Schilbach L, Barisic I, Krall SC, Vogeley K, Fink GR, et al. Look into my eyes: Investigating joint attention using interactive eye-tracking and fMRI in a developmental sample. *Neuroimage* (2016) 130:248–60. doi: 10.1016/j.neuroimage.2016.02.026
49. Leong V, Byrne E, Clackson K, Georgieva S, Lam S, Wass S. Speaker gaze increases information coupling between infant and adult brains. *Proc Natl Acad Sci U S A* (2017) 114:13290–5. doi: 10.1073/pnas.1702493114
50. Schilbach L. Towards a second-person neuropsychiatry. *Philos T R Soc B* (2015) 371:20150081. doi: 10.1098/rstb.2015.0081
51. Kupper Z, Ramseyer F, Hoffmann H, Tschacher W. Nonverbal Synchrony in Social Interactions of Patients with Schizophrenia Indicates Socio-Communicative Deficits. *PloS One* (2015) 10:e0145882. doi: 10.1371/journal.pone.0145882
52. Boker SM, Rotondo JL, Xu M, King K. Windowed cross-correlation and peak picking for the analysis of variability in the association between behavioral time series. *Psychol Methods* (2002) 7:338–55. doi: 10.1037/1082-989X.7.3.338
53. Lachaux JP, Rodriguez E, Martinerie J, Varela FJ. Measuring phase synchrony in brain signals. *Hum Brain Mapp* (1999) 8:194–208. doi: 10.1002/(SICI)1097-0193(1999)8:4<194::AID-HBM4>3.0.CO;2-C
54. Dumas G, Nadel J, Soussignan R, Martinerie J, Garnero L. Inter-brain synchronization during social interaction. *PloS One* (2010) 5:e12166. doi: 10.1371/journal.pone.0012166
55. Goldstein P, Weissman-Fogel I, Dumas G, Shamay-Tsoory SG. Brain-to-brain coupling during handholding is associated with pain reduction. *Proc Natl Acad Sci U S A* (2018) 115:E2528–37. doi: 10.1073/pnas.1703643115
56. Jammalamadaka SR, SenGupta A. *Topics in Circular Statistics*. (2001), (River Edge, NJ: World Scientific). doi: 10.1142/9789812779267
57. Pérez A, Dumas G, Karadag M, Duñabeitia JA. Differential brain-to-brain entrainment while speaking and listening in native and foreign languages. *Cortex* (2019) 111:303–15. doi: 10.1016/j.cortex.2018.11.026
58. Llobera J, Charbonnier C, Chagué S, Preissmann D, Antonietti J-P, Ansermet F, et al. The Subjective Sensation of Synchrony: An Experimental Study. *PloS One* (2016) 11:e0147008. doi: 10.1371/journal.pone.0147008
59. McCall C, Singer T. Facing Off with Unfair Others: Introducing Proxemic Imaging as an Implicit Measure of Approach and Avoidance during Social Interaction. *PloS One* (2015) 10:e0117532. doi: 10.1371/journal.pone.0117532
60. Nozaradan S, Peretz I, Keller PE. Individual Differences in Rhythmic Cortical Entrainment Correlate with Predictive Behavior in Sensorimotor Synchronization. *Sci Rep* (2016) 6:20612. doi: 10.1038/srep20612
61. American Psychiatric Association. *Diagnostic and Statistical Manual of Mental Disorders. 5th ed.* Washington, D.C: American Psychiatric Association (2013).
62. Bruinsma Y, Koegel RL, Koegel LK. Joint attention and children with autism: A review of the literature. *Ment Retard Dev Disabil Res Rev* (2004) 10:169–75. doi: 10.1002/mrdd.20036
63. Nakano T, Kato N, Kitazawa S. Lack of eyeblink entrainments in autism spectrum disorders. *Neuropsychologia* (2011) 49:2784–90. doi: 10.1016/j.neuropsychologia.2011.06.007
64. Oberwelland E, Schilbach L, Barisic I, Krall SC, Vogeley K, Fink GR, et al. Young adolescents with autism show abnormal joint attention network: A gaze contingent fMRI study. *NeuroImage Clin* (2017) 14:112–21. doi: 10.1016/j.nicl.2017.01.006
65. Koehne S, Hatri A, Cacioppo JT, Dziobek I. Perceived interpersonal synchrony increases empathy: Insights from autism spectrum disorder. *Cognition* (2016) 146:8–15. doi: 10.1016/j.cognition.2015.09.007
66. Curioni A, Minio-Paluello I, Sacheli LM, Candidi M, Aglioti SM. Autistic traits affect interpersonal motor coordination by modulating strategic use of role-based behavior. *Mol Autism* (2017) 8:1–13. doi: 10.1186/s13229-017-0141-0
67. Wang Q, Han Z, Hu X, Feng S, Wang H, Liu T, et al. Autism Symptoms Modulate Interpersonal Neural Synchronization in Children with Autism Spectrum Disorder in Cooperative Interactions. *Brain Topogr* (2019) 33:112–22. doi: 10.1007/s10548-019-00731-x
68. Mundy P, Sigman M, Kasari C. A longitudinal study of joint attention and language development in autistic children. *J Autism Dev Disord* (1990) 20:115–28. doi: 10.1007/BF02206861
69. Charman T. Why is joint attention a pivotal skill in autism? *Philos Trans R Soc B Biol Sci* (2003) 358:315–24. doi: 10.1098/rstb.2002.1199
70. Schilbach L, Wilms M, Eickhoff SB, Romanzetti S, Tepest R, Bente G, et al. Minds made for sharing: Initiating joint attention recruits reward-related neurocircuitry. *J Cognit Neurosci* (2010) 22:2702–15. doi: 10.1162/jocn.2009.21401
71. Redcay E, Dodell-Feder D, Mavros PL, Kleiner M, Pearrow MJ, Triantafyllou C, et al. Atypical brain activation patterns during a face-to-face joint attention game in adults with autism spectrum disorder. *Hum Brain Mapp* (2013) 34:2511–23. doi: 10.1002/hbm.22086
72. Tanabe HC, Kosaka H, Saito DN, Koike T, Hayashi MJ, Izuma K, et al. Hard to "tune in": Neural mechanisms of live face-to-face interaction with high-functioning autistic spectrum disorder. *Front Hum Neurosci* (2012) 6:1–15. doi: 10.3389/fnhum.2012.00268
73. Mukai K, Miura A, Kudo K, Tsutsui S. The effect of pairing individuals with different social skills on interpersonal motor coordination. *Front Psychol* (2018) 9:1708. doi: 10.3389/fpsyg.2018.01708
74. Savitz J, Drevets WC. Bipolar and major depressive disorder: Neuroimaging the developmental-degenerative divide. *Neurosci Biobehav Rev* (2009) 33:699–771. doi: 10.1016/j.neubiorev.2009.01.004
75. Takei Y, Suda M, Aoyama Y, Sakurai N, Tagawa M, Motegi T, et al. Near-infrared spectroscopic study of frontopolar activation during face-to-face conversation in major depressive disorder and bipolar disorder. *J Psychiatr Res* (2014) 57:74–83. doi: 10.1016/j.jpsychires.2014.06.009
76. Hooker CI, Bruce L, Lincoln SH, Fisher M, Vinogradov S. Theory of mind skills are related to gray matter volume in the ventromedial prefrontal cortex in schizophrenia. *Biol Psychiatry* (2011) 70:1169–78. doi: 10.1016/j.biopsych.2011.07.027
77. Benedetti F, Bernasconi A, Bosia M, Cavallaro R, Dallaspezia S, Falini A, et al. Functional and structural brain correlates of theory of mind and empathy deficits in schizophrenia. *Schizophr Res* (2009) 114:154–60. doi: 10.1016/j.schres.2009.06.021
78. Takei Y, Suda M, Aoyama Y, Yamaguchi M, Sakurai N, Narita K, et al. Temporal lobe and inferior frontal gyrus dysfunction in patients with schizophrenia during face-to-face conversation: A near-infrared spectroscopy study. *J Psychiatr Res* (2013) 47:1581–9. doi: 10.1016/j.jpsychires.2013.07.029
79. Stegmayer K, Bohlhalter S, Vanbellingen T, Federspiel A, Wiest R, Müri RM, et al. Limbic Interference During Social Action Planning in Schizophrenia. *Schizophr Bull* (2018) 44:359–68. doi: 10.1093/schbul/sbx059
80. Bilek E, Stößel G, Schäfer A, Clement L, Ruf M, Robnik L, et al. State-dependent cross-brain information flow in borderline personality disorder. *JAMA Psychiatry* (2017) 74:949–57. doi: 10.1001/jamapsychiatry.2017.1682
81. Altmann U, Schoenherr D, Paulick J, Deisenhofer AK, Schwartz B, Rubel JA, et al. Associations between movement synchrony and outcome in patients with social anxiety disorder: Evidence for treatment specific effects. *Psychother Res* (2019) 0:1–17. doi: 10.1080/10503307.2019.1630779
82. Paulick J, Rubel JA, Deisenhofer AK, Schwartz B, Thielemann D, Altmann U, et al. Diagnostic Features of Nonverbal Synchrony in Psychotherapy:

Comparing Depression and Anxiety. *Cognit Ther Res* (2018) 42:539–51. doi: 10.1007/s10608-018-9914-9
83. Zhang Y, Meng T, Hou Y, Pan Y, Hu Y. Interpersonal brain synchronization associated with working alliance during psychological counseling. *Psychiatry Res - Neuroimaging* (2018) 282:103–9. doi: 10.1016/j.pscychresns.2018.09.007
84. Bouhuys AL, Sam MM. Lack of coordination of nonverbal behaviour between patients and interviewers as a potential risk factor to depression recurrence: Vulnerability accumulation in depression. *J Affect Disord* (2000) 57:189–200. doi: 10.1016/S0165-0327(99)00093-2
85. Behrends A, Muller S, Dziobek I. Moving in and out of synchrony: A concept for a new intervention fostering empathy through interactional movement and dance. *Arts Psychother* (2012) 39:107–16. doi: 10.1016/j.aip.2012.02.003
86. Scharoun SM, Reinders NJ, Bryden PJ, Fletcher PC. Dance/Movement Therapy as an Intervention for Children with Autism Spectrum Disorders. *Am J Danc Ther* (2014) 36:209–28. doi: 10.1007/s10465-014-9179-0
87. Samaritter R, Payne H. Kinaesthetic intersubjectivity: A dance informed contribution to self-other relatedness and shared experience in non-verbal psychotherapy with an example from autism. *Arts Psychother* (2013) 40:143–50. doi: 10.1016/j.aip.2012.12.004
88. Koch SC, Mehl L, Sobanski E, Sieber M, Fuchs T. Fixing the mirrors: A feasibility study of the effects of dance movement therapy on young adults with autism spectrum disorder. *Autism* (2015) 19:338–50. doi: 10.1177/1362361314522353
89. Koehne S, Behrends A, Fairhurst MT, Dziobek I. Fostering Social Cognition through an Imitation- and Synchronization-Based Dance/Movement Intervention in Adults with Autism Spectrum Disorder: A Controlled Proof-of-Concept Study. *Psychother Psychosom* (2016) 85:27–35. doi: 10.1159/000441111
90. Landa RJ, Holman KC, O'Neill AH, Stuart EA. Intervention targeting development of socially synchronous engagement in toddlers with autism spectrum disorder: A randomized controlled trial. *J Child Psychol Psychiatry Allied Discip* (2011) 52:13–21. doi: 10.1111/j.1469-7610.2010.02288.x
91. Zapata-Fonseca L, Froese T, Schilbach L, Vogeley K, Timmermans B. Sensitivity to social contingency in adults with high-functioning autism during computer-mediated embodied interaction. *Behav Sci (Basel)* (2018) 8:22. doi: 10.3390/bs8020022
92. Novembre G, Knoblich G, Dunne L, Keller PE. Interpersonal synchrony enhanced through 20 Hz phase-coupled dual brain stimulation. *Soc Cognit Affect Neurosci* (2017) 12:662–70. doi: 10.1093/scan/nsw172
93. Szymanski C, Müller V, Brick TR, von Oertzen T, Lindenberger U. Hyper-transcranial alternating current stimulation: Experimental manipulation of inter-brain synchrony. *Front Hum Neurosci* (2017) 11:1–15. doi: 10.3389/fnhum.2017.00539
94. Caria A, Sitaram R, Birbaumer N. Real-time fMRI: A tool for local brain regulation. *Neuroscientist* (2012) 18:487–501. doi: 10.1177/1073858411407205
95. Weiskopf N. Real-time fMRI and its application to neurofeedback. *Neuroimage* (2012) 62:682–92. doi: 10.1016/j.neuroimage.2011.10.009
96. Fovet T, Jardri R, Linden D. Current Issues in the Use of fMRI-Based Neurofeedback to Relieve Psychiatric Symptoms. *Curr Pharm Des* (2015) 21:3384–94. doi: 10.2174/1381612821666150619092540
97. Pan Y, Borragán G, Peigneux P. Applications of Functional Near-Infrared Spectroscopy in Fatigue, Sleep Deprivation, and Social Cognition. *Brain Topogr* (2019) 32:998–1012. doi: 10.1007/s10548-019-00740-w
98. Brigadoi S, Ceccherini L, Cutini S, Scarpa F, Scatturin P, Selb J, et al. Motion artifacts in functional near-infrared spectroscopy: A comparison of motion correction techniques applied to real cognitive data. *Neuroimage* (2014) 85:181–91. doi: 10.1016/j.neuroimage.2013.04.082
99. Cui X, Baker JM, Liu N, Reiss AL. Sensitivity of fNIRS measurement to head motion: An applied use of smartphones in the lab. *J Neurosci Methods* (2015) 245:37–43. doi: 10.1016/j.jneumeth.2015.02.006
100. Zhang X, Noah JA, Hirsch J. Separation of the global and local components in functional near-infrared spectroscopy signals using principal component spatial filtering. *Neurophotonics* (2016) 3:015004. doi: 10.1117/1.nph.3.1.015004
101. Erdfelder E, FAul F, Buchner A, Lang AG. Statistical power analyses using G*Power 3.1: Tests for correlation and regression analyses. *Behav Res Methods* (2009) 41:1149–60. doi: 10.3758/BRM.41.4.1149
102. Grinsted A, Moore JC, Jevrejeva S. Application of the cross wavelet transform and wavelet coherence to geophysical time series. *Nonlinear Process Geophys* (2004) 11:561–6. doi: 10.5194/npg-11-561-2004
103. Seth AK, Barrett AB, Barnett L. Granger causality analysis in neuroscience and neuroimaging. *J Neurosci* (2015) 35:3293–7. doi: 10.1523/JNEUROSCI.4399-14.2015
104. Nastase SA, Gazzola V, Hasson U, Keysers C. Measuring shared responses across subjects using intersubject correlation. *Soc Cognit Affect Neurosci* (2019) 14:669–87. doi: 10.1093/scan/nsz037
105. Bolis D, Schilbach L. Beyond one Bayesian brain: Modeling intra-and inter-personal processes during social interaction: Commentary on "mentalizing homeostasis: The social origins of interoceptive inference" by Fotopoulou & Tsakiris. *Neuropsychoanalysis* (2017) 19:35–8. doi: 10.1080/15294145.2017.1295215
106. Zhou C, Han M, Liang Q, Hu YF, Kuai SG. A social interaction field model accurately identifies static and dynamic social groupings. *Nat Hum Behav* (2019) 3:847–55. doi: 10.1038/s41562-019-0618-2
107. Faraone SV, Doyle AE. Genetic influences on attention deficit hyperactivity disorder. *Curr Psychiatry Rep* (2000) 2:143–6. doi: 10.1007/s11920-000-0059-6

10

Conceptual Analysis: A Social Neuroscience Approach to Interpersonal Interaction in the Context of Disruption and Disorganization of Attachment (NAMDA)

Lars O. White [1†], Charlotte C. Schulz [1,2*†], Margerete J. S. Schoett [1], Melanie T. Kungl [3], Jan Keil [1], Jessica L. Borelli [4] and Pascal Vrtička [5,6*]*

[1] Department of Child and Adolescent Psychiatry, University of Leipzig, Leipzig, Germany, [2] Department of Neurology, Max Planck Institute for Human Cognitive and Brain Sciences, Leipzig, Germany, [3] Department of Psychology, University of Erlangen-Nuremberg, Erlangen, Germany, [4] THRIVE Laboratory, Psychology and Social Behavior, University of California, Irvine, Irvine, CA, United States, [5] Research Group "Social Stress and Family Health", Max Planck Institute for Human Cognitive and Brain Sciences, Leipzig, Germany, [6] Department of Psychology, Centre for Brain Science, University of Essex, Colchester, United Kingdom

***Correspondence:**
Lars O. White
larsotto.white@medizin.uni-leipzig.de
Charlotte C. Schulz
charlotte.schulz@medizin.uni-leipzig.de
Pascal Vrtička
p.vrticka@essex.ac.uk

† These authors have contributed equally to this work and share first authorship

Humans are strongly dependent upon social resources for allostasis and emotion regulation. This applies especially to early childhood because humans—as an altricial species—have a prolonged period of dependency on support and input from caregivers who typically act as sources of co-regulation. Accordingly, attachment theory proposes that the history and quality of early interactions with primary caregivers shape children's internal working models of attachment. In turn, these attachment models guide behavior, initially with the set goal of maintaining proximity to caregivers but eventually paving the way to more generalized mental representations of self and others. Mounting evidence in non-clinical populations suggests that these mental representations coincide with differential patterns of neural structure, function, and connectivity in a range of brain regions previously associated with emotional and cognitive capacities. What is currently lacking, however, is an evidence-based account of how early adverse attachment-related experiences and/or the emergence of attachment disorganization impact the developing brain. While work on early childhood adversities offers important insights, we propose that how these events become biologically embedded crucially hinges on the context of the child–caregiver attachment relationships in which the events take place. Our selective review distinguishes between direct social neuroscience research on disorganized attachment and indirect maltreatment-related research, converging on aberrant functioning in neurobiological systems subserving aversion, approach, emotion regulation, and mental state processing in the wake of severe attachment disruption. To account for heterogeneity of findings, we propose two distinct neurobiological phenotypes characterized by hyper- and hypo-arousal primarily deriving from the caregiver serving either as a threatening or as an insufficient source of co-regulation, respectively.

Keywords: disorganized attachment, neglect and abuse, maltreatment, co-regulation, social interaction, social neuroscience

Disturbances in childhood family functioning account for approximately a quarter to a third of youth- and adult-onset mental disorders (1, 2). Attachment theory and research offer an in-depth theoretical account of how family caregiving relationships from infancy onwards impact development, for better and for worse, across a vast array of psychosocial domains (3). Much work has attempted to leverage attachment theory to shed light on mechanisms underlying the effects of adverse early caregiving experiences on later mental health (4), with most data showing the highest risk to emanate from disorganized attachment (5–7). However, aside from a few recent pioneering empirical studies (8–14), a social neuroscience perspective encompassing disorganized and maltreatment-related disruption of attachment is still notably absent. Recently, a comprehensive functional neuro-anatomical model of human attachment was proposed [NAMA (15–17)]. NAMA describes a prototypical attachment pathway reflecting psychological processes activated in attachment-relevant situations, which is likely to be maintained by four neural modules. It further summarizes the evidence available to date on how inter-individual differences in the three major typical (or "organized") attachment patterns coincide with anatomy and function within, and connectivity between these modules. However, the account of NAMA is notably incomplete in that disorganized attachment is largely omitted due to a paucity of data and the lack of an according conceptual social neuroscience framework. The present paper aims to begin to fill this gap. After providing a brief conceptual overview of organized and disorganized attachment, we extend NAMA to a functional neuro-anatomical model of disrupted attachment (NAMDA). To support our speculations on the putative neurobiological underpinnings of disorganized attachment, we draw on *direct* and *indirect* empirical evidence stemming from studies utilizing samples assessed for attachment disorganization and maltreatment histories, respectively.

ORGANIZED AND DISORGANIZED ATTACHMENT IN A NUTSHELL

Attachment theory claims that children's repeated interactions with their primary caregiver(s) shape their early organization of attachment, thereby guiding behavior in attachment-relevant situations (18–22). Following a developmental sequence, children progress from overt behavioral strategies organized at a procedural level to a later representational organization (23), referred to as internal working models of attachment (24, 25). Children whose caregivers reliably respond in a sensitive manner to their needs tend to adopt an "organized" (i.e., attachment strategy-driven) and secure attachment pattern (19, 26). Thus, they turn to their caregivers in times of distress (safe haven function) and explore in the caregiver's vicinity in times of safety (secure base function), ultimately facilitating a sense of self-efficacy and trust in others, more generally (27).

Conversely, children whose caregivers are merely inconsistently available in times of distress tend to adopt an insecure anxious–ambivalent strategy, involving hyperactivation of the attachment system during distress (e.g., excessive proximity seeking and maintaining), an organized strategy thought to maximize the amount of nurturance elicited from caregivers. In turn, offspring of caregivers who typically thwart their child's bids for contact and are relatively unresponsive to their emotional signals tend to adopt an insecure–avoidant strategy of suppressing (outward signs of) distress, an organized strategy thought to minimize the caregiving burden and odds of further rejection by caregivers (28, 29). These strategies reflect (co-)regulatory mechanisms comprising overdependence on others (anxiety) or overemphasis on self-reliance (avoidance) while they remain expedient (and thus organized), achieving the evolutionarily highly adaptive goal of maintaining sufficient proximity to the caregiver in a given environment (29, 30). Hence, they preserve (limited) co-regulation by caregivers.

By contrast, according to Main (31), disorganized attachment reflects a breakdown of the aforementioned organized strategies and occurs when the child experiences "fright without solution" within the attachment relationship [(32), p. 484]. This state is thought to emerge because the distressed child requires comfort from attachment figures (AFs) which, however, is (felt to be) largely unattainable because the AFs themselves have become associated with alarm (4). The classic case cited in this context is that of caregivers who expose their child to physical abuse so that they simultaneously represent both the primary source of comfort and the primary source of distress for their child. This circumstance is thought to give rise to conflicting motivations on behalf of the child involving co-existing tendencies to approach and avoid their frightened/frightening caregivers, eventuating in a set of apprehensive, disoriented, or contradictory behaviors (e.g., seeking comfort with markedly averted face) (33, 34). It is noteworthy, however, that akin to Ainsworth's early work, Main conceives of fear linked to the AF (e.g., due to maltreatment) as having a disorganizing influence on the child, resulting in a breakdown of organized attachment strategies, i.e., inhibiting bids for co-regulation from caregivers under distress and/or exploration in caregivers' vicinity under calm conditions. Conversely, others consider fear linked to the AF as an organizing force and "disorganization" to be a misnomer (35, 36). In line with Ainsworth's later work, for Crittenden, fear of the AF thus promotes excessive tendencies to either (1) overemphasize cognitive predictability at the expense of negative affect expression or (2) overamplify negative affect at the expense of cognitive predictability (35). While these strategies are thought to result in a lack of integration of cognition and affect, they may serve a self-preserving function, maximizing survival odds (e.g., compulsive compliance with caregivers' demands in the case of physical abuse) (37)[1].

Precursors and Mental Health Sequelae of Disorganized Attachment

As noted above, the state of "fright without solution" is thought to lie at the heart of disorganized attachment. However, "fright without solution" often, though by no means invariably, entails that caregivers act as a *source* of alarm for the child, as in the case of physical abuse (38). Indeed in a meta-analysis on maltreatment and disorganization, the effects of abuse and neglect on disorganization were almost indistinguishable in terms of their effect size and confidence intervals (33). Moreover, disorganization has also been linked to caregivers' withdrawal and dissociative behaviors (39, 40) or hostile–helpless states of mind, possibly due to the caregiver's own traumatic experiences (41, 42). A further case in point is the context of institutionalization or prolonged caregiver separation where the need for a continuously available and reliable caregiver is experienced over a long period without any hope of being met ("activation without assuagement"), resulting in resignation and despair (43, 44). Especially in early childhood, caregivers are the main source of co-regulation of mild to overwhelming affective states (safe haven function). Hence, prolonged absence of or chronically rebuffing caregivers, as well as other major unpredictable discontinuities in the caregiving context (e.g., multiple changing caregivers), bears the potential to disrupt normative development of organized attachment. This dovetails with meta-analytic data showing that over half of institutionalized children are classified as disorganized (31, 45).

Surveying different populations, while disorganization occasionally occurs within middle-class samples (infants:15%, adults: 18%; "unresolved–disorganized state of mind"), prevalence estimates are higher among samples burdened by sociodemographic risks (e.g., offspring of teen mothers: 23%, families with low socioeconomic status: 25%) and yet higher still among samples with clinical or psychosocial risks (clinical adult samples: 43%, children with neurological abnormalities: 35%, adoptees: 31%, offspring of caregivers with substance abuse: 43%, previously institutionalized samples: 54–73%, and children raised by maltreating caregivers: 48–90%) (31, 34, 45–47)[2]. Despite these elevated rates of disorganization in samples exposed to adversity, the mapping of adversity with disorganization is far from perfect, suggesting that disorganization may account for meaningful variance over and above adversity. Thus, for example, in women with a history of childhood abuse, attachment disorganization gave rise to a 7½-fold increase in the odds of being diagnosed with post-traumatic stress disorder (48), stressing its putative role in the aftermath of adversity, where disorganization is thought to act akin to an intermediary factor, signaling how adaptively trauma has been processed (4, 49, 50).

Conceptualizing attachment disorganization as a potential intermediary process may also help explain a salient pattern emerging from recent research—including large-scale studies and meta-analyses (51–55)—documenting unique and especially toxic effects for mental health following emotional maltreatment, in particular [e.g., persistent rejection or absence of support from the caregiver; see (56)]. Mounting evidence thus suggests that the pathogenic effects of emotional maltreatment (e.g., on depression) may exceed and potentially even explain those of other (physical) subtypes of maltreatment. To account for this pattern, many scholars invoke conceptual links between emotional maltreatment and attachment disorganization as well as impaired reflective functioning (54, 55, 57, 58). Supporting these ideas, the maltreatment-related risk for attachment disorganization is mitigated when abuse and neglect transpire in the context of emotionally supportive caregiving relationships (58, 59). In keeping with this, scholars contend that a "pathogenic relational experience" may often lie at the core of child maltreatment (60, 61), potentially reflecting a seedbed for other forms of maltreatment to occur.

Hyper- and Hypo-Arousal Pathways to Disorganization

The brief summary presented above bolsters the view of disorganization as a heterogeneous phenomenon. Thus, many divergent behaviors (e.g., contradictory, freezing, apprehensive behaviors in the presence of caregivers) and narrative indicators (e.g., sudden affective shifts, incompatible affect, interrupted speech, bizarre descriptions, lapses in reasoning when recounting loss or trauma) pertain to the classification of individuals as disorganized in childhood and adulthood (4, 62, 63). Specifically, in the case of narratives, organized strategies for coherently discussing trauma suddenly collapse as the memory of the traumatic experience is thought to become frighteningly imminent and overwhelming (fright without solution), impeding ongoing mental processes (64). Moreover, multiple distinct forms of and pathways to disorganization have been proposed in the

[1] Main's and Crittenden's views are not necessarily mutually exclusive. Thus, fear of the AF can have a disorganizing influence on behavior, especially when the child's own resources are overwhelmed and the caregiver is the only source of comfort available, as may often be the case in the SSP (fright without solution). However, fear of the AF in the same child can also have a highly organizing influence when it comes to compulsively complying with the caregiver's demands in other contexts (e.g., at home) in order to prevent the caregiver from becoming a source of fear in the first place (to which there would be no solution). Thus, fear of the AF can have a disorganizing or organizing influence for the child depending on the context in which it occurs [cf. (37) for evidence and arguments that partly support this line of argument].

[2] An apparent exception to the elevated rates in clinical samples is adult depression, i.e., neither infant disorganization is elevated among depressed mothers nor is unresolved–disorganized status elevated among adults with depression (4, 46, 47). Regarding child depression, while studies assessing attachment in infancy yield a mixed picture, those with post-infancy assessments seem to have established a reliable link between disorganization and depression (6). That said, links to disorganization seem more consistent when considering more serious forms of depression in need of treatment (4), potentially calling for subtype-specific analyses.

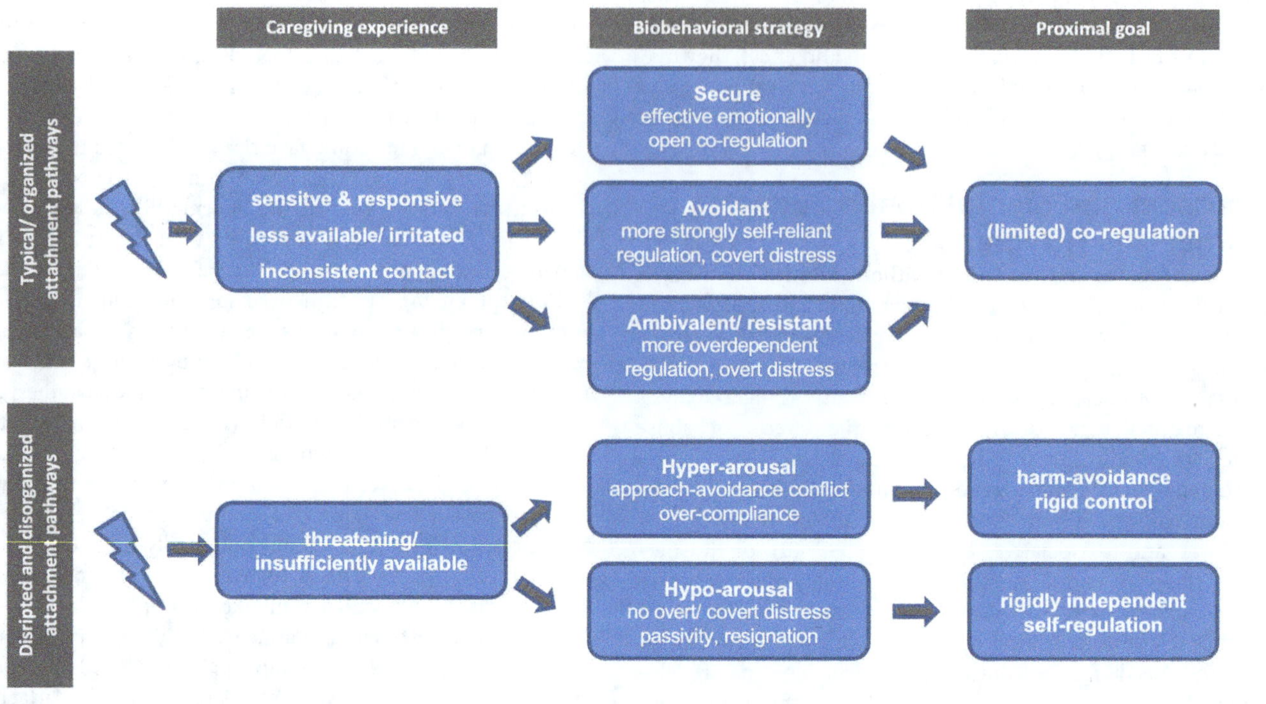

FIGURE 1 | Schematic diagram of the proposed typical vs. disrupted and disorganized attachment pathways.

literature (34, 38, 65) and may even have been anticipated in early unpublished writings of Bowlby (43).

Attempting to come to terms with this heterogeneity, shortly after the notion of disorganization was first introduced, Crittenden and Ainsworth (66)[3] highlighted the added value of distinguishing between abuse and neglect in the context of discussing attachment disorganization. For example, the abused child is "locked into forming an attachment to his primary caregiver and yet his experience teaches him that this attachment figure may be a source of pain and injury" [(66), p. 449]. Conversely, neglected children "desperately need the comfort and support of others [but] rarely seek it or seem comforted by it when they receive it" [(66), p. 450]. In line with these proposals and recent efforts to delineate different pathways to disorganization, **Figure 1** outlines two distinct neurobiological hyper- and hypo-arousal phenotypes in the context of disrupted and disorganized attachment. Importantly, while these pathways are informed by current neural models of adversity, threat, and deprivation (67–70), they remain to be further examined and empirically substantiated, particularly in the case of disrupted and disorganized attachment. Accordingly, the proximate attachment-oriented mechanism of co-regulation by caregivers is thought to be severely impaired for both hyper- and hypo-arousal pathways and subordinated to harm avoidance and rigid self-regulation, respectively. Nevertheless, we believe that these behaviors serve as the best possible solution for promoting survival in the context of insufficiently available or threatening primary caregivers (who exhibit frightened/frightening behaviors).

[3] Although Main and Solomon (33) published their seminal chapter introducing disorganized attachment in the following year, Crittenden and Ainsworth (66) evidently already had access to it and referenced this chapter.

Summary

As a point of departure, we provided a brief overview of disorganized attachment, beginning with key theories and evidence regarding its putative origins and sequelae before turning to its inherent heterogeneity. The heterogeneity of disorganization emerges not only in terms of its phenomenology but also regarding its ontogeny and etiology and may at least partly reflect distinct adaptations upon exposure to abusing and/or neglecting caregivers. Analogous to early and current work on attachment disorganization and recent developments in neuroscience (see below), we consequently propose a distinction between a hypo- and hyper-arousal subtype primarily deriving from the caregiver serving either as a threatening or as an insufficient source of co-regulation, respectively.

In the next section, before elaborating on the possible neurobiological underpinnings of disrupted and disorganized attachment, we offer a brief summary of NAMA's functional neuro-anatomical account of organized human attachment within the field of social neuroscience. Readers familiar with the up-to-date version of NAMA (17) are referred directly to the section on "The Social Neuroscience of Disrupted and Disorganized Attachment."

THE SOCIAL NEUROSCIENCE OF ORGANIZED HUMAN ATTACHMENT

Most theoretical accounts of the neurobiological substrates of interpersonal interactions and relationships derived from social neuroscience thus far only indirectly refer to attachment theory. This likely reflects the fact that only a limited number of social neuroscience studies assess attachment using narrative or self-report measures (71), and extant work has nearly exclusively focused on adult populations. Nevertheless, we recently synthesized all available experimental evidence, suggesting a comprehensive framework of the social neuroscience of (organized) human attachment (functional neuro-anatomical model of human attachment—NAMA; **Figure 2**) (15–17). NAMA draws directly on attachment theory in that it presupposes a prototypical attachment pathway with several sequential components that constitute the proposed underlying neurobiological and brain mechanisms of organized (i.e., secure, avoidant, anxious–ambivalent) human attachment.

Prototypical Attachment Pathways and Neuro-Anatomical Model

In keeping with attachment theory (19–22), we assume that (external or internal) events appraised as threatening reliably activate the attachment behavioral system. Such threat appraisal—and associated appropriate fear response—is thought to challenge homeostasis, necessitating a compensatory physiological and behavioral response to (re-)gain an optimal internal milieu. Following the notion of allostasis (72), this regulatory process helps the organism to adapt to changes in the environment and meet anticipated demands. Accordingly, we postulate the presence of an *aversion module* in NAMA that encodes negative social experiences—from social exclusion or abandonment in times of need to any kind of negative occurrences, including those of a non-social nature—in terms of a neural relevance/salience signal (73), prompting further action (i.e., allostatic regulation). At the level of neurotransmitters/hormones, the primary stress-related hormone cortisol, acting through the hypothalamic–pituitary–adrenocortical (HPA) axis, may underpin such aversion module activation (**Figure 2**).

Once the fear response has been triggered, the next crucial element of a prototypical attachment pathway involves proximity seeking maintained by a fundamental social approach motivation. In other words, we propose a "social flight response" (74), not unlike the tend-and-befriend responses postulated elsewhere (75), but tailored more specifically to AFs. The underlying notion of this approach motivation is that (mutual) social interactions should be subjectively experienced and neurally encoded as intrinsically rewarding. We therefore situate a reward-related *approach module* associated with the action of, among others, dopamine, oxytocin, and endogenous opioids as the second of four modules in NAMA (**Figure 2**).

Both the approach and aversion modules are deemed to be activated by, and represent more automatic, bottom-up biological and neural mechanisms and are thus summarized as *affective evaluation* or *emotional mentalization processes* (76). It should also be noted here that we view the approach and aversion modules as two rather independent—albeit complementary—neurobiological systems that can be de- or hyper-activated to varying degrees in attachment-relevant situations as a function of inter-individual differences in secure vs. insecure attachment orientations (even in opposing directions), that is, we do not equate de- or hyper-activation of the approach module with attachment security and de- or hyper-activation of the aversion module with insecurity as two diametrically opposing ends of one single attachment dimension. Furthermore, we believe that, except during the initial moment of approach module involvement, to motivate a social approach response of support seeking under distress (i.e., during simultaneous aversion module activation), for typical (or organized) attachment patterns, the two emotional modules should not be activated concomitantly for an extensive time period/chronically, as this would lead to conflicting social emotional states.

Once social proximity has been successfully established (and the source of threat has been abolished), NAMA suggests that the next stage in the prototypical attachment pathway can unfold: *emotion regulation.* Initially mainly accomplished by external co-regulation through AFs, this is increasingly supplanted by self-regulation (i.e., by virtue of an internalized source of regulation) with advancing development, with both decelerated and accelerated adoption of self-regulation associated with suboptimal outcomes (69). The primary goal of the emotion regulation module is to down-regulate negative emotional states to re-establish homeostasis and thereby reduce the allostatic load. In the context of attachment, it has been elegantly demonstrated that such regulatory influence of emotion regulation (mainly *via* the aversion module) can encompass both conscious and unconscious mechanisms and relies upon a variety of emotion regulation strategies (77–79).

Provided that emotion regulation is effective and a return to homeostasis is achieved, re-activation of the approach module may occur following NAMA. This is because we assume that the return to the organism's optimal inner milieu and normal range of arousal (entailing a reduced allostatic load) through effective affect co- or self-regulation is experienced as positive *per se.* Such personal positive experience of physically calming down is presumably accompanied by additional socially positive aspects of the interaction with the external co-regulator [e.g., affective touch, soothing verbalizations, etc. (72)] that serve to establish a feeling of safety and security, which further reinforces the rewarding nature particularly of co-regulation and the social interaction as a whole.

Finally, we posit a *mental state representation* module in NAMA. In the context of attachment, the mental state representation module is conceived of as a central part of the neural substrate of internal attachment working models that emerge through repeated interactions with others and comprise predictions about how to approach whom in times of need, how the approached individual(s) will respond, and whether their reaction will be helpful or not. Social neuroscience postulates that a so-called default mode network may maintain such processes [(80), see **Figure 2**].

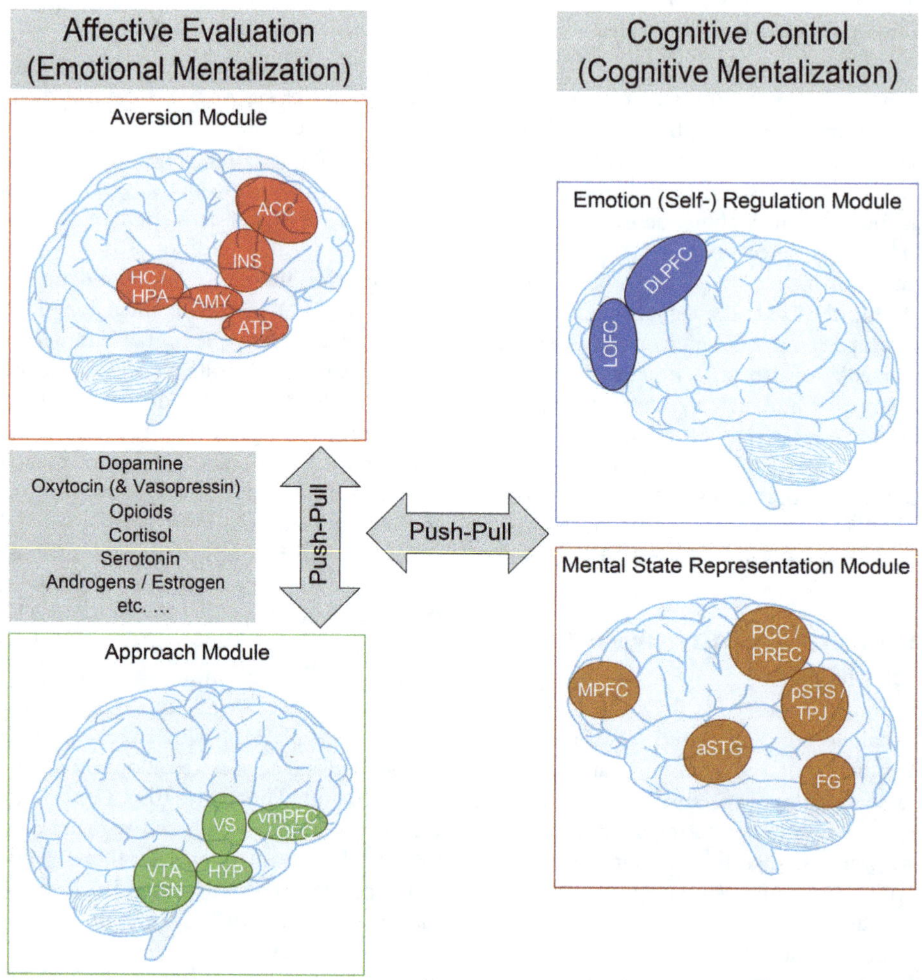

FIGURE 2 | Functional neuro-anatomical model of human (organized) attachment (NAMA). We propose that the (organized) human attachment system can be described by two affective/emotional (left) vs. cognitive/control (right) systems on the neural level, and that these systems can be further separated into two modules each (affective evaluation: aversion—red—and approach—green; cognitive control: emotion regulation—blue—and mental state representation—orange). We further suggest that the aversion and approach modules as part of the affective system, as well as the affective and cognitive systems are in a dynamic "push-pull" balance. Finally, we propose that neural activity within the affective system is mediated by (amongst others) dopamine, oxytocin (and vasopressin), endogenous opioids, cortisol, serotonin, androgens/estrogen, etc. aversion module—ACC, anterior cingulate cortex; INS, insula; HC/HPA, hippocampus/HPA-axis; AMY, amygdala; ATP, anterior temporal pole; approach module—vmPFC/OFC, ventromedial prefrontal/orbitofrontal cortex; HYP, hypothalamus; VTA/SN, ventral tegmental area/substantia nigra; emotion regulation module—DLPFC, dorsolateral prefrontal cortex; LOFC, lateral orbitofrontal cortex; mental state representation module—MPFC, medial prefrontal cortex; PCC/PREC, posterior cingulate cortex/precuneus; pSTS/TPJ, posterior superior temporal sulcus/temporo-parietal junction; aSTG, anterior superior temporal gyrus; FG, fusiform gyrus. For more information, please refer to the main text. Adapted from Long et al. (17) and based on Vrtička (15) and Vrtička and Vuilleumier (16).

Both the emotion regulation and mental state representation modules are summarized as *cognitive control* or *cognitive mentalization* processes in NAMA [see (76)]. They are thought to modulate the perception of social emotional cues and thus emotional mentalization processes through top-down influences by down- and up-regulating emotional states and determining social approach or aversion motivations. Within this context, we refer to mentalization as the imaginative mental activity that enables us to perceive and interpret human behavior in terms of intentional mental states [e.g., needs, desires, feelings, beliefs, and goals; see (51)]. Broadly speaking, it is thought that emotional and cognitive mentalization processes are in a dynamic balance and that the "switch point" between them is determined by the magnitude of affective arousal related to attachment system activation in association with the respective individual attachment-related strategies to maintain successful regulation. Consequently, high affective arousal should push the "switch point" toward emotional mentalization and thus more rigid, fast, and unconscious processing [(76); for neural and behavioral evidence in adults and children see (81, 82), respectively; see **Figure 2**].

Inter-Individual Differences in Organized Attachment

Besides describing the fundamental biological and neural building blocks of human attachment associated with a prototypical attachment pathway (**Figure 2**), we place particular emphasis on how inter-individual differences in the three organized secure vs. insecure—avoidant and anxious–ambivalent—attachment orientations affect the functioning of the four NAMA modules in healthy participants across the lifespan. In so doing, several patterns appear to emerge, which are briefly summarized below and in **Figure 2** [for more details and a comprehensive summary of the evidence base, please see (15–17)].

Firstly, *secure attachment* appears to involve reduced aversion module activation during stressful situations (especially when under threat or in pain) and preserved aversion module structural integrity (comprising the HPA stress axis) in the long term. Both mechanisms are likely propagated *via* a protective effect of initially readily available social resources for co-regulation, eventually translating into more efficient self-regulation (by means of an internalized source of regulation), and enhanced by security priming. This explanation is bolstered by positive representations of others in the approach module and more extensive functional connectivity between the emotional and cognitive mentalization modules of NAMA sustaining self-regulation and mental accessibility of others.

Secondly, *attachment avoidance* and its associated de-activating strategies appear to be most consistently linked to altered approach module functionality because (mutual) social interactions with others are subjectively (i.e., pleasantness ratings), biologically (i.e., oxytocin and opioid signaling), and neurally encoded as less rewarding. Additionally, although aversion module activation during negative social information processing is reduced under specific circumstances (particularly during brief and mild social exclusion in children and adults—likely due to negative expectancy and ensuing disengagement) (83–85), it is typically increased due to inefficient self-regulation (mainly through suppression) (86) and lower availability of social resources to deal with distress (e.g., lengthy social exclusion, especially in adolescence) (87). The latter also manifests by altered aversion module structure and connectivity, epigenetic modification of the HPA stress axis, accelerated biological aging/reduced telomere length, and increased baseline bodily readiness (i.e., higher fasting glucose levels) (88, 89), all indicative of heightened self-reliance and associated chronic stress. The widespread general association between attachment avoidance and the presence of de-activating secondary strategies therefore appears to only partially "succeed" at a neurobiological level.

Finally, *anxious–ambivalent attachment* characterized by hyper-activating strategies also associates with increased aversion module activation during negative social information processing and altered aversion module structure and connectivity. There are, however, no consistent indications of a systematic regulation inefficiency and/or chronic stress on the epigenetic level (HPA stress axis). This pattern related to attachment anxiety therefore rather points to increased saliency processing of social cues, indicating the unavailability of others and a dependence on external (co-)regulation. Such notions are corroborated by increased approach module activation to (unexpected) positive social clues reflecting a sustained wish for social closeness and care when in need.

It should be mentioned here that, in contrast to data on the aversion, approach, and emotion regulation modules, findings implicating the mental state representation module linked to attachment avoidance and anxiety are still too sparse for deriving solid conclusions. We are only aware of one study in adults linking avoidance with neural correlates, reflecting hypo-mentalization during a specific mentalization task, and one study in adolescents associating anxiety with decreases and increases in brain activity during self- and other-representation in a range of areas [also outside the mental state representation module; see (17) for details].

From First- to Second-Person Social Neuroscience of Attachment

Most of the aforementioned patterns of findings draw on data gathered by only obtaining behavioral, biological, and brain measures from one participant (i.e., first-person social neuroscience). During the previous years, however, there has been a paradigm shift toward assessing such measures from two (or more) directly interacting participants (i.e., second-person social neuroscience). In so doing, a special focus is directed toward bio-behavioral synchrony—the time-locked attunement of behavioral, physiological, endocrine, and neural responding—during or immediately after social interaction (90). One prominent social neuroscience method to assess neural attunement in terms of inter-brain coherence is functional near-infrared spectroscopy (fNIRS). In line with the theoretical assumption put forward by Feldman (90), a stronger increase in inter-brain coherence during cooperative tasks is usually found between close interaction partners such as mother–child dyads or romantic couples [as compared to interactions between strangers (91, 92)]. Such results, however, do not allow for directly answering the question whether and, if yes, how, inter-individual differences in relationship quality (i.e., attachment) may influence bio-behavioral synchrony/inter-brain coherence during cooperative tasks within a given interaction partner category. To our knowledge, there are only two fNIRS studies available to date that provide preliminary evidence toward this end.

In a first study, inter-brain coherence during a cooperative button press task within mother–child dyads (child age 8–12 years) was found to be reduced among children with an avoidant attachment toward their mothers (93). These findings, however, did not survive correction for multiple comparison and child gender, age, and attachment anxiety scores. In a second study, inter-brain coherence was assessed during an interactive problem solving task (tangram puzzle) in mothers with their 5 year-old children (94). Besides finding that inter-brain coherence during cooperation was positively associated with task performance, it also correlated positively with behavioral measures reflecting a secure mother–child relationship, such as behavioral reciprocity and child agency. Taken together, these data suggest that a more secure relationship can also manifest itself by increased bio-behavioral synchrony during direct interaction. More research, however, is needed to further extend and replicate these preliminary findings in an attachment context.

Summary

Within NAMA, we propose a prototypical initial attachment pathway and its translation into four fundamental biological and neural building blocks of human attachment—the four aversion, approach, emotion regulation, and mental state representation modules. This framework provides the foundation for the three organized secure, avoidant, and anxious attachment pathway derivatives and how the associated inter-individual differences affect the functioning of the four NAMA modules in healthy participants across the lifespan. As more recent investigations try to establish links between bio-behavioral synchrony and inter-individual differences in attachment in two (or more) interacting individuals, the social neuroscience of attachment is currently entering a new era.

In contrast to the aforementioned emerging patterns relating to organized secure, avoidant, and anxious–ambivalent attachment, much less is known about the social neuroscience of maltreatment-related disruption and disorganization of attachment. One central question is whether attachment disorganization and/or maltreatment may manifest comparably to attachment avoidance and/or anxiety on a biological and brain level. Ideally, the evidence already available from healthy participants summarized in NAMA may serve as a point of reference for interpreting the data thus far available using social neuroscience paradigms in clinical populations and generating future investigations to further characterize the biological and neural signatures of maltreatment-related disruption and disorganization of attachment.

THE SOCIAL NEUROSCIENCE OF DISRUPTED AND DISORGANIZED ATTACHMENT

As outlined above, our aim is to extend NAMA—the model of organized attachment outlined in the previous section—to disrupted and disorganized attachment in the context of maltreatment and adverse attachment-related experiences. To this end, we draw on models of structural and functional brain alterations in the wake of early adversity (67–70). Informed by some of these models (67, 68), we propose distinguishing between a neurobiological *hyper-arousal* phenotype related to primary caregiver(s) as a source(s) of threat (e.g., abuse) and a neurobiological *hypo-arousal* phenotype as a consequence of (early) distress unassuaged by caregiver(s) (e.g., emotional neglect). In so doing, we feel that it is particularly pertinent to point out that we are by no means equating these phenotypes with concrete adverse events, specifically abuse (the presence of threatening/harmful input) and neglect (or deprivation/lack of necessary input), respectively (95). In our view, the fundamental issue rather is if these adversities are mainly attributable to actions by the primary caregivers and the attendant issue of whether the adversities interfere with the function of caregivers as sources of co-regulation. As such, pervasive abuse and neglect may serve as prototypical environmental experiences that often coincide with the expression of these neurobiological phenotypes, yet other dimensions such as timing of adversity [e.g., (96)], child gender (97), neonatal hippocampal volume (11), temperament, or genotype (4, 23) may prove as crucial moderators (see **Figure 3**, row 1).

Thus, as already elegantly outlined by Crittenden and Ainsworth (66), unlike exposure to abuse and neglect, disorganized attachment is conceptualized in terms of a representational model amalgamated from the history of caregiving experiences (i.e., not a singular or set of singular event/s) as well as the individual's adaptive and (co-)regulatory efforts marshaled in response to these experiences. This is not to deny that adversity cannot have a lawful and direct temporary or lasting impact on neurobiological development as a function of the specific patterning of experience regarding, for example, the timing of experience in terms of sensitive periods of brain development (70). However, the recent data from the Bucharest Early Intervention Project (98) and English and Romanian Adoptees study (99) provide first causal evidence in humans that sensitive periods and windows of opportunity regarding the development of the social brain appear to be broader relative to those of other species [see also (100)]. Thus, the impact of severe and chronic deprivation seems at least partly reversible if it is terminated early (101), and puberty may provide yet another window of opportunity for potential recalibration (102). In turn, this suggests that developmental time windows exist, during which effects of even such severe adversities remain highly malleable and under the influence of subsequent caregiving experience.

Informed by the ecophenotype model of Teicher et al. (70, 103), we assert that this perspective on the neural correlates of early adversity may offer a helpful new vantage point, potentially aiding us in understanding the many (initially) adaptive behaviors children and adults show in the face of adversity, including hyper-cooperativeness (104), compulsive compliance (105), and indiscriminate friendliness (106), which would otherwise remain puzzling from a pure perspective of neuro-cognitive dysfunction [see (107) for evolutionary arguments on why these behaviors might be adaptive, for example, in the sense of minimizing the odds of malignant and maximizing the odds of benign interactions]. In particular, we propose distinguishing between neurobiological hyper- and hypo-arousal phenotypes coinciding with disrupted and/or disorganized attachment, primarily based on the available neurobiological data from children with severe adversity. Importantly, these admittedly speculative and preliminary assertions are largely based on *indirect* evidence from samples exposed to severe early-life adversity rather than *direct* evidence from effects of attachment disorganization, a distinction that we will repeatedly return to below (and that is summarized in **Figure 3**, rows 2–5).

Alterations in the Aversion Module

Most neurobiological alterations *directly* associated with disorganized attachment have been documented in neural regions and physiological indices linked to what has been termed the aversion module in NAMA. For example, a number of psychophysiological studies suggest that infants classified as disorganized show increased reactivity of the autonomic nervous system and HPA axis to caregiver separation and reunion

Brain Module	Organized Attachment	Disorganized / Disrupted Attachment	
		Hypo-Arousal	*Hyper-Arousal*
Primary determinants	**SEC:** consistently available caregiver **AV:** consistently less available caregiver **AX:** inconsistently available caregiver	**Caregiving experiences:** • insufficient source of co-regulation • early maltreatment / prenatal risk **Potential moderators:** • fearless temperament • long-term response to chronic stress • male gender	**Caregiving experiences:** • threatening source of co-regulation • later / unpredictable risk **Potential moderators:** • inhibited / negative temperament • short-term response to severe stress • female gender
Aversion 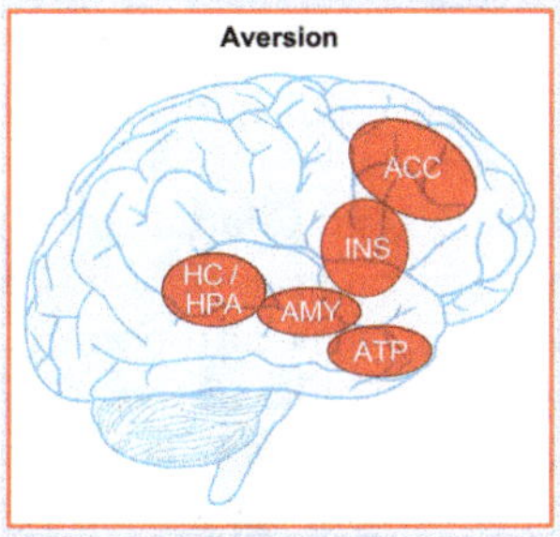 	**SEC:** ↓ activation to negative social information, threat, and pain during secure-based social interactions via (co-) regulation, priming, and representations **AV:** ↑ activation during high level social stressors especially when inhibition / suppression undeployable; ↓ activation to negative expectancy for moderate stress **AX:** ↑ activation during negative social information processing	↓ activation during rejection-related stimuli and threatening faces in early abuse, early separation, and maltreatment ↑ positive connectivity to approach module and ↓ positive connectivity to emotion regulation and mental state representation modules during social exclusion ↓ (re-)activity of HPA axis and ANS	↑ activation during threat cues following (late) maltreatment, and in disorganized/ unresolved attachment ↑ attentional resources allocated to threat cues following physical abuse ↑ (re-)activity of HPA axis and ANS ↑ (and earlier) negative connectivity to mental state and emotion regulation module during fearful faces and social exclusion, respectively
Approach 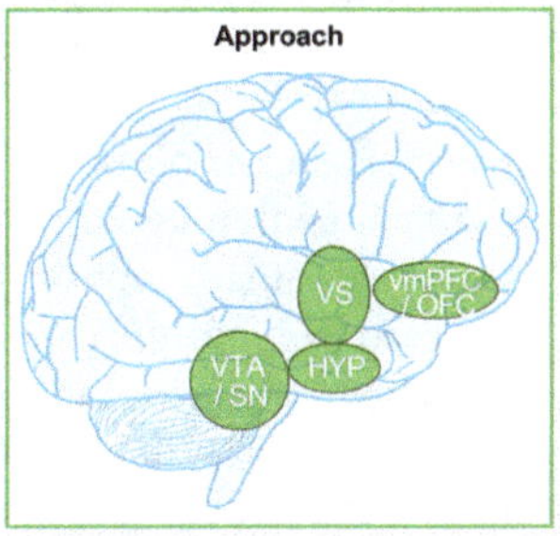 	**SEC:** ↑ activation reflecting positive motivational attributes towards and affective representations of others – also under conditions of threat and stress **AV:** ↓ activation reflecting negative other-model / expectation of unavailability of others when in need (e.g., social exclusion) **AX:** (↑) activation reflecting altered approach module functionality; pattern agrees with a partially positive other-model / wish for closeness and care when in need	↓ activation during reward (anticipation) following institutional deprivation and neglect / abuse ↓ activation during rejection-related stimuli following early separation and maltreatment ↓ activation during social exclusion stimuli in youth with early separation ↑ positive connectivity to aversion module during social exclusion	↑ activation for threatening faces in youth following maltreatment
Emotion (Self-)Regulation 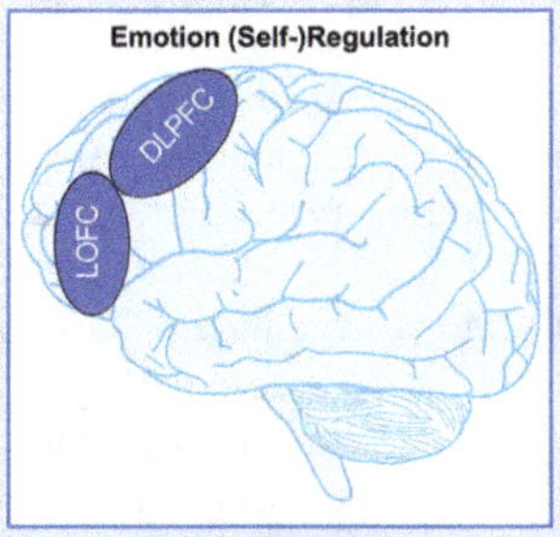 	**SEC:** ↑ functionality / efficiency; ↑ inverse connectivity with aversion module **AV:** ↑ activation during natural viewing reflecting use of suppression but ↓ efficiency of social (co-)regulation when inhibition / suppression undeployable **AX:** no consistent pattern of down-regulation difficulties; potentially (over-) dependence on emotion co-regulation	↓ activation during social exclusion following early separation ↓ positive connectivity to aversion module during social exclusion for youth exposed to early separation and during rest in adults with early neglect	↑ activation during the effortful attempt to reduce an emotional response to negative stimuli in abused adolescents ↑ (and earlier) inverse connectivity to emotion regulation module
Mental State Representation 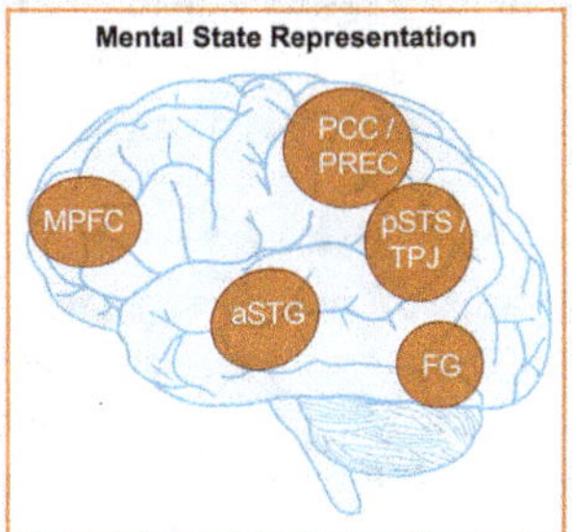 	**SEC:** predominantly positive internal representations of others; ↑ connectivity with the other modules **AV:** (↓) activation during a specific mentalizing task **AX:** (↑) and (↓) activation as a function of mentalization content valence (positive vs. negative) and focus (self vs. close other) during a specific mentalization task in adolescents	↓ activation during rejection-related stimuli in children with early separation and maltreatment experiences ↓ activation during social exclusion for youth with early separation experiences ↓ positive connectivity to aversion module during social exclusion in early separation	↑ activation during threatening faces in maltreated youth and adults, but primarily in regions subserving more automatic forms of mentalizing ↑ (and earlier) inverse connectivity to aversion module

FIGURE 3 | Functional neuro-anatomical model of disrupted attachment (NAMDA). By integrating theoretical models and empirical evidence from the fields of attachment and childhood maltreatment, we propose that disruption and disorganization of attachment manifest in two differential neurobiological phenotypes characterized by hypo-arousal vs. hyper-arousal. Empirical support for these neurobiological phenotypes is summarized focusing on brain function of four neural modules—the aversion, approach, emotion regulation, and mental state representation modules—and compared to the neurobiological underpinnings of organized secure, avoidant, and anxious-ambivalent attachment as formulated in the functional neuro-anatomical model of human (organized) attachment (NAMA). Further, primary determinants of organized and disorganized attachment are listed. aversion module—ACC, anterior cingulate cortex; INS, insula; HC/HPA, hippocampus/hypothalamic-pituitary-adrenal axis; AMY, amygdala; ATP, anterior temporal pole; approach module—vmPFC/OFC, ventromedial prefrontal/orbitofrontal

(Continued)

FIGURE 3 | cortex; HYP, hypothalamus; VTA/SN, ventral tegmental area/substantia nigra; emotion regulation module—DLPFC, dorsolateral prefrontal cortex; LOFC, lateral orbitofrontal cortex; mental state representation module—MPFC, medial prefrontal cortex; PCC/PREC, posterior cingulate cortex/precuneus; pSTS/TPJ, posterior superior temporal sulcus/temporo-parietal junction; aSTG, anterior superior temporal gyrus; FG, fusiform gyrus; ANS, autonomic nervous system; AV, avoidant attachment; AX, anxious-ambivalent attachment; SEC, secure attachment. Adapted from Long et al. (17).

procedures relative to infants classified in one of the organized categories (108–110).

Importantly, these findings, indicative of a hyper-reactive HPA axis, dovetail with the pattern observed in children and adolescents in the wake of severe physical or sexual abuse but not neglect (111, 112). However, by far the largest population-based Generation-R study comparing cortisol responses to the Strange Situation Procedure (SSP) among 72 disorganized to 297 non-disorganized infants failed to confirm this pattern, rather showing that anxious–ambivalent infants exhibited the highest cortisol reactivity relative to other classifications [(113), see (114) for a second non-replication]. That said, although the Generation-R Study is one of the largest of its kind, presumably due to its population-based nature, there was a high proportion of disorganized infants who received a secondary secure classification, potentially suggesting that their disorganized status was less attributable to severe abuse or neglect [see (4, 115, 116)], though this also applied to studies which detected cortisol hyper-responsivity among disorganized infants (110). Moreover, it is noteworthy that Generation-R employed an adapted SSP with shorter (pre)separation episodes, which may have diminished the odds of detecting evidence of HPA axis hyper-reactivity.

Two functional magnetic resonance imaging (fMRI) studies showing distressing attachment-related picture stimuli to unresolved–disorganized adults demonstrated increased amygdala activation compared to their organized counterparts (13, 14). Interestingly, the latter resembles the pattern of increased amygdala activation in response to threatening faces among abused vs. non-abused youth (117), with a recent meta-analysis indicating that this pattern applies across maltreated children and adults alike (118). These data directly implicate the heightened activity and responsivity of threat detection and stress response during activation of the attachment system related to disorganized attachment, which could partly account for the persistent freezing and/or apprehension of these infants in response to their caregivers.

Moreover, in a small study of 18 infants from low-income families followed through adulthood, Lyons-Ruth et al. (9) found that disorganized attachment classified using the SSP in infancy was associated with a larger amygdala volume in adulthood, while a recent study on adults ($N = 74$) showed unresolved attachment to be associated with reduced hippocampal volume (12). Similar morphological changes have again surfaced in human and non-human primate studies showing increased amygdala volume following exposure to physical abuse (119), chronic maternal depression (120), as well as institutional rearing and international adoption (121, 122).

These patterns notwithstanding, there is also some direct support for opposing effects of disorganization, indicating the presence of a hypo-arousal phenotype. Firstly, disorganization coincided with a flattened diurnal cortisol slope in infancy in the aforementioned Generation-R study, with follow-up analyses implicating a hypocortisolism that applied particularly to the disorganized children with an insecure rather than a secure secondary classification (113). Crucially, at the level of the HPA axis, large-scale studies have recently documented that maltreatment, in particular when occurring early and involving neglect by the caregiver, is linked with hypocortisolism (123–126). This tamping down or "blunting" of indices composing the aversion module may reflect the long-term consequences of an "evolutionarily conservative" response involving an excessively self-reliant emotion regulation strategy that is metabolically less costly and minimizes the risk inherent in depending on others as sources of co-regulation (127, 128).

Secondly, the largest recent structural neuroimaging study in over 500 children with infant attachment indexed by the SSP found that disorganized attachment at 14 months was directly linked to 10 year-olds' increased hippocampal volume as well as tentative indications of increased structural integrity of the uncinate fasciculus—the largest white matter tract connecting the prefrontal cortex and the anterior temporal lobe (though the latter finding did not survive correction for multiple testing) (8). Intriguingly, the latter may resemble a stress-dependent acceleration of neural development and prefrontal–amygdala connectivity, in particular, as documented in previously institutionalized youth (69). Potentially in a similar vein, enhanced functional connectivity between anterior medial temporal gyrus and amygdala has also been associated with adverse childhood experiences, with physical and emotional neglect constituting the most important subtypes (129). Moreover, indirect evidence stems from fMRI studies administering rejection–stimuli and a social exclusion task to youth who primarily experienced emotional abuse and neglect, documenting diminished activation of the amygdala and dorsal anterior cingulate (130, 131).

This latter pattern of hypo-arousal may prove particularly distinct compared to the organized insecure attachment classifications outlined in NAMA. Here we also posit a divergent pattern *vis-à-vis* insecure–avoidant individuals whose suppressing strategies primarily are less efficient during excessive, persistent, or inescapable threat (e.g., during the SSP itself or lengthy social exclusion in adolescence). Unlike for avoidance, we predict that the disorganized hypo-arousal phenotype may exhibit reduced aversion/stress responses even during such high-level stressors, such as the Trier Social Stress Test, where early deprivation has been associated with a blunted cortisol response (132). By contrast, we hypothesize that activation in physiological and neural markers of aversion and distress characteristic of the hyper-arousal phenotype will be more pronounced than in the organized attachment classifications as a whole, though the effects are likely to prove least strong *vis-à-vis* organized insecure-ambivalent (i.e., anxious) strategies.

Alterations in the Approach Module

To the best of our knowledge, little or no *direct* evidence exists to date for effects of disorganization on brain regions comprising the approach module in NAMA. However, results from the large-scale Generation-R sample of 626 6 week-old infants of whom 132 were later classified as disorganized (vs. organized) at 14 months in the SSP revealed reduced gangliothalamic ovoid diameter, which may potentially also reflect structural alterations in (early) basal ganglia development (133). Similarly, ample *indirect* evidence suggests the diminished responsiveness of the basal ganglia (mainly ventral striatum) in response to (anticipation of) reward, primarily among youth exposed to severe deprivation or neglect (134, 135) as well as family adversity (136). Though one study also linked childhood abuse to reduction of globus pallidus activation during reward anticipation, the probable concomitant effects of neglect were not assessed in this study (137). Broadly speaking, this blunted approach-related response may reflect a motivational deficit impeding effective engagement with environmental pressures (138) which, we suggest, may also reflect reduced gravitation to sources of co-regulation in childhood. Coupled with the aforementioned blunting of systems involved in the aversion module, diminished reward sensitivity and approach reactivity may account for Crittenden and Ainsworth's (66) prescient observation that neglected children fail to act on the need for co-regulation from their caregivers.

Besides this, it is intriguing that a meta-analysis on maltreated youth and adults specifically suggested increased basal ganglia activation (globus pallidus and lentiform nucleus) during exposure to threatening faces (118). Furthermore, in a sample of children with early caregiver separation experiences (over half of this sample exposed to neglect prior to separation), Puetz and colleagues (130) documented a greater activation of the ventral tegmental area (VTA) and increased functional connectivity of VTA to dACC among youth during social exclusion, though the caudate nucleus showed reduced activation.

Tentatively, we interpret the activation of regions in the approach module during exposure to aversive stimuli as neural evidence of an approach–avoidance conflict, in particular, when it occurs in conjunction with activation of regions linked to aversion [as suggested by VTA–dACC connectivity in (130)]. It will be incumbent on future research to determine whether such patterns are also observable at other physiological levels, such as the potential for co-activation of parasympathetic and sympathetic branches of the autonomic nervous system implicit in the notion of autonomic space proposed by Berntson et al. (139). To the extent that Cyr et al. (34) link the approach–avoidance conflict more specifically with abuse, due to the dual role of the caregiver as safe haven and source of distress, it is conceivable that such patterns will prove more characteristic of the hyper-arousal phenotype of disrupted and disorganized attachment. That said, we noted at the outset that absence of and persistent rebuffs by the caregiver may also coincide with such conflict because the need for the caregiver becomes associated with alarm (even if s/he is not necessarily the source)—which may suggest that an approach–avoidance conflict characterizes both hypo- and hyper-arousal phenotypes.

Alterations in Emotion Regulation and Mental State Representation Modules

Given the paucity of *direct* and *indirect* evidence regarding the effects of attachment disruption on brain regions associated with emotion (self-)regulation and mental state representation modules as well as their structural and functional overlap, we will discuss these jointly. Regarding emotion (self-)regulation, the aforementioned study on youth with early separation experiences showed a diminished activation of the dorsolateral prefrontal cortex (DLPFC) during social exclusion (130). Furthermore, the same and a related study exposing maltreated youth to rejection-related verbal stimuli detected a diminished activation in regions linked to mental state representation [medial PFC (mPFC), temporo-parietal junction, and precuneus], though findings on superior temporal sulcus (STS) were contradictory, with activation increased in one (130) but decreased in another study (131), potentially due to task- or sample-specific factors. Most children in the latter study (131) experienced emotional abuse, followed by neglect and witnessing domestic violence, whereas most children in the former study (130) had been separated from their caregivers, which is usually an indication of severe multiple-subtype maltreatment, but it was only reported that 64% of their sample had experienced some form of neglect. Broadly speaking, we would therefore tentatively link the hypo-arousal phenotype to diminished activation in regions subserving mental state representation, especially during social stress, potentially analogous to the mentalizing deficits often linked with attachment disorganization and related disorders (140, 141).

By contrast, McLaughlin et al. detected increased DLPFC, mPFC, and dACC activation among abused adolescents during the effortful attempt to reduce an emotional response to negative stimuli, potentially indicating a less efficient emotion regulation region, as indicative of the hyper-arousal phenotype (142). Furthermore, the aforementioned meta-analysis by Hein and Monk (118) found an increased activation in posterior STS (pSTS) during exposure to threatening faces among maltreated youth and adults relative to non-maltreated controls. It is noteworthy that while the pSTS is thought to perform a central role across most, if not all, forms of social perception, meta-analytic data suggest an intermediate-level role between automatic/reflexive and effortful/controlled mentalizing, aiding, for example, in the inference of intentions from behavior (143). Notably, this contrasts markedly with the more controlled/effortful forms of higher-order meta-representational mentalizing mediated by the mPFC, subserving, for example, perspective taking when others are thought to be markedly different from oneself (143). Therefore, we concur with Hein and Monk (43), who interpret the maltreatment-related increase in pSTS activation while viewing threatening faces in terms of more rapid (and potentially biased) detection of others' threatening states of mind (e.g., hostile attribution bias), potentially enabling maltreated children to more efficiently navigate socially dangerous or harmful environments—a pattern we would associate more strongly with the hyper-arousal phenotype.

Potential Alterations in Further Brain Regions

In the previous theoretical examination, we focused on four neural systems which are central for inter-individual differences in NAMA. However, there are also other brain regions that could convey differential effects based on early adverse child–caregiver interactions. One such region is the corpus callosum, the white matter structure that connects the brain hemispheres. In both neglected and abused individuals, the reduced integrity and area of the corpus callosum is a well-replicated finding (144). Teicher et al. (70) argue that these alterations might indicate an (at first) adaptive mechanism by which the affected individuals adjust to an enduring approach–avoidance conflict in the relationship to a maltreating caregiver. This notion is supported by research providing evidence for more lateralized and less integrated brain activity in maltreated individuals (145), which could be the functional correlate of reduced callosal integrity.

These functional alterations, in turn, could also underlie the "black and white" thinking as well as "splitting" characteristic of borderline personality disorder, a mental disorder that is often preceded by childhood maltreatment (146) and associated with disorganized attachment (147) and unresolved psychological trauma, as indexed by the Adult Attachment Interview (AAI) (148). Moreover, disorganized attachment has also been associated with the emergence of "segregated systems," a regulatory strategy that entails a diminished integration of affects, expectations, and so on to prevent the individual from feeling overwhelmed in the present but resulting in continuation of mismatched or incompatible fears in the future (43). Therefore, disorganized attachment due to neglect or abuse could also be associated with the reduced integrity or area of the corpus callosum.

Summary

We have offered above a brief overview of the *direct* and *indirect* (i.e., maltreatment-related) evidence in support of the distinction between hyper- and hypo-arousal phenotypes of disorganized attachment (summarized in **Figure 3**). Our proposal receives most direct support in the case of the aversion module where the caregiver primarily serves as a threatening or insufficient source of co-regulation predisposing to hyper- and hypo-arousal profiles, respectively. However, as far as alterations in the approach, emotion regulation, and mentalization modules are concerned, our suggestions remain preliminary and in need of further exploration and confirmation in light of the paucity of direct evidence. In sum, we would like to encourage future research to formulate hypotheses and examine inter-individual differences associated with disorganized attachment regarding regions of interest not only within the proposed four neural modules of NAMA but also within other brain areas implicated in early adverse child–caregiver interactions.

DISCUSSION

We would like to wrap up by reiterating that, unlike most prominent models in the field (67–70), we are not emphasizing alterations in developmental neurobiology across the modules of NAMA as a function of the direct impact of adverse experiences *per se*. We rather contend that the influence of adverse experiences is filtered through the child's self- and co-regulatory efforts with their caregivers. The important implication is that singular maltreatment events in an otherwise nurturing and secure attachment relationship or early adverse events occurring outside the (current) family context should have a much weaker long-term influence in our model relative to these other models (6).

However, the flip-side of this argument is that children are most vulnerable to the occurrence of persistent adversity that occurs within their primary attachment relationships, in particular, before adolescence (69). Here we have proposed the presence of neurobiologically distinct hyper- and hypo-arousal phenotypes prototypically (but not exclusively) emanating from environments characterized by caregiver-related abuse and neglect, respectively. While much *direct* evidence initially accrued in support of a hyper-arousal pattern for disorganized infants (especially regarding cortisol), recent (primarily *indirect*) evidence from severely deprived and neglected samples has increasingly begun to document an opposing hypo-arousal pattern. Furthermore, the latter group also appears to show abnormally low levels of approach- and reward-related neural activity, which may, potentially, serve as a neural substrate for the apparent lack of motivation for interpersonal co-regulation, reflecting an early need that remained largely unmet across childhood.

Our argument, inevitably, raises the issue of adequate characterization of adverse experience. Unfortunately, much neuroimaging work to date has relied on samples with highly heterogeneous and inadequately characterized child caregiving histories. A prominent case in point is that of previously institutionalized samples that are often subsumed under the umbrella term "deprivation" when typically it is very challenging to retrieve information on experiences prior to or during institutionalization. Moreover, the disruption often associated with international adoption and the abrupt shift to (typically) very caring interactions that facilitate catch-up can become sidelined. While this work is ideal for understanding sensitive windows, it is often limited in terms of dissecting differential effects of specific environments because typically too little information on the exact nature of the environments is available, though exceptions exist with considerable effort spent on characterizing the (pre-)institutional (caregiving) environment up to its direct observation [e.g., (149)]. Thus, aside from within-group analyses considering length of institutionalization, extracting more specific dose–response effects of certain attachment-specific environments is exceedingly difficult.

Another issue implicit in our model that deserves more attention in future research is variation within healthy and non-maltreated samples in terms of secure *vs.* insecure (as well as organized and disorganized) attachment[4]. Very little or no research has attempted to take this variation in the "control" group into account when deriving the specific neurobiological sequelae of adversity. What are the distinct patterns of biological measures and neural activity, anatomy and connectivity as compared to these more burdened yet nevertheless normative samples? Actually, a debate within the attachment field that is still ongoing and began with classic attachment theorists, including Main and Ainsworth, implied that disorganization is continuous with the insecure strategies (150).

It is also worth noting that our model is primarily informed by studies relying on Hesse and Main (64) conceptualization of disorganized attachment. Notably, however, an important fMRI study by Strathearn et al. (151) using Crittenden's AAI coding system detected a diminished approach system activation among mothers with increased avoidance (type A) while viewing their own *vs.* other baby's face displaying positive and negative affect[5]. Though this pattern is in keeping with our predictions regarding the hypo-arousal subtype and the Crittenden coding system may have more clinical utility (148), it is important to note that the sample in this study was composed of mothers drawn from the general population. Therefore, it is difficult to judge the extent to which such findings are more applicable to NAMA (with its focus on organized attachment) or NAMDA (with its clinical focus on attachment disruption and disorganization). As noted above, Crittenden's conceptualization of the sequelae of maltreatment or abuse from caregivers holds that children's attachment becomes markedly organized (35, 36). Notably, Crittenden's and Main's attachment categories show a poor empirical overlap (36), cautioning scholars against considering them equivalent. However, Crittenden's system also emphasizes diversity and complexity within the attachment of maltreated children (37, 152), which is consistent with the heterogeneity that we are positing here, and therefore future examination of the extent to which this system conforms to the NAMDA model may be warranted.

One further complicating factor is the question of what happens to disorganization over time. This gets at the complex issue of normative trajectories of brain development (involving proliferation, pruning, etc.) and acceleration or deceleration of brain development due to adversity (69). This cannot be addressed at great length here, but timing of assessment, onset, recency, and chronicity of adversity may be crucial determinants of structural and functional brain alterations and other neurobiological indices. This is a fundamental issue because of well-supported theories that trauma initially leads to up-regulation followed by down-regulation below the initial set-point, resulting in under-responsiveness/blunting of the stress response in the long term (153, 154).

Finally, as mentioned briefly in the introduction when describing NAMA, a paradigm shift is currently underway in social neuroscience emphasizing the assessment of two (or) more directly interacting individuals (i.e., second-person social neuroscience). In the context of attachment, this means that new research is emerging on bio-behavioral synchrony and its association with inter-individual differences in relationship quality, particularly parent–child attachment. Although recent data on organized secure vs. insecure attachment appears promising, more research is necessary to replicate and extend these novel patterns. We are not aware of any direct evidence for effects of attachment disruption and/or disorganization in second-person social neuroscience investigations. However, the first *indirect* evidence on maltreated preschoolers dovetails with our proposal, revealing a positive concordance in parasympathetic activity for abusive, but no concordance for neglectful, mother–child dyads during puzzle tasks (155). It thus remains to be seen whether the proposed dissociation between a hypo-arousal phenotype vs. a hyper-arousal phenotype also extends to patterns of bio-behavioral synchrony among disorganized dyads and, if yes, what the implication of such dissociation may be.

In closing, our focus on co-regulation in the attachment relationship as opposed to the direct impact of early adverse childhood experiences carries important implications for intervention. Thus, to the extent that disorganized attachment is part of a fundamental interpersonal risk mechanism that is self-perpetuating in the sense that it confers deficits in forming and maintaining new relationships, this deserves to be the central focus of intervention (60). Moreover, to the extent that hyper- and hypo-arousal phenotypes can emerge in the wake of early adversity, they may call for differential intervention foci. For example, children exposed to an inaccessible or insufficient source of co-regulation may benefit most from targeting the child's ability to express and the parent's capacity to perceive the child's emotional needs, helping children regain confidence in "being heard." By contrast, in the case of a threatening source of co-regulation, it is crucial to enable children to regain a feeling of emotional and physical safety by providing corrective therapeutic experiences and focusing on the origin and meaning of frightening behaviors for caregivers and children. Analogous to foster care intervention, a central goal may be to establish new trusting relationships by enhancing understanding of children's dysregulated behavior, addressing the caregivers own attachment-related histories, and raising awareness of possibly (often subtle) threatening behaviors (156–158).

It is our hope that our extension of the NAMA to a neuroanatomical model of disrupted attachment (NAMDA) will stimulate further research and debate in the field. With the more widespread availability of advanced biological and neuroimaging techniques, the NAMDA may offer a helpful guide for organizing

[4]In a similar vein, another issue worthy of examination is whether individuals' secondary attachment strategies matter in terms of whether they coincide with hypo- vs. hyper-arousal, that is, if a disorganized child is disorganized/dismissing vs. disorganized/preoccupied will this lead to differential prediction regarding their patterns of neural and physiological activation? These questions are admittedly difficult to examine as they require large samples of children classified with disorganized attachment. However, the use of factor analytically derived scores of preoccupation, dismissal, and disorganization could help researchers gain statistical power to answer some of these research questions.

[5]Please note that Crittenden's coding system, in line with her theoretical perspective, does not include a disorganized category, rendering it conceivable that the findings of Strathearn et al. (151) were driven by what would be classified as higher levels of attachment disruption or disorganization within the Main classification system among what are classified as type A individuals in the Crittenden system.

emerging patterns of data in the field. In turn, this may ultimately help to further advance theory and research on attachment and childhood adversity within the twenty first century and serve as point of departure for the formulation of individualized prevention and intervention strategies.

AUTHOR CONTRIBUTIONS

LW, CS, and PV drafted the initial manuscript. MS, MK, JK, and JB edited and made substantial comments and suggestions for revision of the manuscript. All authors made substantial contributions to the conception/ design/ interpretation of data for the work, help draft and/or revised it critically for important intellectual content and gave final approval of the version to be published as well as agreement to be accountable for all aspects of the work in ensuring that questions related to the accuracy or integrity of any part of the work are appropriately investigated and resolved.

ACKNOWLEDGMENTS

The responsibility for the contents of this publication lies with the authors. We thank Prof. Dr. Gottfried Spangler, Prof. Dr. Kai von Klitzing, and Prof. Dr. Margaret Sheridan for a fruitful exchange of views and for sharing valuable insights on the topic.

REFERENCES

1. McLaughlin KA, Green JG, Gruber MJ, Sampson NA, Zaslavsky AM, Kessler RC. Childhood adversities and adult psychiatric disorders in the National comorbidity survey replication II: associations with persistence of DSM-IV disorders. *Arch Gen Psychiatry.* (2010) 67:124–32. doi: 10.1001/archgenpsychiatry.2009.187
2. Green JG, McLaughlin KA, Berglund PA, Gruber MJ, Sampson NA, Zaslavsky AM, et al. Childhood adversities and adult psychiatric disorders in the national comorbidity survey replication i: associations with first onset of dsm-iv disorders. *Arch Gen Psychiatry.* (2010) 67:113–23. doi: 10.1001/archgenpsychiatry.2009.186
3. Bowlby J. *A Secure Base.* New York, NY: Basic Books (1988).
4. Lyons-Ruth K, Jacobvitz D. Attachment disorganization from infancy to adulthood: neurobiological correlates, parenting contexts, and pathways to disorder. In: Cassidy J, Shaver PR, editors. *Handbook of Attachment: Theory, Research, and Clinical Applications.* New York, NY: Guilford (2016). p. 667–95.
5. Groh AM, Fearon RMP, van Ijzendoorn MH, Bakermans-Kranenburg MJ, Roisman GI. Attachment in the early life course: meta-analytic evidence for its role in socioemotional development. *Child Dev Perspect.* (2017) 11:70–6. doi: 10.1111/cdep.12213
6. DeKlyen M, Greenberg MT. Attachment and psychopathology in childhood. In: Cassidy J, Shaver PR, editors. *Handbook of Attachment: Theory, Research, and Clinical Applications.* 3rd ed. New York, NY: Guildford Press (2016). p. 639–66.
7. Stovall-McClough KC, Dozier M. Attachment states of mind and psychopathology in adulthood. In: Shaver PR, Cassidy J, editors. *Handbook of Attachment: Theory, Research, and Clinical Applications.* 3rd ed. New York, NY: Guilford (2016) p. 715–38.
8. Cortes Hidalgo AP, Muetzel R, Luijk MPCM, Bakermans-Kranenburg MJ, El Marroun H, Vernooij MW, et al. Observed infant-parent attachment and brain morphology in middle childhood– a population-based study. *Dev Cogn Neurosci.* (2019) 40:100724. doi: 10.1016/j.dcn.2019.100724
9. Lyons-Ruth K, Pechtel P, Yoon SA, Anderson CM, Teicher MH. Disorganized attachment in infancy predicts greater amygdala volume in adulthood. *Behav Brain Res.* (2016) 308:83–93. doi: 10.1016/j.bbr.2016.03.050
10. Riem MME, van Hoof MJ, Garrett AS, Rombouts SARB, van der Wee NJA, van Ijzendoorn MH, et al. General psychopathology factor and unresolved-disorganized attachment uniquely correlated to white matter integrity using diffusion tensor imaging. *Behav Brain Res.* (2019) 359:1–8. doi: 10.1016/j.bbr.2018.10.014
11. Rifkin-Graboi A, Tan HM, Shaun GKY, Sim LW, Sanmugam S, Chong YS, et al. An initial investigation of neonatal neuroanatomy, caregiving, and levels of disorganized behavior. *Proc Natl Acad Sci USA.* (2019) 116:16787. doi: 10.1073/pnas.1900362116
12. van Hoof M-J, Riem M, Garrett A, Pannekoek N, van der Wee N, van Ijzendoorn M, et al. Unresolved–Disorganized attachment is associated with smaller hippocampus and increased functional connectivity beyond psychopathology. *J Traumatic Stress.* (2019) 32:742–52. doi: 10.1002/jts.22432
13. Buchheim A, Erk S, George C, Kächele H, Kircher T, Martius P, et al. Neural correlates of attachment trauma in borderline personality disorder: a functional magnetic resonance imaging study. *Psychiatry Res.* (2008) 163:223–35. doi: 10.1016/j.pscychresns.2007.07.001
14. Buchheim A, Erk S, George C, Kächele H, Ruchsow M, Spitzer M, et al. Measuring attachment representation in an fMRI environment: a pilot study. *Psychopathology.* (2006) 39:144–52. doi: 10.1159/000091800
15. Vrtička P. The social neuroscience of attachment. In: Ibáñez A, Sedeño L, García AM, editors. *Neuroscience and Social Science: The Missing Link.* Cham: Springer International Publishing (2017). p. 95–119.
16. Vrtička P, Vuilleumier P. Neuroscience of human social interactions and adult attachment style. *Front Hum Neurosci.* (2012) 6:212. doi: 10.3389/fnhum.2012.00212
17. Long M, Verbeke W, Ein-Dor T, Vrtička P. A functional neuro-anatomical model of human attachment (NAMA): insights from first- and second-person social neuroscience. *Cortex.* (2020) 126:281–321. doi: 10.1016/j.cortex.2020.01.010
18. Cassidy J, Shaver PR. *Handbook of Attachment.* 3rd ed. New York, NY: Guilford; (2016).
19. Ainsworth MDS, Blehar MC, Waters E, Wall S. *Patterns of Attachment: A Psychological Study of the Strange Situation.* Hillsdale, NJ: Erlbaum (1978).
20. Bowlby J. *Attachment and Loss: Vol. 1. Attachment.* London: Hogarth (1969).
21. Bowlby J. *Separation: Anxiety and Anger.* London: Hogarth (1973).
22. Bowlby J. *Attachment and Loss: Vol. 3. Loss: Sadness and Depression.* London: Hogarth (1980).
23. Spangler G, Zimmermann P. Attachment representation and emotion regulation in adolescents: a psychobiological perspective on internal working models. *Attachment Hum Dev.* (1999) 1:270–90. doi: 10.1080/14616739900134151
24. Bretherton I, Munholland KA. Internal working models in attachment relationships: elaborating a central construct in attachment theory. In: Cassidy J, Shaver PR, editors. *Handbook of Attachment: Theory, Research, and Clinical Implications.* 2nd ed. New York, NY: Guilford (2008). p. 102–27.
25. Bretherton I, Munholland KA. The internal working model construct in light of contemporary neuroimaging research. In: Cassidy J, Shaver PR, editors. *Handbook of Attachment: Theory, Research, and Clinical Implications.* 3rd ed. New York, NY: Guilford (2016) p. 63–88.
26. Solomon J, George C. The measurement of attachment security and related constructs in infancy and early childhoo. In: Cassidy J, Shaver PR, editors. *Handbook of Attachment: Theory, Research, and Clinical Implications.* 2nd ed. New York, NY: Guiford (2016). p. 366–98.
27. Thompson RA. Early attachment and later development: reframing the questions. *Handbook of Attachment: Theory, Research, and Clinical Applications. 3rd ed.* New York, NY: Guilford (2016). p. 330–48.

28. Main M. Avoidance in the service of attachment: a working paper. In: Immelmann K, Barlow GW, Petrinovich L, Main M, editors. *Behavioral Development: The Bielefeld Interdisciplinary Project*. New York, NY: Cambridge University Press (1981). p. 651–93.
29. Simpson JA, Belsky J. Attachment theory within a modern evolutionary framework. In: Cassidy J, Shaver PR, editors. *Handbook of Attachment: Theory, Research, and Clinical Implications*. New York, NY: Guilford (2008). p. 131–57.
30. Cassidy J. Emotion regulation: influences of attachment relationships. *Monographs Soc Res Child Dev.* (1994) 59:228–49. doi: 10.1111/j.1540-5834.1994.tb01287.x
31. Lionetti F, Pastore M, Barone L. Attachment in institutionalized children: a review and meta-analysis. *Child Abuse Neglect.* (2015) 42:135–45. doi: 10.1016/j.chiabu.2015.02.013
32. Hesse E, Main M. Second-generation effects of unresolved trauma in nonmaltreating parents: dissociated, frightened, and threatening parental behavior. *Psychoanal Inquiry.* (1999) 19:481–540. doi: 10.1080/07351699909534265
33. Main M, Solomon J. Procedures for identifying infants as disorganized/disoriented attachment pattern. In: Greenberg MT, Cicchetti D, Cummings EM, editors. *Attachment in the Preschool Years: Theory, Research, and Intervention*. Chicago, IL: University of Chicago (1990). p. 121–60.
34. Cyr C, Euser EM, Bakermans-Kranenburg MJ, Van Ijzendoorn MH. Attachment security and disorganization in maltreating and high-risk families: a series of meta-analyses. *Dev Psychopathol.* (2010) 22:87–108. doi: 10.1017/S0954579409990289
35. Crittenden PM. *Raising Parents: Attachment, Representation, and Treatment*. Oxon: Routledge (2016).
36. Baldoni F, Minghetti M, Craparo G, Facondini E, Cena L, Schimmenti A. Comparing main, goldwyn, and hesse (Berkeley) and Crittenden (DMM) coding systems for classifying adult attachment interview transcripts: an empirical report. *Attach Hum Dev.* (2018) 20:423–38. doi: 10.1080/14616734.2017.1421979
37. Crittenden PM. Children's strategies for coping with adverse home environments: an interpretation using attachment theory. *Child Abuse Neglect.* (1992) 16:329–43. doi: 10.1016/0145-2134(92)90043-Q
38. Duschinsky R. Disorganization, fear and attachment: working towards clarification. *Infant Mental Health J.* (2018) 39:17–29. doi: 10.1002/imhj.21689
39. Abrams KY, Rifkin A, Hesse E. Examining the role of parental frightened/frightening subtypes in predicting disorganized attachment within a brief observational procedure. *Dev Psychopathol.* (2006) 18:345–61. doi: 10.1017/S0954579406060184
40. Lyons-Ruth K, Bureau J-F, Easterbrooks MA, Obsuth I, Hennighausen K, Vulliez-Coady L. Parsing the construct of maternal insensitivity: distinct longitudinal pathways associated with early maternal withdrawal. *Attach Hum Dev.* (2013) 15:562–82. doi: 10.1080/14616734.2013.841051
41. Fonagy P. The transgenerational transmission of holocaust trauma. *Attach Hum Dev.* (1999) 1:92–114. doi: 10.1080/14616739900134041
42. Lyons-Ruth K, Yellin C, Melnick S, Atwood G. Childhood experiences of trauma and loss have different relations to maternal unresolved and Hostile-Helpless states of mind on the AAI. *Attach Hum Dev.* (2003) 5:330–52. doi: 10.1080/14616730310001633410
43. Reisz S, Duschinsky R, Siegel DJ. Disorganized attachment and defense: exploring John Bowlby's unpublished reflections. *Attach Hum Dev.* (2018) 20:107–34. doi: 10.1080/14616734.2017.1380055
44. Bowlby J. Processes of mourning. *Int J Psycho-Anal.* (1961) 42:317–40.
45. van den Dries L, Juffer F, van Ijzendoorn MH, Bakermans-Kranenburg MJ. Fostering security? A meta-analysis of attachment in adopted children. *Child Youth Serv Rev.* (2009) 31:410–21. doi: 10.1016/j.childyouth.2008.09.008
46. van Ijzendoorn MH, Schuengel C, Bakermans–Kranenburg MJ. Disorganized attachment in early childhood: meta-analysis of precursors, concomitants, and sequelae. *Dev Psychopathol.* (1999) 11:225–50. doi: 10.1017/S0954579499002035
47. Bakermans-Kranenburg MJ, van Ijzendoorn MH. The first 10,000 adult attachment interviews: distributions of adult attachment representations in clinical and non-clinical groups. *Attach Hum Dev.* (2009) 11:223–63. doi: 10.1080/14616730902814762
48. Stovall-McClough KC, Cloitre M. Unresolved attachment, PTSD, and dissociation in women with childhood abuse histories. *J Consult Clin Psychol.* (2006) 74:219–28. doi: 10.1037/0022-006X.74.2.219
49. Berthelot N, Ensink K, Bernazzani O, Normandin L, Luyten P, Fonagy P. Intergenerational transmission of attachment in abused and neglected mothers: the role of trauma-specific reflective functioning. *Infant Mental Health J.* (2015) 36:200–12. doi: 10.1002/imhj.21499
50. Borelli JL, Cohen C, Pettit C, Normandin L, Target M, Fonagy P, et al. Maternal and child sexual abuse history: an intergenerational exploration of children's adjustment and maternal trauma-reflective functioning. *Front Psychol.* (2019) 10:1062. doi: 10.3389/fpsyg.2019.01062
51. Humphreys KL, LeMoult J, Wear JG, Piersiak HA, Lee A, Gotlib IH. Child maltreatment and depression: a meta-analysis of studies using the childhood trauma questionnaire. *Child Abuse Neglect.* (2020) 102:104361. doi: 10.1016/j.chiabu.2020.104361
52. Infurna MR, Reichl C, Parzer P, Schimmenti A, Bifulco A, Kaess M. Associations between depression and specific childhood experiences of abuse and neglect: a meta-analysis. *J Affective Disord.* (2016) 190:47–55. doi: 10.1016/j.jad.2015.09.006
53. LeMoult J, Humphreys KL, Tracy A, Hoffmeister J-A, Ip E, Gotlib IH. Meta-analysis: exposure to early life stress and risk for depression in childhood and adolescence. *J Am Acad Child Adolesc Psychiatry.* (2020) 59:842–55. doi: 10.1016/j.jaac.2019.10.011
54. Ross ND, Kaminski PL, Herrington R. From childhood emotional maltreatment to depressive symptoms in adulthood: the roles of self-compassion and shame. *Child Abuse Neglect.* (2019) 92:32–42. doi: 10.1016/j.chiabu.2019.03.016
55. Sekowski M, Gambin M, Cudo A, Wozniak-Prus M, Penner F, Fonagy P, et al. The relations between childhood maltreatment, shame, guilt, depression and suicidal ideation in inpatient adolescents. *J Affective Disord.* (2020) 276:667–77. doi: 10.1016/j.jad.2020.07.056
56. Barnett D, Manly JT, Cicchetti D. Defining child maltreatment: the interface between policy and research. In: Cicchetti D, Toth SL, editors. *Child Abuse, Child Development, and Social Policy*. 8th ed. New York, NY: Ablex (1993). p. 7–73.
57. Wright MOD, Crawford E, Del Castillo D. Childhood emotional maltreatment and later psychological distress among college students: the mediating role of maladaptive schemas. *Child Abuse Neglect.* (2009) 33:59–68. doi: 10.1016/j.chiabu.2008.12.007
58. Riggs SA. Childhood emotional abuse and the attachment system across the life cycle: what theory and research tell Us. *J Aggress Maltreatment Trauma.* (2010) 19:5–51. doi: 10.1080/10926770903475968
59. Murphy A, Steele M, Dube SR, Bate J, Bonuck K, Meissner P, et al. Adverse childhood experiences (ACEs) questionnaire and adult attachment interview (AAI): implications for parent child relationships. *Child Abuse Neglect.* (2014) 38:224–33. doi: 10.1016/j.chiabu.2013.09.004
60. Valentino K. Relational interventions for maltreated children. *Child Dev.* (2017) 88:359–67. doi: 10.1111/cdev.12735
61. Cicchetti D, Toth SL. Child maltreatment. *Annu Rev Clin Psychol.* (2005) 1:409–38. doi: 10.1146/annurev.clinpsy.1.102803.144029
62. George C, Kaplan N, Main M. *Adult Attachment Interview, 3rd Edn.* Department of Psychology, University of California, Berkeley (1996).
63. Shmueli-Goetz Y, Target M, Datta A, Fonagy P. *Child Attachment Interview (CAI) Coding and Classification Manual, Version V.* Unpublished Manuscript, The Sub-Department of Clinical Health Psychology, University College London (2004).
64. Hesse E, Main M. Disorganized infant, child, and adult attachment: collapse in behavioral and attentional strategies. *J Am Psychoanal Assoc.* (2000) 48:1097–127. doi: 10.1177/00030651000480041101
65. Lyons-Ruth K. The interface between attachment and intersubjectivity: perspective from the longitudinal study of disorganized attachment. *Psychoanal Inquiry.* (2007) 26:595–616. doi: 10.1080/07351690701310656
66. Crittenden PM, Ainsworth MDS. Child maltreatment and attachment theory. In: Cicchetti D, Carlson V, editors. *Child Maltreatment: Theory and*

Research on the Causes and Consequences of Child Abuse and Neglect. New York, NY: Cambridge University Press (1989) p. 432–63.

67. Sheridan MA, McLaughlin KA. Dimensions of early experience and neural development: deprivation and threat. *Trends Cogn Sci.* (2014) 18:580–5. doi: 10.1016/j.tics.2014.09.001
68. Humphreys KL, Zeanah CH. Deviations from the expectable environment in early childhood and emerging psychopathology. *Neuropsychopharmacology.* (2015) 40:154–70. doi: 10.1038/npp.2014.165
69. Callaghan BL, Tottenham N. The neuro-environmental loop of plasticity: a cross-species analysis of parental effects on emotion circuitry development following typical and adverse caregiving. *Neuropsychopharmacology.* (2016) 41:163–76. doi: 10.1038/npp.2015.204
70. Teicher MH, Samson JA, Anderson CM, Ohashi K. The effects of childhood maltreatment on brain structure, function and connectivity. *Nat Rev Neurosci.* (2016) 17:652–66. doi: 10.1038/nrn.2016.111
71. Jewell T, Gardner T, Susi K, Watchorn K, Coopey E, Simic M, et al. Attachment measures in middle childhood and adolescence: a systematic review of measurement properties. *Clin Psychol Rev.* (2019) 68:71–82. doi: 10.1016/j.cpr.2018.12.004
72. Atzil S, Gao W, Fradkin I, Barrett LF. Growing a social brain. *Nat Hum Behav.* (2018) 2:624–36. doi: 10.1038/s41562-018-0384-6
73. Menon V. Salience network. In: Toga AW, editor. *Brain Mapping: An Encyclopedic Reference, 2th ed.* London: Academic Press, Elsevier (2015). p. 597–611.
74. Ein-Dor T, Hirschberger G. Rethinking attachment theory: from a theory of relationships to a theory of individual and group survival. *Curr Direct Psychol Sci.* (2016) 25:223–7. doi: 10.1177/0963721416650684
75. Taylor SE, Master SL. Social responses to stress: the tend-and-befriend model. In: Contrada R, Baum A, editors. The Handbook of Stress Science: *Biology, Psychology, and Health*. New York, NY: Springer Publishing (2011). p. 101–9.
76. Fonagy P, Luyten P. A developmental, mentalization-based approach to the understanding and treatment of borderline personality disorder. *Dev Psychopathol.* (2009) 21:1355–81. doi: 10.1017/S0954579409990198
77. Canterberry M, Gillath O. Neural evidence for a multifaceted model of attachment security. *Int J Psychophysiol.* (2013) 88:232–40. doi: 10.1016/j.ijpsycho.2012.08.013
78. Gillath O, Karantzas GC, Fraley RC. What can neuroscience, genetics, and physiology tell us about attachment? In: Karantzas GC, Fraley RC, editors. *Adult Attachment: A Concise Introduction to Theory and Research.* New York, NY: Academic Press (2016). p. 219–41
79. Ochsner KN, Silvers JA, Buhle JT. Functional imaging studies of emotion regulation: a synthetic review and evolving model of the cognitive control of emotion. *Ann N Y Acad Sci.* (2012) 1251:E1–24. doi: 10.1111/j.1749-6632.2012.06751.x
80. Raichle ME. The brain's default mode network. *Ann Rev Neurosci.* (2015) 38:433–47. doi: 10.1146/annurev-neuro-071013-014030
81. Nolte T, Bolling D, Hudac C, Fonagy P, Mayes L, Pelphrey K. Brain mechanisms underlying the impact of attachment-related stress on social cognition. *Front Hum Neurosci.* (2013) 7:816. doi: 10.3389/fnhum.2013.00816
82. White LO, Klein A, von Klitzing K, Graneist A, Otto Y, Hill J, et al. Putting ostracism into perspective: young children tell more mentalistic stories after exclusion, but not when anxious. *Front Psychol.* (2016) 7:1926. doi: 10.3389/fpsyg.2016.01926
83. DeWall CN, Masten CL, Powell C, Combs D, Schurtz DR, Eisenberger NI. Do neural responses to rejection depend on attachment style? An fMRI study. *Soc Cogn Affective Neurosci.* (2012) 7:184–92. doi: 10.1093/scan/nsq107
84. White LO, Bornemann B, Crowley MJ, Sticca F, Vrtička P, Stadelmann S, et al. Exclusion expected? Cardiac slowing upon peer exclusion links preschool parent representations to school-age peer relationships. *Child Dev.* (in press). doi: 10.1111/CDEV.13494
85. White LO, Wu J, Borelli JL, Mayes LC, Crowley MJ. Play it again: neural responses to reunion with excluders predicted by attachment patterns. *Dev Sci.* (2013) 16:850–63. doi: 10.1111/desc.12035
86. Zilverstand A, Parvaz MA, Goldstein RZ. Neuroimaging cognitive reappraisal in clinical populations to define neural targets for enhancing emotion regulation. A systematic review. *NeuroImage.* (2017) 151:105–16. doi: 10.1016/j.neuroimage.2016.06.009
87. White LO, Wu J, Borelli JL, Rutherford HJV, David DH, Kim-Cohen J, et al. Attachment dismissal predicts frontal slow-wave ERPs during rejection by unfamiliar peers. *Emotion.* (2012) 12:690–700. doi: 10.1037/a0026750
88. Ein-Dor T, Coan JA, Reizer A, Gross EB, Dahan D, Wegener MA, et al. Sugarcoated isolation: evidence that social avoidance is linked to higher basal glucose levels and higher consumption of glucose. *Front Psychol.* (2015) 6:492. doi: 10.3389/fpsyg.2015.00492
89. Dagan O, Asok A, Steele H, Steele M, Bernard K. Attachment security moderates the link between adverse childhood experiences and cellular aging. *Dev Psychopathol.* (2018) 30:1211–23. doi: 10.1017/S0954579417001705
90. Feldman R. The neurobiology of human attachments. *Trends Cogn Sci.* (2017) 21:80–99. doi: 10.1016/j.tics.2016.11.007
91. Pan Y, Cheng X, Zhang Z, Li X, Hu Y. Cooperation in lovers: an fNIRS-based hyperscanning study. *Hum Brain Mapp.* (2017) 38:831–41. doi: 10.1002/hbm.23421
92. Reindl V, Gerloff C, Scharke W, Konrad K. Brain-to-brain synchrony in parent-child dyads and the relationship with emotion regulation revealed by fNIRS-based hyperscanning. *Neuroimage.* (2018) 178:493–502. doi: 10.1016/j.neuroimage.2018.05.060
93. Miller JG, Vrtička P, Cui X, Shrestha S, Hosseini SMH, Baker JM, et al. Inter-brain synchrony in mother-child dyads during cooperation: an fNIRS hyperscanning study. *Neuropsychologia.* (2019) 124:117–24. doi: 10.1016/j.neuropsychologia.2018.12.021
94. Nguyen T, Schleihauf H, Kayhan E, Matthes D, Vrtička P, Hoehl S. The effects of interaction quality on neural synchrony during mother-child problem solving. *Cortex.* (2020) 124:235–49. doi: 10.1016/j.cortex.2019.11.020
95. Granqvist P, Sroufe LA, Dozier M, Hesse E, Steele M, van Ijzendoorn M, et al. Disorganized attachment in infancy: a review of the phenomenon and its implications for clinicians and policy-makers. *Attach Hum Dev.* (2017) 19:534–58. doi: 10.1080/14616734.2017.1354040
96. Zhu J, Lowen SB, Anderson CM, Ohashi K, Khan A, Teicher MH. Association of prepubertal and postpubertal exposure to childhood maltreatment with adult amygdala function. *JAMA Psychiatry.* (2019) 76:843–53. doi: 10.1001/jamapsychiatry.2019.0931
97. Del Giudice M. Sex, attachment, and the development of reproductive strategies. *Behav Brain Sci.* (2009) 32:1–21. doi: 10.1017/S0140525X09000016
98. Zeanah CH, Gunnar MR, McCall RB, Kreppner JM, Fox NA. VI. Sensitive periods. *Monog Soc Res Child Dev.* (2011) 76:147–62. doi: 10.1111/j.1540-5834.2011.00631.x
99. Rutter M, Kumsta R, Schlotz W, Sonuga-Barke E. Longitudinal studies using a "natural experiment" design: the case of adoptees from romanian institutions. *J Am Acad Child Adolesc Psychiatry.* (2012) 51:762–70. doi: 10.1016/j.jaac.2012.05.011
100. O'Connor TG. Developmental models and mechanisms for understanding the effects of early experiences on psychological development. In: Cicchetti D, editor. *Developmental Psychopathology. 1: Theory and Method.* 3rd ed. New York, NY: John Wiley & Sons, Inc. (2016). p. 156–98.
101. Zeanah CH, Humphreys KL, Fox NA, Nelson CA. Alternatives for abandoned children: insights from the bucharest early intervention project. *Curr Opin Psychol.* (2017) 15:182–8. doi: 10.1016/j.copsyc.2017.02.024
102. Gunnar MR, DePasquale CE, Reid BM, Donzella B. Pubertal stress recalibration reverses the effects of early life stress in postinstitutionalized children. *Proc Natl Acad Sci USA.* (2019) 116:23984. doi: 10.1073/pnas.1909699116
103. Teicher MH, Samson JA. Childhood maltreatment and psychopathology: a case for ecophenotypic variants as clinically and neurobiologically distinct subtypes. *Am J Psychiatry.* (2013) 170:1114–33. doi: 10.1176/appi.ajp.2013.12070957
104. Keil J, Perren S, Schlesier-Michel A, Sticca F, Sierau S, Klein AM, et al. Getting less than their fair share: maltreated youth are hyper-cooperative yet vulnerable to exploitation in a public goods game. *Dev Sci.* (2019) 22:e12765. doi: 10.1111/desc.12765
105. Crittenden PM, DiLalla DL. Compulsive compliance: the development of an inhibitory coping strategy in infancy. *J Abnormal Child Psychol.* (1988) 16:585–99. doi: 10.1007/BF00914268
106. Zeanah CH, Gleason MM. Annual research review: attachment disorders in

early childhood – clinical presentation, causes, correlates, and treatment. *J Child Psychol Psychiatry.* (2015) 56:207–22. doi: 10.1111/jcpp.12347

107. Sloman L, Taylor P. Impact of child maltreatment on attachment and social rank systems. *Trauma Violence Abuse.* (2016) 17:172–85. doi: 10.1177/1524838015584354
108. Bernard K, Dozier M. Examining infants' cortisol responses to laboratory tasks among children varying in attachment disorganization: stress reactivity or return to baseline? *Dev Psychol.* (2010) 46:1771–8. doi: 10.1037/a0020660
109. Hertsgaard L, Gunnar M, Erickson MF, Nachmias M. Adrenocortical responses to the strange situation in infants with disorganized/disoriented attachment relationships. *Child Dev.* (1995) 66:1100–6. doi: 10.2307/1131801
110. Spangler G, Grossmann KE. Biobehavioral organization in securely and insecurely attached infants. *Child Dev.* (1993) 64:1439–50. doi: 10.2307/1131544
111. De Bellis MD, Baum AS, Birmaher B, Keshavan MS, Eccard CH, Boring AM, et al. Developmental traumatology part I: biological stress systems. *Biol Psychiatry.* (1999) 45:1259–70. doi: 10.1016/S0006-3223(99)00044-X
112. De Bellis MD, Chrousos GP, Dorn LD, Burke L, Helmers K, Kling MA, et al. Hypothalamic-pituitary-adrenal axis dysregulation in sexually abused girls. *J Clin Endocrinol Metab.* (1994) 78:249–55. doi: 10.1210/jcem.78.2.8106608
113. Luijk MPCM, Saridjan N, Tharner A, van Ijzendoorn MH, Bakermans-Kranenburg MJ, Jaddoe VWV, et al. Attachment, depression, and cortisol: deviant patterns in insecure-resistant and disorganized infants. *Dev Psychobiol.* (2010) 52:441–52. doi: 10.1002/dev.20446
114. Spangler G, Schieche M. Emotional and adrenocortical responses of infants to the strange situation:the differential function of emotional expression. *Int J Behav Dev.* (1998) 22:681–706. doi: 10.1080/016502598384126
115. Lyons-Ruth K, Spielman E. Disorganized infant attachment strategies and helpless-fearful profiles of parenting: integrating attachment research with clinical intervention. *Infant Mental Health J.* (2004) 25:318–35. doi: 10.1002/imhj.20008
116. Lyons-Ruth K, Melnick S, Bronfman E, Sherry S, Llanas L. Hostile-helpless relational models and disorganized attachment patterns between parents and their young children: review of research and implications for clinical work. In: *Attachment Issues in Psychopathology and Intervention.* Mahwah, NJ: Lawrence Erlbaum Associates Publishers (2004). p. 65–94.
117. McCrory EJ, De Brito SA, Sebastian CL, Mechelli A, Bird G, Kelly PA, et al. Heightened neural reactivity to threat in child victims of family violence. *Curr Biol.* (2011) 21:R947–R8. doi: 10.1016/j.cub.2011.10.015
118. Hein TC, Monk CS. Research review: neural response to threat in children, adolescents, and adults after child maltreatment – a quantitative meta-analysis. *J Child Psychol Psychiatry.* (2017) 58:222–30. doi: 10.1111/jcpp.12651
119. Howell BR, Grand AP, McCormack KM, Shi Y, LaPrarie JL, Maestripieri D, et al. Early adverse experience increases emotional reactivity in juvenile rhesus macaques: relation to amygdala volume. *Dev Psychobiol.* (2014) 56:1735–46. doi: 10.1002/dev.21237
120. Lupien SJ, Parent S, Evans AC, Tremblay RE, Zelazo PD, Corbo V, et al. Larger amygdala but no change in hippocampal volume in 10-year-old children exposed to maternal depressive symptomatology since birth. *Proc Natl Acad Sci USA.* (2011) 108:14324. doi: 10.1073/pnas.1105371108
121. Mehta MA, Golembo NI, Nosarti C, Colvert E, Mota A, Williams SCR, et al. Amygdala, hippocampal and corpus callosum size following severe early institutional deprivation: the english and romanian adoptees study pilot. *J Child Psychol Psychiatry.* (2009) 50:943–51. doi: 10.1111/j.1469-7610.2009.02084.x
122. Tottenham N, Hare TA, Quinn BT, McCarry TW, Nurse M, Gilhooly T, et al. Prolonged institutional rearing is associated with atypically large amygdala volume and difficulties in emotion regulation. *Dev Sci.* (2010) 13:46–61. doi: 10.1111/j.1467-7687.2009.00852.x
123. Bruce J, Fisher PA, Pears KC, Levine S. Morning cortisol levels in preschool-aged foster children: differential effects of maltreatment type. *Dev Psychobiol.* (2009) 51:14–23. doi: 10.1002/dev.20333
124. Schalinski I, Teicher MH, Rockstroh B. Early neglect is a key determinant of adult hair cortisol concentration and is associated with increased vulnerability to trauma in a transdiagnostic sample. *Psychoneuroendocrinology.* (2019) 108:35–42. doi: 10.1016/j.psyneuen.2019.06.007
125. White LO, Ising M, von Klitzing K, Sierau S, Michel A, Klein AM, et al. Reduced hair cortisol after maltreatment mediates externalizing symptoms in middle childhood and adolescence. *J Child Psychol Psychiatry.* (2017) 58:998–1007. doi: 10.1111/jcpp.12700
126. Reilly EB, Gunnar MR. Neglect, HPA axis reactivity, and development. *Int J Dev Neurosci.* (2019) 78:100–8. doi: 10.1016/j.ijdevneu.2019.07.010
127. Fisher PA. Commentary: is there a there there in hair? A reflection on child maltreatment and hair cortisol concentrations in White et al. 2017. *J Child Psychol Psychiatry.* (2017) 58:1008–10. doi: 10.1111/jcpp.12719
128. White LO, Ising M, von Klitzing K, Sierau S, Michel A, Klein AM, et al. Commentary: the importance of exploring dose-dependent, subtype-specific, and age-related effects of maltreatment on the HPA axis and the mediating link to psychopathology. A response to Fisher 2017. *J Child Psychol Psychiatry.* (2017) 58:1011–3. doi: 10.1111/jcpp.12770
129. Krause AL, Borchardt V, Li M, van Tol M-J, Demenescu LR, Strauss B, et al. Dismissing attachment characteristics dynamically modulate brain networks subserving social aversion. *Front Hum Neurosci.* (2016) 10:77. doi: 10.3389/fnhum.2016.00077
130. Puetz VB, Kohn N, Dahmen B, Zvyagintsev M, Schüppen A, Schultz RT, et al. Neural response to social rejection in children with early separation experiences. *J Am Acad Child Adolesc Psychiatry.* (2014) 53:1328–37.e8. doi: 10.1016/j.jaac.2014.09.004
131. Puetz VB, Viding E, Palmer A, Kelly PA, Lickley R, Koutoufa I, et al. Altered neural response to rejection-related words in children exposed to maltreatment. *J Child Psychol Psychiatry.* (2016) 57:1165–73. doi: 10.1111/jcpp.12595
132. McLaughlin KA, Sheridan MA, Tibu F, Fox NA, Zeanah CH, Nelson CA. Causal effects of the early caregiving environment on development of stress response systems in children. *Proc Natl Acad Sci USA.* (2015) 112:5637–42. doi: 10.1073/pnas.1423363112
133. Tharner A, Herba CM, Luijk MPCM, van Ijzendoorn MH, Bakermans-Kranenburg MJ, Govaert PP, et al. Subcortical structures and the neurobiology of infant attachment disorganization: a longitudinal ultrasound imaging study. *Soc Neurosci.* (2011) 6:336–47. doi: 10.1080/17470919.2010.538219
134. Mehta MA, Gore-Langton E, Golembo N, Colvert E, Williams SCR, Sonuga-Barke E. Hyporesponsive reward anticipation in the basal ganglia following severe institutional deprivation early in life. *J Cogn Neurosci.* (2010) 22:2316–25. doi: 10.1162/jocn.2009.21394
135. Takiguchi S, Fujisawa TX, Mizushima S, Saito DN, Okamoto Y, Shimada K, et al. Ventral striatum dysfunction in children and adolescents with reactive attachment disorder: functional MRI study. *BJPsych Open.* (2015) 1:121–8. doi: 10.1192/bjpo.bp.115.001586
136. Holz NE, Boecker R, Hohm E, Zohsel K, Buchmann AF, Blomeyer D, et al. The long-term impact of early life poverty on orbitofrontal cortex volume in adulthood: results from a prospective study over 25 years. *Neuropsychopharmacology.* (2015) 40:996–1004. doi: 10.1038/npp.2014.277
137. Dillon DG, Holmes AJ, Birk JL, Brooks N, Lyons-Ruth K, Pizzagalli DA. Childhood adversity is associated with left basal ganglia dysfunction during reward anticipation in adulthood. *Biol Psychiatry.* (2009) 66:206–13. doi: 10.1016/j.biopsych.2009.02.019
138. Carroll D, Ginty AT, Whittaker AC, Lovallo WR, de Rooij SR. The behavioural, cognitive, and neural corollaries of blunted cardiovascular and cortisol reactions to acute psychological stress. *Neurosci Biobehav Rev.* (2017) 77:74–86. doi: 10.1016/j.neubiorev.2017.02.025
139. Berntson GG, Cacioppo JT, Quigley KS. Cardiac psychophysiology and autonomic space in humans: empirical perspectives and conceptual implications. *Psychol Bull.* (1993) 114:296–322. doi: 10.1037/0033-2909.114.2.296
140. Fonagy P, Leigh T, Steele M, Steele H, Kennedy R, Mattoon G, et al. The relation of attachment status, psychiatric classification, and response to psychotherapy. *J Consult Clin Psychol.* (1996) 64:22–31. doi: 10.1037/0022-006X.64.1.22
141. Katznelson H. Reflective functioning: a review. *Clin Psychol Rev.* (2014) 34:107–17. doi: 10.1016/j.cpr.2013.12.003
142. McLaughlin KA, Peverill M, Gold AL, Alves S, Sheridan MA. Child

maltreatment and neural systems underlying emotion regulation. *J Am Acad Child Adolesc Psychiatry.* (2015) 54:753–62. doi: 10.1016/j.jaac.2015.06.010
143. Yang DYJ, Rosenblau G, Keifer C, Pelphrey KA. An integrative neural model of social perception, action observation, and theory of mind. *Neurosci Biobehav Rev.* (2015) 51:263–75. doi: 10.1016/j.neubiorev.2015.01.020
144. Rinne-Albers MAW, van der Wee NJA, Lamers-Winkelman F, Vermeiren RRJM. Neuroimaging in children, adolescents and young adults with psychological trauma. *Eur Child Adolesc Psychiatry.* (2013) 22:745–55. doi: 10.1007/s00787-013-0410-1
145. Schiffer F, Teicher MH, Papanicolaou AC. Evoked potential evidence for right brain activity during the recall of traumatic memories. *J Neuropsychiatr Clin Neurosci.* (1995) 7:169–75. doi: 10.1176/jnp.7.2.169
146. Johnson JG, Cohen P, Brown J, Smailes EM, Bernstein DP. Childhood maltreatment increases risk for personality disorders during early adulthood. *Archives of General Psychiatry.* (1999) 56:600–6. doi: 10.1001/archpsyc.56.7.600
147. Dozier M, Stovall-McClough KC, Albus KE. Attachment and psychopathology in adulthood. In: Cassidy J, Shaver PR, editors. *Handbook of Attachment: Theory, Research, and Clinical Applications*, 2nd ed. New York, NY: The Guilford Press (2008). p. 718–44.
148. Crittenden PM, Newman L. Comparing models of borderline personality disorder: mothers' experience, self-protective strategies, and dispositional representations. *Clinical Child Psychol Psychiatry.* (2010) 15:433–51. doi: 10.1177/1359104510368209
149. Zeanah CH, Nelson CA, Fox NA, Smyke AT, Marshall P, Parker SW, et al. Designing research to study the effects of institutionalization on brain and behavioral development: the bucharest early intervention project. *Dev Psychopathol.* (2003) 15:885–907. doi: 10.1017/S0954579403000452
150. Duschinsky R. The emergence of the disorganized/disoriented (D) attachment classification, 1979–1982. *History Psychol.* (2015) 18:32–46. doi: 10.1037/a0038524
151. Strathearn L, Fonagy P, Amico J, Montague PR. Adult attachment predicts maternal brain and oxytocin response to infant cues. *Neuropsychopharmacology.* (2009) 34:2655–66. doi: 10.1038/npp.2009.103
152. Crittenden PM. Distorted patterns of relationship in maltreating families: The role of internal representation models. *J Reprod Infant Psychol.* (1988) 6:183–99. doi: 10.1080/02646838808403555
153. Miller GE, Chen E, Zhou ES. If it goes up, must it come down? Chronic stress and the hypothalamic-pituitary-adrenocortical axis in humans. *Psychol Bull.* (2007) 133:25–45. doi: 10.1037/0033-2909.133.1.25
154. Steudte-Schmiedgen S, Kirschbaum C, Alexander N, Stalder T. An integrative model linking traumatization, cortisol dysregulation and posttraumatic stress disorder: insight from recent hair cortisol findings. *Neurosci Biobehav Rev.* (2016) 69:124–35. doi: 10.1016/j.neubiorev.2016.07.015
155. Lunkenheimer E, Busuito A, Brown KM, Skowron EA. Mother–child coregulation of parasympathetic processes differs by child maltreatment severity and subtype. *Child Maltreatment.* (2018) 23:211–20. doi: 10.1177/1077559517751672
156. Lieberman AF, Ghosh Ippen C, van Horn P. Child-parent psychotherapy: 6-month follow-up of a randomized controlled trial. *J Am Acad Child Adolesc Psychiatry.* (2006) 45:913–8. doi: 10.1097/01.chi.0000222784.03735.92
157. Lieberman AF, Ghosh Ippen C, van Horn P. "Don't Hit My Mommy!": a manual for child-parent psychotherapy with young children exposed to violence and other trauma. Washington, DC: Zero to Three (2015).
158. Dozier M, Bick J, Bernard K. Intervening with foster parents to enhance biobehavioral outcomes among infants and toddlers. *Zero Three.* (2011) 31:17–22.

11

Imaging Real-Time Tactile Interaction with Two-Person Dual-Coil fMRI

Ville Renvall[1,2], *Jaakko Kauramäki*[1], *Sanna Malinen*[1], *Riitta Hari*[1,3] *and Lauri Nummenmaa*[1,4*]

[1] Department of Neuroscience and Biomedical Engineering, Aalto University School of Science, Espoo, Finland, [2] Advanced Magnetic Imaging Centre, Aalto University School of Science, Espoo, Finland, [3] Department of Art, Aalto University School of Arts, Design and Architecture, Espoo, Finland, [4] Turku PET Centre and Department of Psychology, University of Turku, Turku, Finland

***Correspondence:**
Lauri Nummenmaa
latanu@utu.fi

Studies of brain mechanisms supporting social interaction are demanding because real interaction only occurs when persons are in contact. Instead, most brain imaging studies scan subjects individually. Here we present a proof-of-concept demonstration of two-person blood oxygenation dependent (BOLD) imaging of brain activity from two individuals interacting inside the bore of a single MRI scanner. We developed a custom 16-channel (8 + 8 channels) two-helmet coil with two separate receiver-coil pairs providing whole-brain coverage, while bringing participants into a shared physical space and realistic face-to-face contact. Ten subject pairs were scanned with the setup. During the experiment, subjects took turns in tapping each other's lip versus observing and feeling the taps timed by auditory instructions. Networks of sensorimotor brain areas were engaged alternatingly in the subjects during executing motor actions as well as observing and feeling them; these responses were clearly distinguishable from the auditory responses occurring similarly in both participants. Even though the signal-to-noise ratio of our coil system was compromised compared with standard 32-channel head coils, our results show that the two-person fMRI scanning is feasible for studying the brain basis of social interaction.

Keywords: functional magnetic resonance imaging, touch, somatosensory, motor, two-person neuroscience

INTRODUCTION

Humans are embedded in complex social networks where individuals interact at different temporal scales. Most social interactions, such as verbal and nonverbal communication, occur in dyads or groups, where people constantly strive to predict, understand, and influence each other. During the interaction, sensory, cognitive, and emotional information is constantly remapped in the observers' brain and used for motor actions as responses attuned to the received input (1). Thus the interlocutors' minds are intertwined into a shared system facilitating reciprocation (2–4) as well as anticipation of the other person's acts, allowing distribution of neural processing across brains to aid, for example, problem solving.

Some aspects of human social behavior—in particular perceptual and decision-making processes —can be studied by measuring single brains in isolation. Conventional BOLD-fMRI experiments allow to locate brain processes related to different social functions, while intersubject correlation (ISC) analysis based on voxelwise temporal correlation of BOLD-fMRI time series (5–7) or neuromagnetic activity with higher temporal resolution (8) across subject pairs can be used to index similarity of sensory and socioemotional information processing across subjects (9, 10). Recently this approach has also been extended to quantifying but also similarity of person preferences and social relationships (11). Although such data-driven analyses can be used to map brain basis of social perception with high-dimensional stimulus spaces, they are still essentially based on measurement of extrinsic, fixed stimuli and lack the very definition of social interaction, as the subjects have no influence whatsoever on other peoples' minds during the experiment. This is a critical limitation as social interaction cannot be reduced to sequential, partially parallel processing of the input of the interacting brains, because social interaction only emerges when the two brains (*via* their owners) are hooked up together (4, 8, 12). Simply put, real-time social interaction does not exist when two or more individuals are not engaged in the same physical or virtual space (13).

Reciprocal social cognitive processes cannot thus be understood completely without studying the complete interaction unit consisting of two individuals (14). Behavioral work suggests that social interaction tunes the individuals into a self-organizing, interactive state. For example, humans automatically mimic other's emotional expressions (15), gaze direction (16), and postures (17). Social signals, such as laughter, also automatically attune individual not just at the level of motor responses, but also in terms of activation of specific neurotransmitter systems (18). Moreover, many social processes, such as gaze following (19, 20) and turn taking during conversation (21), take place with gaps less than 250 ms, and social interaction may lead to episodes of two-person flow without neither of them consciously leading or following (22). Yet, most of what we know about human social brain functions comes from "spectator" studies where the brains are assumed to generate responses to pre-defined stimulation (8). Even though this approach has been successful in delineating the brain basis of social perception, and on some occasions of social communication, it tells relatively little about the actual mechanisms of dynamic social interaction. Consequently, several researchers have suggested that the spectator paradigm and offline social cognition studies should be complemented with real-time two-person paradigms, where two interacting individuals constantly generate "stimuli" for each other (1, 2, 4, 23, 24).

Some aspects of human communication can be investigated using alternated scanning of the subjects sending and receiving information. In such an approach, the senders convey some social information *via*, for example, speech or gestures, while their brain activity as well as the communicative information are recorded. The communicative information can then be presented to the receiver subjects as stimuli during brain imaging, allowing joint analysis of the brain activity of the sender and receiver subjects. This line of work has revealed how successful communication *via* speech (25, 26), hand gestures (3, 27), and facial expressions (28) enhances similarity of neural activation patterns across the interlocutors in a task-specific manner. This approach however lacks any interactivity, as the receiver subjects are essentially viewing pre-recorded stimuli, and need not to generate any responses to them. Recently different neuroimaging techniques have been proposed for studying dynamic "live" interaction. In the hyperscanning approach, two individuals are scanned with two MRI (29–31) or MEG (32) devices connected with an audio-video link, thus enabling interaction of two subjects in independent devices. Furthermore, with EEG recordings real face-to-face to interaction can be achieved in reasonably unconstrained social interaction tasks (33).

Such natural sense of presence of another individual might be critical for understanding the brain basis of social interaction. For example, resting-state brain activity in nonhuman primates is different when conspecifics are present versus absent (34). In humans, interaction with real rather than recorded persons elicits stronger hemodynamic responses (35), and even early electrophysiological responses such as the face-sensitive N170 responses are amplified for real human faces versus those of a human-like dummy (36). These findings highlight the importance of co-presence with other people, and the consequent changes in the way the brain processes both internal and external cues. Consequently, to understand the intricacies of the brain basis of human social interaction and communication, we need techniques that allow simultaneous recording of two individuals in the same physical space. This has already been technically achieved with simultaneous EEG (e.g. 37) and NIRS (e.g. 38, 39) recordings, as these devices can be easily attached to subjects measured in a conventional face-to-face settings. Nevertheless, neither of these techniques allows volumetric measurements of the deep brain structures, many of which are critical for human social processes (40–42).

The Current Study

One potentially powerful approach for studying brain basis of social interaction involves simultaneous blood oxygenation dependent (BOLD) imaging of two persons within one magnetic resonance imaging scanner. Such an approach would bring both subjects into the same physical space whilst allowing tomographic imaging of hemodynamic brain activation. Currently, one such solution has been published, based on decoupled circular-polarized volume coil for two heads (43, 44). We have, in turn, developed a custom-built 16-channel (8 + 8 channels) two-helmet coil with two separate receiving elements (45), allowing experimental setups where the subjects were facing each other so that their feet pointed to opposite directions in the magnet bore. In the present proof-of-concept study we demonstrate how hemodynamic signals can be recorded during real-time social interaction using this a novel MRI setup so that the subject can lie parallel to each other while sharing the same physical space in a realistic face-to-face contact. The setup thereby allows seamless interaction between the members of the dyad, while providing whole-brain coverage.

Because this was the very first proof-of-concept human experiment done with our dual-coil design, we wanted to benchmark the feasibility of the setup with a robust and simple social interaction task, rather than setting up an overly complex design without knowing the potential limitations of the coil setup. Consequently, we used social touching as the model task, as touching is an intimate way of conveying affect and trust in social relationships (46–48). During the fMRI experiments, subjects took turns in tapping each other's lip *versus* observing and feeling the taps. We show that overlapping networks of sensorimotor brain areas are engaged during executing motor actions as well as observing and feeling social touching, suggesting that the two-person fMRI recordings are feasible for studying the brain basis of social interaction.

MATERIALS AND METHODS

Subjects

We scanned 10 pairs of volunteers with a mean age of 23 ± 3 years (20 subjects; 7 female–male pairs and 3 female–female pairs). One further pair was scanned but excluded due to excessive head motions: one of the subjects moved so that the detector array's sensitivity was compromised, and repositioning was not possible due to time constraints. All subjects were right-handed per self-report, and none of them reported any history of neurological illness. All pairs were friends or romantic partners. The study was approved by the Aalto University Institutional Review Board. All subjects gave written informed consent and were screened for MRI exclusion criteria prior to scanning.

MRI Acquisition

Data were acquired with 3-T whole body MRI system (MAGNETOM Skyra 3.0 T, Siemens Healthcare, Erlangen, Germany) with both a vendor-provided 32-channel receive head coil (reference scans) and a custom-built 16-channel (8 + 8 channels) two-head, two-helmet receive coil (anatomical images, task-based fMRI, and resting state scan). With both receive coils, the integrated body coil was used for transmit. **Figure 1** shows an overview of the coil and subject setup. We originally experimented with a setup where subjects were lying either sideways or in a supine position, while entering the gantry from the opposite ends so that a second custom MRI bed was used for the backwards entry. This setup was however discarded due to subject discomfort and concomitant motion-related artifacts.

Every scanning session consisted of two parts. First both subjects were scanned one-by-one using normal one-person setup (head-first supine, 32-channel coil). T1-weighted MP-RAGE images were acquired for anatomical reference, and gradient echo (GRE) echo-planar imaging (EPI) data were acquired for evaluating the temporal signal-to-noise ratio (tSNR), especially in comparison with the two-person data. Imaging parameters for the MP-RAGE scans were as follows: repetition time (TR) = 2.53 s, echo time (TE) = 28 ms, readout flip angle (α) = 7°, 256 × 256 × 176 imaging matrix, isotropic 1-mm^3 resolution, and GRAPPA reduction factor (R) = 2. The parameters for the GRE-EPI were: TR = 3 s, TE = 28 ms, α = 80°, fat saturation was used, in-plane imaging matrix (frequency encoding × phase encoding) = 70 × 70, field-of-view (FOV) = 21 × 21 cm^2, in-plane resolution 3 × 3 mm^2, R = 2, effective echo spacing (esp) = 0.26 ms, bandwidth = 2380 Hz/pixel (total bandwidth = 167 kHz), phase encoding in anterior–posterior direction, slice thickness = 3 mm with 10% slice gap, interleaved slice-acquisition order. Altogether 126 volumes, with 49 oblique axial slices in each, were

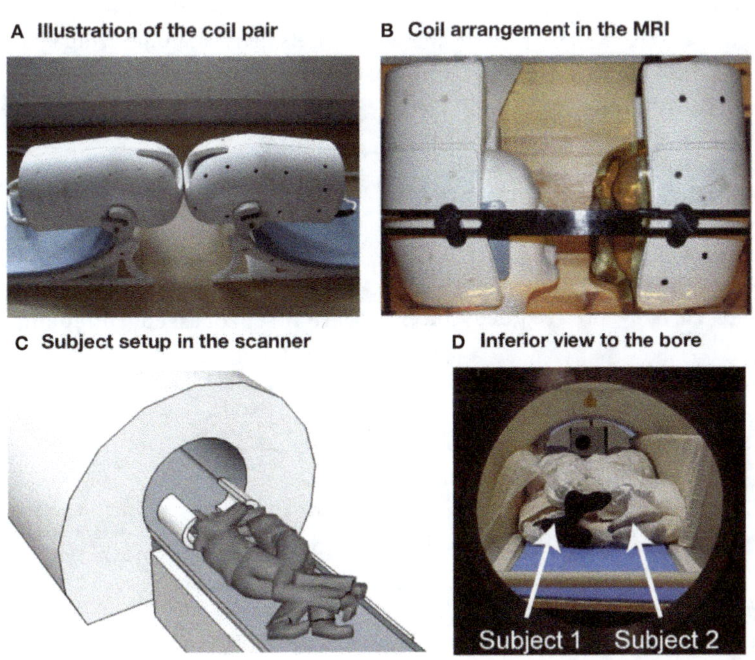

FIGURE 1 | Coil and subject setup. **(A, B)** Illustration of the dual coil and its arrangement in the scanner. **(C, D)** Subject setup inside the scanner.

acquired during the 6 min 18 s data-collection period. Three "dummy" scans were acquired at the beginning of each acquisition to stabilize the longitudinal magnetization.

Next the subjects were positioned in the scanner together with the two-head coil; the subjects were lying on their sides, facing each other at a close distance. Localizer and GRE-EPI data were acquired after shimming the magnet, using the semi-automated workflow by iteratively acquiring B_0 field maps and calculating the shims for as long as the shim was deemed unacceptable. In this phase, the subjects could be repositioned if the their field maps appeared excessively dissimilar. The scan parameters were the same as in the one-person setup, with the following exceptions: in-plane matrix = 160 × 70, FOV = 48.6 × 20.1 cm^2, and bandwidth = 2404 Hz/pixel (total bandwidth = 385 kHz). Moreover, the phase encoding was in subjects' left–right direction to avoid aliasing ghosts from one subject's brain into the other, and to reduce distortion and scan time by limiting the number of phase encoding steps (to 35 per slice). The 49 slices were oriented axially and tilted only to maximize the symmetry of the acquisition of the two brains. During the two-person measurements, the bodies of the subjects were in contact (without direct skin contact) and pillows and foam mattresses were used to make the subjects as comfortable as possible. The subjects' heads were stabilized using small pillows with non-slippery surface and additional support was provided using a large vacuum pillow that once deflated retained its shape throughout the session.

Touching Task

Figure 2 summarizes the touching task. The subjects took turns in repeatedly tapping ("actor" subject) the lower lip of their partner ("receiver" subject) with the tip of the index finger, so that both partners could also clearly see the finger movement. This site was chosen so that that the finger movements would be clearly visible to both subjects. Self-paced (~2 Hz) tapping was performed throughout the 30-s task blocks. Subjects were stressed to minimize finger movements, because motion near the imaging volume perturbs the magnetic field and can interfere with the spatial encoding and introduce head motion. During the rest blocks the subjects were instructed to hold their finger close by but not touching the lower lip of their partner. Each task run contained six rest–task block cycles with an additional rest block at the end of the run. Except for the initial rest condition, transitions between blocks were cued by pre-recorded voice command "Touch" and "Rest." These were delivered to the participants by connecting the stimulus computer's audio output to the magnet console to use the intercom system of the MRI scanner. Presentation software (Neurobehavioral Systems, Berkeley, CA, USA) controlled stimulus presentation. After the first task run we confirmed that the subjects could hear the voice commands. For any given run, only one of the subjects performed the active touching task while the other focused on feeling the taps. The roles were switched between runs. Both subjects were always scanned twice in both roles so that altogether four task runs with 126 EPI volumes in each were acquired.

Resting-State Scans

Resting state scans were obtained for inspecting signal quality. During the single-subject GRE-EPI data acquisition, the subjects were instructed to keep their eyes open and still. Eye-blinking was allowed. The two-person resting-state scans were always acquired prior to the task scans, asking the subjects to lie still with eyes open without actively looking at each other.

Image Preprocessing—One-Person Scans

The fMRI data were preprocessed in Matlab utilizing custom code and FSL functions (49). The one-person fMRI data were motion-corrected using FSL MCFLIRT (50). Next, slice-timing correction was applied and the frame-wise motion within each fMRI run was corrected using FSL function MCFLIRT after brain extraction using BET (51) and smoothed with structure-preserving smoothing with SUSAN (52) that employed a 6-mm (full-width-at-half-maximum, FWHM) Gaussian smoothing kernel. The data were rigidly (six free parameters) aligned to the anatomical MP-RAGE scans, with narrow search space for the alignment because the receiver intensity was spatially atypical and prohibited the use of the standard options for several datasets. The anatomical images were normalized to the MNI space, and the resulting warps were then applied to the EPI images. Data were finally smoothed using a Gaussian kernel with 8 mm FWHM.

Image Preprocessing—Two-Person Scans

Individual heads were first separated and rotated to standard head-first supine orientation using a fixed coordinate transformation without resampling. Next both subjects' data were preprocessed independently as described above.

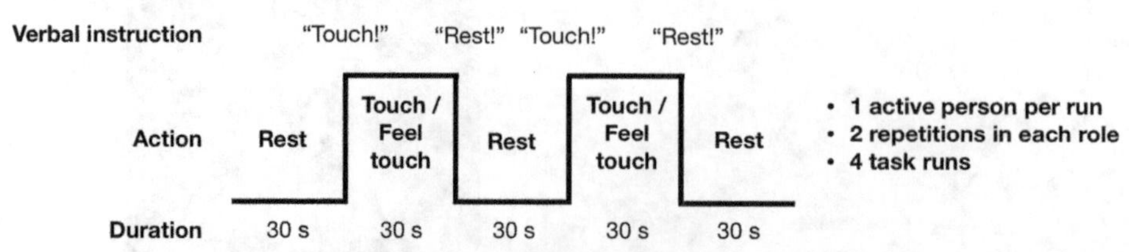

FIGURE 2 | Experimental design. Subjects took 30-s turns in tapping the top of each other's lip with their index finger, resulting in alternating tapping-feeling boxcar design with complete antiphase across the subjects. Turns were indicated with commands relayed *via* headphones.

Preprocessing was concluded by recombining the data of each pair so that one subject's data were in MNI space, and the other subject's data were placed nose-to-nose with that to mimic the actual positioning during the scanning.

Signal-to-Noise Ratios

Coil performance was assessed with temporal signal-to-noise ratio (tSNR) of resting-state fMRI scans comprising of 126 time points. The FSL BET program was used to extract the brain voxels from the images, after which the data were motion-corrected using FSL MCFLIRT. Next, voxelwise tSNR values were calculated as the ratio of the mean signal over the measurement, divided by the standard deviation (std) at each voxel. For comparison, similar analysis was carried out for the one-person resting-state data.

Task-Evoked BOLD Responses

Task-evoked BOLD responses were analyzed in FSL using the General Linear Model (GLM). The main blocks were modeled at the stimulus periodicity, and the voice instructions were modeled as 3-s events at the beginning and end of each block (see **Figure 2**). A canonical double-gamma hemodynamic response function (HRF) was convolved with the timeseries of tactile stimulus blocks and voice events. Also, the motion parameter estimates of both of the simultaneously scanned heads were included as nuisance regressors for both heads individually; in other words, both subjects' models had their own as well as the other subjects' motion parameters as nuisance covariates. The other head's motion estimates were included to gain resilience against motion-related field or signal fluctuations extending from one head to the location of the other. The analyses included the entire two-head volumes, allowing quantification and visualization of subject-specific and shared activation patterns across the dyad. In a complementary methodological approach, we used independent-component analysis with the GIFT toolbox (http://icatb.sourceforge.net/) on the joint dual-head EPI data, and we assessed the temporal profile of the top extracted components against the experimental stimulus model.

RESULTS

Dual-Coil Performance

Figures 3A, B show a representative dyad's normalized data for T1 and EPI sequences. tSNR was compared between resting-state scans of the two subjects imaged simultaneously with the two-person coil and the same subjects imaged alone with standard 32-channel head coil. **Figure 3C** shows the mean tSNR in a sagittal plane of a representative dyad and in a roughly corresponding plane of one of the subjects of this dyad measured individually. The scales of the color bars are different by a factor of 1.5, corresponding to the theoretical scaling factor of SNR resulting from the differences in acquisition bandwidth (inversely proportional to the square-root of the bandwidth). As expected, the tSNRs of the two-person measurements were almost 50% lower than those of the single-subject measurements, with most salient drop of signal in the frontal cortices.

Regional Effects in the GLM

The voice cues modeled as 3-s events elicited reliable bilateral auditory-cortex activations similarly in both subjects regardless of their role as the actor or the receiver (**Figure 4A**). In turn, the touching task resulted in differential activation patterns in the

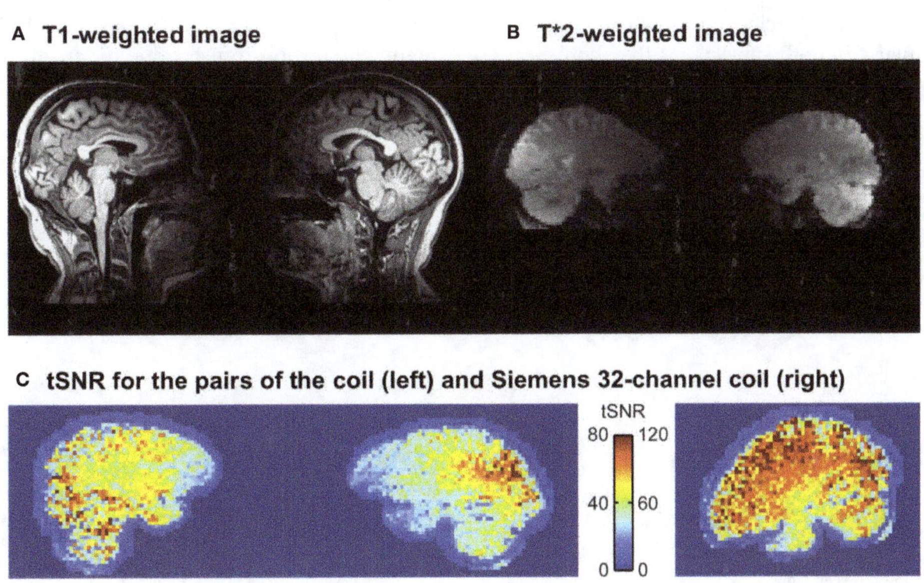

FIGURE 3 | Representative single-dyad T1 **(A)** and T*2 **(B)** -weighted images acquired with the dual coil. **(C)** tSNR for the dual coil and **(D)** conventional Siemens 32-channel head coil. Note that in due to preprocessing, the data from the dual coil pairs in panel **(C)** are further away from each other than they actually are (c.f. panel B).

somatosensory and motor cortices depending on whether the subject was tapping or receiving taps (**Figure 4B** and **Figure S1**).

We next evaluated the consistency of the auditory and somatosensory activations across individual subjects. To that end, we binarized the first-level activation maps for the verbal instructions and tactile tasks, and generated cumulative activation maps where voxels indicated in how many subjects task-dependent activations were detected at the a priori threshold (**Figure 5**). This analysis confirmed that the evoked auditory responses could be detected practically in all the subjects, while the magnitude and detectability of the somatosensory responses was significantly more variable.

Independent-Component Analysis (ICA)

ICA (**Figure 6**) applied on the combined data of the two subjects revealed two clear components during the task: IC1 centrally involving the sensorimotor network, and the IC2 involving the auditory cortices and lateral frontal cortices. Both these components were shared with the subjects, implying that similar auditory and somatomotor activity patterns were present in both subjects, irrespectively of whether they were currently executing *versus* feeling the touches.

DISCUSSION

Our results show that hemodynamic activity can be reliably measured from two interacting subjects' brains within one scanner using a dual-helmet setup with two separate coil arrays, and that this technique can be used for studying elementary social cognitive functions, such as interpersonal communication *via* touching. Although the SNR of the dual-helmet coil was compromised (see **Figure 3**) compared with a conventional 32-channel head coil (53), the task-dependent BOLD responses were task- and region-specific: auditory cues activated the auditory cortex similarly in both subjects (as they both heard the same cues), while the somatosensory and motor activations varied depending on which subject was actively tapping the other. The cues however appeared to alert the acting subject more than the reacting subject, as reflected by activation of the parieto-occipital cortex (precuneus). ICA also revealed activation of sensorimotor and auditory networks in both subjects. Altogether our results highlight how sensorimotor networks "resonate" across individuals during tactile interaction and confirm that fMRI with our novel dual-coil design is a potentially useful tool for studying brain basis of social interaction.

Performance of the Dual Coil

GLM revealed that specific task-dependent fluctuations in hemodynamic activity can be picked up with the setup. Despite relatively modest sample size, the contrasts of interest (tactile, motor, and auditory activations) were significant at the a priori FDR-corrected statistical threshold. However, SNR of the dual coil was clearly inferior to a conventional 32-channel head coil. An important source of discrepancy in the tSNR between the two- and the single-subject setups is the smaller number of coil elements in each of the helmets in the two-person coil in comparison to the one-person coil (8 vs. 32). The overall quality and geometry of the coil also matters: while the two-person coil is a working prototype, the 32-channel coil is the state-of-the-art product of the magnet vendor. The homogeneity of the main magnetic field (B_0) is another important factor. The second-order shim coils cannot achieve the same degree of homogeneity for the two heads than for a single round object, and the B_0 at the edges of the imaging volume is, to begin with, less homogeneous than in the center of the magnet. For these reasons, the water peak is wider in the two-person case.

Also, as the two heads are typically of somewhat different size, the flip angles differ between the heads. Moreover, as the heads after shimming remain in different magnetic fields (and often result in a two-peaked water spectrum; the phase maps of the individual brains are relatively even, but have different offsets), the magnetization transfer due to fat saturation tends to reduce

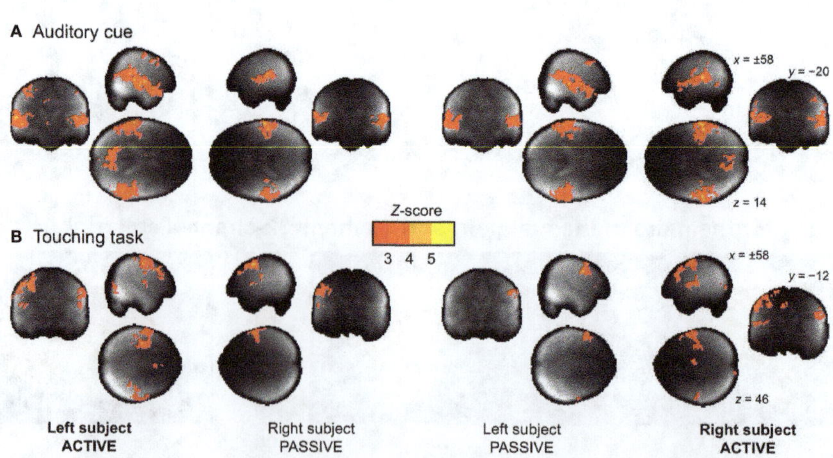

FIGURE 4 | Main effects of auditory cue **(A)** and the touching task **(B)** for the actor and receiver subjects. The data are thresholded at $p < 0.05$, FDR corrected.

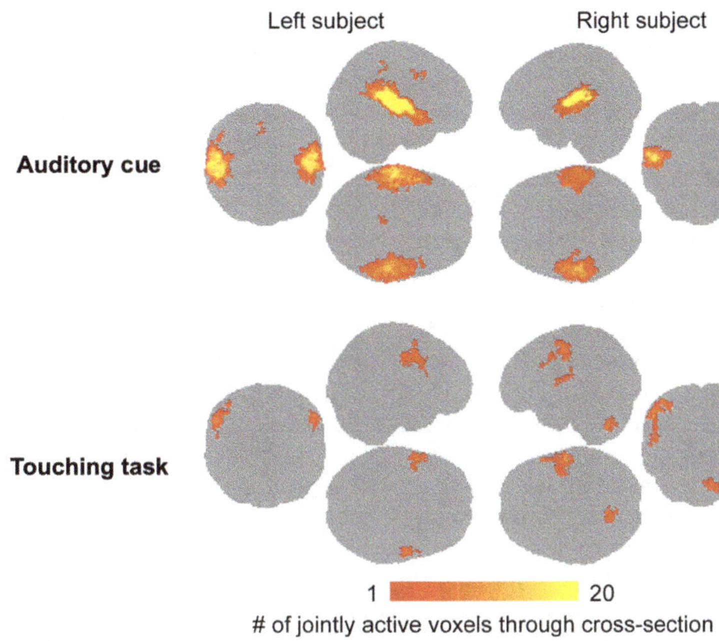

FIGURE 5 | Cumulative map of the binarized (active / inactive) single-pair level activation maps for the auditory cues and touching task. Color bar indicates the number of subjects where significant activations were observed in the first-level analyses. Note that this analysis does not differentiate which subject was active in the tapping task.

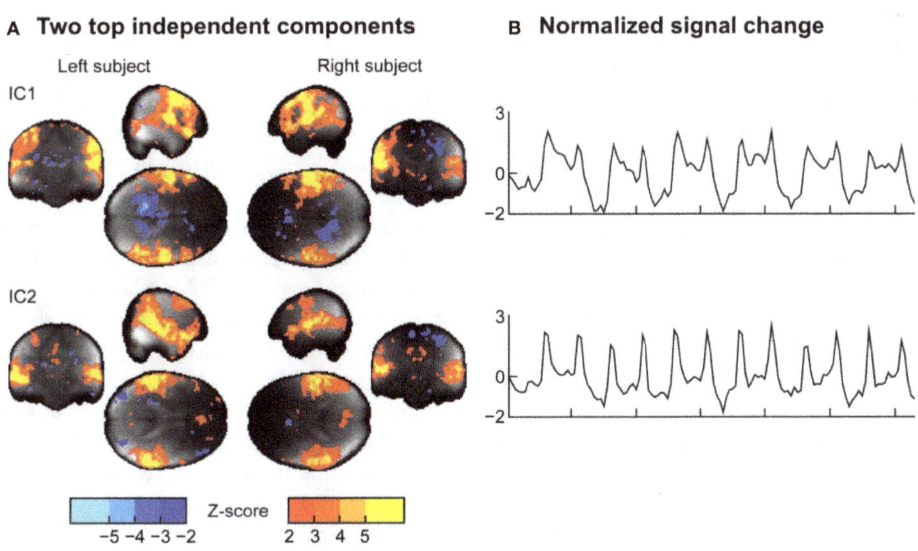

FIGURE 6 | (A) Two representative independent components (ICs) and **(B)** their time courses extracted from the data.

the signal of one head more than of the other, with fat saturation performance varying correspondingly. The homogeneity of the tSNR in the brain is also compromised due to the absence of coil elements in the anterior parts of the brains (see **Figures 1** and **3**). This drop is similar to what occurs when the anterior part of the 32-channel coil is removed and only the posterior elements are used for imaging. A final reason that influences the tSNR is the subject comfort and stability, which in the two-person setup are worse than in the normal setup, further compromised because the subjects need to be scanned in close proximity and in a sideways position. We tried to alleviate this problem by keeping the experimental runs short and by padding the subjects well, as well as using both subjects' motion parameters as nuisance regressors in the analysis. It is however obvious that future studies need to implement more effective prospective means for motion control, such as neck or head restraints.

Simultaneous Measurement of Interacting Individuals

In contrast to conventional single-person MR imaging, the present two-person functional imaging approach provides novel means for understanding the neural basis of human social interaction. During social interaction, the interaction partners' brains need to continuously anticipate as well as respond and adjust to incoming signals. A critical question is whether these sensorimotor loops function only recursively, as a cascade of third-person action-response processes? For example, a dialogue between two persons becomes fully incomprehensible if one persons' speech fragments are removed from the recording. Brains are coupled with each other *via* behavior, and they influence each other *via* extracranial loops: Motor actions conveyed by one individual are interpreted by means of the sensory systems of another, and converted to sensorimotor format for promoting action understanding (1). The present 2-person fMRI setup provides means for studying how these loops are established during real-time interaction, as the evolving temporal cascade of sender-receiver operations in the social interaction can be measured continuously.

Intuitively two-person neuroimaging sounds like an outstanding means for analyzing social interaction, because it allows quantifying the dynamic interaction between two brains similarly as such interaction occurs in real life. Yet after initial demonstrations of the feasibility of the two-person hyperscanning fMRI technique (30), it is surprising how little work has been conducted in this domain given the prominence of other individuals to practically all aspects of our lives (54). For example, by the time of writing this article, searching Web of Science for "fMRI and hyperscanning" yields only 52 hits (of which 15 are original articles actually using fMRI hyperscanning), whereas searching for "fMRI" yields no less than 70,460 hits. One likely reason for the paucity of fMRI hyperscanning studies is that such experiments are inherently difficult to carry out and analyze. The two-person approach adds significantly to the complexity of the data—not just due to the doubled number of analyzed voxels, but due to the interactive and temporally evolving nonlinear nature of real social interaction. It is thus possible that this line of work has not increased our knowledge on social interaction as much as the extra complexity would warrant. But it is also possible that we have not yet asked the best questions with the two-person neuroimaging setups, and maybe we need to adopt a new theoretical framework for measuring and analyzing brain signals emerging from social interaction, rather than just scanning two brains at the same time using traditional approach with pre-determined stimulus models. During social interaction, the interlocutors constantly generate "stimuli" for each other in an adaptive fashion, meaning that one potentially powerful approach involves careful recording and annotation of the behavioral dimensions of the social interaction as it occurs during the experiment, and using that data for post-experiment generation of the subject-specific stimulus models. This approach obviously leads to a high-dimensional stimulus space that again can be capitalized in the analysis: we do not necessarily know which features of social interaction form the most important dimensions when generating a classic stimulation model (55). On the contrary, when the stimulus model is generated based on the subject behavior during the experiment, the critical dimensions do not need to be known in advance but the research may aim at constructing them based on the data.

Practicality of the Two-Person Imaging Setup

We had to position our subjects into close proximity with each other due to the limited size of the transmitting body coil but also to provide a shared interpersonal space, allowing, for example, joint manipulation of objects. However, this intimate setting likely led to breaching the subjects' peripersonal spaces, potentially influencing social processes because close social proximity may feel uncomfortable (56, 57). Accordingly, this setup is best suited for scanning subjects who know each other well enough, and the intimacy may also yield biases in subject selection. For the same reasons, this type of dual-coil imaging might be impossible for patient populations with disorders involving social interaction. An optimized version of the coil design could involve a setup comparable to two conventional head coils with subjects' vertices aligned against each other, so that both subjects can be scanned in supine position while they enter the scanner from opposite ends of the bore. Although subjects cannot directly see each other, eye contact can be arranged using a mirror system. Our setup only had external auditory stimulus delivery system for the subjects. In theory, it would also be possible to project visual stimuli to the subjects, but due to the close proximity of the subjects' faces this is deemed impractical. Our proof-of-concept study also revealed that the dual-coil setup is significantly less comfortable than conventional 32-channel head coil. Subject setup and shimming are slow, and the scanning position is difficult to maintain over prolonged periods of time. Interlocking of the head coils and close proximity of subjects also increased susceptibility to motion. Accordingly, we tried to maximize subject comfort by limiting the scanning time into short blocks; in our experience the current scanning time (four 6-min sessions plus anatomical images and preparations) was close to the maximum that subjects can comfortably do.

Limitations and Future Directions

In this study we resorted to conventional moderately accelerated fMRI acquisitions. However, recent advances in multi-band excitation, to improve temporal resolution, and parallel transmit, to even out the flip angles in the two potentially very different sized heads, could greatly benefit the two-person MRI setup. The SNR for the dual coil was significantly worse than that of the conventional 32-channel head coil, particularly in the frontal cortex due to multiple factors pertaining to coil geometry and the low number of channels. This lacking signal in frontal cortex is a limiting factor when it comes to investigating social interaction, for which the frontal cortex acts as a central hub region (58). However, many social processes emerge in regions where the coil system has adequate signal [such as posterior temporal and parietal cortices (16, 40, 59)], thus care must be taken when deciding what sort of social tasks can be studied with the present setup. Additionally, future benchmarking with variable tasks and experimental setups should be conducted to evaluate what types of tasks are ultimately feasible for this type of dual-coil imaging setup. Future developments of the coil setup should strive to maximize coil coverage of the scalp more evenly, and with higher-density coil arrangements. Such new devices would also allow more efficient control of subject motion: the limited contact of the current coil design with the scalp, combined with the sideways scanning position makes the setup sensitive to head motion.

CONCLUSIONS

We conclude that two-person fMRI is a feasible and potentially powerful tool for studying brain dynamics of real-time social interaction. Even though the signal quality was compromised compared with state-of-the art head coils, our results show that our dual-head coil yields sufficient SNR for quantifying the dynamics of the real-time two-person interaction. This proof-of-concept study revealed that it is possible to measure good-quality hemodynamic signals simultaneously from two brains with one scanner. The two-person fMRI approach presented in this study complements the existing fMRI and MEG hyperscanning and face-to-face EEG and fNIRS techniques by allowing tomographic imaging of brain activations of two interacting subjects in face-to-face settings. Even though both subjects generated tactile stimuli to each other in the experiment, the task was still externally controlled. Our data however suggest that in the future this methodology can be used for quantifying brain activation in dyadic, unconstrained, and naturalistic social interaction.

AUTHOR CONTRIBUTIONS

VR, JK, RH, and LN designed research. VR, SM, and RH developed instruments. VR and JK acquired data. VR and JK analyzed data. VR, JK, RH, and LN interpreted data. VR, JK, SM, RH, and LN wrote the paper.

ACKNOWLEDGMENTS

We thank Ms. Anna Anttalainen, Dr. Toni Auranen, Ms. Marita Kattelus, Mr. Veli-Matti Saarinen, and Mr. Tuomas Tolvanen for assistance, and Insight MRI for the development of the dual coil. The research was made possible by the Advanced Magnetic Imaging Centre, Aalto University School of Science, Espoo, Finland. VR is grateful to the funding provided by the Swedish Cultural Foundation in Finland, Instrumentarium Science Foundation, and Kalle and Dagmar Välimaa Fund of the Finnish Cultural Foundation. The funding support of the Academy of Finland (grant #218072 to RH, grant #265917 to LN) and European Research Council ("Brain2Brain" grant #232946 to RH and "SocialBrain" grant #313000 to LN) is thankfully acknowledged.

SUPPLEMENTARY MATERIAL

FIGURE S1 | (A) Alternating responses to active touching by left and right subjects. **(B)** Overlapping activations for touching and feeling touch.

REFERENCES

1. Hari R, Kujala MV Brain Basis of Human Social Interaction: From Concepts to Brain Imaging. *Physiol Rev* (2009) 89:453–79. doi: 10.1152/physrev.00041.2007
2. Hasson U, Ghazanfar AA, Galantucci B, Garrod S, Keysers C Brain-To-Brain Coupling: a Mechanism for Creating and Sharing a Social World. *Trends Cognit Sci* (2012) 16:114–21. doi: 10.1016/j.tics.2011.12.007
3. Smirnov D, Lachat F, Peltola T, Lahnakoski JM, Koistinen O-P, Glerean E, et al. Brain-To-Brain Hyperclassification Reveals Action-Specific Motor Mapping of Observed Actions in Humans. *PloS One* (2017) 12:E0189508. doi: 10.1371/journal.pone.0189508
4. Nummenmaa L, Lahnakoski JM, Glerean E Sharing the Social World Via Intersubject Neural Synchronisation. *Curr Opin Psychol* (2018) 24:7–14. doi: 10.1016/j.copsyc.2018.02.021
5. Bartels A, Zeki S. The Chronoarchitecture of the Human Brain—Natural Viewing Conditions Reveal a Time-Based Anatomy of the Brain. *Neuroimage* (2004) 22:419–33. doi: 10.1016/j.neuroimage.2004.01.007
6. Hasson U, Nir Y, Levy I, Fuhrmann G, Malach R. Intersubject Synchronization of Cortical Activity During Natural Vision. *Science* (2004) 303:1634–40. doi: 10.1126/science.1089506
7. Wilson SM, Molnar-Szakacs I, Iacoboni M. Beyond Superior Temporal Cortex: Intersubject Correlations in Narrative Speech Comprehension. *Cereb Cortex* (2008) 18:230–42. doi: 10.1093/cercor/bhm049
8. Hari R, Henriksson L, Malinen S, Parkkonen L. Centrality of Social Interaction in Human Brain Function. *Neuron* (2015) 88:181–93. doi: 10.1016/j.neuron.2015.09.022
9. Lahnakoski JM, Glerean E, Jääskeläinen IP, Hyönä J, Hari R, Sams M. Synchronous Brain Activity Across Individuals Underlies Shared Psychological Perspectives. *Neuroimage* (2014) 100:316–24. doi: 10.1016/j.neuroimage.2014.06.022
10. Nummenmaa L, Glerean E, Viinikainen M, Jaaskelainen IP, Hari R, Sams M. Emotions Promote Social Interaction by Synchronizing Brain Activity Across Individuals. *Proc Natl Acad Sci U S A* (2012) 109:9599–604. doi: 10.1073/pnas.1206095109
11. Parkinson C, Kleinbaum AM, Wheatley T. Similar Neural Responses Predict Friendship. *Nat Commun* (2018) 9:332. doi: 10.1038/s41467-017-02722-7
12. Hari R, Sams M, Nummenmaa L. Attending to and Neglecting People: Bridging Neuroscience, Psychology and Sociology. *Phil Trans B* (2016) 371:1–9. doi: 10.1098/rstb.2015.0365

13. De Jaegher H, Di Paolo E, Gallagher S. Can Social Interaction Constitute Social Cognition? *Trends Cognit Sci* (2010) 14:441–7. doi: 10.1016/j.tics.2010.06.009
14. Konvalinka I, Roepstorff A. The Two-Brain Approach: How Can Mutually Interacting Brains Teach Us Something About Social Interaction? *Front Hum Neurosci* (2012) 6:1–10. doi: 10.3389/fnhum.2012.00215
15. Dimberg U, Thunberg M, Elmehed K. Unconscious Facial Reactions to Emotional Facial Expressions. *Psychol Sci* (2000) 11:86–9. doi: 10.1111/1467-9280.00221
16. Nummenmaa L, Calder AJ. Neural Mechanisms of Social Attention. *Trends Cognit Sci* (2009) 13:135–43. doi: 10.1016/j.tics.2008.12.006
17. Lakin JL, Jefferis VE, Cheng CM, Chartrand TL. The Chameleon Effect as Social Glue: Evidence for the Evolutionary Significance of Nonconscious Mimicry. *J Nonverbal Behav* (2003) 27:145–62. doi: 10.1023/A:1025389814290
18. Manninen S, Tuominen L, Dunbar RIM, Karjalainen T, Hirvonen J, Arponen E, et al. Social Laughter Triggers Endogenous Opioid Release in Humans. the. *J Neurosci* (2017) 37:6125–31. doi: 10.1523/JNEUROSCI.0688-16.2017
19. Frischen A, Bayliss AP, Tipper SP. Gaze Cueing of Attention: Visual Attention, Social Cognition, and Individual Differences. *Psychol Bull* (2007) 133:694–724. doi: 10.1037/0033-2909.133.4.694
20. Pfeiffer UJ, Vogeley K, Schilbach L. From Gaze Cueing to Dual Eye-Tracking: Novel Approaches to Investigate the Neural Correlates of Gaze in Social Interaction. *Neurosci Biobehav Rev* (2013) 37:2516–28. doi: 10.1016/j.neubiorev.2013.07.017
21. Stivers T, Enfield NJ, Brown P, Englert C, Hayashi M, Heinemann T, et al. Universals and Cultural Variation in Turn-Taking in Conversation. *Proc Nat Acad Sci USA* (2009) 106:10587–92. doi: 10.1073/pnas.0903616106
22. Noy L, Dekel E, Alon UT. The Mirror Game as a Paradigm for Studying the Dynamics of Two People Improvising Motion Together. *Proc Natl Acad Sci* (2011) 108:20947–52. doi: 10.1073/pnas.1108155108
23. Redcay E, Schilbach L. Using Second-Person Neuroscience to Elucidate the Mechanisms of Social Interaction. *Nat Rev Neurosci* (2019) 20:495–505. doi: 10.1038/s41583-019-0179-4
24. Schilbach L, Timmermans B, Reddy V, Costall A, Bente G, Schlicht T, et al. Toward a Second-Person Neuroscience. *Behav Brain Sci* (2013) 36:393–414. doi: 10.1017/S0140525X12000660
25. Smirnov D, Saarimäki H, Glerean E, Hari R, Sams M, Nummenmaa L. Emotions Amplify Speaker–Listener Neural Alignment. *Hum Brain Mapp* (2019) 40:4777–88. doi: 10.1002/hbm.24736
26. Stephens GJ, Silbert LJ, Hasson U. Speaker-Listener Neural Coupling Underlies Successful Communication. *Proc Natl Acad Sci U S A* (2010) 107:14425–30. doi: 10.1073/pnas.1008662107
27. Schippers MB, Roebroeck A, Renken R, Nanetti L, Keysers C. Mapping the Information Flow From One Brain to Another During Gestural Communication. *Proc Natl Acad Sci U S A* (2010) 107:9388–93. doi: 10.1073/pnas.1001791107
28. Anders S, Heinzle J, Weiskopf N, Ethofer T, Haynes JD. Flow of Affective Information Between Communicating Brains. *Neuroimage* (2011) 54:439–46. doi: 10.1016/j.neuroimage.2010.07.004
29. King-Casas B, Sharp C, Lomax-Bream L, Lohrenz T, Fonagy P, Montague PR. the Rupture and Repair of Cooperation in Borderline Personality Disorder. *Science* (2008) 321:806–10. doi: 10.1126/science.1156902
30. Montague PR, Berns GS, Cohen JD, McClure SM, Pagnoni G, Dhamala M, et al. Hyperscanning: Simultaneous Fmri During Linked Social Interactions. *Neuroimage* (2002) 16:1159–64. doi: 10.1006/nimg.2002.1150
31. Saito DN, Tanabe HC, Izuma K, Hayashi MJ, Morito Y, Komeda H, et al. "Stay Tuned": Inter-Individual Neural Synchronization During Mutual Gaze and Joint Attention. *Front Integr Neurosci* (2010) 4:1–12. doi: 10.3389/fnint.2010.00127
32. Baess P, Zhdanov A, Mandel A, Parkkonen L, Hirvenkari L, Mäkelä JP, et al. Meg Dual Scanning: a Procedure to Study Real-Time Auditory Interaction Between Two Persons. *Front Hum Neurosci* (2012) 6:1–7. doi: 10.3389/fnhum.2012.00083
33. Babiloni F, Astolfi L. Social Neuroscience and Hyperscanning Techniques: Past, Present and Future. *Neurosci Biobehav Rev* (2014) 44:76–93. doi: 10.1016/j.neubiorev.2012.07.006
34. Monfardini E, Redoute J, Hadj-Bouziane F, Hynaux C, Fradin J, Huguet P, et al. Others' Sheer Presence Boosts Brain Activity in the Attention (But Not the Motivation) Network. *Cereb Cortex* (2016) 26:2427–39. doi: 10.1093/cercor/bhv067
35. Redcay E, Dodell-Feder D, Pearrow MJ, Mavros PL, Kleiner M, Gabrieli JDE, et al. Live Face-To-Face Interaction During Fmri: a New Tool for Social Cognitive Neuroscience. *Neuroimage* (2010) 50:1639–47. doi: 10.1016/j.neuroimage.2010.01.052
36. Ponkanen LM, Hietanen JK, Peltola MJ, Kauppinen PK, Haapalainen A, Leppanen JM. Facing a Real Person: an Event-Related Potential Study. *Neuroreport* (2008) 19:497–501. doi: 10.1097/WNR.0b013e3282f7c4d3
37. Dumas G, Nadel J, Soussignan R, Martinerie J, Garnero L. Inter-Brain Synchronization During Social Interaction. *PloS One* (2010) 5:E12166. doi: 10.1371/journal.pone.0012166
38. Cui X, Bryant DM, Reiss AL. Nirs-Based Hyperscanning Reveals Increased Interpersonal Coherence in Superior Frontal Cortex During Cooperation. *Neuroimage* (2012) 59:2430–7. doi: 10.1016/j.neuroimage.2011.09.003
39. Funane T, Kiguchi M, Atsumori H, Sato H, Kubota K, Koizumi H. Synchronous Activity of Two People's Prefrontal Cortices During a Cooperative Task Measured by Simultaneous Near-Infrared Spectroscopy. *J Biomed Opt* (2011) 16:1–10. doi: 10.1117/1.3602853
40. Lahnakoski JM, Glerean E, Salmi J, Jaaskelainen I, Sams M, Hari R, et al. Naturalistic Fmri Mapping Reveals Superior Temporal Sulcus as the Hub for the Distributed Brain Network for Social Perception. *Front Hum Neurosci* (2012) 6:14. doi: 10.3389/fnhum.2012.00233
41. Saarimaki H, Ejtehadian LF, Glerean E, Jaaskelainen IP, Vuilleumier P, Sams M, et al. Distributed Affective Space Represents Multiple Emotion Categories Across the Human Brain. *Soc Cognit Affect Neurosci* (2018) 13:471–82. doi: 10.1093/scan/nsy018
42. Saarimäki H, Gotsopoulos A, Jääskeläinen IP, Lampinen J, Vuilleumier P, Hari R, et al. Discrete Neural Signatures of Basic Emotions. *Cereb Cortex* (2016) 6:2563–73. doi: 10.1093/cercor/bhv086
43. Lee RF. Dual Logic and Cerebral Coordinates for Reciprocal Interaction in Eye Contact. *PloS One* (2015) 10. doi: 10.1371/journal.pone.0121791
44. Lee RF, Dai W, Jones J. Decoupled Circular-Polarized Dual-Head Volume Coil Pair for Studying Two Interacting Human Brains With Dyadic Fmri. *Magn Reson Med* (2012) 68:1087–96. doi: 10.1002/mrm.23313
45. Renvall V, Malinen S. Setup and apparatus for two-person fMRI. (Beijing China: Poster presented at the 18th annual meeting of the Organization for Human Brain Mapping). (2012).
46. Nummenmaa L, Suvilehto JM, Glerean E, Santtila P, Hietanen JK. Topography of Human Erogenous Zones. *Arch Sex Behav* (2016). 1207–16 doi: 10.1007/s10508-016-0745-z
47. Suvilehto J, Glerean E, Dunbar RIM, Hari R, Nummenmaa L. Topography of Social Touching Depends on Emotional Bonds Between Humans. *Proc Natl Acad Sci U S A* (2015) 112:13811–6. doi: 10.1073/pnas.1519231112
48. Suvilehto J, Nummenmaa L, Harada T, Dunbar RIM, Hari R, Turner R, et al. Cross-Cultural Similarity in Relationship-Specific Social Touching. *Proc R Soc Ser B-Biol Sci* (2019). 1–10 doi: 10.1098/rspb.2019.0467
49. Jenkinson M, Beckmann CF, Behrens TE, Woolrich MW, Smith SM. Fsl. *Neuroimage* (2012) 62:782–90. doi: 10.1016/j.neuroimage.2011.09.015
50. Jenkinson M, Bannister P, Brady M, Smith S. Improved Optimization for the Robust and Accurate Linear Registration and Motion Correction of Brain Images. *Neuroimage* (2002) 17:825–41. doi: 10.1006/nimg.2002.1132
51. Smith SM. Fast Robust Automated Brain Extraction. *Hum Brain Mapp* (2002) 17:143–55. doi: 10.1002/hbm.10062
52. Smith SM, Brady JM. Susan - a new approach to low level image processing. *Int J Comput Vis* (1997) 23:45–78. doi: 10.1023/A:1007963824710
53. Kaza E, Klose U, Lotze M. Comparison of a 32-Channel With a 12-Channel Head Coil: Are There Relevant Improvements for Functional Imaging? *J Magn Reson Imaging* (2011) 34:173–83. doi: 10.1002/jmri.22614
54. Dunbar RIM. the Social Brain Hypothesis. *Evol Anthropol* (1998) 6:178–90. doi: 10.1002/(SICI)1520-6505(1998)6:5<178::AID-EVAN5>3.0.CO;2-8
55. Adolphs R, Nummenmaa L, Todorov A, Haxby JV. Data-Driven Approaches in the Investigation of Social Perception. *Phil Trans B* (2016), 371. doi: 10.1098/rstb.2015.0367
56. Kennedy DP, Glascher j, Tyszka JM, Adolphs R. Personal Space Regulation by the Human Amygdala. *Nat Neurosci* (2009) 12:1226–7. doi: 10.1038/nn.2381
57. Tsakiris M. My Body in the Brain: a Neurocognitive Model of Body-Ownership. *Neuropsychologia* (2010) 48:703–12. doi: 10.1016/j.neuropsychologia.2009.09.034

12

Social Attention in Autism: Neural Sensitivity to Speech Over Background Noise Predicts Encoding of Social Information

Leanna M. Hernandez[1,2]*, Shulamite A. Green*[1,2]*, Katherine E. Lawrence*[1,2]*, Marisa Inada*[1]*, Janelle Liu*[1,2]*, Susan Y. Bookheimer*[1,3] *and Mirella Dapretto*[1,2]*

[1] *Ahmanson-Lovelace Brain Mapping Center, University of California, Los Angeles, Los Angeles, CA, United States,*
[2] *Department of Psychiatry and Biobehavioral Sciences, University of California, Los Angeles, Los Angeles, CA, United States,*
[3] *Staglin IMHRO Center for Cognitive Neuroscience, University of California, Los Angeles, Los Angeles, CA, United States*

Correspondence:
Mirella Dapretto
mirella@ucla.edu

Autism spectrum disorder (ASD) is a neurodevelopmental disorder characterized by lack of attention to social cues in the environment, including speech. Hypersensitivity to sensory stimuli, such as loud noises, is also extremely common in youth with ASD. While a link between sensory hypersensitivity and impaired social functioning has been hypothesized, very little is known about the neural mechanisms whereby exposure to distracting sensory stimuli may interfere with the ability to direct attention to socially-relevant information. Here, we used functional magnetic resonance imaging (fMRI) in youth with and without ASD (N=54, age range 8–18 years) to (1) examine brain responses during presentation of brief social interactions (i.e., two-people conversations) shrouded in ecologically-valid environmental noises, and (2) assess how brain activity during encoding might relate to later accuracy in identifying what was heard. During exposure to conversation-in-noise (*vs*. conversation or noise alone), both neurotypical youth and youth with ASD showed robust activation of canonical language networks. However, the extent to which youth with ASD activated temporal language regions, including voice-selective cortex (i.e., posterior superior temporal sulcus), predicted later discriminative accuracy in identifying what was heard. Further, relative to neurotypical youth, ASD youth showed significantly greater activity in left-hemisphere speech-processing cortex (i.e., angular gyrus) while listening to conversation-in-noise (*vs*. conversation or noise alone). Notably, in youth with ASD, increased activity in this region was associated with higher social motivation and better social cognition measures. This heightened activity in voice-selective/speech-processing regions may serve as a compensatory mechanism allowing youth with ASD to hone in on the conversations they heard in the context of non-social distracting stimuli. These findings further suggest that focusing on social and non-social stimuli simultaneously may be more challenging for youth with ASD requiring the recruitment of additional neural resources to encode socially-relevant information.

Keywords: speech, autism, voice-selective, attention, conversation, noise, aversive, sensory

INTRODUCTION

Autism spectrum disorder (ASD) is a common neurodevelopmental disorder characterized by difficulties in social interaction and communication, the presence of repetitive behaviors and restricted interests, as well as sensory processing atypicalities (1). Research in infants who later go on to get an ASD diagnosis has consistently shown that allocation of attention to social stimuli is disrupted early in development [for a review, see (2)]. For instance, young children with ASD fail to show a preference for listening to their mothers' voice (3), as well as to child-directed speech (4); disrupted attention to language early in life may set the stage for subsequent atypical language acquisition, as well as altered development of the neural systems responsible for language processing. Importantly, the ability to selectively attend to and learn from social interactions in one's environment often requires the simultaneous filtering out competing non-social stimuli. As heightened sensory sensitivity to mildly aversive auditory stimuli (e.g., loud noises) is observed in a significant number of children with ASD (5), we hypothesize that this may be one potential mechanism through which attention may be drawn away from social input in favor of other non-social stimuli present in the environment. Despite growing interest in the relationship between sensory processing and social impairments in ASD (6–8), little research to date has investigated how individual variability in neural responses to *simultaneous* social and non-social sensory stimuli may relate to the ability to "hone in" on socially-relevant input.

Converging neuroimaging data indicate altered brain responses to language in individuals with ASD. While ASD is characterized by a great deal of heterogeneity (9), young children with ASD who go on to have poorer language skills show hypoactivity in temporal cortex during language listening (10), as well as reduced functional connectivity between nodes of the language network (11). In children and adolescents with ASD, functional MRI (fMRI) studies have found reduced functional lateralization and increased rightward asymmetry during a variety of language processing tasks, as compared to the leftward asymmetry observed in neurotypical individuals (12–17), as well as reduced connectivity between voice-selective cortex and reward-related brain regions (18).

Importantly, however, in most real-life situations language is not heard in isolation but against the background of other competing sensory distractors (e.g., a buzzing fan, a barking dog). In neurotypical adults, the bilateral posterior superior temporal sulcus (pSTS) responds selectively to vocal stimuli, and activity in this region is reduced when voice stimuli are degraded or masked by background noise (19, 20). In contrast, individuals with ASD fail to activate voice-selective regions in the pSTS during exposure to vocal stimuli (12) and show increased recruitment of right hemisphere language homologues (21). Furthermore, the ability to detect speech-in-noise appears reduced in individuals with ASD, who are poorer at identifying speech heard in the context of background noise (22, 23). Interestingly, a recent study showed that sensory processing atypicalities modulate brain activity during language processing in youth with ASD during simultaneous processing of sarcastic remarks and distracting tactile stimulation (24). However, it has yet to be examined how sensory distractors in the *same sensory modality* as speech may affect the allocation of attention to language processing during social interactions. This type of study has implications for understanding how auditory filtering deficits may affect encoding of social information in everyday life where conversations commonly occur in the context of background noises.

In adults with ASD, heightened sensory over-responsivity (SOR)—characterized by extreme behavioral response to everyday sensory stimuli—is related to higher autism traits (25). Importantly, roughly 65% of children with ASD show atypical sensory responsivity to non-social auditory stimuli (26, 27), including a lower tolerance for loud noises (28, 29) and hypersensitivity to certain environmental noises, such as the sound of a dog barking or a vacuum cleaner (30). A growing body of neuroimaging research also suggests that children with ASD who have high levels of SOR display neural hyper-responsivity to aversive visual, tactile, and auditory stimuli in primary sensory brain regions and areas important for salience detection (31, 32), suggesting that there may be an over-allocation of attentional resources to sensory stimuli in youth with ASD. Together, these data suggest that language processing within social contexts in which there are other competing sensory stimuli—such as those that occur in the natural environment—may be particularly challenging for some individuals with ASD.

Here, we examined brain responses to auditory social and non-social stimuli in a paradigm where participants heard brief conversations between two people which were shrouded in competing environmental noises. Ecologically valid stimuli were developed to examine the effects of ASD diagnosis on neural processing of commonly encountered environmental noise, conversation, and conversation-in-noise (i.e., noise and conversation presented simultaneously). In addition, participants completed a post-scan computerized test that probed recognition of the noises and topics of conversation presented during the fMRI paradigm, thus providing a measure of attention to, and encoding of social and non-social information. We hypothesized that, relative to neurotypical youth, youth with ASD would show reduced activity in left hemisphere language cortices when listening to conversation alone, as well as increased activity in sensory cortices when exposed to aversive noise. Further, we expected that the presence of distracting noises during speech processing would result in greater activation of subcortical and cortical brain regions involved in sensory processing in youth with ASD relative to neurotypical youth. Finally, we expected that the ability to recognize details from the conversations heard in presence of background noises would be associated with increased activity in canonical left hemisphere language regions and voice-selective cortex in the pSTS in both groups, reflecting the recruitment of additional neural resources to "hone in" on social stimuli in the context of non-social distractors; to the extent that some youth with ASD may show hypersensitivity to auditory stimuli, we expect this effect would be more pronounced in this group.

MATERIALS AND METHODS

Participants

Participants were 26 youth with ASD and 28 age-matched typically-developing (TD) youth who were recruited through referrals from the University of California, Los Angeles (UCLA) Child and Adult Neurodevelopmental (CAN) Clinic, as well as from posted advertisements throughout the greater Los Angeles area. Exclusionary criteria included any diagnosed neurological or genetic disorders, as well as structural brain abnormalities, or metal implants. ASD participants had a prior clinical diagnosis, which was confirmed using the Autism Diagnostic Observation Schedule—2nd Edition (ADOS-2) (33) and Autism Diagnostic Interview-Revised (ADI-R) (34) by licensed clinicians at the UCLA CAN Clinic. All participants had full-scale IQ above 70 as assessed by the Wechsler Abbreviated Scale of Intelligence (35) (**Table 1**). Data were originally acquired for 30 ASD and 30 TD youth, 4 ASD participants, and 2 TD participants were excluded from the final sample due to excessive head motion during fMRI data acquisition (i.e., greater than 3.5 mm of maximum relative motion; see **Table 1** for mean motion parameters in the final sample). Study procedures were approved by the UCLA Institutional Review Board and informed consent and assent to participate in this research were obtained in writing from legal guardians and study participants.

TABLE 1 | Descriptive statistics.

	ASD mean (SD)	TD mean (SD)	t or x^2	
Demographics				
Sex (N male)	19	17	0.93	
Age	13.75 (2.98)	13.78 (2.66)	−0.04	
Full IQ	102.42 (14.92)	113.11 (13.05)	−2.79	**
Nonverbal IQ	107.96 (17.61)	112.61 (12.69)	−1.11	
Verbal IQ	97.42 (14.30)	110.64 (13.42)	−3.50	***
SRS Total T-Score	68.77 (12.06)	44.46 (5.90)	9.30	***
SRS Social Awareness T-Score	67.50 (11.19)	45.18 (6.98)	8.72	***
SRS Social Cognition T-Score	67.27 (12.54)	44.54 (7.30)	8.06	***
SRS Social Communication T-Score	67.58 (12.75)	44.57 (5.76)	8.44	***
SRS Social Motivation T-Score	61.77 (11.80)	47.01 (7.41)	5.44	***
Motion				
Mean absolute motion (mm)	0.44 (0.28)	0.42 (0.28)	0.36	
Max absolute motion (mm)	1.76 (1.65)	1.39 (1.23)	0.92	
Mean relative motion (mm)	0.14 (0.07)	0.14 (0.06)	−0.02	
Max relative motion (mm)	1.21 (1.08)	0.92 (0.78)	1.11	
Post-scan test: percent correct				
Conversations, alone condition				
Easy questions	75.76% (20.77)	81.95% (17.35)	−1.18	
Hard questions	79.58% (16.92)	76.02% (22.82)	0.65	
Conversations, conversation-in-noise condition				
Easy questions	66.43% (16.36)	69.59% (16.36)	−0.60	
Hard questions	61.73% (25.46)	73.16% (25.46)	−1.60	
Post-Scan Test: discriminative accuracy (d')				
Conversations, alone condition	1.73 (0.97)	1.92 (1.01)	−0.71	
Conversations, conversation-in-noise condition	1.28 (0.86)	1.59 (0.99)	−1.21	

$^{**}p < 0.01$, $^{***}p < 0.001$

ASD, autism spectrum disorder; TD, typically developing; IQ, intelligence quotient.

Behavioral Measures

Social functioning was assessed in both ASD and TD youth using the Social Responsiveness Scale—2nd Edition (SRS-2) (36). The SRS-2 is intended for use in both neurotypical populations and individuals with ASD and provides a measure of the severity of social impairment associated with autism. In the current study, we examined the relationship between t-scores for the socially-relevant subscales of the SRS-2 (i.e., social awareness, social cognition, social communication, and social motivation) and neural activity during conversation-in-noise listening.

Experimental Design

During the fMRI scan, auditory stimuli were presented according to a canonical block design (**Figure 1A**) using E-Prime 2.0 Software on a Dell Latitude E6430 laptop computer. Each block consisted of 15 s of auditory stimulus presentation alternating with 7.5 s of rest. A crosshair was presented at the center of a white screen throughout the duration of the scan. Blocks consisted of three types: conversation (C), noise (N), and conversation-in-noise (CIN; i.e., conversation and noise presented simultaneously). Stimuli were ecologically valid and mimicked those encountered in everyday life, whereby one overhears two people engaged in a conversation that is shrouded by competing auditory stimuli, thus forcing the listener to "hone in" on the socially relevant speech. Inspiration for conversation topics were taken from scripted television series focusing on childhood/adolescence (**Figure 1B**). Speech passages were recorded by two actors (one male, one female) using GarageBand 6.0.5 and an Apogee MiC digital microphone connected to a Macintosh computer. Noise stimuli were downloaded from Freesound.org. Selection of noise stimuli ensured that they were ecologically valid (i.e., commonly encountered in everyday life). The aversive nature of the selected noises was rated in an independent sample (N=30) using a 7-point Likert scale (1=not aversive, 7=extremely aversive); the final 12 noise stimuli used in the fMRI paradigm were rated as moderately aversive (rating M=4.7, range 3.6–5.5) and included such sounds as a jackhammer, a police siren, and a blender. Root-mean-square amplitude was normalized across all stimuli to control for loudness. Stimuli were counterbalanced such that half of the participants heard a given conversation without noise, whereas the other half of participants heard the same conversation masked by noise (i.e., in the CIN condition). Likewise, for any given noise, half of participants heard the noise alone, while the other half heard the noise in the CIN condition. Each block type (C, N, CIN) was presented six times; order was counterbalanced across subjects. The total run time was 7 min and 7.5 s. Prior to the fMRI scan, participants were told that they

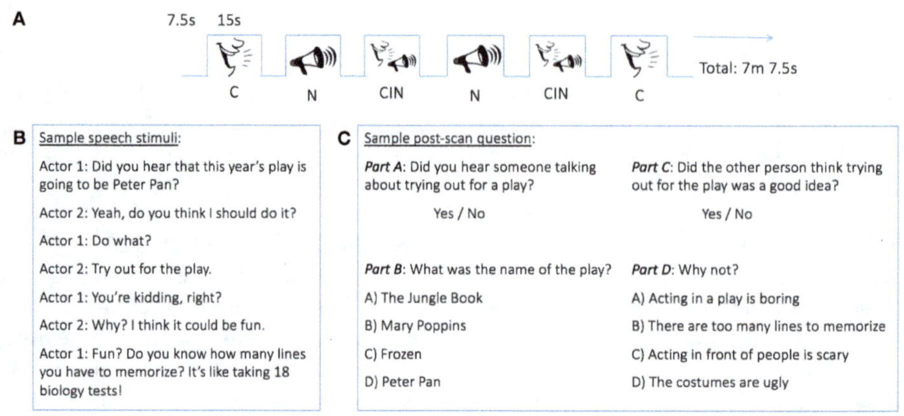

FIGURE 1 | Experimental design. **(A)** Block design functional MRI (fMRI) task. **(B)** Example of a conversation heard during fMRI data acquisition. **(C)** Sample of post-scan questions. CIN, conversation-in-noise; C, conversation; N, noise.

would hear some people talking and some noises; they were instructed to just listen and look at the crosshair on the screen. Participants were not specifically instructed to pay attention to what was said, as we wanted the paradigm to have high ecological validity by mimicking situations encountered in everyday life when we may overhear others talking and are not explicitly asked to pay attention or remember what was said.

To assess the participants' ability to recognize stimuli presented in the three experimental conditions, and thus gain a proximal measure of in-scanner attention, a brief post-MRI scanning questionnaire was administered using E-Prime 2.0 Software on a Dell Latitude E6430 laptop computer. During this post-scanning test, participants heard and read questions about the conversations and noises they were exposed to during the fMRI data acquisition, interspersed with foils (i.e., with questions about conversations and noises they did not hear). For each conversation and noise stimulus presented during the fMRI scan, participants were first asked to answer a question about whether they heard such a particular conversation topic or noise. For the conversations, the post-scan test was tiered such that if a participant's yes/no response to this initial question was correct (**Figure 1C**, top), a more nuanced question about that conversation was then presented (**Figure 1C**, bottom). Incorrect responses to the initial yes/no questions resulted in being presented the next set of questions about a different conversation topic. Participant responses were recorded in E-Prime. A sensitivity index (d') was calculated to assess the ability of youth to discriminate between topics of conversation heard during MRI scanning and foils. d' was calculated as the standardized (i.e., z-transformed) proportion of hits minus the standardized proportion of false alarms.

MRI Data Acquisition

MRI data were collected on a 3.0 Tesla Siemens Prisma MRI Scanner using a 64-channel head coil. For each subject, a multi-slice echo-planar (EPI) sequence was used to acquire functional data: 595 volumes; repetition time (TR) = 720 ms; multiband acceleration factor = 8; matrix size = 104 x 104; field of view (FOV) = 208 × 208 mm; in-plane resolution = 2 × 2 mm; slice thickness = 2 mm, no gap; 72 slices; bandwidth = 2,290 Hz per pixel; echo time (TE) = 37 ms. Visual and auditory stimuli were presented *via* magnetic resonance compatible goggles and headphones (Optoacoustics LTD, Or Yehuda, Israel). Subjects wore earplugs and headphones to lessen scanner noise.

Functional MRI Data Analysis

Data were processed using FSL (FMRIB's Software Library, www.fmrib.ox.ac.uk/fsl) (37) and AFNI (Analysis of Functional NeuroImages) (38). Functional data were motion corrected to the average functional volume with FSL's Motion Correction Linear Registration Tool (MCFLIRT) (39) using sinc interpolation and skull stripped using FSL's Brain Extraction Tool (BET) (40). Time series statistical analyses were run in FSL's FMRI Expert Analysis Tool (FEAT) version 6.0. Functional images were spatially smoothed [full width at half maximum (FWHM) 5 mm] and a temporal high pass filter of 67.5 s was applied. Functional data were linearly registered to the Montreal Neurological Institute (MNI) 2 mm standard brain with 12° of freedom. Motion outliers were identified using FSL's motion outliers tool (comparing the root mean square intensity difference from the center volume to identify outliers) and were included as a confound explanatory variable in the single subject analyses; there was no difference in the mean number of volumes censored between ASD and TD participants (p=0.31). Condition effects were estimated by convolving a box-function for each condition with a double-gamma hemodynamic response function, along with the temporal derivative. Each condition was modeled with respect to resting baseline (C, N, CIN); single-subject models were combined into a group-level mixed effects model (FLAME1+2). Verbal IQ was entered as a covariate in all group-level analyses. Within-group and between-group maps were pre-threshold masked by grey matter and thresholded at $z > 3.1$ ($p < 0.001$), cluster-corrected for multiple comparisons at $p < 0.05$. Between-group comparisons (i.e., ASD *vs.* TD) were masked by the sum of within-group activity for each condition of interest.

Statistical Analysis

Two-tailed t-tests were performed to assess between-group differences in age, IQ, and motion parameters. To test whether participant's discriminative accuracy (d') for identifying the topics of conversation varied as a function of diagnostic group, condition, or question, a repeated measures ANOVA was conducted with group (i.e., ASD *vs.* TD) as the between-subjects factor and condition (i.e., N, C, CIN) as within-subjects factors. To further examine differences in behavioral performance, we also ran separate repeated measures ANOVAs comparing percent of correct responses for easy (yes/no) and hard (multiple-choice) questions separately with group (i.e., ASD *vs.* TD) as the between-subjects factor and condition (i.e., C *vs.* CIN) as the within-subjects factor.

RESULTS

Demographics

There were no statistically significant differences between ASD and TD youth in sex, age, and non-verbal IQ, or across any of the four motion parameters tested (**Table 1**). Two-sample t-tests revealed significant differences in full-scale and verbal IQ between ASD and TD youth, whereby TD youth had higher IQ relative to their ASD counterparts. As expected, ASD and TD youth also had significantly different t-scores on the social awareness, social cognition, social communication, and social motivation subscales of the Social Responsiveness Scale (SRS), as well as differences in SRS Total t-scores, indicative of poorer parent-reported social functioning in youth with ASD.

Post-Scan Recognition Test

To assess participants' ability to discriminate between what was actually heard *vs.* foils (i.e., correctly identifying a conversation, or noise, that was heard—"hits"—*vs.* incorrectly endorsing a conversation or noise that was not heard—"false alarms"), we calculated a sensitivity index (d') for each participant. In ASD youth, mean d' was 0.64, 0.59, 1.73, 1.28, for noises heard in the alone condition, noises heard in the conversation-in-noise condition, conversations head in the alone condition, and conversations heard in the conversation-in-noise condition, respectively. Likewise, mean d' in TD youth was 0.65, 0.67, 1.92, and 1.59 for noises heard in the alone condition, noises heard in the conversation-in-noise condition, conversations head in the alone condition, and conversations heard in the conversation-in-noise condition, respectively. A repeated-measures ANOVA was performed to test the interaction between group x condition. This analysis revealed no significant group x condition interaction [$F(3,156)=0.56$, $p=0.64$)] or main effect of Group [$F(1,52)=0.83$, $p=0.37$)]. However, the main effect of condition was significant [$F(3,156)=46.46$, $p < 0.001$)]; pairwise comparisons showed that both ASD and TD participants had higher accuracy (d') for conversations heard in the alone condition as compared to noises heard in the alone condition, as well as higher accuracy for conversations than noises when these were heard in the conversation-in-noise condition.

In order to further examine differences in behavioral performance, we also compared subjects' percent accuracy using separate repeated measures ANOVAs for easy (yes/no) and hard (multiple-choice) questions. For the easy questions, the main effect of condition was significant [$F(1,52)=19.77$, $p < 0.001$], whereby both groups were more accurate at identifying topics of conversation heard in the conversation alone condition than in the conversation-in-noise condition. However, there was no significant group x condition interaction [$F(1,52)=0.38$, $p=0.54$] or main effect of group [$F(1,52)=1.02$, $p=0.32$)]. For the hard (multiple-choice) questions, there was also a main effect of condition [$F(1,52)=10.00$, $p < 0.01$)], whereby both groups were more accurate at identifying topics of conversation heard in the conversation alone condition. However, while there was no main effect of group [$F(1,52)=0.51$, $p=0.48$)], there was a significant group x condition interaction [$F(1,52)=5.53$, $p=0.02$)]. *Post hoc* tests showed that while the ASD and TD groups did not differ in percent accuracy for the conversation alone or conversation-in-noise conditions, the ASD group was significantly more accurate for the conversation alone condition than for the conversation-in-noise ($p < 0.01$); this was not the case for TD youth ($p > 0.05$).

Functional MRI Results

Within-Condition Analyses

Across each of the three conditions, both youth with ASD and TD youth showed the expected activity in bilateral Heschl's gyrus, superior temporal gyrus, planum temporal, and planum polare (**Figure 2**, **Table 2**). During exposure to conversation-in-noise (CIN) and conversation alone (C), both groups showed robust activation in auditory and language cortices, including bilateral superior temporal gyrus (STG), middle temporal gyrus, temporal pole, left angular gyrus, and superior frontal gyrus. Activity in ventromedial prefrontal cortex, a region involved in theory of mind and mentalizing, was observed in TD youth in the CIN condition, and in ASD youth in the C condition. In contrast to the extended network of regions activated during conditions in which speech was presented (i.e., CIN and C), brain activity during the noise condition (N) was restricted to primary and secondary auditory cortices; ASD youth showed additional activation in right inferior frontal gyrus and pars triangularis. No between-group differences were observed for any of the three experimental conditions at this statistical threshold ($z > 3.1$, $p < 0.05$).

Between-Condition Analyses

Here we compared brain activity between experimental conditions. First, we examined differences in brain activity when listening to conversation-in-noise relative to listening to noise alone (CIN > N). For this contrast, both TD and ASD youth showed increased activity in bilateral temporal pole, superior temporal gyrus, Heschl's gyrus, superior frontal gyrus, and medial prefrontal cortex (**Figure 3**, **Table 3**), consistent with increased attention to language stimuli in the CIN condition. TD youth also showed activation in the right angular gyrus and bilateral hippocampus, whereas ASD youth showed significant activation in the precuneus. No regions

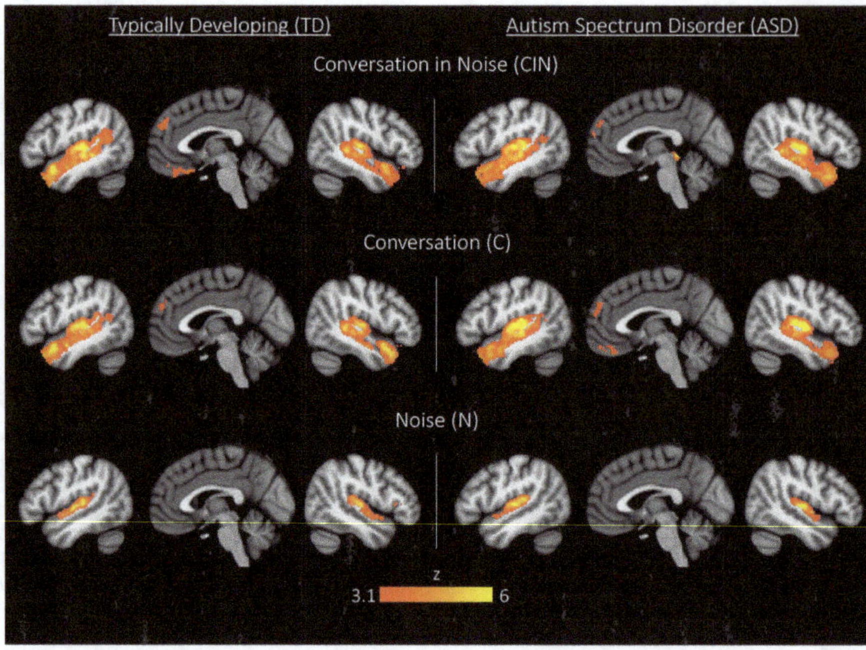

FIGURE 2 | Whole-brain activation in typically developing (TD) youth and youth with autism spectrum disorder (ASD) during exposure to conversation-in-noise (CIN), conversation (C), and noise (N). Maps are thresholded at $z > 3.1$, corrected for multiple comparisons at the cluster level ($p < 0.05$).

showed significant between-group differences when comparing CIN and N conditions.

Next, we assessed differences in brain activity when listening to conversation-in-noise *versus* conversation alone (CIN > C). For this contrast, TD youth showed increased activity in lateral occipital cortex, whereas ASD youth had increased activity in right frontal pole, precuneus, and occipital pole (**Figure 3**, **Table 3**). Between-group comparisons revealed that the ASD group had greater activity in primary visual cortex and precuneus relative to TD youth for the contrast of CIN > C; there were no brain regions where TD youth showed greater activity relative to ASD youth (**Table 4**). No brain regions showed greater activity when listening to conversation alone *vs.* conversation-in-noise (i.e., C > CIN).

Lastly, to tap into the neural correlates of social attention (i.e., selective attention to speech in the context of background noise), we examined brain activity specifically associated with listening to conversation-in-noise, above and beyond activity observed for the conversation and noise alone conditions (CIN > C+N). For this contrast, both TD and ASD youth displayed activity in brain regions involved in auditory and language processing as well as theory of mind (i.e., angular gyri, superior frontal gyrus, and superior temporal regions); ASD youth displayed additional activity in the precuneus whereas TD youth showed activity in ventral medial frontal cortex (**Figure 3**, **Table 3**). No significant between-group differences were observed for this contrast.

Brain Activity Predicting Post-Scan Performance

In an attempt to identify the neural substrates of social attention, we assessed how brain activity during the fMRI scan might predict accuracy in the post-scan test by entering d' as a regressor of interest in bottom-up regression analyses. We focused these analyses on our primary contrast of interest—CIN > C+N—in order to examine how d' related to brain activity specifically associated with processing conversation-in-noise *above and beyond* brain activity associated with processing conversation and noise alone. Whereas TD youth with higher d' showed selective activation of left posterior superior temporal sulcus (pSTS; i.e., voice-selective cortex), ASD youth with higher d' showed widespread increased activity primarily in language areas (**Figure 4**, **Table 5**). Direct between-group comparisons showed that, relative to TD youth, ASD youth with higher d' showed significantly greater activity in speech-processing cortex in the left angular gyrus; there were no significant results for the reverse contract. To interpret the ASD > TD effect, we examined how activity in this speech-processing region while listening to conversation-in-noise might be related to social functioning in ASD youth. Parameter estimates of activity during the CIN condition were extracted from this region and correlated with scores from the SRS subscales. Higher activity in this left speech-processing region in ASD youth was associated with lower scores on the social motivation ($r=-0.51$, $p=0.009$) and social cognition ($r=-0.41$, $p=0.04$) SRS subscales, indicating more typical patterns of behavior.

DISCUSSION

Here, we examined neural activity in response to *ecologically valid* social and non-social stimuli in youth with and without ASD to elucidate the neural mechanisms through which

TABLE 2 | Montreal Neurological Institute (MNI) coordinates for each condition (conversation-in-noise, CIN; conversation, C; noise, N) compared to baseline.

		Conversation-in-noise (CIN)								Conversation (C)								Noise (N)							
		ASD				TD				ASD				TD				ASD				TD			
		Max z	MNI peak (mm)			Max z	MNI peak (mm)			Max z	MNI peak (mm)			Max z	MNI peak (mm)			Max z	MNI peak (mm)			Max z	MNI peak (mm)		
			X	Y	Z		X	Y	Z		X	Y	Z		X	Y	Z		X	Y	Z		X	Y	Z
Angular gyrus	L	3.57	−60	−58	22	5.27	−58	−56	20	3.66	−60	−58	22	3.83	−58	−58	16								
Central opercular cortex	L	4.39	−52	−12	10	4.12	−58	−10	8	4.79	−60	−20	14	4.21	−58	−10	8	3.85	−60	−16	12	3.59	−50	−20	14
Central opercular cortex	R	4.63	50	−12	10	4.24	56	−6	6	4.81	48	−12	10	4.00	54	−10	8	3.58	50	−10	8	3.55	56	−6	6
Frontal operculum cortex																						3.51	40	24	2
Frontal orbital cortex	R					4.48	40	30	−18					3.26	40	26	−20								
Frontal pole	L	3.54	−2	60	20	5.06	−12	50	34	3.88	−10	58	28	4.83	−12	52	32								
Frontal pole	R	3.77	4	60	20									4.01	12	50	36								
Frontal medial cortex	L					3.48	−2	36	−24	4.07	−4	38	−20												
Frontal medial cortex	R					4.41	2	44	−16	4.10	4	38	−20												
Heschl's gyrus	L	5.78	−50	−22	8	6.79	−40	−24	10	6.73	−38	−26	12	7.15	−40	−24	10	6.13	−44	−18	4	6.03	−44	−18	4
Heschl's gyrus	R	6.43	44	−16	6	5.75	50	−20	8	6.71	48	−14	6	5.62	42	−22	10	6.21	46	−14	6	5.49	44	−18	8
Insular cortex	L					3.74	−40	−16	6	3.68	−42	−12	4	3.69	−40	−16	6	3.88	−40	−4	−12	3.82	−42	−6	−6
Insular cortex	R									3.20	42	−12	6					3.17	40	−6	−10				
Lateral occipital cortex	L	3.11	−58	−64	24																				
Middle temporal gyrus	L	5.01	−58	−2	−16	5.58	−52	−28	−6	5.55	−56	−2	−18	5.59	−66	−16	−16								
Middle temporal gyrus	R	5.32	50	−24	−6	5.26	58	−32	−2	4.98	50	−24	−6	5.16	64	−12	−10								
Paracingulate gyrus	L					3.79	−4	48	26																
Paracingulate gyrus	R	3.78	4	52	20									3.30	4	50	22								
Parietal operculum cortex	L	5.22	−48	−28	14	3.54	−46	−30	14	5.59	−48	−28	14	3.70	−58	−30	16	5.59	−46	−30	14	3.93	−48	−28	14
Parietal operculum cortex	R	4.31	44	−24	16	3.77	46	−26	16	3.87	44	−24	16	3.84	48	−26	16					4.12	54	−24	16
Planum polare	L	4.82	−44	−18	−4	4.08	−48	0	−12	4.65	−42	2	−20	4.06	−48	0	−12	4.47	−46	0	−12	5.40	−46	−8	−6
Planum polare	R	4.25	46	−12	−4	3.97	48	2	−14	4.10	58	2	0	4.26	46	4	−16	4.19	44	4	−16	4.47	46	−4	−10
Planum temporale	L	6.55	−56	−28	8	6.25	−52	−26	6	7.23	−56	−28	8	6.01	−62	−20	8	6.27	−44	−32	10	5.74	−52	−26	8
Planum temporale	R	6.18	58	−24	10	6.02	62	−20	8	6.00	44	−30	12	6.00	62	−20	8	4.65	60	−22	10	6.64	58	−26	12
Postcentral gyrus	L	3.25	−64	−16	16					3.63	−64	−16	16												
Postcentral gyrus	R	3.10	66	−14	16					3.13	66	−14	16												
Subcallosal cortex	L					4.39	−2	20	−24																
Subcallosal cortex	R					4.71	2	20	−24																
Superior frontal gyrus	L	3.43	−2	52	34	4.59	−4	52	28	5.54	−4	50	32	4.70	−6	52	30								
Superior frontal gyrus	R	5.77	4	52	30					3.35	2	48	36	3.66	6	50	36								
Superior temporal gyrus	L	6.65	−66	−28	10	6.23	−66	−24	0	6.39	−66	−28	10	6.13	−66	−18	4	4.10	−66	−26	10	4.89	−66	−26	10
Superior temporal gyrus	R	6.25	68	−18	4	6.72	66	−20	2	6.71	68	−18	4	6.96	66	−20	2	5.18	68	−20	2	7.17	70	−24	2
Supramarginal gyrus	L	4.38	−58	−46	22	3.99	−64	−46	16	3.93	−64	−46	16	3.17	−64	−48	16								
Supramarginal gyrus	R	3.63	66	−40	10	3.65	66	−40	10																
Temporal pole	L	5.69	−44	16	−20	6.10	−46	10	−20	5.90	−58	6	−16	5.88	−50	10	−20	4.50	−52	6	−8	3.81	−52	6	−6
Temporal pole	R	7.08	42	14	−22	5.51	56	10	−20	5.38	52	12	−26	6.63	52	14	−18	3.60	58	8	−8	3.52	56	8	−6
Thalamus	L	3.63	−10	−32	0																				
Thalamus	R	3.70	10	−32	0																				

Region labels refer to Harvard Oxford Atlas, thresholded at 50%.

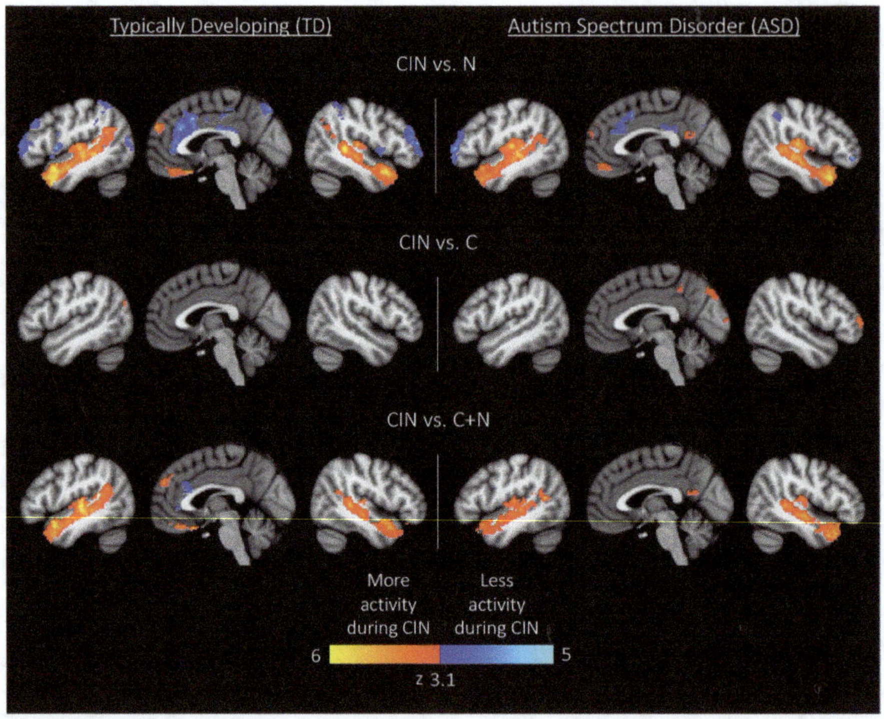

FIGURE 3 | Within-group results for comparisons between experimental conditions. Maps are thresholded at z > 3.1, corrected for multiple comparisons at the cluster level ($p < 0.05$). CIN, conversation-in-noise; N, noise; C, conversation.

attention may be drawn away from socially-relevant information in the presence of distracting sensory stimulation in individuals with ASD. To do so, we employed a novel paradigm whereby participants heard naturalistic conversations in the context of common environmental noises that are often in the background of everyday social interactions. Overall, both youth with ASD and typically-developing youth showed a similar pattern of brain activity in auditory and language networks when listening to conversations presented alone and conversations presented with background noise; further, minimal differences were observed between diagnostic groups when comparing brain activity during listening to conversations alone *versus* conversations shrouded in noise. When we honed in on neural mechanisms underlying the ability to later recognize the topics of conversations that were heard in the presence of background noise, we found that higher recognition accuracy was associated with greater activity in left hemisphere voice-selective cortex in typically-developing youth. In contrast, in youth with ASD, better recognition accuracy was associated with increased activity in a larger network of regions subserving language processing, with significantly greater activity observed in left speech-processing cortex relative to typically-developing youth. Furthermore, we found that increased activity in this left-hemisphere speech-processing region when listening to conversations masked in noise was related to better social motivation and social cognition in ASD youth.

At the behavioral level, youth with and without ASD were equally accurate at discriminating noises *vs.* foils (d'), regardless of whether these were presented alone or simultaneously with conversations. As expected, accuracy in discriminating what was heard during the conversations (*vs.* foils) was overall higher in typically-developing youth, compared to youth with ASD, both when the conversations were presented alone or in the context of background noise; however, these differences were not statistically significant. Notably, we deliberately did not alert participants to pay attention to what was heard in the MRI scanner, as we wanted our paradigm to have high ecological validity by mimicking situations encountered in everyday life, when we may overhear a conversation and are not asked to explicitly pay attention or remember what was said. By explicitly asking participants to carefully listen and try to remember the conversations, any differences in overall discriminative accuracy between diagnostic groups would have likely been further reduced. Indeed, previous studies where direct attentional cues were provided to ASD youth have shown increased brain activity and improved behavioral performance as compared to conditions where such instructions were not given (24, 41). Importantly, both neurotypical youth and youth with ASD had higher discriminative accuracy for conversations than noises when these were each presented alone, as well as higher discriminative accuracy when identifying conversations than noises when conversations and noises were presented simultaneously. In addition, both neurotypical and ASD youth showed the expected pattern whereby accuracy in identifying topics of conversation was poorer for conversations presented

TABLE 3 | Montreal Neurological Institute (MNI) coordinates for between-condition contrasts.

		CIN > N								*CIN > C*								*CIN > C+N*							
		ASD				TD				ASD				TD				ASD				TD			
		Max z	MNI peak (mm)			Max z	MNI peak (mm)			Max z	MNI peak (mm)			Max z	MNI peak (mm)			Max z	MNI peak (mm)			Max z	MNI peak (mm)		
			X	Y	Z		X	Y	Z		X	Y	Z		X	Y	Z		X	Y	Z		X	Y	Z
Amygdala	L					4.78	−28	−6	−20																
Amygdala	R					4.74	24	−6	−20																
Angular gyrus	L	3.89	−62	0	20	4.64	−58	−56	20									3.32	−62	−54	20	5.92	−56	−54	20
Angular gyrus	R					5.39	52	−54	20									4.35	62	−48	22	4.15	54	−50	18
Central opercular cortex	L	3.95	−52	−12	10	4.52	−58	−10	8									3.64	−50	−8	6	3.96	−52	−10	8
Central opercular cortex	R	4.33	48	−16	12	3.19	62	−8	8									3.57	48	−16	12	4.25	62	−8	8
Cingulate gyrus posterior	L	3.83	−2	−50	22													4.26	−2	−50	18				
Cingulate gyrus posterior	R	3.68	2	−50	20													3.24	2	−48	18				
Cuneal cortex	L									3.77	−2	−82	34												
Frontal medial cortex	L	4.46	−4	42	−16	4.45	−2	38	−22													4.6	−2	36	−22
Frontal medial cortex	R	4.93	2	44	−16	6.46	2	42	−22													5.05	4	40	−22
Frontal orbital cortex	L	3.65	−38	20	−20																				
Frontal orbital cortex	R					3.14	40	26	−20													3.19	44	28	−18
Frontal pole	L	3.57	−4	64	24	3.7	−10	58	28																
Frontal pole	R	4.11	12	42	48					4.84	38	44	6					4.03	12	48	46				
Fusiform cortex	L					3.69	−40	−18	−24																
Heschl's gyrus	L	5.11	−48	−18	8	5.09	−40	−22	8									4.45	−50	−22	8	6.35	−46	−24	10
Heschl's gyrus	R	5.25	48	−20	10	5.67	50	−20	8									4.04	48	−20	10	4.66	50	−20	8
Hippocampus	L					4.85	−26	−8	−22																
Hippocampus	R					4.66	26	−8	−20																
Inferior temporal gyrus	L					3.61	−56	−18	−28													3.58	−56	−20	−26
Lateral occipital cortex	L	3.86	−56	−64	24	4.2	−50	−62	26	3.7	−12	−82	46	4.41	−48	−74	26	3.57	−56	−62	26				
Lateral occipital cortex	R																	4.79	54	−64	18				
Middle temporal gyrus	R	5.26	50	−24	−6	6.31	−54	−26	−8									4.02	−56	−32	−4	5.84	−54	−28	−6
Middle temporal gyrus	L	5.55	−56	0	−28	4.99	64	−12	−10									5.16	52	−20	−8	4.9	62	−30	−4
Occipital pole	L									4.74	−12	−96	−2												
Occipital pole	R									3.51	2	−96	6												
Paracingulate gyrus	L	3.26	−6	50	20	3.32	−2	48	26													3.31	−2	48	26
Paracingulate gyrus	R	3.18	4	52	20													3.27	4	42	34				
Parahippocampal gyrus	L					4.16	−20	−26	−18																
Parietal operculum Cortex	L	4.11	−42	−34	16													3.18	−42	−34	16				
Parietal operculum Cortex	R	3.45	48	−22	16	3.75	44	−24	16																
Planum polare	L	3.43	−54	−2	0	3.99	−44	−2	−18									3.18	−48	−4	−8	4.04	−44	0	−18
Planum polare	R	3.56	58	2	0	4.07	46	4	−16									3.62	46	0	−16	4.54	48	2	−14
Planum temporale	L	5.61	−54	−28	8	5.92	−62	−20	8									5.24	−54	−28	8	6.15	−62	−20	8
Planum temporale	R	4.39	62	−20	8	4.39	62	−18	8									3.86	62	−20	8	4.19	62	−18	8
Precuneus cortex	L	3.59	−2	−60	22					4.05	−12	−64	22					3.75	−2	−58	18				
Precuneus cortex	R	4.07	4	−56	22					4.06	8	−54	50					4.07	2	−58	18				
Subcallosal cortex	L					5.07	−2	20	−24													4.84	−2	20	−24
Subcallosal cortex	R					5.61	2	24	−26													4.66	2	20	−24
Superior frontal gyrus	L	3.12	−4	54	24	5.57	−4	54	24													4.69	−4	42	38
Superior frontal gyrus	R	4.79	2	50	36													4.03	2	42	40	3.29	4	50	32

(Continued)

TABLE 3 | Continued

		CIN > N								*CIN > C*								*CIN > C+N*							
		ASD				TD				ASD				TD				ASD				TD			
		Max z	MNI peak (mm)			Max z	MNI peak (mm)			Max z	MNI peak (mm)			Max z	MNI peak (mm)			Max z	MNI peak (mm)			Max z	MNI peak (mm)		
			X	Y	Z		X	Y	Z		X	Y	Z		X	Y	Z		X	Y	Z		X	Y	Z
Superior temporal gyrus	L	5.7	-62	-26	0	6.59	-64	-18	-4									5.47	-64	-26	2	6.01	-64	-18	-4
Superior temporal gyrus	R	5.31	54	-18	-6	6.34	58	-18	-4									5.26	52	-12	-10	6.06	58	-20	-2
Supramarginal gyrus	L	4.33	-64	-46	16	3.22	-64	-48	16									4.08	-58	-46	22	4.25	-64	-46	16
Supramarginal gyrus	R																	3.46	66	-38	18	3.37	66	-40	10
Temporal pole	L	5.19	-32	14	-28	6.47	-50	12	-36									5.74	-46	16	-20	6.52	-50	8	-22
Temporal pole	R	5.84	48	18	-30	5.63	50	14	-22									7.31	50	18	-30	6.04	58	8	-18

Region labels refer to Harvard Oxford Atlas, thresholded at 50%.

TABLE 4 | Montreal Neurological Institute (MNI) coordinates for between-condition between-group contrasts.

		CIN > C ASD > TD			
		Max z	MNI peak (mm)		
			X	Y	Z
Cuneal cortex	L	3.47	−2	−86	34
Occipital pole	L	3.6	−10	−94	0
Precuneus cortex	L	3.51	−6	−64	30

Region labels refer to Harvard Oxford Atlas, thresholded at 50%.

over background noise than for conversations presented alone. Although this latter difference was not statistically significant when using d' collapsed across the easy (yes/no) and hard (multiple-choice) questions, when looking at percent accuracy for the harder multiple-choice questions, ASD youth performed significantly worse in the conversation-in-noise condition than in the conversation alone condition, a pattern not observed in TD youth. Overall, these findings are in agreement with previous work in adults and adolescents with ASD showing that recall is poorer for sentences presented simultaneously with background sounds (22, 23). However, our findings of similar discriminative accuracy (d') between typically-developing and ASD youth when identifying conversations heard in the context of background noises are in contrast to previous work suggesting that individuals with ASD are poorer at discriminating speech-in-noise relative to their neurotypical counterparts (22, 23). This difference may in part be explained by our choice of noise stimuli, which were deliberately chosen to be only mildly aversive and, unlike those used in prior studies, also easily recognizable. Indeed, this methodological choice may also explain why we did not observe between-group differences in brain regions previously implicated in processing aversive auditory stimuli (e.g., amygdala, thalamus, auditory cortex), which have previously been documented in ASD participants (24, 31, 32, 42). Importantly, the lack of significant between-group differences in brain responses to mildly aversive noises in this study may also in part reflect the more stringent statistical threshold employed in the current study, in keeping with evolving standards in the neuroimaging field (43). Indeed, at more liberal thresholds we too observed greater activity in the amygdala and primary auditory cortex during exposure to mildly aversive noise in ASD youth as compared to TD youth.

At the neural level, typically-developing and ASD youth showed overall similar patterns of brain activity when listening to conversations alone, noises alone, and conversations shrouded in noise. The only significant between-group difference was detected when comparing brain activity observed when youth were presented with conversations and environmental noises simultaneously *versus* conversations alone. Here, the addition of background noise to conversations elicited greater activity in the precuneus and primary visual cortex in ASD relative to TD youth. The precuneus is a canonical hub of the default mode network, a network of brain regions implicated in thinking about the self and others (44) and narrative comprehension in

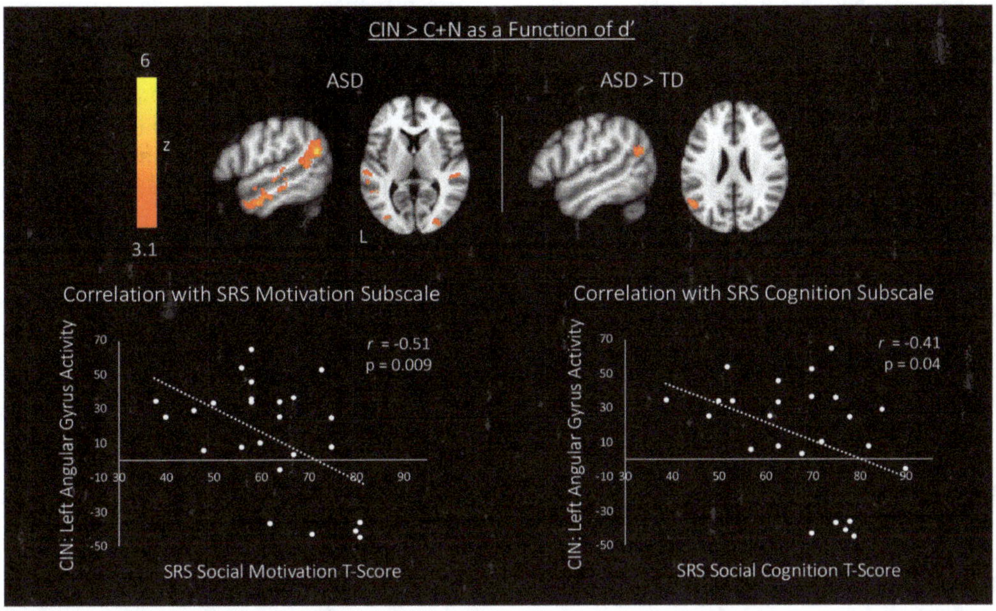

FIGURE 4 | Top: associations between brain activity (CIN > C+N) and discriminative accuracy (i.e., d') for topics of conversation heard in the CIN condition. Maps are thresholded at z > 3.1, corrected for multiple comparisons at the cluster level (p < 0.05). Bottom: correlations between blood oxygen level dependent (BOLD) signal response for the CIN condition and scores on two subscales of the SRS in autism spectrum disorder (ASD) youth. CIN, conversation-in-noise; N, noise; C, conversation; SRS, Social Responsiveness Scale.

TABLE 5 | Montreal Neurological Institute (MNI) coordinates for brain activity associated with discriminative accuracy (d') for topics of conversation heard in the conversation-in-noise (CIN) condition.

		CIN > C+N															
		ASD + TD				ASD				TD				ASD > TD			
		Max z	MNI peak (mm)			Max z	MNI peak (mm)			Max z	MNI peak (mm)			Max z	MNI peak (mm)		
			X	Y	Z		X	Y	Z		X	Y	Z		X	Y	Z
Angular gyrus	L	4.98	-52	-60	20	5.37	-56	-58	26					4.07	-50	-60	24
Angular gyrus	R					3.82	46	-50	28								
Frontal orbital cortex	R	4.44	44	24	−14	4.26	44	24	−14								
Fusiform cortex	L													3.86	−34	−58	−16
Lateral occipital cortex	L	3.16	-54	-64	26	5.48	-54	-64	20					4.74	-48	-64	26
Lateral occipital cortex	R					4.09	42	-84	-2								
Middle temporal gyrus	L	4.95	-62	-10	-8	5.15	-54	-4	-28	3.74	-52	-34	-4				
Middle temporal gyrus	R	4.79	56	2	-20	5.02	56	2	-30								
Occipital pole	L					4.07	-32	-94	-10								
Occipital pole	R					4.47	36	-92	-2								
Parietal operculum cortex	R					4.19	44	-32	20								
Planum temporale	L	4.00	-60	-26	6	4.37	-62	-24	10								
Planum temporale	R	4.34	52	-30	16	4.82	60	-30	16								
Precentral gyrus	R					4.17	54	-2	42								
Superior temporal gyrus	L	5.47	-62	-26	2	3.62	-58	-38	6	3.13	-60	-44	8				
Superior temporal gyrus	R	4.52	46	-32	4	3.55	52	-32	4								
Supramarginal gyrus	L	5.31	-56	-46	10	3.89	-60	-46	22								
Temporal pole	L	4.71	−44	4	−20	4.43	−44	14	−38								
Temporal pole	R	5.17	58	8	−20	4.7	56	10	−30								

Region labels refer to Harvard Oxford Atlas, thresholded at 50%.

neurotypical adults (45, 46). Our finding of increased activity in visual cortex during auditory stimulation in ASD youth, relative to typically-developing youth, is consistent with previous findings in individuals with ASD showing increased brain activity in the visual system during semantic decision making (47) as well as auditory pitch discrimination (48), suggesting atypical integration of auditory and visual sensory systems in ASD (42, 49). Our findings thus suggest that similar behavioral profiles may in part reflect processing differences at the neural level whereby the challenging task of listening to social interactions over background noise requires activation of additional brain regions in youth with ASD, relative to neurotypical controls.

The ability to deploy attention to socially meaningful information rests on being able to divert attention away from less relevant distracting stimuli; accordingly, in an attempt to hone in on the neural substrates of social attention, we next sought to identify brain activity that was related to the successful encoding of the topics of conversation. More specifically, we examined how brain responses while participants listened to conversations in the context of background noise (above and beyond brain responses associated with attending to conversations and noises alone) predicted later recognition of what was heard. In both neurotypical youth and youth with ASD, greater accuracy in identifying the topics of conversations heard in the context of background noise was predicted by greater activity in left hemisphere voice-selective cortex. Previous work in neurotypical adults has shown that this voice-selective region preferentially responds to vocal stimuli, and that activity in this region decreases when voice stimuli are masked by background noise (19, 20). Thus, heightened activity in this region when listening to conversations shrouded in common environmental noises may serve as a compensatory mechanism, allowing both youth with and without ASD to focus their attention on the socially-relevant information in the presence of distracting auditory stimuli. Importantly, better recognition accuracy in youth with ASD was also associated with greater activity in a wider network of brain regions implicated in language processing. Indeed, relative to typically-developing youth, ASD youth showed significantly greater activity in left-hemisphere angular gyrus. This region plays an important role in language comprehension (50–52) and prior work shows that disrupting activity in this area reduces the ability to comprehend speech under difficult listening conditions (53). The angular gyrus is also an important region for theory of mind (TOM)—the ability to understand the actions and thoughts of others (54, 55). TOM is a critical skill in reasoning about others' state of mind and plays a role in high-level language processing including the use and understanding of language within a social environment (56). Thus, similar to the heightened response in the voice-selective-region observed in both neurotypical and ASD youth, this increased activity in speech processing cortex in youth with ASD could reflect compensatory processes resulting in improved sensitivity to speech stimuli, thereby boosting youths' ability to encode and later accurately discriminate between conversation topics heard over background noise. If this interpretation is correct, individual differences in responsivity observed in this region in the context of our paradigm should be associated with the more general ability to hone in on socially-relevant information, and ultimately result in less severe social impairments. Consistent with this hypothesis, neural activity in this speech-processing region while participants listened to conversations shrouded in noise was associated with better social motivation and social cognition in youth with ASD.

This study has several limitations. First, due to the correlational nature inherent to all neuroimaging studies, while we hypothesized that the increased activity in language-related and TOM regions allowed ASD youth to hone in on socially relevant information, we cannot rule out the alternative account that greater activity in these brain regions merely resulted from more successful processing of language through noise. Second, atypical heightened sensitivity to sensory stimuli (known as sensory over-responsivity; SOR) affects over half of children with ASD (26, 27) and is an important contributor to altered processing of both social and non-social stimuli in youth with ASD (24, 31, 32, 42); however, given our small sample size, we were unable to directly compare groups of ASD youth with and without SOR. More work is needed to understand how SOR may mediate neural responses to ecologically valid social and non-social stimuli in the environment. Importantly, recent work also suggests that there may be sex-differences in the development of multisensory speech processing in TD and ASD youth (57); thus, examining the interaction between sex, sensory processing, and social cognition is an important direction for future research. In addition, participants in our study were all high-functioning individuals who developed language and had verbal IQ in the normal range, making it more likely that our participants would have the ability to hone in on social stimuli compared to more affected individuals. In future studies it will be crucial replicate these findings and to extend this work to individuals with more severe ASD phenotypes, as well as to younger children on the autism spectrum. To this end, prospective studies of infants at high risk for developing ASD will be essential to track the longitudinal co-development of sensory responsivity, language acquisition, and ASD symptomatology.

To conclude, using a novel and ecologically valid paradigm, here we sought to better understand the neural correlates of social attention. Our findings indicate youth with ASD who successfully encoded socially-relevant information in the presence of distracting stimuli did so by up-regulating activity in neural systems supporting speech and language processing, thus suggesting that focusing on both social and non-social stimuli simultaneously may be more of a challenge for ASD youth relative to their neurotypical counterparts. This work buttresses the importance of further examining the relationship between social attention and sensory processing atypicalities, particularly early in development, to shed new light on the onset of autism symptomatology, as well as to inform the design of novel interventions.

AUTHOR CONTRIBUTIONS

This study was conceived of and designed by LH, SG, KL, JL, SB, and MD. Data acquisition was performed by LH, KL, and JL. Data analysis was completed by LH and MI. All authors contributed to data interpretation and drafting of the manuscript, and provided critical feedback on the manuscript and its intellectual content.

FUNDING

This work was supported by the National Institute of Mental Health (grants R01MH100028 and K08 MH112871) and the Simons Foundation Autism Research Initiative (grant 345389). Some of the authors were supported by training grants/fellowships from the National Institute of Neurological Disorders and Stroke (F99 NS105206 to LH, T32 NS048004 to LH and KL), the National Institute of Mental Health (F32 MH105167 to SG, F31 MH110140 to KL), the National Institute of Child Health and Human Development (F31 HD088102 to JL), and the Roche/ARCS Foundation Scholar Award Program in the Life Sciences (KL and JL). The project was also in part supported by grants RR12169, RR13642, and RR00865 from the NIH National Center for Research Resources. We are also grateful for generous support from the Brain Mapping Medical Research Organization, Brain Mapping Support Foundation, Pierson-Lovelace Foundation, The Ahmanson Foundation, the William M. and Linda R. Dietel Philanthropic Fund at the Northern Piedmont Community Foundation, the Tamkin Foundation, the Jennifer Jones-Simon Foundation, the Capital Group Companies Charitable Foundation, the Robson Family, and the Northstar Fund. The contents of this paper are solely the responsibility of the authors and do not necessarily represent the official views of the National Institutes of Health.

REFERENCES

1. American Psychiatric Association. *Diagnostic and Statistical Manual of Mental Disorders. 5th ed.* Arlington, VA: American Psychiatric Publishing (2013).
2. Shultz S, Klin A, Jones W. Neonatal Transitions in Social Behavior and Their Implications for Autism. *Trends Cogn Sci* (2018) 22:452–69. doi: 10.1016/j.tics.2018.02.012
3. Klin A. Young Autistic Children's Listening Preferences in Regard to Speech: A Possible Characterization of the Symptom of Social Withdrawal. *J Autism Dev Disord* (1991) 21:29–42. doi: 10.1007/bf02206995
4. Kuhl PK, Coffey-Corina S, Padden D, Dawson G. Links between social and linguistic processing of speech in preschool children with autism: behavioral and electrophysiological measures. *Dev Sci* (2005) 8:F1–F12. doi: 10.1111/j.1467-7687.2004.00384.x
5. Ben-Sasson A, Hen L, Fluss R, Cermak SA, Engel-Yeger B, Gal EA. Meta-Analysis of Sensory Modulation Symptoms in Individuals with Autism Spectrum Disorders. *J Autism Dev Disord* (2009) 39:1–11. doi: 10.1007/s10803-008-0593-3
6. Piven J, Elison JT, Zylka MJ. Toward a conceptual framework for early brain and behavior development in autism. *Mol Psychiatry* (2017) 23:165. doi: 10.1038/mp.2017.131
7. Thye MD, Bednarz HM, Herringshaw AJ, Sartin EB, Kana RK. The impact of atypical sensory processing on social impairments in autism spectrum disorder. *Dev Cogn Neurosci* (2017) 29:151–67. doi: 10.1016/J.DCN.2017.04.010
8. Hamilton A. Sensory and social features of autism – can they be integrated? *Dev Cogn Neurosci* (2018) 29:1–3. doi: 10.1016/J.DCN.2018.02.009
9. Hernandez LM, Rudie JD, Green SA, Bookheimer S, Dapretto M. Neural signatures of autism spectrum disorders: Insights into brain network dynamics. *Neuropsychopharmacology* (2015) 40:171–89. doi: 10.1038/npp.2014.172
10. Lombardo MV, Pierce K, Eyler LT, Carter Barne C, Ahrens-Barbeau C, Solso S, et al. Different Functional Neural Substrates for Good and Poor Language Outcome in Autism. *Neuron* (2015) 86:567–77. doi: 10.1016/J.NEURON.2015.03.023
11. Dinstein I, Pierce K, Eyler L, Solso S, Malach R, Behrmann M, et al. Disrupted Neural Synchronization in Toddlers with Autism. *Neuron* (2011) 70:1218–25. doi: 10.1016/J.NEURON.2011.04.018
12. Gervais H, Belin P, Boddaert N, Leboyer M, Coez A, Sfaello I, et al. Abnormal cortical voice processing in autism. *Nat Neurosci* (2004) 7:801–2. doi: 10.1038/nn1291
13. Kleinhans NM, Müller RA, Cohen DN, Courchesne E. Atypical functional lateralization of language in autism spectrum disorders. *Brain Res* (2008) 1221:115–25. doi: 10.1016/J.BRAINRES.2008.04.080
14. Lai G, Pantazatos SP, Schneider H, Hirsch J. Neural systems for speech and song in autism. *Brain: A J Neurol* (2012) 135:961–75. doi: 10.1093/brain/awr335
15. Eyler LT, Pierce K. Courchesne E. A failure of left temporal cortex to specialize for language is an early emerging and fundamental property of autism. *Brain* (2012) 135:949–60. doi: 10.1093/brain/awr364
16. Mody M, Belliveau JW. Speech and Language Impairments in Autism: Insights from Behavior and Neuroimaging. *North Am J Med Sci* (2013) 5:157–61. doi: 10.7156/v5i3p157
17. Tryfon A, Foster NEV, Sharda M, Hyde KL. Speech perception in autism spectrum disorder: An activation likelihood estimation meta-analysis. *Behav Brain Res* (2018) 338:118–27. doi: 10.1016/J.BBR.2017.10.025
18. Abrams DA, Lynch CJ, Cheng KM, Phillips J, Supekar K, Ryali S, et al. Underconnectivity between voice-selective cortex and reward circuitry in children with autism. *Proc Natl Acad Sci United States America* (2013) 110:12060–65. doi: 10.1073/pnas.1302982110
19. Belin P, Zatorre RJ, Lafaille P, Ahad P , Pike B. Voice-selective areas in human auditory cortex. *Nature* (2000) 403(6767), 309–12. doi: 10.1038/35002078
20. Vander Ghinst M, Bourguignon M, Op de Beeck M, Wens V, Marty B, Hassid S, et al. Left Superior Temporal Gyrus Is Coupled to Attended Speech in a Cocktail-Party Auditory Scene. *J Neuroscie: Off J Soc Neurosci* (2016) 36:1596–606. doi: 10.1523/JNEUROSCI.1730-15.2016
21. Redcay E, Courchesne E. Deviant Functional Magnetic Resonance Imaging Patterns of Brain Activity to Speech in 2–3-Year-Old Children with Autism Spectrum Disorder. *Biol Psychiatry* (2008) 64:589–98. doi: 10.1016/J.BIOPSYCH.2008.05.020
22. Alcantara JI, Weisblatt EJL, Moore BCJ, Bolton PF. Speech-in-noise perception in high-functioning individuals with autism or Asperger's syndrome. *J Child Psychol Psychiatry* (2004) 45:1107–14. doi: 10.1111/j.1469-7610.2004.t01-1-00303.x
23. Dunlop WA, Enticott PG, Rajan R. Speech Discrimination Difficulties in High-Functioning Autism Spectrum Disorder Are Likely Independent of Auditory Hypersensitivity. *Front Hum Neurosci* (2016) 10:401. doi: 10.3389/fnhum.2016.00401
24. Green SA, Hernandez LM, Bowman HC, Bookheimer SY, Dapretto M. Sensory over-responsivity and social cognition in ASD: Effects of aversive sensory stimuli and attentional modulation on neural responses to social cues. *Dev Cogn Neurosci* (2018) 29:127–39. doi: 10.1016/j.dcn.2017.02.005
25. Tavassoli T, Miller LJ, Schoen SA, Nielsen DM, Baron-Cohen S. Sensory over-responsivity in adults with autism spectrum conditions. *Autism* (2014) 18:428–32. doi: 10.1177/1362361313477246
26. Bishop SL, Hus V, Duncan A, Huerta M, Gotham K, Pickles A, et al. Subcategories of restricted and repetitive behaviors in children with autism

spectrum disorders. *J Autism Dev Disord* (2013) 43:1287–97. doi: 10.1007/s10803-012-1671-0

27. Marco EJ, Hinkley LBN, Hill SS, Nagarajan SS. Sensory processing in autism: a review of neurophysiologic findings. *Pediatr Res* (2011) 69:48R–54R. doi: 10.1203/PDR.0b013e3182130c54
28. Rosenhall U, Nordin V, Sandström M, Ahlsén G, Gillberg C. Autism and hearing loss. *J Autism Dev Disord* (1999) 29:349–57. doi: 10.1023/a:1023022709710
29. Khalfa S, Bruneau N, Rogé B, Georgieff N, Veuillet E, Adrien JL, et al. Increased perception of loudness in autism. *Hearing Res* (2004) 198:87–92. doi: 10.1016/J.HEARES.2004.07.006
30. O'Connor K. Auditory processing in autism spectrum disorder: A review. *Neurosci Biobehav Rev* (2012) 36:836–54. doi: 10.1016/J.NEUBIOREV.2011.11.008
31. Green SA, Hernandez L, Tottenham N, Krasileva K, Bookheimer SY, Dapretto M. Neurobiology of sensory overresponsivity in youth with autism spectrum disorders. *JAMA Psychiatry* (2015) 72:778–86. doi: 10.1001/jamapsychiatry.2015.0737
32. Green SA, Rudie JD, Colich NL, Wood JJ, Shirinyan D, Hernandez L, et al. Overreactive brain responses to sensory stimuli in youth with autism spectrum disorders. *J Am Acad Child Adolesc Psychiatry* (2013) 52:1158–72. doi: 10.1016/j.jaac.2013.08.004
33. Lord C, Rutter M, DiLavore P, Risi S, Gotham K, Bishop S. *Autism Diagnostic Observation Schedule. 2nd ed.* Torrance, CA, USA: Western Psychological Services (2012).
34. Lord C, Rutter M, Le Couteur A. Autism Diagnostic Interview-Revised: A revised version of a diagnostic interview for caregivers of individuals with possible pervasive developmental disorders. *J Autism Dev Disord* (1994) 24:659–85. doi: 10.1007/BF02172145
35. Wechsler D. *Wechsler Abbreviated Scale of Intelligence*. New York, NY, USA: The Psychological Corporation, Harcourt Brace & Company (1999).
36. Constantino JN, Gruber CP. *Social Responsiveness Scale–Second Edition (SRS-2)*. Torrance, CA, USA: Western Psychological Services (2012). p. 2nd ed.
37. Smith SM, Jenkinson M, Woolrich MW, Beckmann CF, Behrens TEJ, Johansen-Berg H, et al. Advances in functional and structural MR image analysis and implementation as FSL. *NeuroImage* (2004) 23:S208–19. doi: 10.1016/J.NEUROIMAGE.2004.07.051
38. Cox RW. AFNI: Software for Analysis and Visualization of Functional Magnetic Resonance Neuroimages. *Comput Biomed Res* (1996) 29:162–73. doi: 10.1006/cbmr.1996.0014
39. Jenkinson M, Bannister P, Brady M, Smith S. Improved Optimization for the Robust and Accurate Linear Registration and Motion Correction of Brain Images. *NeuroImage* (2002) 17:825–41. doi: 10.1006/NIMG.2002.1132
40. Smith SM. Fast robust automated brain extraction. *Hum Brain Mapp* (2002) 17:143–55. doi: 10.1002/hbm.10062
41. Wang TA, Lee SA, Sigman M, Dapretto M. Reading affect in the face and voice: Neural correlates of interpreting communicative intent in children and adolescents with autism spectrum disorders. *JAMA Psychiatry* (2007) 64:698–708. doi: 10.1001/archpsyc.64.6.698
42. Green SA, Hernandez L, Lawrence KE, Liu J, Tsang T, Yeargin J, et al. Distinct Patterns of Neural Habituation and Generalization in Children and Adolescents With Autism With Low and High Sensory Overresponsivity. *Am J Psychiatry* (2019) 176:1010–20. doi: 10.1176/appi.ajp.2019.18121333
43. Eklund A, Nichols TE, Knutsson H. Cluster failure: Why fMRI inferences for spatial extent have inflated false-positive rates. *Proc Natl Acad Sci United States America* (2016) 113:7900–05. doi: 10.1073/pnas.1602413113
44. Raichle ME, MacLeod AM, Snyder AZ, Powers WJ, Gusnard DA, Shulman GL. A default mode of brain function. *Proc Natl Acad Sci United States America* (2001) 98:676–82. doi: 10.1073/pnas.98.2.676
45. Lerner Y, Honey CJ, Silbert L, Hasson U. Topographic mapping of a hierarchy of temporal receptive windows using a narrated story. *J Neurosci* (2011) 31:2906–15. doi: 10.1523/JNEUROSCI.3684-10.2011
46. Xu J, Kemeny S, Park G, Frattali C, Braun A. Language in context: Emergent features of word, sentence, and narrative comprehension. *NeuroImage* (2005) 25:1002–15. doi: 10.1016/j.neuroimage.2004.12.013
47. Gaffrey MS, Kleinhans NM, Haist F, Akshoomoff N, Campbell A, Courchesne E. A typical participation of visual cortex during word processing in autism: An fMRI study of semantic decision. *Neuropsychologia* (2007) 45:1672–84. doi: 10.1016/j.neuropsychologia.2007.01.008
48. Jao Keehn RJ, Sanchez SS, Stewart CR, Zhao W, Grenesko-Stevens EL, Keehn B, et al. Impaired downregulation of visual cortex during auditory processing is associated with autism symptomatology in children and adolescents with autism spectrum disorder. *Autism Res* (2017) 10:130–43. doi: 10.1002/aur.1636
49. Stevenson RA, Segers M, Ferber S, Barense MD, Wallace MT. The impact of multisensory integration deficits on speech perception in children with autism spectrum disorders. *Front Psychol* (2014) 5:379. doi: 10.3389/fpsyg.2014.00379
50. Binder JR, Desai RH, Graves WW, Conant LL. Where is the semantic system? A critical review and meta-analysis of 120 functional neuroimaging studies. *Cereb Cortex* (2009) 19:2767–96. doi: 10.1093/cercor/bhp055
51. Obleser J, Kotz SA. Expectancy Constraints in Degraded Speech Modulate the Language Comprehension Network. *Cereb Cortex* (2010) 20:633–40. doi: 10.1093/cercor/bhp128
52. Seghier ML, Fagan E, Price CJ. Functional subdivisions in the left angular gyrus where the semantic system meets and diverges from the default network. *J Neurosci* (2010) 30:16809–17. doi: 10.1523/JNEUROSCI.3377-10.2010
53. Hartwigsen G, Golombek T, Obleser J. Repetitive transcranial magnetic stimulation over left angular gyrus modulates the predictability gain in degraded speech comprehension. *Cortex* (2015) 68:100–10. doi: 10.1016/j.cortex.2014.08.027
54. Barron-Cohen S. The development of a theory of mind in autism: deviance and delay? *Psychiatr Clinics North America* (1991) 14(1):33–51. doi: 10.1016/S0193-953X(18)30323-X
55. Frith U, Happé F. Theory of mind and self-consciousness: What is it like to be autistic? *Mind Lang* (2002) 14:82–9. doi: 10.1111/1468-0017.00100
56. Boucher J. Language development in autism. *Int J Pediatr Otorhinolaryngol* (2003) 67:S159–163. doi: 10.1006/cbmr.1996.0014
57. Ross LA, Del Bene VA, Molholm S, Frey HP, Foxe JJ. Sex differences in multisensory speech processing in both typically developing children and those on the autism spectrum. *Front Neurosci* (2015) 9:185. doi: 10.3389/fnins.2015.00185

13

Evidence of an Own-Age Bias in Facial Emotion Recognition for Adolescents with and without Autism Spectrum Disorder

Kathryn M. Hauschild[1*], *Peter Felsman*[1,2], *Cara M. Keifer*[1] *and Matthew D. Lerner*[1,3]

[1] *Social Competence and Treatment Laboratory, Department of Psychology, Stony Brook University, Stony Brook, NY, United States,* [2] *Alan Alda Center for Communicating Science, Stony Brook University, Stony Brook, NY, United States,* [3] *Department of Psychology, University of Virginia, Charlottesville, VA, United States*

***Correspondence:**
Kathryn M. Hauschild
kathryn.hauschild@stonybrook.edu

A common interpretation of the face-processing deficits associated with autism spectrum disorder (ASD) is that they arise from a failure to develop normative levels of perceptual expertise. One indicator of perceptual expertise for faces is the own-age bias, operationalized as a processing advantage for faces of one's own age, presumably due to more frequent contact and experience. This effect is especially evident in domains of face recognition memory but less commonly investigated in social-emotional expertise (e.g., facial emotion recognition; FER), where individuals with ASD have shown consistent deficits. In the present study, we investigated whether a FER task would elicit an own-age bias for individuals with and without ASD and explored how the magnitude of an own-age bias may differ as a function of ASD status and symptoms. Ninety-two adolescents (63 male) between the ages of 11 and 14 years completed the child- and adult-face subtests of a standardized FER task. Overall FER accuracy was found to differ by ASD severity, reflecting poorer performance for those with increased symptoms. Results also indicated that an own-age bias was evident, reflecting greater FER performance for child compared to adult faces, for all adolescents regardless of ASD status or symptoms. However, the strength of the observed own-age bias did not differ by ASD status or severity. Findings suggest that face processing abilities of adolescents with ASD may be influenced by experience with specific categories of stimuli, similar to their typically developing peers.

Keywords: face processing, perceptual expertise, own-age bias, emotion recognition, autism spectrum disorder, adolescents

INTRODUCTION

Individuals with autism spectrum disorder (ASD) demonstrate impaired categorization of the emotional facial expressions of others (1–3). Some have hypothesized that this characteristic deficit may arise from a failure to develop normative levels of face-relevant perceptual expertise (4–6). Face-relevant expertise develops with frequent and recent experience (7–9), resulting in improved performance on behavioral tasks of recognition memory and emotion identification for faces of one's own age compared to faces of another age, known as the own-age bias [OAB; (10–12)]. Thus, if

ASD-related deficits in FER can be explained by a failure to develop normative levels of face-relevant perceptual expertise, then people with ASD may not be expected to demonstrate an OAB to the same extent as their peers. However, whether such a bias occurs among individuals with ASD to the same extent as their peers has not been tested. The current study addresses this question.

Although the magnitude and universality of emotion perception deficits associated with ASD have been debated [see (1, 13) for review], recent meta-analyses support the presence of behavioral deficits in facial emotion recognition (2, 3). Early accounts of these deficits posited that observed group differences in performance may have been driven by difficulty in processing negative (14) or threat-relevant (i.e. fearful) emotions (15, 16). However, more recent work indicates that individuals with ASD perform worse than typically developing individuals on tasks of facial emotion identification and recognition across all six basic emotions (2, 17). These deficits appear to be particularly pronounced during the completion of tasks that require judgments related to more subtle expressions of emotion [(5, 18); but also see (19)]. Additionally, eye tracking, electrophysiological, and neuroimaging data suggest atypical attentional and cognitive processing of emotional faces by individuals with ASD (20–22).

One explanation of FER deficits in ASD is that those with ASD fail to develop normative levels of face-relevant perceptual expertise (4, 6). For typically developing individuals, increased experience with categories of face stimuli, such as human faces compared to macaque faces (23), confers an expert level processing advantage for stimuli of that category (8, 24). This advantage is related to the ability to integrate previously experienced exemplars into prototypic mental representations (9, 25) and engage in configural processing (26). Individuals with ASD, on the other hand, have failed to demonstrate many of these same markers (27, 28). Moreover, developmental studies of facial emotion recognition have noted that deficits in FER for individuals with ASD increase with age, observing the greatest divergence between group performance trajectories in adulthood (5, 29, 30), when typically developing individuals demonstrate expert performance levels. Together these patterns of findings suggest that face-relevant perceptual representations of individuals with ASD may not be as sensitive to experience as those of their typically developing peers.

The idea that face-relevant perceptual experience leads to expertise is demonstrated in the own-age bias (OAB). The OAB constitutes a processing advantage for own- compared to other-aged faces that is contingent upon greater contact with individuals of one's own age (11, 12). This bias is dependent upon differential experience with face age (31, 32), is reduced by visual exposure training of other-aged faces (33), and has been reliably observed in both tasks of face recognition memory (11) and FER (10, 34). As is true of many indicators of perceptual expertise, the OAB is also reflected in differential patterns of visual attention to own-age faces (35–39) and the recruitment of specialized cortical networks when processing own-age faces (36, 40).

The OAB likely reflects the influence of increased contact and visual experience with faces of one's age cohort (11; for an alternate account see 41); thus, signaling ongoing plasticity in perceptual representations as they adapt to the changing facial structures of peers over time. This is in contrast to a processing advantage for adult faces regardless of one's own current age that would be predicted if age biases in FER were due to cumulative lifetime visual experience. Exceptions to OAB in the literature support this account; for example, infants who spend most of their time with adults show a processing advantage for adult faces (42) and teachers working with young children are equally accurate in identifying child and adult faces (33).

The same principle underlying the OAB is demonstrated in the other-race effect (ORE). The ORE constitutes a processing advantage for own- compared to other-race faces that is contingent upon greater contact with individuals of one's own race (see 43 for review). However, unlike the OAB, the ORE likely reflects a summation of visual experience across development, not merely the most recently encountered exemplars (43). Findings from the ORE literature suggest that individuals with ASD may indeed be sensitive to cumulative visual experience with faces, reflected in greater performance accuracy for own- compared to other-race in tasks of facial recognition memory (44, 45). Although, this has not always been replicated (46, 47). Furthermore, it remains unknown whether such effects extend to tasks of FER, where individuals with ASD demonstrate increased impairment (1).

To date, no work has examined whether the strength or direction of the OAB varies for individuals with ASD. In order to better understand the role of experience in face processing for individuals with ASD, the present study aimed to explore whether adolescents with and without ASD would evidence an OAB while completing a task of FER; that is, demonstrate greater performance accuracies in emotion identification for own-age compared to other-age faces. Given the well-documented deficits in FER (1–3), we predicted that individuals with ASD would demonstrate poorer FER accuracy compared to controls regardless of the stimulus face age or emotion. We also predicted that individuals with ASD would demonstrate greater performance deficits across all four emotions compared to their typically developing peers, regardless of stimulus face age. Based on previous findings (11), it was predicted that adolescents without ASD would demonstrate an own-age bias. Due to conflicting evidence on whether individuals with ASD are as sensitive to visual experience with faces (27, 44, 45, 47), analyses related to how the magnitude of any observed OAB would be attenuated by ASD status and severity or differ by emotion were considered exploratory in order to support future hypothesis generation; thus, no specific predictions were made at this time.

Previous quantitative work has found that social deficits associated with ASD are not clearly diagnostically differentiable and may thus be best modeled continuously rather than categorically (48–50). This effect is well illustrated in work examining the broader autism phenotype, an occurrence of sub-clinical ASD-like traits often observed in the genetic relatives of individuals with ASD (51). Therefore, the relationships between FER and OAB were also tested against a dimensional measure of ASD symptom severity, the ADOS-2 comparison score (ADOS-2 CS). It was hypothesized that if an overall deficit in FER or magnitude of any observed OAB did not differ by diagnostic group, these measures may vary by symptom severity assessed across the full sample.

MATERIALS AND METHODS

Participants

One hundred adolescents between the ages of 11 and 14 years were recruited from the greater Long Island area (**Table 1**). Eight individuals (non-ASD $n = 1$; ASD $n = 7$) were ineligible following initial screening due to a full-scale intelligence quotient (FSIQ) <70 (presence of intellectual disability) as determined by the Kaufman Brief Intelligence Test-Second Edition (KBIT-2; 52). The remaining 92 eligible participants were assessed and classified into one of two groups: ASD ($n = 52$, 38 male) or non-ASD ($n = 40$, 25 male), using cutoffs determined by the Autism Diagnostic Observation Schedule-Second Edition (ADOS-2; 53) administered by research-reliable examiners. ADOS-2 Comparison Scores (CS) were computed for all participants as a dimensional measure of ASD symptom severity (54). Groups did not differ by age ($t(90) = .90$, $p = .37$) or IQ ($t(90) = .29$, $p = .77$). Informed consent was obtained from the guardians of all study participants and all participants assented to study procedures prior to participation. All study procedures were approved by the Institutional Review Board of Stony Brook University and conform to Common Rule standards.

TABLE 1 | Descriptive Statistics and Independent Samples t-Tests Comparing Age, Full-Scale IQ, and ADOS-2 CS Across Participants in the ASD and Non-ASD Groups.

	ASD (N = 52, 38 male)	Non-ASD (N = 40, 25 male)	t	df
Racial or Ethnic Minority (*n*, %)	7, 13.5%	10, 25%	–	–
Parental Education (*n*, %)			–	–
High School Degree	3, 5.8%	3, 7.5%		
Some College	15, 28.8%	10, 25%		
College Graduate	21, 40.4%	14, 35%		
Graduate or Professional Degree	13, 25%	13, 32.5%		
Yearly Household Income (*n*, %)			–	–
Less than $30,000	4, 7.7%	1, 2.5%		
$30,000–$75,000	6, 11.5%	7, 17.5%		
$75,000–$120,000	19, 36.5%	17, 42.5%		
$120,000–$165,000	5, 9.6%	5, 12.5%		
Greater than $165,000	14, 26.9%	8, 20.0%		
Declined to Answer	4, 7.7%	2, 5.0%		
Age (*M, SD*)	12.64, 1.10	12.85, 1.07	.90	90
Full-Scale IQ (*M, SD*)	105.67, 14.08	106.55, 14.79	.29	90
ADOS-2 CS (*M, SD*)	7.58, 2.05	1.83,.87	−16.59***	90

****p* <.001. *ADOS-2 CS, Autism Diagnostic Observation Schedule–Second Edition Comparison Score.*

Facial Emotion Recognition Task

Participants completed a computerized version of the adult and child facial expression subtests from the Diagnostic Analyses of Nonverbal Accuracy 2 (DANVA-2; 55), a standardized measure of facial emotion recognition that has been previously validated in typically developing and ASD samples (55, 56). Stimuli included 48 naturalistic color photographs of males (24) and females (24), depicting one of four emotions (12 happy, 12 sad, 12 angry, and 12 fearful, **Figure 1**). Within each subtest, presentation order of the four emotions is randomized; however, all participants viewed the photographs in the same, standardized order. All participants completed the task in a blocked fashion: adult face subtest, followed by the child face subtest. Images included in the adult subtest (24) were of individuals above the age of 18 years while images in the child subtest (24) were of individuals between the ages of 6 and 12 years. All faces were displayed in a frontal view and included the neck and torso of the individual photographed in front of either a chalkboard (the adult subtest) or a white brick wall (the child subtest).

During the task, participants were asked to view each face and make a behavioral determination of the emotion displayed (happy, sad, angry, or fearful) *via* button press. Stimulus presentation time varied from 1 to 3 s with trial advancement dependent upon participant response. In the event that a participant did not provide a response within the maximum 3 s time window, the face was removed from the screen, but the response options remained requiring the selection of a response to advance to the next trial.

Data Analytic Plan

Percent accuracy of emotion recognition for adult and child face stimuli was calculated by dividing the total number of correct responses by the total number of stimuli (24) in the subtest. In order to ensure that all participant groups were able to perform above chance, one-sample t-tests were then carried out comparing the percent accuracy of FER for adult and child faces to the chance value of 25% (1/4 possible responses) separately for both the Non-ASD and ASD groups.

To test for an OAB and any attenuation by emotion or ASD status, a 2 (face age: adult, child) × 4 (emotion: happy, sad, angry, fearful) × 2 (diagnostic group: Non-ASD, ASD) mixed-design ANOVA was calculated. Pearson's correlations were used to test for a relationship between a measure of ASD symptom severity, ADOS-2 CS, and FER accuracy across the entire sample as well as in each diagnostic group separately. Following the proposed procedures of Edwards (1994; 57), a moderated regression model was used to probe the relationship between the magnitude of the own-age bias and ASD symptom severity in each group separately and then combined. All findings with $p < .05$ were considered to be statistically significant while findings of $p = .05$ to $p = .08$ were considered marginal and reported as such.

Post-hoc power analyses were conducted using G*Power 3.1 (58, 59) to determine whether the sample size recruited was sufficient to detect main effects of diagnostic group, face age, and emotion as well as the potential two-way interactions between the three primary variables of interest. Given the expected effect

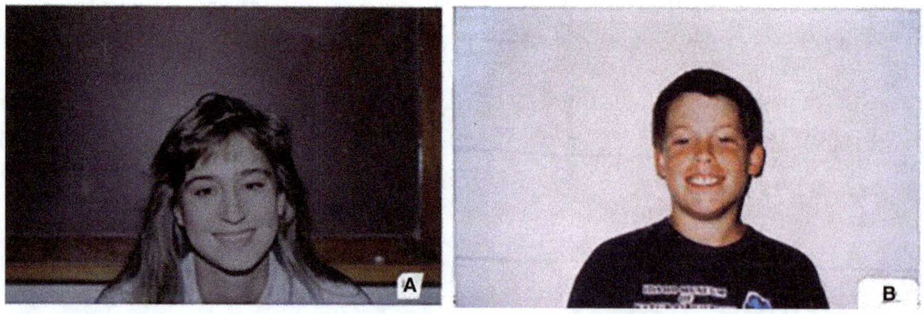

FIGURE 1 | Example images from the Diagnostic Analysis of Nonverbal Accuracy-2 depicting happy expressions from the **(A)** adult face subtest and **(B)** child face subtest.

size (d =.40) for the main effect of diagnostic status on FER task accuracy reported by Uljarevic and Hamilton (3), an alpha of.05, and sample of 92 participants, the power for main effects was at least 0.66. Assuming an equivalent medium effect size of η_p^2 = .06, an alpha of .05, and sample of 92 participants, the power to detect interaction effects was at least .99. Analyses pertaining to the three-way interaction between diagnostic groups, stimulus age, and emotion were exploratory; therefore, power analyses could not be carried out.

Shapiro-Wilk's tests of normality indicated that our primary dependent variables of interest were not normally distributed. Therefore, we ran all follow-up paired comparisons bootstrapped as well as re-tested any significant differences nonparametrically. Additionally, as the distributions of our primary variables of interest were found to be skewed, we removed outliers more than two standard deviations outside of the mean performance accuracy for either the adult or child subtest (n = 4) and re-ran all analyses with no substantial changes in findings. Results from these additionally analyses were consistent with our primary findings; therefore, in order to best represent the FER ability observed in our sample, findings reported here reflect the full sample, including identified outliers.

RESULTS

Results indicated that, regardless of diagnostic group, all adolescents performed above chance levels (ps <.05) on both the adult and child subtests of the FER task (see **Table 2**).

The three-way ANOVA testing for effects of face age, emotion, and diagnostic group indicated a main effect of face age (F(1,90) = 47.51, p <.001, η_p^2 = .35, **Figure 2**), such that all participants were more accurate in identifying child compared to adult facial expressions of emotion. A main effect of emotion was also identified (F(3,270) = 95.80, p <.001, η_p^2 = .52). *Post-hoc* pairwise comparisons using Bonferroni correction revealed an ordinal relationship of performance accuracy between the four emotions such that accuracy was greater for happy than sad (p <.001), sad than fearful (p <.001), and fearful than angry (p <.001). A main effect of diagnostic group was not identified (F(1,90) = 1.06, p =.31, η_p^2 = .01). Similarly, there was no evidence of an interaction between face age and diagnostic group (F(1,90) =.01, p =.93, η_p^2 <.001) or emotion and diagnostic group (F(3,270) = 0.66, p =.58, η_p^2 =.007). However; an interaction between face age and emotion was observed (F(3,270) = 5.77, p =.001, η_p^2 =.06, **Figure 3**). *Post-hoc* paired samples t-tests indicated that participants demonstrated greater accuracy for child compared to adult faces for happy (t (91) = 3.61, p <.001), sad (t(91) = 4.98, p <.001), and fearful (t(91) = 6.46, p <.001), but not angry faces (t(91) =.84, p =.41). Evidence for a three-way interaction between face age, emotion, and diagnostic group was not observed (F(3,270) = 0.426, p =.73, η_p^2 =.005).

Results of Person's correlations for the combined sample indicated a significant relationship between ADOS-2 CS and total FER accuracy (r(90) = −.23, p =.03) as well as child accuracy (r(90) = −.21, p =.04), but only a marginal relationship with adult accuracy (r (90) = −.20, p =.06, see **Figure 4**). When examined separately by group, child accuracy (r(38) = −.34, p =.03) but not adult accuracy (r (38) = −.16, p =.31) or overall FER accuracy (r(38) = −.27, p =.09) was significantly associated with ADOS-2 CS for the non-ASD group. Conversely, for the ASD group, ADOS-2 CS was significantly associated with overall FER accuracy (r(50) = −.32, p =.02) and marginally associated with child accuracy (r(50) = −.27, p =.052) and adult accuracy (r(50) = −.27, p =.054).

Moderated regression models predicting ADOS-2 CS from adult and child accuracy indicated that the difference between FER performance on the adult and child subtest (e.g. strength of the OAB) did not predict ASD symptom severity for the non-ASD group (B = 4.59, p =.42), ASD group (B = −5.01, p =.72), or the two groups combined (B = −21.52, p =.16).

DISCUSSION

General Discussion

The present study investigated whether a task of facial emotion recognition (FER) would elicit a performance advantage for own-age compared to other-age faces, known as an own-age bias (OAB) for individuals with and without ASD. In doing so, it was the first to explore whether the magnitude of an OAB is attenuated by ASD status or severity. Findings indicated that an

TABLE 2 | Descriptive Statistics and One-Sample t-Tests for Facial Emotion Accuracy on the DANVA-2.

	DANVA-2 Subtest	Mean Accuracy (SD)	N	Comparison Value	95% CI for Mean Difference	*t*	df
ASD	Adult Faces	72.76% (11.08)	52	.25	44.67–50.84	31.07***	51
	Adult Happy Faces	89.74% (12.42)					
	Adult Sad Faces	78.85% (24.72)					
	Adult Angry Faces	59.29% (20.46)					
	Adult Fearful Faces	63.14% (20.96)					
	Child Faces	81.41% (12.66)	52	.25	52.89–59.94	32.128***	51
	Child Happy Faces	94.55% (11.30)					
	Child Sad Faces	89.10% (14.34)					
	Child Angry Faces	63.46% (29.34)					
	Child Fearful Faces	78.53% (17.57)					
Non-ASD	Adult Faces	75.10% (12.39)	40	.25	46.14–54.07	25.57***	39
	Adult Happy Faces	89.58% (14.95)					
	Adult Sad Faces	80.83% (18.32)					
	Adult Angry Faces	61.25% (20.81)					
	Adult Fearful Faces	68.75% (20.74)					
	Child Faces	83.54% (11.40)	40	.25	54.90–62.19	32.48***	39
	Child Happy Faces	95.83% (11.79)					
	Child Sad Faces	94.17% (9.66)					
	Child Angry Faces	61.67% (26.74)					
	Child Fearful Faces	82.50% (18.47)					

****p <.001. 95% CI for Mean Difference = 95% Confidence Interval for Mean Difference. As there are four face options for every trial, ¼ (or.25) is the comparison (chance) value against which response rates are compared. DANVA-2 Adult Face Accuracy, percentage of facial emotions correctly identified on the Diagnostic Analysis of Nonverbal Accuracy–Second Edition adult subtest; DANVA-2 Child Face Accuracy, percentage of facial emotions correctly identified on the Diagnostic Analysis of Nonverbal Accuracy–Second Edition child subtest.*

OAB was elicited by the FER task for both adolescents with and without ASD and that the magnitude of the effect did not differ across groups. Similarly, overall accuracy differed ordinally by emotional expression such that recognition performance was best for happy, followed by sad, fearful, and angry. FER accuracy for individual expressions did not significantly differ by ASD group status. However, an interaction was observed between stimulus face age and emotion such that all participants demonstrated greater FER accuracy for child compared to adult faces for all emotions tested with the exception of anger. An examination of the relationship between FER accuracy and ASD symptom severity across the entire sample indicated a significant negative relationship between symptom severity and overall task accuracy as well as child accuracy, and a marginal negative relationship with adult accuracy. Follow-up analyses were all in the same direction, indicating that symptom severity was significantly associated with overall task accuracy and marginally associated with both child accuracy and adult accuracy for the ASD group. Symptom severity was significantly associated with poorer performance on only the child subtest for the non-ASD group. In line with the overall diagnostic status findings, results of a moderated regression approach indicated that the magnitude of the OAB was unrelated to ASD symptom severity in the individual groups as well as the combined sample.

In the present work, adolescents were observed to demonstrate greater performance accuracies for child

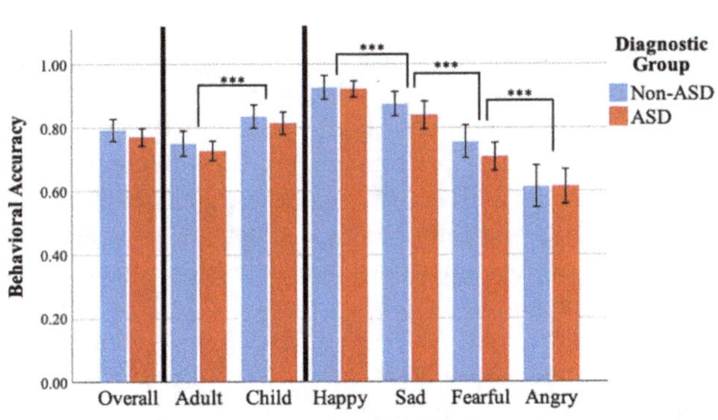

FIGURE 2 | FER percent accuracy for the non-ASD and ASD diagnostic groups on the DANVA-2 by stimulus face age and emotion. Observed main effects of face age and emotion are denoted. A stepwise relationship was observed for comparisons between emotions such that accuracy for happy was significantly greater than sad, fearful, and angry; accuracy for sad was significantly greater than fearful and angry; and accuracy for angry was significantly greater than fearful, all at the *p* <.001 level. *** *p* <.001.

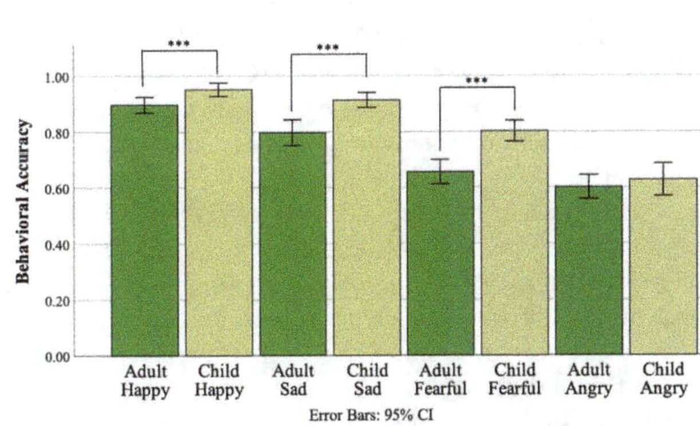

FIGURE 3 | Percent FER accuracy for the adult and child subtests of the DANVA-2 by emotion. *** *p* <.001.

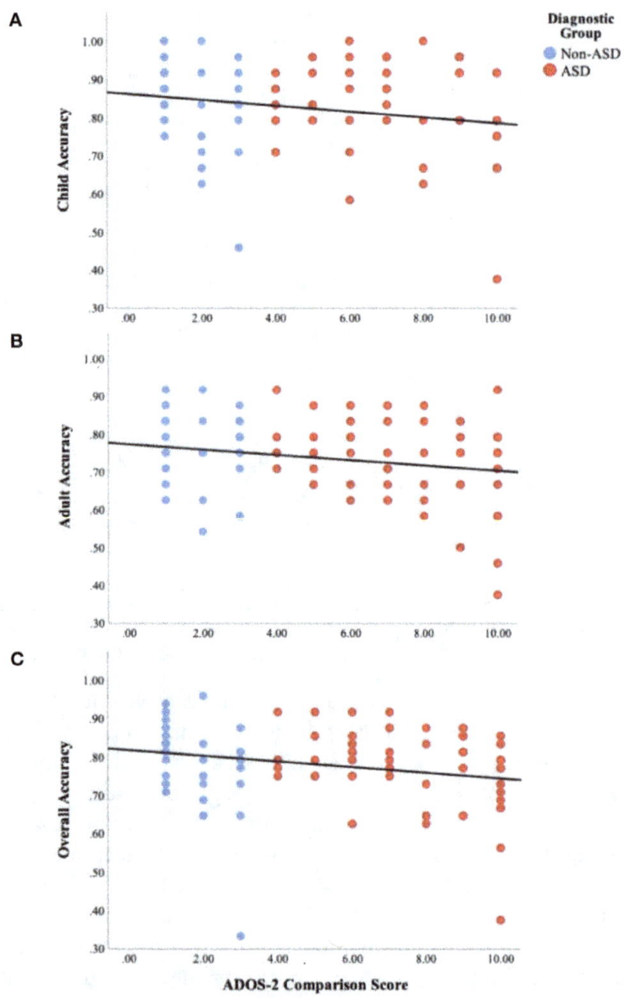

FIGURE 4 | Scatter plots displaying the relationship between ASD symptom severity, as measured by the ADOS-2 Comparison Scores, and behavioral facial emotion recognition accuracy on the **(A)** child subtest ($r(90) = -.21$, $p = .04$), **(B)** adult subtest ($r(90) = -.20$, $p = .06$), and **(C)** overall task ($r(90) = -.23$, $p = .03$).

compared to adult faces as hypothesized, regardless of ASD diagnostic status. This replicates previous findings that own-age biases are elicited by tasks of FER (10, 34), suggesting that increased contact with and exposure to peer faces during this developmental period, presumably through interactions with similarly-aged siblings, friends, and schoolmates, incurs a processing advantage for own-age faces (60). Alternatively, this processing advantage may not be due to an overall increase in visual experience with own-age faces, but rather increased social saliency and importance of peer interactions in adolescence (37, 61). Integrative accounts of the OAB, such as the categorization-individuation model (CIM; 62), posit that the processing advantage for own- compared to other-age faces reflects both an increase in perceptual expertise as well as a greater tendency to individuate, rather than categorize, faces of ingroup members. However, evidence in support of social-cognitive and integrative accounts of the OAB remains limited, with the majority of research findings substantiating experience-based accounts (11).

Interestingly, the presence of the OAB observed in this sample did not differ by ASD group. That is, adolescents with ASD demonstrated a robust performance advantage for child faces compared to adult faces that was no different than that of their peers without ASD. In conjunction with findings from the other-race effect (ORE) literature (44, 45), these results indicate that adolescents with ASD may be sensitive to both cumulative and more recent visual experience with faces.

Contrary to prediction, the diagnostic groups also did not differ on overall FER performance. Regardless of ASD status, adolescents demonstrated an ordinal relationship in their ability to accurately recognize specific emotional expressions such that performance was greatest for happy, followed by sad, fearful, and angry. This pattern of recognition accuracies replicates findings from the typical literature demonstrating that the ability to identify happy and sad facial expressions develops earlier than the ability to identify either fearful or angry facial expression (63). In addition to a main effect of expression type, an interaction between expression type and stimulus face age was also identified such that adolescents were better at identifying the expressions of child compared to adult faces for all emotions with the exception of anger. Interestingly, anger was also the expression that adolescents had the most difficulty in accurately identifying. Therefore, it may be the case that a processing advantage for own compared to other-aged faces may only become evident once a threshold level of expression specific accuracy is reached. Alternatively, this may be an artifact of the specific FER task, the DANVA-2, used in the present study.

In addition to examining differences in OAB and FER by diagnostic status, the present study also examined the impact of a continuous measure of ASD symptom severity. When diagnostic groups were combined, ASD symptom severity was found to be negatively associated with performance across the entirety of the task and the child subtest as well as marginally associated with poorer performance on the adult subtest. Although FER ability was not found to differ by diagnostic status, follow-up, group-specific correlational analyses indicated that the observed relationships between ASD symptom severity and overall performance as well as performance on the adult subtest may have been primarily driven by the ASD group. That is, ASD symptom severity was found to be significantly associated with overall task performance and marginally associated with performance on the adult subtest for individuals in the ASD group but not the non-ASD group. However, ASD symptom severity was found to be either significantly or marginally related to poorer performance on the child subtest for both individuals in the non-ASD and ASD diagnostic groups respectively. This suggests that the observed relationship between ASD symptom severity and performance on the child subtest was not primarily driven by adolescents that met diagnostic criteria for ASD. Overall, these findings replicate that of the existing literature which has identified broad deficits in FER for individuals with ASD (1–3). However, it should be noted that in the present sample impaired FER performance was only found when treating ASD symptom severity continuously, not categorically. This provides support for the argument that FER deficits associated with ASD may vary more subtly along dimensions of severity rather than being categorically distinct (48–50). It is also likely the case that measuring ASD symptom severity continuously afforded more power to detect differences in FER.

While ASD symptom severity was associated with overall FER performance, it did not predict the magnitude of the OAB (e.g. the discrepancy between performance on the child and adult subtests). This suggests that while ASD symptom severity may impact overall ability to recognize facial expressions it may not be due to an inability to incorporate more recent visual experiences into perceptual judgments. Many models of face-relevant perceptual expertise posit that exposure to exemplars of a face category results in the formation of a prototypic mental representation of that category. As exposure to a face category increases, its prototypic representation becomes more refined and more accurately reflects the distinguishing features of that category (9, 25). While these models were developed in the context of facial identity recognition tasks, it is likely the case that emotion identification also requires individuals to abstract and store prototypical representations of the basic emotions that can then be generalized across individuals.

Studies examining the development of prototype formation suggest that individuals with ASD demonstrate difficulty in abstracting prototypic representations of natural categories such as faces (27, 64, 65). If the OAB is a reflection of more refined prototypic representations for own- compared to other-age faces, then deficits in prototype formation should preclude individuals from demonstrating the effect. Findings here suggest that individuals with ASD may indeed be sensitive to increases in visual experience with own-age faces. However, given the relatively high performance accuracies observed for this task, it is possible that the impact of underlying deficits in prototype formation may only become apparent during more difficult tasks of FER (5, 18).

Limitations and Future Directions

This work is the first to explore the impact of ASD status and symptom severity on the magnitude of an OAB. As such, there are notable limitations. First, the present study did not include an adult comparison group. Although a robust OAB was observed, without an adult comparison group, the possibility that this effect was due to systematic differences between the adult and child subtests cannot be definitively eliminated. Potential task specific factors include an imbalance in the difficulty of the adult- and child-subtests, differences in perceptual features between images in each subtest (e.g. luminance, contrast, and background), and the failure to randomize presentation order of adult and child faces. However, given the extensive literature demonstrating the reliability of this bias (11, 12), we can be relatively confident that this was not, in fact, the case. The lack of an adult comparison group may have also limited our ability to identify differences in the magnitude of an OAB associated with ASD. While deficits in FER are associated with ASD across the lifespan, evidence suggests that the greatest levels of impaired performance are observed in adulthood (5, 22, 29, 30). Thus, while ASD status and symptom severity appear unrelated to the strength of an OAB for adolescents, this may not hold at older ages, when deficits in FER are more pronounced.

Second, while the stimuli in the child-face subtest overlapped our participants in age, they were not perfectly age-matched. Given that our oldest adolescents were still in middle school, it is reasonable to presume they likely encountered children of younger ages during their typical school days and through engagement in extracurricular activities or time spent with siblings. However, this presumption of increased experience with peer faces may be less true of adolescents with ASD whom may experience greater ostracization from peers (66) and/or demonstrate less selective attention to peer faces in their daily environment (67, 68). Future work should take care to match ages of participants to stimuli more precisely as well as include a direct measure of visual facial experience. Ideally, future work will also incorporate experimental training-based designs into study methodologies to allow for direct manipulations of experience with faces of a target age as well as take into account additional characteristics of the sample that may impact task performance such as overall cognitive ability and adaptive functioning.

Conclusions

Findings indicate the presence of an OAB, reflected in greater FER performance for child compared to adult faces, for adolescents, regardless of ASD diagnostic status or symptom severity. Although overall FER performance was poorer as a function of ASD symptom severity, the strength of the OAB was not influenced by either ASD categorical group membership or symptom severity. This suggests that recent visual experiences may not differentially influence the face processing abilities of adolescents with ASD and their typically developing peers. This work highlights the importance of leveraging theoretical perspectives established in the extant face processing literature on typically developing individuals in order to better understand the mechanisms underlying face processing deficits associated with ASD.

AUTHOR CONTRIBUTIONS

KH, PF, CK, and ML contributed to the conceptualization and refining of research ideas. KH, CK, and ML contributed to the acquisition of the data. KH and ML contributed to the analysis and interpretations of data. KH, PF, CK, and ML contributed to the drafting and revising of the manuscript for important intellectual content. KH, CF, and ML contributed to the creation of tables and figures. ML contributed to the creation of the research design and selection of measures. All authors contributed to manuscript revision, read and approved the submitted version.

REFERENCES

1. Harms MB, Martin A, Wallace GL. Facial emotion recognition in autism spectrum disorders: A review of behavioral and neuroimaging studies. *Neuropsychol Rev* (2010) 20(3):290–322. doi: 10.1007/s11065-010-9138-6
2. Lozier LM, Vanmeter JW, Marsh AA. Impairments in facial affect recognition associated with autism spectrum disorders: A meta-analysis. *Dev Psychopathol* (2014) 26(4pt1):933–45. doi: 10.1017/S0954579414000479
3. Uljarevic M, Hamilton A. Recognition of emotions in autism: A formal meta-analysis. *J Autism Dev Disord* (2013) 43(7):1517–26. doi: 10.1007/s10803-012-1695-5
4. Dawson G, Webb SJ, McPartland J. Understanding the nature of face processing impairment in autism: Insights from behavioral and electrophysiological studies. *Dev Neuropsychol* (2005) 27:403–24. doi: 10.1207/s15326942dn2703_6
5. Rump KM, Giovannelli JL, Minshew NJ, Strauss MS. The development of emotion recognition in individuals with autism. *Child Dev* (2009) 80:1434–47. doi: 10.1111/j.1467-8624.2009.01343.x
6. Webb SJ, Neuhaus E, Faja S. Face perception and learning in autism spectrum disorders. *Q J Exp Psychol* (2017) 70:970–86. doi: 10.1080/17470218.2016.1151059
7. Gauthier I, Nelson CA. The development of face expertise. *Curr Opin Neurobiol* (2001) 11:219–24. doi: 10.1016/S0959-4388(00)00200-2
8. Nelson CA. The Development and Neural Bases of Face Recognition. *Infant Child Dev* (2001) 10:3–18. doi: 10.1002/icd.239
9. Valentine T. A Unified Account of the Effects of Distinctiveness, Inversion, and Race in Face Recognition. *Q J Exp Psychol Sect A* (1991) 43:161–204. doi: 10.1080/14640749108400966
10. Ebner NC, Johnson MK. Young and Older Emotional Faces: Are There Age Group Differences in Expression Identification and Memory? *Emotion* (2009) 9:329–39. doi: 10.1037/a0015179
11. Rhodes MG, Anastasi JS. The own-age bias in face recognition: A meta-analytic and theoretical review. *Psychol Bull* (2012) 138:146–74. doi: 10.1037/a0025750
12. Wiese H, Komes J, Schweinberger SR. Ageing faces in ageing minds: A review on the own-age bias in face recognition. *Vis Cognit* (2013) 21:1337–63. doi: 10.1080/13506285.2013.823139
13. Jemel B, Mottron L, Dawson M. Impaired face processing in autism: Fact or artifact? *J Autism Dev Disord* (2006) 36(1):91–106. doi: 10.1007/s10803-005-0050-5
14. Ashwin C, Chapman E, Colle L, Baron-Cohen S. Impaired recognition of negative basic emotions in autism: A test of the amygdala theory. *Soc Neurosci* (2006) 1:349–63. doi: 10.1080/17470910601040772
15. Howard MA, Cowell PE, Boucher J, Broks P, Mayes A, Farrant A, et al. Convergent neuroanatomical and behavioural evidence of an amygdala hypothesis of autism. *Neuroreport* (2000) 11:2931–5. doi: 10.1097/00001756-200009110-00020
16. Pelphrey K, Sasson N, Goldman BD, Piven J. Visual Scanning of Faces in Autism Neural mechanisms of CBT for anxiety in children with autism View project Imaging studies in ASD View project. *Artic J Autism Dev Disord* (2002) 32(4):249–61. doi: 10.1023/A:1016374617369
17. Ekman P, Friesen W, Ellsworth P. *Emotion in the human face: Guidelines for research and an integration of findings* Vol. 11. (New York: Pergamon Press Inc.,) (2013).
18. Humphreys K, Minshew N, Leonard GL, Behrmann M. A fine-grained analysis of facial expression processing in high-functioning adults with autism. *Neuropsychologia* (2007) 45(4):685–95. doi: 10.1016/j.neuropsychologia.2006.08.003
19. Griffiths S, Jarrold C, Penton-Voak IS, Woods AT, Skinner AL, Munafò MR. Impaired Recognition of Basic Emotions from Facial Expressions in Young People with Autism Spectrum Disorder: Assessing the Importance of Expression Intensity. *J Autism Dev Disord* (2019) 49:2768–78. doi: 10.1007/s10803-017-3091-7
20. Aoki Y, Cortese S, Tansella M. Neural bases of atypical emotional face processing in autism: A meta-analysis of fMRI studies. *World J Biol Psychiatry* (2015) 16:291–300. doi: 10.3109/15622975.2014.957719
21. Black MH, Chen NTM, Iyer KK, Lipp OV, Bölte S, Falkmer M, et al. Mechanisms of facial emotion recognition in autism spectrum disorders: Insights from eye tracking and electroencephalography. *Neurosci Biobehav Rev* (2017) 80:488–515. doi: 10.1016/j.neubiorev.2017.06.016
22. Kang E, Keifer CM, Levy EJ, Foss-Feig JH, McPartland JC, Lerner MD. Atypicality of the N170 Event-Related Potential in Autism Spectrum Disorder: A Meta-analysis. *Biol Psychiatry Cognit Neurosci Neuroimaging* (2018) 3:657–66. doi: 10.1016/j.bpsc.2017.11.003
23. Scott LS, Monesson A. The Origin of Biases in Face Perception. *Psychol Sci* (2009) 20:676–80. doi: 10.1111/j.1467-9280.2009.02348.x
24. Tanaka J, Gauthier I. Expertise in object and face recognition. *Psychol Learn Motiv* (1997) 36:83–125. doi: 10.1016/S0079-7421(08)60282-0
25. Valentine T, Endo M. Towards an Exemplar Model of Face Processing: The Effects of Race and Distinctiveness. *Q J Exp Psychol Sect A* (1992) 44:671–703. doi: 10.1080/14640749208401305
26. Maurer D, Le Grand R, Mondloch CJ. The many faces of configural processing. *Trends Cognit Sci* (2002) 6:255–60. doi: 10.1016/S1364-6613(02)01903-4
27. Gastgeb HZ, Wilkinson DA, Minshew NJ, Strauss MS. Can individuals with autism abstract prototypes of natural faces? *J Autism Dev Disord* (2011) 41:1609–18. doi: 10.1007/s10803-011-1190-4
28. Weigelt S, Koldewyn K, Kanwisher N. Face identity recognition in autism spectrum disorders: A review of behavioral studies. *Neurosci Biobehav Rev* (2012) 36:1060–84. doi: 10.1016/j.neubiorev.2011.12.008
29. Gepner B, Deruelle C, Grynfeltt S. Motion and emotion: a novel approach to the study of face processing by young autistic children. *J Autism Dev Disord* (2001) 31(1):37–45. doi: 10.1023/A:1005609629218
30. Greimel E, Schulte-Rüther M, Kamp-Becker I, Remschmidt H, Herpertz-Dahlmann B, Konrad K. Impairment in face processing in autism spectrum disorder: A developmental perspective. *J Neural Transm* (2014) 121(9):1171–81. doi: 10.1007/s00702-014-1206-2
31. Proietti V, Pisacane A, Macchi Cassia V. Natural Experience Modulates the Processing of Older Adult Faces in Young Adults and 3-Year-Old Children. *PloS One* (2013) 8(2):e57499. doi: 10.1371/journal.pone.0057499
32. Fölster M, Werheid K. ERP evidence for own-age effects on late stages of processing sad faces. *Cognit Affect Behav Neurosci* (2016) 16:635–45. doi: 10.3758/s13415-016-0420-9
33. Harrison V, Hole GJ. Evidence for a contact-based explanation of the own-age bias in face recognition. *Psychon Bull Rev* (2009) 16:264–9. doi: 10.3758/PBR.16.2.264
34. Riediger M, Voelkle MC, Ebner NC, Lindenberger U. Beyond "Happy, angry, or sad?": Age-of-poser and age-of-rater effects on multi-dimensional emotion perception. *Cognit Emot* (2011) 25:968–82. doi: 10.1080/02699931.2010.540812
35. Ebner NC, He Y, Johnson MK. Age and emotion affect how we look at a face: Visual scan patterns differ for own-age versus other-age emotional faces. *Cognit Emot* (2011) 25:983–97. doi: 10.1080/02699931.2010.540817
36. Ebner NC, Johnson MK, Fischer H. Neural mechanisms of reading facial emotions in young and older adults. *Front Psychol* (2012) 3:223. doi: 10.3389/fpsyg.2012.00223
37. He Y, Ebner NC, Johnson MK. What predicts the own-age bias in face recognition memory? *Soc Cognit* (2011) 29:97–109. doi: 10.1521/soco.2011.29.1.97
38. Hills PJ, Willis SFL. Children view own-age faces qualitatively differently to other-age faces. *J Cognit Psychol* (2016) 28:601–10. doi: 10.1080/20445911.2016.1164710
39. Proietti V, Macchi Cassia V, dell'Amore F, Conte S, Bricolo E. Visual scanning behavior is related to recognition performance for own- and other-age faces. *Front Psychol* (2015) 6:1684. doi: 10.3389/fpsyg.2015.01684
40. Ebner NC, Johnson MR, Rieckmann A, Durbin KA, Johnson MK, Fischer H. Processing own-age vs. other-age faces: Neuro-behavioral correlates and effects of emotion. *Neuroimage* (2013) 78:363–71. doi: 10.1016/j.neuroimage.2013.04.029
41. Macchi Cassia V. Age biases in face processing: The effects of experience across development. *Br J Psychol* (2011) 102:816–29. doi: 10.1111/j.2044-8295.2011.02046.x
42. Macchi Cassia V, Bulf H, Quadrelli E, Proietti V. Age-related face processing bias in infancy: Evidence of perceptual narrowing for adult faces. *Dev Psychobiol* (2014) 56:238–48. doi: 10.1002/dev.21191
43. Meissner CA, Brigham JC. Thirty Years of Investigating the Own-Race Bias in Memory for Faces: A Meta-Analytic Review. *Psychol Public Pol Law* (2001) 7:3–35. doi: 10.1037/1076-8971.7.1.3

44. Wilson CE, Palermo R, Burton AM, Brock J. Recognition of own- and other-race faces in autism spectrum disorders. *Q J Exp Psychol* (2011) 64:1939–54. doi: 10.1080/17470218.2011.603052
45. Yi L, Quinn PC, Feng C, Li J, Ding H, Lee K. Do individuals with autism spectrum disorder process own- and other-race faces differently? *Vision Res* (2015) 107:124–32. doi: 10.1016/j.visres.2014.11.021
46. Chien SHL, Wang LH, Chen CC, Chen TY, Chen HS. Autistic children do not exhibit an own-race advantage as compared to typically developing children. *Res Autism Spectr Disord* (2014) 8(11):1544–51. doi: 10.1016/j.rasd.2014.08.005
47. Hadad BS, Schwartz S, Binur N. Reduced perceptual specialization in autism: Evidence from the other-race face effect. *J Exp Psychol Gen* (2019) 148:588–94. doi: 10.1037/xge0000550
48. Constantino JN. The quantitative nature of autistic social impairment. *Pediatr Res* (2011) 69(8):55–62. doi: 10.1203/PDR.0b013e318212ec6e
49. Constantino JN, Gruber CP, Davis S, Hayes S, Passanante N, Przybeck T. The factor structure of autistic traits. *J Child Psychol Psychiatry* (2004) 45:719–26. doi: 10.1111/j.1469-7610.2004.00266.x
50. Robinson EB, Munir K, Munaf MR, Hughes M, McCormick MC, Koenen KC. Stability of autistic traits in the general population: Further evidence for a continuum of impairment. *J Am Acad Child Adolesc Psychiatry* (2011) 50:376–84. doi: 10.1016/j.jaac.2011.01.005
51. Wilson CE, Freeman P, Brock J, Burton AM, Palermo R. Facial identity recognition in the broader autism phenotype. *PloS One* (2010) 5:1–7. doi: 10.1371/journal.pone.0012876
52. Kaufman AS. Kaufman Brief Intelligence Test–Second Edition (KBIT-2). *Circ Pines MN Am Guid Serv* (2004).
53. Lord C, Rutter M, DiLavore P, Risi S, Gotham K, Bishop S. Autism diagnostic observation schedule–2nd edition (ADOS-2). *Los Angeles CA West Psychol Corp* (2012).
54. Hus V, Lord C. The autism diagnostic observation schedule, module 4: revised algorithm and standardized severity scores. *J Autism Dev Disord* (2014) 44:1996–2012. doi: 10.1007/s10803-014-2080-3
55. Nowicki S, Duke, MP. Manual for the receptive tests of the diagnostic analysis of nonverbal accuracy 2 (DANVA2). Atlanta, GA: Department of Psychology, Emory University (2008).
56. Booth AJ, Rodgers JD, Volker MA, Lopata C, Thomeer ML. Psychometric Characteristics of the DANVA-2 in High-Functioning Children with ASD. *J Autism Dev Disord* (2019) 49(10):4147–58. doi: 10.1007/s10803-019-04130-w
57. Edwards JR. Regression analysis as an alternative to difference scores. *J Manag Stud* (1994) 20(3):683–9. doi: 10.1177/014920639402000311
58. Faul F, Erdfelder E, Lang AG, Buchner A. G*Power 3: A flexible statistical power analysis program for the social, behavioral, and biomedical sciences. *Behav Res Methods* (2007) 39:175–91. doi: 10.3758/BF03193146
59. Erdfelder E, FAul F, Buchner A, Lang AG. Statistical power analyses using G*Power 3.1: Tests for correlation and regression analyses. *Behav Res Methods* (2009) 41:1149–60. doi: 10.3758/BRM.41.4.1149
60. Hills PJ, Lewis MB. Rapid communication: The own-age face recognition bias in children and adults. *Q J Exp Psychol* (2011) 64:17–23. doi: 10.1080/17470218.2010.537926
61. Sporer SL. Recognizing Faces of Other Ethnic Groups: An Integration of Theories. *Psychol Public Pol Law* (2001) 7:36–97. doi: 10.1037/1076-8971.7.1.36
62. Hugenberg K, Young SG, Bernstein MJ, Sacco DF. The Categorization-Individuation Model: An Integrative Account of the Other-Race Recognition Deficit. *Psychol Rev* (2010) 117:1168–87. doi: 10.1037/a0020463
63. Durand K, Gallay M, Seigneuric A, Robichon F, Baudouin JY. The development of facial emotion recognition: The role of configural information. *J Exp Child Psychol* (2007) 97:14–27. doi: 10.1016/j.jecp.2006.12.001
64. Gastgeb HZ, Rump KM, Best CA, Minshew NJ, Strauss MS. Prototype formation in autism: Can individuals with autism abstract facial prototypes? *Autism Res* (2009) 2:279–84. doi: 10.1002/aur.93
65. Klinger LG, Dawson G. Prototype formation in autism. *Dev Psychopathol* (2001) 13:111–24. doi: 10.1017/S0954579401001080
66. Schroeder JH, Cappadocia MC, Bebko JM, Pepler DJ, Weiss JA. Shedding light on a pervasive problem: A review of research on bullying experiences among children with autism spectrum disorders. *J Autism Dev Disord* (2014) 44:1520–34. doi: 10.1007/s10803-013-2011-8
67. Wilson CE, Brock J, Palermo R. Attention to social stimuli and facial identity recognition skills in autism spectrum disorder. *J Intellect Disabil Res* (2010) 54:1104–15. doi: 10.1111/j.1365-2788.2010.01340.x
68. Chita-tegmark M. Research in Developmental Disabilities Review article Social attention in ASD : A review and meta-analysis of eye-tracking studies. *Res Dev Disabil* (2016) 48:79–93. doi: 10.1016/j.ridd.2015.10.011

14

Interactive Psychometrics for Autism with the Human Dynamic Clamp: Interpersonal Synchrony from Sensorimotor to Sociocognitive Domains

Florence Baillin[1,2†], *Aline Lefebvre*[1,2†], *Amandine Pedoux*[2], *Yann Beauxis*[1], *Denis A. Engemann*[3], *Anna Maruani*[2], *Frédérique Amsellem*[2], *J. A. Scott Kelso*[4,5], *Thomas Bourgeron*[1], *Richard Delorme*[1,2†] and *Guillaume Dumas*[1,4,6,7*†]

[1] Human Genetics and Cognitive Functions, Institut Pasteur, UMR3571 CNRS, Université de Paris, Paris, France, [2] Child and Adolescent Psychiatry Department, Robert Debré Hospital, Paris, France, [3] Parietal Project-Team, INRIA Saclay – Île de France, Palaiseau, France, [4] Human Brain and Behavior Laboratory, Center for Complex Systems and Brain Sciences, Florida Atlantic University, Boca Raton, FL, United States, [5] Intelligent Systems Research Centre, University of Ulster, Derry Londonderry, United Kingdom, [6] Department of Psychiatry, Université de Montréal, Montreal, QC, Canada, [7] CHU Sainte-Justine Centre de Recherche, Precision Psychiatry and Social Physiology Laboratory, Montreal, QC, Canada

Correspondence:
Guillaume Dumas
guillaume.dumas@centraliens.net

† These authors have contributed equally to this work

The human dynamic clamp (HDC) is a human–machine interface designed on the basis of coordination dynamics for studying realistic social interaction under controlled and reproducible conditions. Here, we propose to probe the validity of the HDC as a psychometric instrument for quantifying social abilities in children with autism spectrum disorder (ASD) and neurotypical development. To study interpersonal synchrony with the HDC, we derived five standardized scores following a gradient from sensorimotor and motor to higher sociocognitive skills in a sample of 155 individuals (113 participants with ASD, 42 typically developing participants; aged 5 to 25 years; IQ > 70). Regression analyses were performed using normative modeling on global scores according to four subconditions (HDC behavior "cooperative/competitive," human task "in-phase/anti-phase," diagnosis, and age at inclusion). Children with ASD had lower scores than controls for motor skills. HDC motor coordination scores were the best candidates for stratification and diagnostic biomarkers according to exploratory analyses of hierarchical clustering and multivariate classification. Independently of phenotype, sociocognitive skills increased with developmental age while being affected by the ongoing task and HDC behavior. Weaker performance in ASD for motor skills suggests the convergent validity of the HDC for evaluating social interaction. Results provided additional evidence of a relationship between sensorimotor and sociocognitive skills. HDC may also be used as a marker of maturation of sociocognitive skills during real-time social interaction. Through its standardized and objective evaluation, the HDC not only represents a valid paradigm for the study of interpersonal synchrony but also offers a promising, clinically relevant psychometric instrument for the evaluation and stratification of sociomotor dysfunctions.

Keywords: computational psychiatry, human-machine interface (HMI), psychometric, interpersonal synchrony, autism spectrum disorder, coordination dynamics

INTRODUCTION

Autism spectrum disorder (ASD) is a complex neurodevelopmental disorder (1) defined by the co-occurrence of social communication problems, repetitive behaviors, and restricted interests. The prevalence of ASD has increased in recent years from <1 in 1,000 individuals to 1 in 58 (2, 3). With different levels of severity of symptoms, ASD is highly heterogeneous, both phenotypically (4) and genetically (5). More than 50% of patients suffer from at least four other psychiatric comorbid conditions (6). This strong heterogeneity complicates the development of psychometric assessment tools that allow for a personalized and thorough evaluation of a child's skills (7). Identification of robust, valid, and quantitative biomarkers of social communication disability, a key symptom of ASD, is thus a major societal challenge for improving early diagnosis and individualized care.

As a keystone of social communication, interpersonal synchrony (IS) is a fundamental aspect to explore in order to better understand and apprehend ASD. IS can be defined as a rhythmic matching of actions in time and in phase with another person based on nonverbal behaviors (8). IS comprises multiple components, involving sociocognitive, sensory motor, and motor skills, as well as adaptive capacities (9, 10). At the behavioral level, IS can be measured through microlevel detection of bonding-related behaviors (11), frame-by-frame analysis of video (12), or even using machine learning tools (13).

In this context, the human dynamic clamp (HDC) is a new paradigm of human–machine interaction based on the science of coordination (coordination dynamics) that enables the study of the neurobehavioral processes involved in IS (14–16). Controlled using empirically grounded models of coordination dynamics (17), the HDC allows a dynamic bidirectional interaction in real time between a human and a virtual avatar. The HDC paradigm has already been validated empirically in adults (15, 18, 19). Using high-resolution electroencephalography, it recently revealed how distributed neural dynamics integrate information from "low-level" sensorimotor mechanisms and "high-level" sociocognitive processes such as intention attribution or judgment of humanness (18). Using skin potential responses, we demonstrated that HDC is able to induce emotional reaction, especially when human participants believed that their partner was human and when movement coordination was stable (19). Finally, we also introduced the virtual teacher (VT) configuration that allows human participants to change their behavioral repertoire by internalizing new interpersonal coordination patterns (e.g., nontrivial relative phase between movements of the two interacting partners), thereby opening possibilities of applying HDC to rehabilitation (15).

IS seems to be substantially impaired in children and adolescents with ASD (20, 21). A few studies among children (6–11 years old) (22) and adolescents (10–16.5 years old) (23) have explored IS in automated motion analysis to quantify movements of body parts. Still, the exploratory paradigms are mainly rhythmic in children with ASD (3.5–10 years old) (24–27) and in adolescents (12–17 years old) (28, 29). However, even if children with ASD face difficulties in movement coordination during a social exchange, social embodiment seems preserved and appears to correlate with social cognitive ability (22).

One hypothesis currently under investigation suggests that motor and sensory motor skill development are linked to social cognition and cognitive development (25, 30). ASD is frequently found to be associated with difficulties in attributing mental states to oneself and to others (31), where intention attribution is characterized by an appraisal based on the intention underlying someone else's action (32). In addition to primary dysfunctions in social communication skills, deficits in perceptual–motor performance are found in between 50 and 80% of children diagnosed with ASD (moving with awareness, integrated self, proprioceptive feedback, visuo-perceptual performance, sensory integration) (23, 25, 33–37). About 80% also show motor skill impairments such as praxis, basic motor control, postural control, gait abnormalities, motor coordination, manual dexterity, gross and fine motor skills, and gestures in complex movement sequences (20, 25, 38).

Interventions targeting the development of IS are promising and show evidence for plasticity (39–41). Early detection and intervention directly focusing on the development of IS showed preliminary evidence of positive effects on motor and communication skills (42), especially later in both language and social abilities (39). Such evidence supports IS as a potent tool for the diagnosis and care of ASD children.

Up to now, language, cognitive ability, social engagement, and motor skills have emerged as the most robust predictors of ASD among toddlers (43–45) and during childhood and adolescence (46). Thus, early dysfunction in IS could have cascading consequences and even participate in explaining the heterogeneity of ASD. Such observations reflect the difficulty of assessment by means of reliable and age-scalable markers of IS and the need for personalized analysis [as has been done, for example, in studies of skill learning, cf. (47)].

In the present work, we first validate how the HDC measures different behavioral processes involved in social dynamic interactions in children with neurotypical development, and then evaluate how the HDC can assess IS alterations in children with ASD. A secondary objective is to standardize the test and develop indicators that measure and identify sociocognitive and sensorimotor markers. In order to highlight the specific heterogeneity of ASD compared to typical neurodevelopment, developmental trajectories are integrated into our analysis using normative modeling (48), and HDC behavioral measures are tested as reproducible and reliable clinical markers.

METHODS

Sample

We enrolled in the study a sample of 156 individuals composed of 114 participants with ASD and 42 participants with typical development (**Table 1**). All participants were recruited at the Child Psychiatry Department of the Robert Debré University Hospital, Paris (France).

Patients with ASD were included after a systematic clinical and medical examination, including negative blood test results for Fragile-X and the exclusion of participants carrying a

TABLE 1 | Demographic and clinical characteristics of the participants enrolled in the study.

	Children with ASD ($n = 113$)	Children with typical development ($n = 42$)	Group test; p value
Gender (m/f)	96/18	25/17	$\chi^2 = 9.37$; $p = 0.002$
Age at inclusion	11.2 ± 3.2	16 ± 4.4	$t = -7.51$; $p = 4.6e-12$
SRS *t* score	74.2 ± 12	45 ± 5.4	$t = 14.20$; $p = 1.5e-28$
Full-scale intellectual quotient	101.2 ± 18.5	107.4 ± 13.2	$t = -1.88$; $p = 0.06$
Right handedness	92/21	38/11	$\chi^2 = 1.47$; $p = 0.23$

Mean values and respective standard deviations for continuous variables. n, sample size; ASD, autism spectrum disorder; IQ, intellectual quotient; SRS t score, Social Responsiveness Scale t score.

large deletion over 2 Mb as detected by the Illumina 700 SNPs array. The final diagnosis of ASD was based on DSM-5 criteria and outcomes from the Autism Diagnostic Observation Schedule-Second Edition (ADOS-II) (49), the Autism Diagnostic Interview-Revised (ADI-R) (50), and the Social Responsiveness Scale—2nd edition (SRS-2) (51) for the dimensional diagnosis of social skills and data from experts in the field. Intellectual functioning for all participants was estimated using the Wechsler Intelligence Scale for Children and Adolescents—5th edition (WISC-V) (52). The current threshold for intellectual disability (i.e., IQ <70) was used, following international standards (DSM-5). Among participants, 14 children (controls = 2, ASD = 12) were below 85 and 33 (controls = 14, ASD = 19) were above 115. Participants with normal neurotypical development were from the general population and reported no personal or familial history of ASD or axis I psychiatric conditions requiring specific needs.

An assessment of dexterity and motor coordination of hands and fingers was made using the Purdue Pegboard (53). For the present study, we used the versions with charts defined on a population aged 5 to 15 years 11 months and beyond the age of 16 years (54, 55). Only the "preferred hand score," viz. place the most items using the preferred hand in a row in 30 s, was conserved. A *z* score was calculated according to age and gender. Children were also assessed with the Child Neuropsychological Assessment—second edition (NEPSY-II) (56) to specifically explore affect recognition (AF) and theory of mind (TOM).

The research was carried out in accordance with the recommendations of the local ethics committee of Hospital Robert Debré. All the parents of participants gave written informed consent in accordance with the Declaration of Helsinki. The protocol was approved by the INSERM Ethics Committee (study approval no. 08-029).

The Human Dynamic Clamp Paradigm

The HDC system (14–16) is a human-machine interface consisting of three parts: (1) a sensor measuring the movement of the participant's index finger which is fed into (2) a mathematical model integrating the position and velocity of the human's movement to simulate in real time [*via* the HKB model; (57)] the behavior of a virtual partner or avatar and 3) a screen facing the participant where the resulting finger movements of the virtual partner (VP) appear as a human hand. The HDC software computes in real time the corresponding position of the VP (**Figure 1**). At the beginning of each trial, an instruction was given to the participant to synchronize her/his movement in-phase (i.e., synchronize her/his movements to those of the VP) or anti-phase (i.e., synchronize her/his movements with a half-period offset with the VP's phase). In this experiment, while the partner is a virtual partner throughout, all participants were instructed that half the time the partner is virtual (i.e., movements are computer-driven) and half the time the partner is a real sex- and age-matched human performing the same task in another room of the hospital. The protocol was composed of 40 trials, divided into four blocks. The instructions to the participant stayed the same within each block. The instruction for the first block was randomly assigned at the beginning of the experiment. During the trials, the VP could adopt a "cooperative" or "competitive" behavior, meaning that it shares the same goal or the opposite goal to the one assigned to the participant (i.e., VP aims to move its finger in in-phase coordination when the participant aims to move his finger in anti-phase and vice versa, exactly as if the partner was not cooperating with but in opposition to the participant). Behavior of the VP was randomized across all trials, disregarding block structure. At the end of each trial, the participant was asked if s/he felt like s/he was playing with a human or a VP and to quantify the level of cooperativeness or competitiveness of the partner (see also 88).

HDC Behavioral Measures

In the present study, five normalized scores (between 0 and 1, 0 being the worst) of the HDC paradigm were automatically aimed at evaluating dimensions of social cognition, ranging from sensory motor to representational aspects: (1) a motor score which measures the difference of amplitude of imitative gestures between the participant and the VP; (2) a coordination score which corresponds to the temporal index of imitation; (3) a task score which is based on how well the ongoing relative phase of the VP and the participant match, taking into account the task condition; (4) an intention score which evaluates the ability

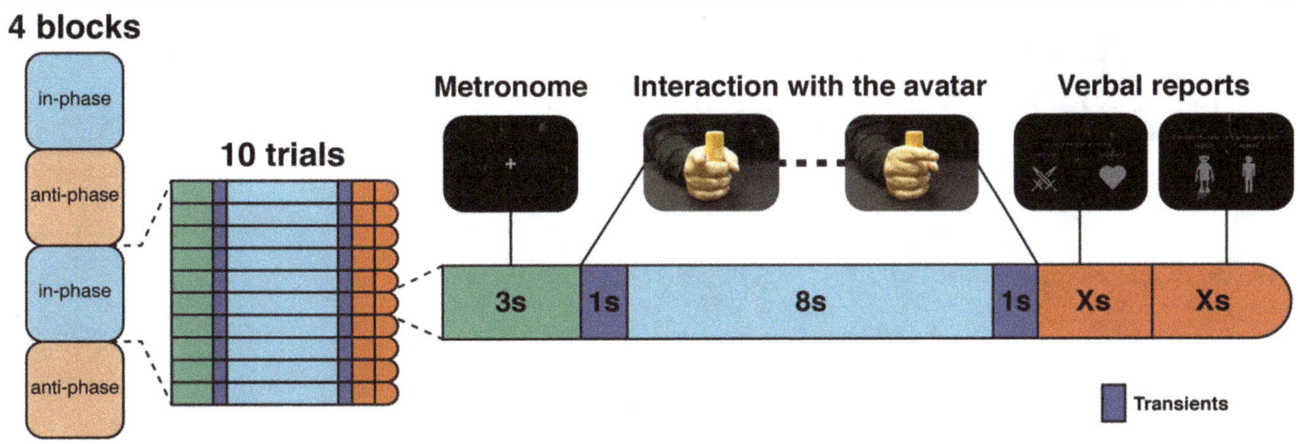

FIGURE 1 | Experimental design. Structure of the protocol with four blocks alternating "in-phase/anti-phase." Each block is divided into 10 trials (left). Each trial starts with the participant instructed to synchronize with the sound of a metronome for 3 s. Then, the participant interacts with the avatar according to the instruction (e.g., "in-phase"). At the end of the trial, two questions appear directly on the screen. First, the impression of the participant on the competitive or cooperative behavior of the avatar, and second regarding the humanness of the avatar (right). Shown are screenshots of what participants could see (top). In-phase refers to synchronized movements using homologous muscles of the limbs and anti-phase to alternating movements (180° out of phase). Cooperative and competitive refer respectively to the behavior of the virtual partner when it has shared or conflicting goals with the human participant.

of the participant to properly attribute intention toward the "cooperative" or "competitive" behavior of the VP; and (5) a humanness score which reflects quantitatively the impression of the participant on the human or robotic character of the partner (see **Supplementary Material** for more details).

Data Analysis Using Normative Modeling

All statistical data analyses were performed using Python 3.7 (58) [numpy 1.17.2 (59, 60) and scipy 1.3.1 (61)]. Normative modeling (NM) provides a metric similar to a z score, but accounts for the underlying structure of the population across multiple covariates. NM uses Gaussian processes (GP) to model the distribution of control group measures while estimating separately the overall trajectory in the covariate space, the heterogeneity in the population, and the uncertainty of the fit (62). The Python code is available in open access at https://github.com/GHFC/SoNeTAA/.

RESULTS

Sociodemographic and Group Comparative Analyses

Overall, participants with ASD were younger than the control group [$t(154) = 2.6$, $p = 2.6\text{e-}11$], with a larger male/female ratio (Fisher exact, $p = 0.002$) than the control group. No statistically significant differences were found for IQ and handedness. As expected, the group with ASD scored higher in the SRS [$t(154) = 14.3$, $p = 7.4\text{e-}29$]. No statistically significant differences were found for IQ and handedness. The group with ASD scored lower on all the standardized psychometric instruments assessing social skills: NEPSY-II TOM total score (Mann–Whitney $U = 104.5$, $p = 0.0005$), NEPSY-II AF raw ($U = 114$, $p = 0.0017$), and the Purdue Pegboard, the validated task assessing motor coordination skills ($U = 138$, $p = 0.0006$).

Developmental Trajectories of HDC Scores

Within the entire cohort (both groups of participants with ASD and with typical development), a developmental trajectory was found with a statistically significant correlation of age with task comprehension ($r = 0.33$; $p = 2.7\text{e-}05$) (**Figure 2A**), intention attribution ($r = 0.30$; $p = 0.00011$) (**Figure 2B**), and humanness ($r = 0.27$; $p = 0.00057$) (**Figure 2C**). Only a few children with ASD diagnosis answered systematically the same rating of humanness across the whole experiment ($N = 3$ always human, i.e., humanness score $= 1$; $N = 3$ always robot, i.e., humanness score $= 0$). A significant interaction was observed between chronological age and comprehension score only in the control group ($r = 0.40$; $p = 0.0084$) (**Figure 2A**) (the older the participant is, the better the skills are) and with intention attribution ($r = 0.21$; $p = 0.024$) and humanness ($r = 0.38$; $p = 3.8\text{e-}0.5$) in the group with ASD.

Comparison With Standardized Tests Using Normative Models

Using normative modeling allows us to correct any developmental bias on the HDC scores. We were then able to observe how these "age-controlled HDC scores" related to standard neuropsychological tests (**Table 2**).

We observed a significant interaction effect between the SRS-2 and motor score ($r = -0.22$; $p = 0.01$) (**Figure 3A**); high SRS scores (in favor of the diagnosis of ASD) are correlated with low motor scores. The NEPSY-II test showed a significant interaction effect between AF score and the HDC task comprehension score ($r = 0.33$; $p = 0.02$) (**Figure 3B**); good skills in the AF task of the NEPSY-II are associated with good scores at the HDC task comprehension score. The **Supplementary Data Sheet** contain the details of the correlation per group, along with the HDC scores before normative modeling correction.

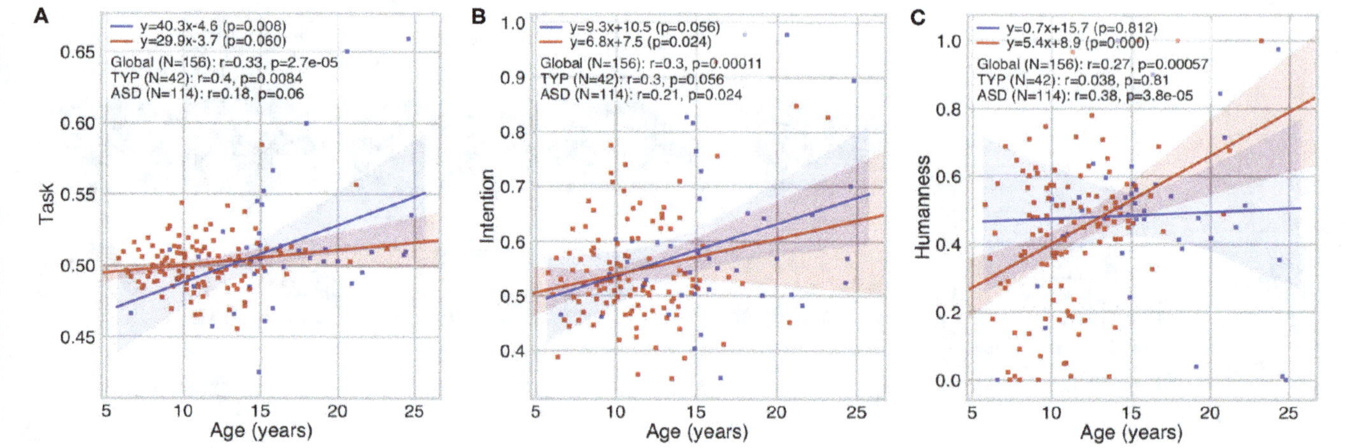

FIGURE 2 | Developmental aspect of higher-level correlates of interpersonal synchrony (IS). Correlations between age at inclusion and task comprehension **(A)**, intention attribution **(B)**, and humanness **(C)** scores. The three scores show a remarkable positive correlation with age, suggesting a developmental trajectory of sociocognitive skills. No outliers were removed.

TABLE 2 | Summary of the main correlations between HDC scores and those from the NEPSY-II [affect recognition (AF) and theory of mind (TOM) subdomains], the Social Responsiveness Scale—second edition (SRS-2), and the Purdue Pegboard.

	Motor (NM)	Coordination (NM)	Task (NM)	Intention (NM)	Humanness (NM)
SRS-2	$r = -0.22$; $p = 0.01$*	$r = 0.0031$; $p = 0.97$	$r = -0.22$; $p = 0.0086$	$r = -0.15$; $p = 0.076$	$r = -0.045$; $p = 0.6$
NEPSY-II TOM	$r = -0.081$; $p = 0.59$	$r = -0.35$; $p = 0.016$*	$r = -0.26$; $p = 0.08$	$r = 0.17$; $p = 0.24$	$r = -0.09$; $p = 0.55$
NEPSY-II AF	$r = 0.2$; $p = 0.18$	$r = -0.043$; $p = 0.78$	$r = 0.33$; $p = 0.023$*	$r = 0.16$; $p = 0.3$	$r = 0.11$; $p = 0.48$
Purdue Pegboard	$r = 0.14$; $p = 0.31$	$r = -0.2$; $p = 0.16$	$r = -0.015$; $p = 0.91$	$r = -0.25$; $p = 0.07$	$r = 0.13$; $p = 0.34$

*$p < 0.05$.

Global Comparative Analysis Between Participants With ASD and Typical Development Groups Using Normative Models

Comparative analysis between the two groups revealed a statistically significant decrease of the motor score ($d = -0.5$; $p = 0.0029$) in individuals with an ASD diagnosis compared with individuals with typical development. We also observed evidence of better understanding of the task among participants with ASD diagnosis compared with those with typical development ($d = 0.23$; $p = 0.0077$). Interactions between the two groups for the other scores (coordination: $d = -0.21$, $p = 0.12$; intention: $d = -0.12$, $p = 0.49$; humanness: $d = 0.12$, $p = 0.19$) were not significant (**Figure 4**).

HDC Scores Analysis by Subconditions

Different subconditions are associated with the HDC paradigm: the diagnosis, the age, the avatar behavior, and the humanness or robotic character of the HDC (see **Figure 5** for a summary). Multiple regression was thus calculated to predict the different normalized HDC scores based on the diagnosis (coded as 0 = ASD and 1 = CTR), age (in years), avatar behavior (coded as 0 = competitive and 1 = cooperative), and the humanness or robotic character discrimination task (coded as 0 = anti-phase and 1 = in-phase).

We found a significant regression equation for the motor score [$F_{(5, 618)} = 7.634$, $p = 5.64\text{e-}07$]. Both the diagnostic and the human task were significant predictors of the motor score, with the control group having higher scores (coeff = 0.44, $p < 0.001$), as well as the in-phase task (coeff = 0.27, $p = 0.016$). There was also a significant regression equation for the coordination score [$F_{(5, 618)} = 3.252$, $p = 0.006$], with age, as might be expected, a significant predictor (coeff = 0.0272, $p = 0.02$). A significant regression equation for task score [$F_{(5, 618)} = 409.1$, $p = 2.42\text{e-}193$] revealed that avatar behavior was a significant predictor, with a cooperative behavior of the VP having a huge effect on the task comprehension of participants (coeff = 6.96, $p < 0.001$). Further analysis of a significant regression equation for the intention score [$F_{(5, 618)} = 28.84$, $p = 2.46\text{e-}26$] showed that

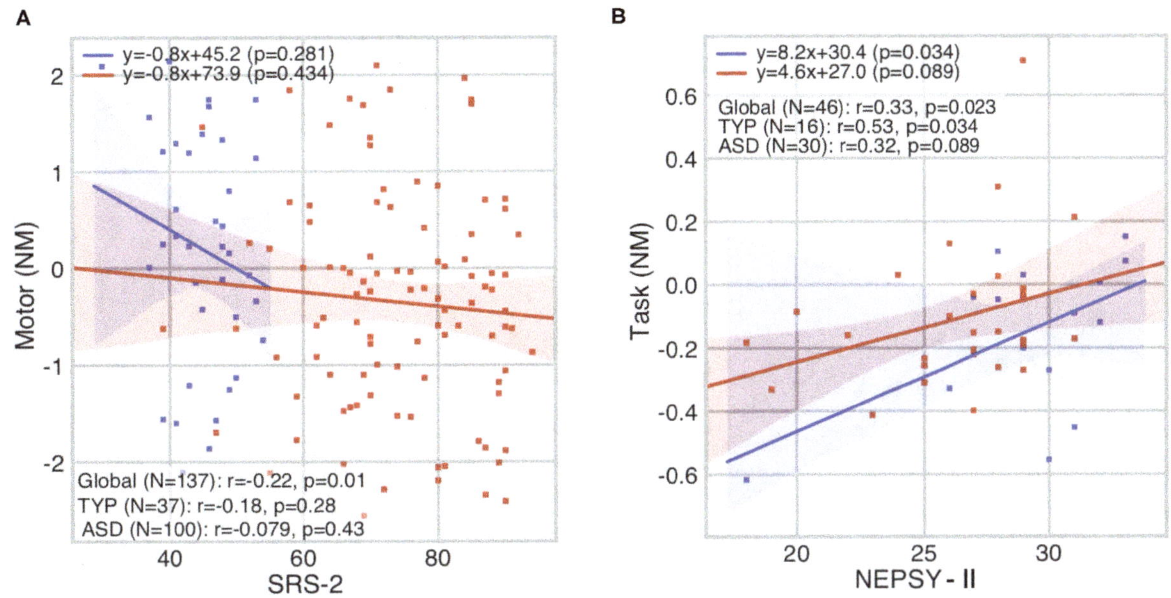

FIGURE 3 | Significant correlations between sociocognitive and motor skills in children with (in red) autism spectrum disorder (ASD) or with typical development (TYP) (in blue): **(A)** SRS-2 vs. motor score: a dimensional diagnosis of ASD correlates with lower levels of motor skills; and **(B)** NEPSY-II affect recognition (AF) vs. HDC task score: greater cognitive abilities correlate with higher levels of affect recognition skill; NM, normative models.

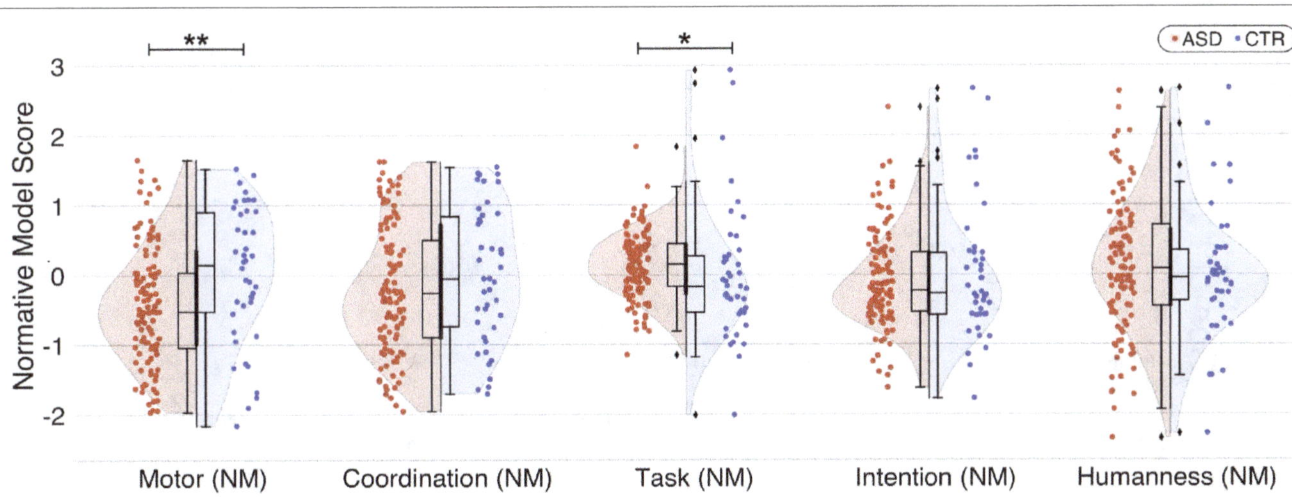

FIGURE 4 | Comparison between the two groups with ASD and typical development for different behavioral scores derived from the HDC protocol and corrected with normative modeling (NM). Only the motor score really discriminates between the two populations ($d = -0.5$; $p < 0.005$**), with significantly lower results among ASD. The lines represent linear regressions. Colored areas: 95% confidence intervals (CI). Neurotypical participants: blue; participants with ASD: red. *$p < 0.05$; **$p < 0.005$.

both human task and avatar behavior were significant predictors of VP intention. Participants tended to better detect the intention of the VP while "anti-phase" (coeff $= -1.27$, $p < 0.001$), and "in-phase" if the VP takes on a cooperative behavior (coeff $= 2.31$, $p < 0.001$).

For the motor score, detailed analysis indicates that during both VP "cooperative" ("in-phase": $d = -0.51$; $p = 0.006$ and "anti-phase": $d = -0.59$; $p = 0.002$) and "competitive" behavior ("in-phase": $d = -0.34$; $p = 0.025$ and "anti-phase": $d = -0.35$; $p = 0.025$), the task allows to distinguish the two groups (cf. **Table 3**).

DISCUSSION

Aim of the Study

The main objective of the study was to identify which HDC scores distinguish our two populations of children with and without a diagnosis of ASD and, thus, provide potential predictors of the condition. A particularly interesting aspect is that our results show the motor score discriminates between the two groups. Motor abnormalities in the disorder are widely described. However, they are still currently little taken into account in the diagnosis. As a reminder, the HDC is validated in adults as an

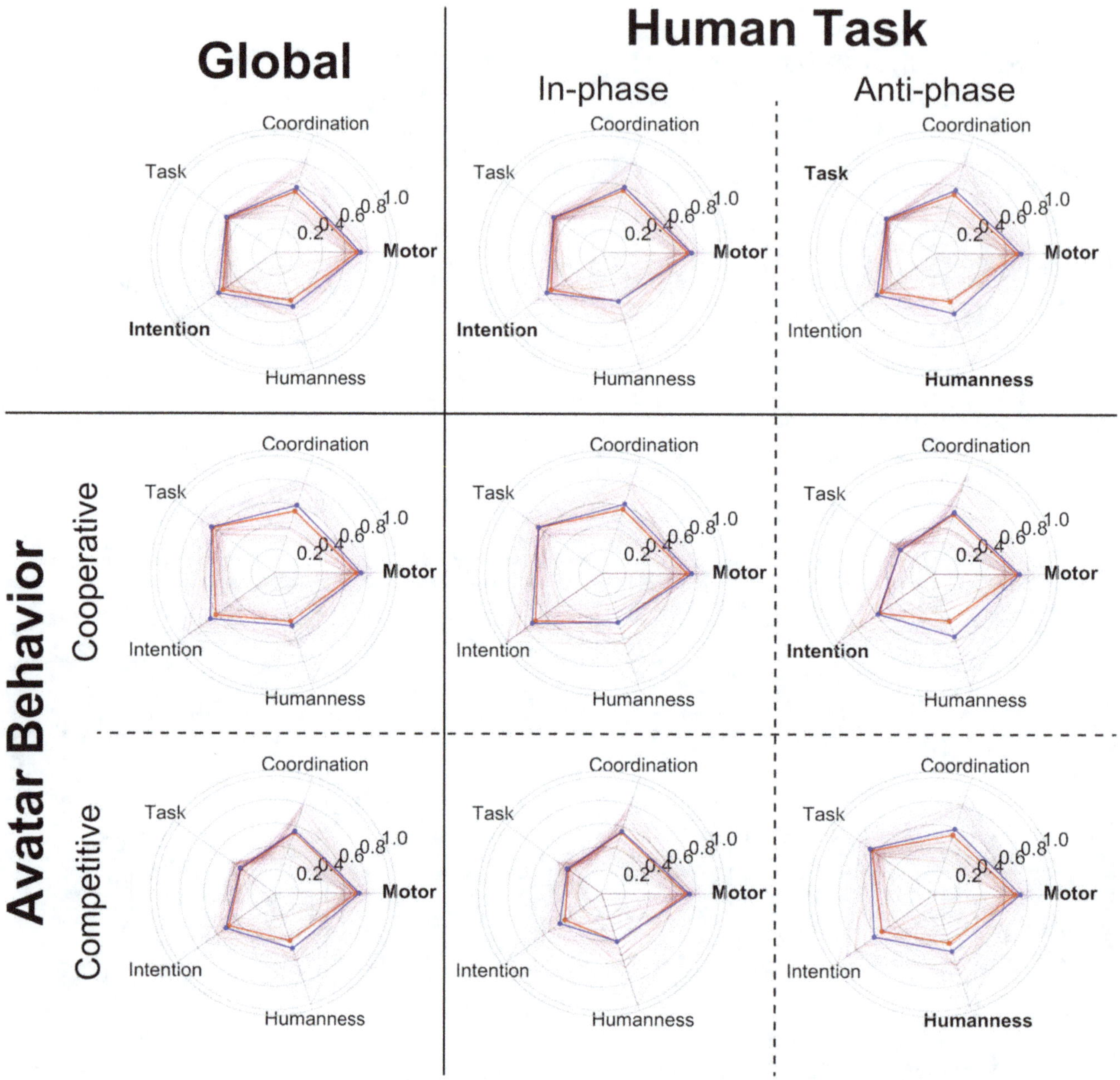

FIGURE 5 | Score analysis by subcondition of the two groups (human task: in-phase/anti-phase and avatar behavior: cooperation/competition). Both the global and the human task were significant predictors of the motor score, with the control group having greater scores (coeff = 0.4413, $p < 0.001$**) and "in-phase" task also leading to higher scores (coeff = 0.2726, $p = 0.016$*). Controls are in blue and participants with ASD in red. Scores with statistically significant differences between participants with ASD and participants with typical development are in bold typeface. *$p < 0.05$; **$p < 0.005$.

instrument to artificially recreate a social interaction, from low-level (motor and coordination scores) to higher-level domains of social coordination [intention attribution to another and human (/or robotic) judgment of an interaction]. Our secondary objective was to study the developmental trajectory of HDC scores and to demonstrate by a valid scientific approach that interpersonal synchrony captures the coupling between low-level sensorimotor and high-level sociocognitive skills in a population of children.

Developmental Aspects of Sociocognitive Skills and Intervention Based on Interpersonal Synchrony in Children With ASD

The literature on interpersonal synchrony attests to the significance of development and plasticity in affording therapeutic detection and action (39, 41, 43). The present HDC results are in line with this developmental aspect of

TABLE 3 | HDC score analysis by subconditions.

	Motor (NM)		Coordination (NM)		Task (NM)		Intention (NM)		Humanness (NM)	
	Coop	**Comp**	**Coop**	**Comp**	**Coop**	**Comp**	**Coop**	**Comp**	**Coop**	**Comp**
In-phase	$d = -0.51$ ($p = 0.0059^*$)	$d = -0.34$ ($p = 0.025^*$)	$d = -0.26$ ($p = 0.098$)	$d = -0.087$ ($p = 0.35$)	$d = 0.12$ ($p = 0.17$)	$d = 0.067$ ($p = 0.47$)	$d = -0.018$ ($p = 0.47$)	$d = -0.084$ ($p = 0.35$)	$d = 0.34$ ($p = 0.014^*$)	$d = 0.3$ ($p = 0.046^*$)
Anti-phase	$d = -0.59$ ($p = 0.0015^{**}$)	$d = -0.35$ ($p = 0.025^*$)	$d = -0.3$ ($p = 0.054$)	$d = -0.11$ ($p = 0.29$)	$d = -0.067$ ($p = 0.41$)	$d = 0.16$ ($p = 0.23$)	$d = -0.2$ ($p = 0.14$)	$d = 0.067$ ($p = 0.31$)	$d = 0.012$ ($p = 0.49$)	$d = -0.25$ ($p = 0.058$)

*Coop, cooperative behavior of the VP, Comp, competitive behavior of the VP, d, Cohen's d, p, p value, *p < 0.05, **p < 0.005.*

sociocognitive skills, with significant effects of intention attribution, humanness, and task comprehension in children and adolescents with and without ASD. Interventions targeting early development of socially synchronous interactions in toddlers with ASD attest to its effectiveness (39), with improvement in child language comprehension being linked to the severity of ASD symptoms (63). The neurodevelopmental trajectory observed here only in the group with ASD is fully in line with this picture.

Coupling Between Low-Level Sensorimotor and High-Level Sociocognitive Skills

The present findings also show that affect recognition may be associated with better task comprehension. Greater cognitive abilities are correlated with a higher level of affect recognition skill hinting at the possibility of a mediating effect of IQ on the recognition of emotions. At the same time, we found that lower motor skills are associated with a higher probability of a dimensional diagnosis of ASD. Motricity in ASD will be discussed further, but this result suggests a linkage between the so-called "lower-level" motor skills and "higher-level" social–cognitive skills in this population. Some support already exists for a strong pairing between the mirror and mentalizing systems during communicative gestures, suggesting a cognitive–motor coupling in children (64). The mechanisms involved range from the release of endogenous opioids (dopamine, endorphins, serotonin, and oxytocin) (65, 66) to the recruitment of now well-described neural processes (67, 68). From an evolutionary perspective, IS is thought to play a role in shared common goals that lead to: a) cooperative expectations and joint action behaviors (69); b) shared basic affective states and emotions; c) better attribution ability of one's self and others; and d) in general, better comprehension of social situations (70).

Motor Skills as a Developmental Marker of Children and Adolescents at Risk With ASD

The motor score is the only HDC measure that allows a distinction between the two groups. In overall terms, this motor low-level score is found to be statistically lower among participants with ASD, confirming current data finding altered motor skills in ASD. Despite the small sample size, it is interesting to note that the HDC motor score is also one of the two scores (together with the motor coordination score) on which the classification into two clusters is essentially based—a classification that significantly respects the status of participants (see **Supplementary Material**) (71). These results demonstrate the essential nature of motor assessment, including the use of HDC, in participants with ASD, suggesting a major role in ASD diagnosis (72). Alterations in motor control (38), and particularly of executive motor control (73), have been widely demonstrated in children with ASD. However, although motor disorders are associated with the diagnosis of children with ASD in 50 to 80% (74), their prevalence apparently increasing with age (75), they remain underdiagnosed in clinical practice (1.34%) (75). On the other hand, the estimated prevalence of motor disorders (36%) makes them almost as frequent as cognitive disorders (38%) among children under 6 years (75). Children and adolescents with ASD tend to have difficulties in planning and sequencing movements (76), which are also associated with higher levels of neuromotor noise (77) [i.e., disturbing action (motor commands) and perception (sensory feedback) (20)]. Such variability can have multiple substrates but relies on hypotheses that can be explained using Bayesian models, namely an imbalance between prediction, inputs, and expectations (78). Indeed, ASD is associated with alterations in the ability to integrate social stimuli (79) and a reduced ability to incorporate somatosensory and visual information into accurate motor responses (37). Moreover, some studies now describe deficits in joint-attention as an endophenotype of ASD (80, 81). Vis-à-vis our results, children with ASD may have difficulties in sustaining attention long enough to perceive the stimulus. Further analysis showed that the instruction given to the participant (human task: "in-phase") is associated with a better motor score among the control group (coeff $= 0.2726$, $p = 0.016^*$). Also, we observed interactions by subcondition. Children with ASD tend to have lower results than children with typical development in all the conditions, i.e., "in-phase" as well as "anti-phase" during both competitive and cooperative behavior of the avatar (**Table 3**). This result accords with Wang et al. (82) who reported that during a cooperative task of synchronization (i.e., "in-phase"), children with severe diagnosis of ASD tend to exhibit lower neural activity.

Sociocognitive Skills Based on Interpersonal Synchrony

Mentalizing deficits have repeatedly been described in the population with ASD (83). Mentalizing requires preserved metacognitive skills, yet metacognitive monitoring is found diminished in children with ASD (84). Higher-level scores (intention attribution and task comprehension) demand efficient use of metacognitive processes. However, for both scores, we did not observe a group effect: it seemed easier for participants to detect the intention of the VP when it takes on a cooperative behavior whether "anti-phase" or "in-phase". Furthermore, comprehension of the task is better if the avatar is cooperative. A result that seems difficult to interpret is that participants with an ASD diagnosis appear to have a better understanding of the task than controls. This could be due to the tendency of ASD children to generate mainly the same movement "in-phase" with the avatar without taking the instruction into account–or it could be due to the lack of a real-time social context (85). Such a possibility of bias may produce a false positive result.

In addition, only children with a diagnosis of ASD showed a persistence of the same response in the assessment of the attribution of humanness (or robotic) judgment to the avatar. This result reinforces the previous observation of an insistence on sameness in ASD (86, 87) and may be consistent with the repetitive behaviors that are part of the diagnosis (DSM-5).

Implications of Findings for Clinical Practice and Public Health

One of the challenges of the present approach is to develop an application of HDC that can be used for the early assessment and training of motor coordination and interpersonal synchrony in order to improve social skills (42). The aim of our study was also to offer standardized ways to assess the efficacy of the HDC. We were able to generate percentile ranks for each HDC score from the results obtained in control patients (see **Supplementary Table 1**). This step made it possible to estimate a child's skills for each assessment.

Research has tried to identify clinical markers in ASD ranging from early signs of regression patterns (44, 88) to atypical neural responses of gaze (89). Later possibilities include neurological soft signs (90), abnormalities of sensorimotor priors (34), and anomalies in proprioceptive and sensory motor development (including alteration of motor priors, micromovements, and the presence of noise in sensory motor variables that may be associated with lack of embodiment) (34).

Systematic and reliable metrics of the HDC, normalized across developmental trajectories by means of normative models (91), could help predict phenotypic profiles and, thus, refine the diagnosis, associated comorbidities, and stratification of the disorder. Here, we highlighted how HDC measures can provide new markers of ASD, either alone or in combination with psychometric scales for assessing social and motor coordination skills. Despite the limited sample size, exploratory analyses of stratification and multivariate predictive diagnosis (see **Supplementary Material** for more details on the methodology and the preliminary results) tend to confirm the potential of the HDC paradigm for ASD diagnostics with the motor and coordination scores, individually, and/or combined with other clinical evidence of ASD, appearing as the most promising candidates. Clearly, there is a need to develop dedicated HDC-based predictive models and for further data collection and analyses to be carried out to assess them rigorously (92). Many studies have reported divergences in the core symptoms of ASD by gender (93) and level of intellectual disability (94). Future studies in larger cohorts will allow disentangling such key factors in the development of interpersonal synchrony.

CONCLUSION

The HDC is an effective means to evaluate interpersonal synchrony at both low and high levels of social cognition during live interactions. It can also probe the developmental aspects of their evolving relationship. On the other hand, the psychometric evaluation of HDC provides reliable, reproducible, objective, and standardized scores, derived from a natural movement. As a new psychometric test, HDC provides motor and social markers that help to improve the early detection of neurobehavioral abnormalities during human interaction. The HDC paradigm also provides a dynamical basis for the development of further therapeutic approaches, for instance in the area of serious games (e.g., in mixed reality: https://vimeo.com/277085489).

AUTHOR CONTRIBUTIONS

FB, AL, and AP collected all the data. FB, AL, FA, and AM worked on the inclusion of patients and their clinical exploration. FB, AL, YB, and DE participated in both analysis and writing. RD and TB participated in the design and relecture. GD participated in the design, analysis, and writing. All authors contributed to the article and approved the submitted version.

ACKNOWLEDGMENTS

The authors would like to thank the participants and their families who participated in this study. They also thank Benjamin Landman, Anna Banki, and Ramon Aparicio-Garcia for their early help in the project.

SUPPLEMENTARY MATERIAL

Supplementary Data Sheet | Additional methods regarding the calculation of the HDC scores, the stratification using clustering analysis, and the supervised learning with logistic regression.

Supplementary Figure 1 | Stratification based on HDC scores. **(A)** Optimal number of clusters between k = 2 to k = 20 obtained by NbClust with 26 indices. The majority vote (9 of 26) indicates k = 2 as the optimal cluster configuration. **(B)** Corresponding Hierarchical Clustering using Euclidian distance and the Ward method.

Supplementary Table 1 | HDC percentile ranks by age group.

Supplementary Table 2 | Comparison of HDC and clinical scores between the two clusters identified.

REFERENCES

1. American Psychiatric Association. *Diagnostic and Statistical Manual of Mental Disorders (DSM-5).* American Psychiatric Association (APA). (2013). doi: 10.1176/appi.books.9780890425596
2. Baxter AJ, Brugha TS, Erskine HE, Scheurer RW, Vos T, Scott JG. The epidemiology and global burden of autism spectrum disorders. *Psychol Med.* (2015) 45:601. doi: 10.1017/S003329171400172X
3. Fombonne E. The prevalence of autism. *JAMA.* (2003) 289:87–9. doi: 10.1001/jama.289.1.87
4. Georgiades S, Szatmari P, Boyle M, Hanna S, Duku E, Zwaigenbaum L, et al. Investigating phenotypic heterogeneity in children with autism spectrum disorder: a factor mixture modeling approach. *J Child Psychol Psychiatry.* (2013) 54:206–15. doi: 10.1111/j.1469-7610.2012.02588.x
5. Huguet G, Ey E, Bourgeron T. The genetic landscapes of autism spectrum disorders. *Ann Rev Genom Hum Genet.* (2013) 14:191–213. doi: 10.1146/annurev-genom-091212-153431
6. Soke GN, Maenner MJ, Christensen D, Kurzius-Spencer M, Schieve LA. Prevalence of co-occurring medical and behavioral conditions/symptoms among 4-and 8-year-old children with autism spectrum disorder in selected areas of the United States in 2010. *J Aut Dev Disord.* (2018) 48:2663–76. doi: 10.1007/s10803-018-3521-1
7. Vivanti G, Trembath D, Dissanayake C. Mechanisms of imitation impairment in autism spectrum disorder. *J abnormal child psychol.* (2014) 42:1395–405. doi: 10.1007/s10802-014-9874-9
8. Mogan R, Fischer R, Bulbulia JA. To be in synchrony or not? A meta-analysis of synchrony's effects on behavior, perception, cognition and affect. *J Exp Soc Psychol.* (2017) 72:13–20. doi: 10.1016/j.jesp.2017.03.009
9. Nebel MB, Eloyan A, Nettles CA, Sweeney KL, Ament K, Ward RE, et al. Intrinsic visual-motor synchrony correlates with social deficits in autism. *Biol Psychiatry.* (2016) 79:633–41. doi: 10.1016/j.biopsych.2015.08.029
10. Xavier J, Magnat J, Sherman A, Gauthier S, Cohen D, Chaby L. A developmental and clinical perspective of rhythmic interpersonal coordination: From mimicry toward the interconnection of minds. *J Physiol.* (2016) 110:420–6. doi: 10.1016/j.jphysparis.2017.06.001
11. Atzil S, Hendler T, Feldman R. Specifying the neurobiological basis of human attachment: brain, hormones, and behavior in synchronous and intrusive mothers. *Neuropsychopharmacology.* (2011) 36:2603–15. doi: 10.1038/npp.2011.172
12. Dumas G, Nadel J, Soussignan R, Martinerie J, Garnero L. Inter-Brain synchronization during social interaction. Édité par Jan Lauwereyns. *PLoS ONE.* (2010) 5:e12166. doi: 10.1371/journal.pone.0012166
13. Delaherche E, Chetouani M, Mahdhaoui A, Saint-Georges C, Viaux S, Cohen D. Interpersonal synchrony: a survey of evaluation methods across disciplines. *IEEE Trans Affect Comp.* (2012) 3:349–65. doi: 10.1109/T-AFFC.2012.12
14. Dumas G, de Guzman GC, Tognoli E, Kelso JAS. The human dynamic clamp as a paradigm for social interaction. *Proc Natl Acad Sci USA.* (2014) 111:E3726–34. doi: 10.1073/pnas.1407486111
15. Kostrubiec V, Dumas G, Zanone PG, Kelso JAS. The virtual teacher (VT) paradigm: learning new patterns of interpersonal coordination using the human dynamic clamp. *PLoS ONE.* (2015) 10:e0142029. doi: 10.1371/journal.pone.0142029
16. Kelso JAS, de Guzman GC, Reveley C, Tognoli E. Virtual partner interaction (VPI): exploring novel behaviors via coordination dynamics. *PLoS ONE.* (2009) 4:e5749. doi: 10.1371/journal.pone.0005749
17. Kelso JAS. Coordination dynamics. In: Meyers RA, editors. *Encyclopedia of Complexity and System Science.*Heidelberg: Springer (2009/2013). p. 1537–64. doi: 10.1007/978-0-387-30440-3_101
18. Dumas GQ, Moreau E, Kelso JAS. The human dynamic clamp reveals the fronto-parietal network linking real-time social coordination and cognition. Cerebral Cortex, (2019) 30:3271–85. doi: 10.1101/651232
19. Zhang M, Dumas G, Kelso JAS, Tognoli E. Enhanced emotional responses during social coordination with a virtual partner. *Int J Psychophysiol.* (2016) 104:33–43. doi: 10.1016/j.ijpsycho.2016.04.001
20. Xavier J, Gauthier S, Cohen D, Zahoui M, Chetouani M, Villa F, et al. Interpersonal synchronization, motor coordination, and control are impaired during a dynamic imitation task in children with autism spectrum disorder. *Front Psychol.* (2018) 9:1467. doi: 10.3389/fpsyg.2018.01467
21. McNaughton KA, Redcay E. Interpersonal synchrony in autism. *Curr Psychiatry Rep.* (2020) 22:12. doi: 10.1007/s11920-020-1135-8
22. Romero V, Fitzpatrick P, Roulier S, Duncan A, Richardson MJ, Schmidt RC. Evidence of embodied social competence during conversation in high functioning children with autism spectrum disorder. *PLoS ONE.* (2018) 13:e0193906. doi: 10.1371/journal.pone.0193906
23. Noel JP, De Niear MA, Lazzara NS, Wallace MT. Uncoupling between multisensory temporal function and nonverbal turn-taking in autism spectrum disorder. *IEEE Trans Cogn Dev Syst.* (2017) 10:973–82. doi: 10.1109/TCDS.2017.2778141
24. Marsh KL, Isenhower RW, Richardson MJ, Helt M, Verbalis AD, Schmidt RC, et al. Autism and social disconnection in interpersonal rocking. *Front Integr Neurosci.* (2013) 7:4. doi: 10.3389/fnint.2013.00004
25. Kaur M, Srinivasan SM, Bhat AN. Comparing motor performance, praxis, coordination, and interpersonal synchrony between children with and without Autism Spectrum Disorder (ASD). *Res Dev Dis.* (2018) 72:79–95. doi: 10.1016/j.ridd.2017.10.025
26. Fitzpatrick P, Romero V, Amaral JL, Duncan A, Barnard H, Richardson MJ, et al. Social motor synchronization: insights for understanding social behavior in autism. *J Aut Dev Disord.* (2017) 47:2092–107. doi: 10.1007/s10803-017-3124-2
27. Fitzpatrick P, Romero V, Amaral JL, Duncan A, Barnard H, Richardson MJ, et al. Evaluating the importance of social motor synchronization and motor skill for understanding autism. *Autism Res.* (2017) 10:1687–99. doi: 10.1002/aur.1808
28. Marchena A, de, Eigsti AM. Conversational gestures in autism spectrum disorders: asynchrony but not decreased frequency. *Aut Res.* (2010) 3:311–22. doi: 10.1002/aur.159
29. Fitzpatrick P, Frazier JA, Cochran DM, Mitchell T, Coleman C, Schmidt RC. Impairments of social motor synchrony evident in autism spectrum disorder. *Front Psychol.* (2016) 7:1323. doi: 10.3389/fpsyg.2016.01323
30. Bhat AN, Srinivasan SM, Woxholdt C, Shield A. Differences in praxis performance and receptive language during fingerspelling between deaf children with and without autism spectrum disorder. *Autism.* (2018) 22:271–82. doi: 10.1177/1362361316672179
31. Zalla T, Korman J. Prior knowledge, episodic control and theory of mind in autism: toward an integrative account of social cognition. *Front Psychol.* (2018) 9:752. doi: 10.3389/fpsyg.2018.00752
32. Hilton BC, Kuhlmeier VA. Intention attribution and the development of moral evaluation. *Front Psychol.* (2019) 9:2663. doi: 10.3389/fpsyg.2018.02663
33. Bhat AN, Landa RJ, Galloway JC. Current perspectives on motor functioning in infants, children, and adults with autism spectrum disorders. *Phys Ther.* (2011) 91:1116–29. doi: 10.2522/ptj.20100294
34. Torres EB, Nguyen J, Suresh C, Yanovich P, Kolevzon A. Noise from the periphery in autism spectrum disorders of idiopathic origins and of known etiology. In: *Paper Presentation at the Annual Meeting of the Society for Neuroscience SFN.* (2013).
35. Righi G, Tenenbaum EJ, McCormick C, Blossom M, Amso D, Sheinkopf SJ. Sensitivity to audio-visual synchrony and its relation to language abilities in children with and without ASD. *Aut Res.* (2018) 11:645–53. doi: 10.1002/aur.1918
36. Greenfield K, Ropar D, Smith AD, Carey M, Newport R. Visuo-tactile integration in autism: atypical temporal binding may underlie greater reliance on proprioceptive information. *Mol Aut.* (2015) 6:51. doi: 10.1186/s13229-015-0045-9
37. Lim YH, Partridge K, Girdler S, Morris SL. Standing postural control in individuals with autism spectrum disorder: systematic review and meta-analysis. *J Aut Dev Disord.* (2017) 47:2238–53. doi: 10.1007/s10803-017-3144-y
38. Fournier KA, Hass CJ, Naik SK, Lodha N, Cauraugh JH. Motor coordination in autism spectrum disorders: a synthesis and meta-analysis. *J Aut Dev Disord.* (2010) 40:1227–40. doi: 10.1007/s10803-010-0981-3

39. Landa RJ, Holman KC, O'Neill AH, Stuart EA. Intervention targeting development of socially synchronous engagement in toddlers with autism spectrum disorder: a randomized controlled trial. *J Child Psychol Psychiatry.* (2011) 52:13–21. doi: 10.1111/j.1469-7610.2010.02288.x
40. Zhou B, Xu Q, Li H, Zhang Y, Wang Y, Rogers SJ, et al. Effects of parent-implemented Early Start Denver Model intervention on Chinese Toddlers with autism spectrum disorder: A non-randomized controlled trial. *Aut Res.* (2018) 11:654–66. doi: 10.1002/aur.1917
41. Franz L, Dawson G. Implementing early intervention for autism spectrum disorder: a global perspective. *Pediatr Med.* (2019) 2:44. doi: 10.21037/pm.2019.07.09
42. Eapen V, Crnčec R, Walter A. Clinical outcomes of an early intervention program for preschool children with Autism Spectrum Disorder in a community group setting. *BMC Pediatr.* (2013) 13:3. doi: 10.1186/1471-2431-13-3
43. Landa RJ, Gross AL, Stuart EA, Faherty A. Developmental trajectories in children with and without autism spectrum disorders: the first 3 years. *Child Dev.* (2013) 84:429–2. doi: 10.1111/j.1467-8624.2012.01870.x
44. Ozonoff S, Gangi D, Hanzel EP, Hill A, Hill MM, Miller M, et al. Onset patterns in autism: Variation across informants, methods, and timing. *Aut Res.* (2018) 11:788–97. doi: 10.1002/aur.1943
45. Iverson JM, Shic F, Wall CA, Chawarska K, Curtin S, Estes A, et al. Early motor abilities in infants at heightened versus low risk for ASD: A Baby Siblings Research Consortium (BSRC) study. *J Abnorm Psychol.* (2019) 128:69. doi: 10.1037/abn0000390
46. Stahmer AC, Akshoomoff N, Cunningham AB. Inclusion for toddlers with autism spectrum disorders: the first ten years of a community program. *Autism.* (2011) 15:625–41. doi: 10.1177/1362361310392253
47. Kostrubiec V, Zanone PG, Fuchs A, Kelso JAS. Beyond the blank slate: routes to learning new coordination patterns depend on the intrinsic dynamics of the learner:experimental evidence and theoretical model. *Front Hum Neurosci.* (2012) 6:222 doi: 10.3389/fnhum.2012.00222
48. Marquand AF, Rezek I, Buitelaar J, Beckmann CF. Understanding heterogeneity in clinical cohorts using normative models: beyond case-control studies. *Biol Psychiatry.* (2016) 80:552–61. doi: 10.1016/j.biopsych.2015.12.023
49. Lord C, Rutter M, DiLavore PC, Risi S, Gotham K, Bishop SL. *Autism Diagnostic Observation Schedule. 2nd (ADOS-2).* Torrance, CA: Western Psychological Services (2012).
50. Lord C, Rutter M, Le Couteur. A. Autism diagnostic interview-revised: a revised version of a diagnostic interview for caregivers of individuals with possible pervasive developmental disorders. *J Aut Dev Disord.* (1994) 24:659–85. doi: 10.1007/BF02172145
51. Constantino JN. Social responsiveness scale. In: Volkmar FR, editor. *Encyclopedia of Autism Spectrum Disorders.* New York, NY: Springer New York (2013). p. 2919–29. doi: 10.1007/978-1-4419-1698-3_296
52. Wechsler D, Pearson Education Inc, Psychological Corporation. *WISC-V: Wechsler Intelligence Scale for Children.* San Antonio, TX: NCS Pearson, Inc. (2014).
53. Tiffin J, Asher EJ. The Purdue Pegboard: norms and studies of reliability and validity. *J Appl Psychol.* (1948) 32:234. doi: 10.1037/h0061266
54. Gardner RA, Broman M. The Purdue Pegboard: Normative data on 1334 school children. *J Clin Child Adolesc Psychol.* (1979) 8:156–62. doi: 10.1080/15374417909532912
55. Yeudall LT, Fromm D, Reddon JR, Stefanyk WO. Normative data stratified by age and sex for 12 neuropsychological tests. *J Clin Psychol.* (1986) 42:918–46. doi: 10.1002/1097-4679(198611)42:6<918::AID-JCLP2270420617>3.0.CO;2-Y
56. Kemp SL, Korkman M. *Essentials of NEPSY-II Assessment (Vol. 69).* San Diego, CA: John Wiley and Sons (2010).
57. Haken H, Kelso JAS, Bunz H. A theoretical model of phase transitions in human hand movements. *Biol Cybern.* (1985) 51:347–56. doi: 10.1007/BF00336922
58. Millman KJ, Aivazis M. Python for scientists and engineers. *Comput Sci Engin.* (2011) 13:9–12. doi: 10.1109/MCSE.2011.36
59. Oliphant TE. *A Guide to NumPy (Vol. 1).* Provo, UT: Trelgol Publishing (2006).
60. Walt SVD, Colbert SC, Varoquaux G. The NumPy array: a structure for efficient numerical computation. *Comp Sci Engin.* (2011) 13:22–30. doi: 10.1109/MCSE.2011.37
61. Virtanen P, Gommers R, Oliphant TE, Haberland M, Reddy T, Cournapeau D, et al. SciPy 1.0: fundamental algorithms for scientific computing in Python. *Nat Methods.* (2020) 17:261–72. doi: 10.1038/s41592-019-0686-2
62. Zabihi M, Oldehinkel M, Wolfers T, Frouin V, Goyard D, Loth E, et al. Dissecting the heterogeneous cortical anatomy of autism spectrum disorder using normative models. *Biol Psychiatry.* (2019) 4:567–78. doi: 10.1016/j.bpsc.2018.11.013
63. Tachibana Y, Miyazaki C, Ota E, Mori R, Hwang Y, Kobayashi E, et al. A systematic review and meta-analysis of comprehensive interventions for pre-school children with autism spectrum disorder (ASD). *PLoS ONE.* (2017) 12:e0186502. doi: 10.1371/journal.pone.0186502
64. Nadel J. Perception-action coupling and imitation in autism spectrum disorder. *Dev Med Child Neurol.* (2015) 57:55–8. doi: 10.1111/dmcn.12689
65. Mu Y, Guo C, Han S. Oxytocin enhances inter-brain synchrony during social coordination in male adults. *Soc Cogn Affect Neurosci.* (2016) 11:1882–93. doi: 10.1093/scan/nsw106
66. Lang M, Bahna V, Shaver JH, Reddish P, Xygalatas D. Sync to link: Endorphin-mediated synchrony effects on cooperation. *Biol Psychol.* (2017) 127:191–7. doi: 10.1016/j.biopsycho.2017.06.001
67. Bhat AN, Michael D, Hoffman SL, McKenzie TL, Culotta EJ, Daisuke T, et al. Cortical activation during action observation, action execution, and interpersonal synchrony in adults: a functional near-infrared spectroscopy (FNIRS) study. *Front Hum Neurosci.* (2017) 11:431. doi: 10.3389/fnhum.2017.00431
68. Valencia A, Froese T. What binds us? Inter-brain neural synchronization and its implications for theories of human consciousness. *Neurosci. Conscious.* (2020) 2020, niaa010. doi: 10.1093/niaa010
69. Valdesolo P, Ouyang J, DeSteno D. The rhythm of joint action: Synchrony promotes cooperative ability. *J Exp Soc Psychol.* (2010) 46:693–5. doi: 10.1016/j.jesp.2010.03.004
70. Valdesolo P, DeSteno D. Synchrony and the social tuning of compassion. *Emotion.* (2011) 11:262. doi: 10.1037/a0021302
71. Malika C, Ghazzali N, Boiteau V, Niknafs A. NbClust: an R package for determining the relevant number of clusters in a data Set. *J Stat Softw.* (2014) 61:1–36. doi: 10.18637/jss.v061.i06
72. Chukoskie L, Townsend J, Westerfield M. Motor skill in autism spectrum disorders: a subcortical view. In: *International Review of Neurobiology.* San Diego, CA: Academic Press. (2013). p. 207–49. doi: 10.1016/B978-0-12-418700-9.00007-1
73. Demetriou EA, Lampit A, Quintana DS, Naismith SL, Song YJC, Pye JE, et al. Autism spectrum disorders: a meta-analysis of executive function. *Mol Psychiatry.* (2018) 23:1198–204. doi: 10.1038/mp.2017.75
74. Green D, Charman T, Pickles A, Chandler S, Loucas TOM, Simonoff E, et al. Impairment in movement skills of children with autistic spectrum disorders. *Dev Med Child Neurol.* (2009) 51:311–6. doi: 10.1111/j.1469-8749.2008.03242.x
75. Licari MK, Alvares GA, Varcin K, Evans KL, Cleary D, Reid SL, et al. Prevalence of motor difficulties in autism spectrum disorder: analysis of a population-based cohort. *Aut Res.* (2019) 2019:2230. doi: 10.1002/aur.2230
76. Grace N, Johnson BP, Rinehart NJ, Enticott PG. Are motor control and regulation problems part of the ASD motor profile? A handwriting study. *Dev Neuropsychol.* (2018) 43:581–94. doi: 10.1080/87565641.2018.1504948
77. Torres EB, Mistry S, Caballero C, Whyatt CP. Stochastic signatures of involuntary head micro-movements can be used to classify females of ABIDE into different subtypes of neurodevelopmental disorders. *Front Integr Neurosci.* (2017) 11:10. doi: 10.3389/fnint.2017.00010
78. Bolis D, Schilbach L. Beyond one Bayesian brain: Modeling intra-and inter-personal processes during social interaction: Commentary on "Mentalizing homeostasis: the social origins of interoceptive inference" by Fotopoulou and Tsakiris. *Neuropsychoanalysis.* (2017) 19:35–8. doi: 10.1080/15294145.2017.1295215
79. Thye MD, Bednarz HM, Herringshaw AJ, Sartin EB, Kana RK. The impact of atypical sensory processing on social impairments in autism spectrum disorder. *Dev Cogn Neurosci.* (2018) 29:151–67. doi: 10.1016/j.dcn.2017.04.010
80. Mundy P, Novotny S, Swain-Lerro L, McIntyre N, Zajic M, Oswald T. Joint-

attention and the social phenotype of school-aged children with ASD. *J Aut Dev Disord.* (2017) 47:1423–35. doi: 10.1007/s10803-017-3061-0

81. Jones EJ, Venema K, Earl RK, Lowy R, Webb SJ. Infant social attention: an endophenotype of ASD-related traits? *J Child Psychol Psychiatry.* (2017) 58:270–81. doi: 10.1111/jcpp.12650
82. Wang Q, Han Z, Hu X, Feng S, Wang H, Liu T, et al. Autism symptoms modulate interpersonal neural synchronization in children with autism spectrum disorder in cooperative interactions. *Brain Topogr.* (2020) 33:112–22. doi: 10.1007/s10548-019-00731-x
83. Bliksted V, Ubukata S, Koelkebeck K. Discriminating autism spectrum disorders from schizophrenia by investigation of mental state attribution on an on-line mentalizing task: A review and meta-analysis. *Schizophr Res.* (2016) 171:16–26. doi: 10.1016/j.schres.2016.01.037
84. Grainger C, Williams DM, Lind SE. Metacognitive monitoring and control processes in children with autism spectrum disorder: Diminished judgement of confidence accuracy. *Conscious Cogn.* (2016) 42:65–74. doi: 10.1016/j.concog.2016.03.003
85. Forgeot d'Arc B, Devaine M, Daunizeau J. Social behavioural adaptation in Autism. *PLoS Comp Biol.* (2020) 16:e1007700. doi: 10.1371/journal.pcbi.1007700
86. Gotham K, Bishop SL, Hus V, Huerta M, Lund S, Buja A, et al. Exploring the relationship between anxiety and insistence on sameness in autism spectrum disorders. *Aut Res.* (2013) 6:33–41. doi: 10.1002/aur.1263
87. Kanner L. Early infantile autism. *J Pediatr.* (1944) 25:211–7. doi: 10.1016/S0022-3476(44)80156-1
88. Ozonoff S, Iosif AM. Changing conceptualizations of regression: what prospective studies reveal about the onset of autism spectrum disorder. *Neurosci Biobehav Rev.* (2019) 100:296–304. doi: 10.1016/j.neubiorev.2019.03.012
89. Jones EJ, Gliga T, Bedford R, Charman T, Johnson MH. Developmental pathways to autism: a review of prospective studies of infants at risk. *Neurosci Biobehav Rev.* (2014) 39:1–33. doi: 10.1016/j.neubiorev.2013.12.001
90. Tani P, Lindberg N, Appelberg B, Nieminen-von Wendt T, Wendt von L, Porkka-Heiskanen T. Clinical neurological abnormalities in young adults with Asperger syndrome. *Psychiatry Clin Neurosci.* (2006) 60:253–5. doi: 10.1111/j.1440-1819.2006.01494.x
91. Lefebvre A, Delorme R, Delano, C, Amsellem F, Beggiato A, Germanaud D, et al. Alpha waves as a neuromarker of autism spectrum disorder: the challenge of reproducibility and heterogeneity. *Front Neurosci.* (2018) 12:662. doi: 10.3389/fnins.2018.00662
92. Poldrack RA, Huckins G, Varoquaux G. Establishment of best practices for evidence for prediction: a review. *JAMA Psychiatry.* (2020) 77:534–40. doi: 10.1001/jamapsychiatry.2019.3671
93. Beggiato A, Peyre H, Maruani A, Scheid I, Rastam M, Amsellem F, et al. Gender differences in autism spectrum disorders : Divergence among specific core symptoms. *Aut Res.* (2017) 10:680–9. doi: 10.1002/aur.1715
94. Martos-Perez J, Freire-Prudencio S, Llorente-Comi M, Ayuda-Pascual R, Gonzalez-Navarro A. [Autism and intelligence quotient : Stability?]. *Revista De Neurol.* (2018) 66:S39–44. doi: 10.33588/rn.66S01.2018011

15

Social Cognition and Obsessive-Compulsive Disorder: A Review of Subdomains of Social Functioning

Myrthe Jansen[1,2]*, *Sandy Overgaauw*[1,2] *and Ellen R. A. De Bruijn*[1,2]

[1] *Department of Clinical Psychology, Institute of Psychology, Leiden University, Leiden, Netherlands,* [2] *Leiden Institute for Brain and Cognition (LIBC), Leiden University, Leiden, Netherlands*

Correspondence:
Myrthe Jansen
m.jansen@fsw.leidenuniv.nl

Disturbances in social cognitive processes such as the ability to infer others' mental states importantly contribute to social and functional impairments in psychiatric disorders. Yet, despite established social, emotional, and cognitive problems, the role of social cognition in obsessive-compulsive disorder is largely overlooked. The current review provides a first comprehensive overview of social (neuro)cognitive disturbances in adult patients with obsessive-compulsive disorder. Results of our review indicate various social cognitive alterations. Patients with obsessive-compulsive disorder show deficits in the recognition of affective social cues, specifically facial expressions of disgust, and more general deficits in theory of mind/mentalizing. Additionally, patients show heightened affective reactions and altered neural responding to emotions of self and others, as well as poor emotion regulation skills, which may contribute to poor social functioning of patients. However, the discrepancies in findings and scarcity of studies make it difficult to draw firm conclusions with regard to the specificity of social cognitive disturbances. The review offers directions for future research and highlights the need to investigate obsessive-compulsive disorder from an interactive social neurocognitive perspective in addition to the prevalent passive spectator perspective to advance our understanding of this intricate and burdensome disorder.

Keywords: social cognition, obsessive-compulsive disorder, social cue perception, facial emotion recognition, mentalizing / theory of mind, empathy, emotion experience, emotion regulation

INTRODUCTION

Essentially, almost all psychiatric disorders are characterized by disturbances in the ability to have successful and meaningful interactions with others. As such, a novel suggestion has been to reconstruct the social difficulties observed in psychiatric disorders as disorders of social cognition (1). Social cognition is a broad term that includes a wide variety of interrelated cognitive processes that enable successful and adaptive behavior in a social context [e.g., (2, 3)]. It includes, among other things, the ability to recognize social cues such as facial emotions, the ability to understand others' mental states [known as theory of mind (ToM) or mentalizing], the ability to share the experiences and emotions of others, as well as the capacity to regulate one's emotional responses to others (4). Disturbances in these social cognitive abilities are important predictors of social and functional impairments in psychiatric disorders [e.g., (5)].

Obsessive-compulsive disorder (OCD) is a burdensome psychiatric illness with a lifetime prevalence of 1%–3% (6). The disorder is characterized by the presence of unwanted, persistent obsessions that cause significant anxiety or distress, often in combination with compulsions, which are repetitive ritualistic behaviors or mental acts carried out in response to obsessions to ease distress or anxiety (7). Obsessions can range from a fear of contamination to the experience of intrusive violent or sexually explicit thoughts or images, while compulsions may include repeated checking, washing, cleaning, and counting (7). These symptoms carry a great emotional and social burden on patients as well as their relatives. Indeed, quality of life is significantly impaired in OCD patients, with social and emotional functioning being among the most greatly affected quality of life domains (8). Scores on psychosocial functioning are also lower compared to most other psychiatric disorders, and similar to schizophrenia, which is considered one of the most severe psychiatric disorders in terms of social impairments (9). Moreover, higher symptom severity has been found to be associated with poorer social adjustment (10). The extent to which these self-reported social impairments of patients with OCD simply result as a consequence of the invalidating nature of the disorder, e.g., when a patient is not able to establish or maintain meaningful relations with others because their compulsions take up too much time, or whether factors more directly related to their symptomatology such as social-cognitive problems may play a role as well, is currently unknown.

Despite these acknowledged social difficulties in OCD, research up to date has been largely limited to nonsocial cognition. This research has demonstrated that patients with OCD are characterized by meta-cognitive biases such as (moral) thought-action fusion, which is the belief that having unwanted and intrusive thoughts is (morally) equivalent to acting on these thoughts [see, e.g., (11)]. Furthermore, neuropsychological research has described that patients show cognitive deficits in a wide range of domains, including response inhibition, interference control, cognitive flexibility, and executive functioning, although findings are somewhat inconsistent [for a recent review, see (12)]. More consistently, increased performance or error monitoring has been demonstrated in OCD [for a recent review see (13)]. Given that cognitive abilities are thought to be integral aspects of social cognitive skills such as mentalizing [e.g., (14)], impairments in these abilities may also have important implications for the social cognitive functioning of patients.

Neuroimaging studies in patients with OCD suggest that dysfunctions in cortical-striatal-thalamic-cortical circuitry underlie aforementioned cognitive deficits [e.g., (15)]. More recent work specifically implicates the lateral and medial orbitofrontal cortices, (dorsal) anterior cingulate cortex (ACC), and amygdala-cortical circuitry in the psychopathology of the disorder (16, 17). The insular cortex, a brain area involved in, among other things, the processing of disgust (18), is also implicated in the disorder. Hyperactivity of this region is commonly reported during symptom provocation, especially in those with contamination-related obsessions (19–21). The performance monitoring account of OCD also proposes a central role for both the ACC and the insular cortex. This account suggests that these brain areas are involved in producing persistent high error or conflict signals which patients are unable to reduce by behavioral action, resulting in repeated actions (i.e., compulsions) in an attempt to temper such signals (22). This theory is supported by findings of enhanced amplitudes of an event-related potential (ERP) component related to error detection called the error-related negativity [ERN; (23, 24)] in patients with OCD [see (13)]. This component is thought to be generated in the ACC (25), thus highlighting the importance of this area in the psychopathology of the disorder.

Importantly, many of the brain areas known to be implicated in the psychopathology of OCD, such as the amygdala, ACC, and insula, are also areas known to be involved in social cognitive processes and are considered to be part of the social brain in general (26–29). ToM abilities for example, have been shown to involve a network of brain regions also implicated in OCD including the amygdala, ACC, as well as other prefrontal regions (29). The amygdala and insula are both implicated in the perception of facial expressions of emotions as well (28). Furthermore, social influences have been shown to importantly modulate electrophysiological measures and brain regions involved in cognitive processes such as performance monitoring [for a review see (30)]. Yet, while research shows that many cognitive functions and brain areas involved in social behavior and cognition are affected in patients with OCD, research has largely overlooked the implications of these anomalies for social cognitive functioning and associated symptomatology in this disorder.

Identifying social cognitive disturbances has great functional relevance, as this may advance our understanding of altered social functioning of patients with OCD and lead to an improved characterization of the phenotype of this disorder. It may also have important therapeutic implications, as recent studies are increasingly starting to recognize the potential of social cognition as a target for clinical intervention [see, e.g., (31–33)]. A previous meta-analysis focusing on various anxiety disorders showed social cognitive deficits with small to moderate effect sizes for patients with OCD (34). This however concerned an exclusively quantitative analysis covering a limited number of studies (N=14, of which 12 concerned facial emotion recognition). As a result, to this date, social cognition in OCD is still poorly understood. The current review therefore aims to advance our understanding of social cognition in this disorder by qualitatively reviewing existing studies on this topic. As there are many different perspectives on what processes or domains can be considered as social cognition, we decided to adopt the framework used by Green et al. (4) in their widely cited review paper on social cognition in schizophrenia. The authors of this paper divided subdomains of social cognition according to "recent organizational models of neural systems in social neuroscience" (4 p. 620). We will therefore focus on these same domains: "social cue perception," "mentalizing/ToM," "experience sharing and empathy," and "emotion experience and regulation."

SOCIAL CUE PERCEPTION

The way people act, move, speak, gesture, and express their emotions conveys important social information. How we perceive, identify or interpret these social cues expressed by other people essentially determines how we interact with others. The following section will focus on how patients with OCD perceive affective (*Affective Social Cues*) as well as nonaffective social cues (*Nonaffective Social Cues*). **Table 1** contains an overview of the studies discussed in this section.

Affective Social Cues

Studies on how patients with OCD process affective social cues have mainly focused on our ability to identify the affective states of others from facial cues, which is generally referred to as facial emotion recognition. Other cues, such as emotion expressed in voice or body language, have received less attention. The current section will discuss research on the recognition of facial emotions (*Facial Emotion Recognition*) in adult patients (*Facial Emotion Recognition in Patients With OCD*), studies on the role of symptom severity (*The Role of Symptom Severity in Facial Emotion Recognition*), and subtype (*The Role of Symptom Subtype in Facial Emotion Recognition*), facial emotion perception biases (*Biases in Facial Emotion Recognition*) as well as on how adults with OCD process facial emotions on a neural level (*Neural Correlates of Facial Emotion Processing*). Only one study investigating nonfacial affective cues was identified, which will be discussed in the section *Affective Prosody*.

Facial Emotion Recognition

Studies assessing facial emotion recognition have typically assessed the recognition of what are believed to be the six basic emotions, i.e., anger, fear, sadness, disgust, happiness, and surprise. Most emotion recognition studies in patients with OCD originated from an interest in the emotional expression of disgust. Many patients are characterized by a fear of contamination, which is associated with behavioral compulsions such as washing and cleaning. Because facial expressions of disgust convey potential contamination, this emotional expression is thought to be particularly relevant to the symptomatology of OCD (56). The expression of fear seems relevant to OCD as well, since patients with OCD are characterized by high levels of anxiety, and previous studies have among others demonstrated that anxious individuals show increased attentional bias to fear- or threat-related stimuli [see (57)] including facial expressions of fear [e.g., (58)].

Facial Emotion Recognition in Patients With OCD

The first investigation of facial emotion recognition in patients with OCD was conducted by Sprengelmeyer and colleagues (50), over 20 years ago. Despite their small sample (12 patients), this study reported striking deficits in the recognition of the facial expression of disgust in two tests: an emotional hexagon and static test. Both tests asked patients to label the facial emotional expressions portrayed, but while one test focused on static expressions (e.g., 100% disgust), the other test using emotional hexagons, in which distinct emotional expressions were morphed (e.g., 70% disgust and 30% anger). Patients with OCD showed specific deficits in the recognition of disgust compared to healthy controls. The emotional hexagon test also indicated a marginal deficit in the recognition of anger in the patient group but not for any other emotional expressions. Parker, McNally, Nakayama, and Wilhelm (48) attempted to replicate the findings by Sprengelmeyer et al. (50) using the same tasks in a marginally larger sample (15 patients), yet failed to find any facial emotion recognition deficits in patients. In contrast, a later study in 40 patients conducted by Corcoran, Woody and Tolin (40) followed a similar procedure as the two aforementioned studies and found that overall, patients showed a specific deficit in the recognition of static expressions of disgust, but not in any other emotion.

Other studies investigated the identification of static (37, 47) or morphed emotional facial expressions (36, 42, 43) using similar tasks, yet did not reveal any significant differences between patients and healthy controls. Lawrence et al. (44) specifically investigated fear and disgust recognition, but did not observe differences in accuracy between patients and controls, despite observing differences in neural responsiveness to facial expressions of disgust (see below in *Neural Correlates of Facial Emotion Processing*). Cardoner et al. (39) and Via et al. (52) both used an active matching task in which happy and fearful target faces had to be matched with happy, fearful or angry probe faces. Although Cardoner et al. found a main group effect, showing that patients suffering from OCD were less accurate in matching both emotional faces as well as nonemotional shapes, a similar study by Via et al. found no behavioral differences between groups, in the presence of neural differences (see below in *Neural Correlates of Facial Emotion Processing*).

Two studies specifically investigated the effect of treatment on facial emotion recognition, which suggest that medication or therapy may improve or remediate disgust recognition. Lochner et al. (45) administered a single dose of the selective serotonin reuptake inhibitor (SSRI) escitalopram to OCD patients, which is an antidepressant considered as a first-line option in the treatment of OCD (59). Compared to controls, patients showed no significant deficits in the recognition of disgust in the placebo condition, although patients were significantly more accurate after a single administration of escitalopram, especially when they were already receiving SSRI treatment. Rector, Daros, Bradbury, and Richter (49) compared patients receiving cognitive-behavioral therapy (CBT) with patients not receiving CBT. Results showed that patients not receiving CBT showed significant disgust recognition deficits, whereas patients receiving therapy showed disgust recognition scores comparable to a normative sample and also showed significantly higher accuracy of anger compared to the untreated patient group.

In an attempt to clarify inconsistencies between studies, Daros, Zakzanis, and Rector (41) conducted a meta-analytic review on facial emotion recognition including ten studies in adolescent (60) and adult OCD patients (36, 37, 40, 42, 45, 48–50, 61) (not discussed in the current review as the article was not available in

TABLE 1 | Overview of studies investigating the perception of social cues in obsessive-compulsive disorder.

Domain	Author	Method	Participants	Comorbid diagnoses?	Concurrent medication/ therapy?	Task description	Subdomain	Emotions assessed	Diagnosis/ symptom assessment	Main results
Affective cues										
	Aigner et al. (35)	Case-control Outpatients	OCD = 40 [34.8 ± 10.4, 24M:16F]; HC = 40 [34.7 ± 8.7, 24M:16F]	None.	All patients were treated with SSRIs. Therapy not reported.	Static tasks (EMODIFF (differentiate emotions) and PEAT (rate valence from very sad – very happy)	Facial emotion recognition	Happiness, sadness, neutral	DSM-IV, SCID/Y-BOCS	OCD patients less accurate in identifying sad faces on the PEAT, but only of females (p=0.034). They also showed a bias to recognize neutral as sad (p=0.029), happy faces as neutral (p=0.022) and happy as sad (p=0.024).
	Bozikas et al. (36)	Case-control Outpatients	OCD = 25 [32.7 ± 9.0, 10M:15F]; HC = 25 [33.4 ± 7.3, 14M:11F]	Depression (n=4), PD (n=2).	Antidepressants without (n=11) and with (n=5) atypical antipsychotics, antipsychotics only (n=1). All patients were receiving CBT.	KAMT; Static matching task	Facial emotion recognition + affective prosody	Happiness, surprise, sadness, anger, fear, disgust	DSM-IV, MINI (4.4)/Y-BOCS	Compulsion subscale correlated significantly with sadness recognition (p=0.006). Total Y-BOCS scores correlated significantly with fear recognition (p=0.042). Associations did not survive Bonferroni correction.
	Buhlmann et al. (37)	Case-control Outpatients	OCD = 20 [31.0 ± 10.5, 8M:12F]; HC = 20 [32.9 ± 11.7, 7M:13F]	Not reported.	Not reported.	Static labelling task	Facial emotion recognition	Happiness, surprise, sadness, anger, fear, disgust, neutral	SCID	No differences between OCD and HC.
	Cannistraro et al. (38)	Case-control fMRI	OCD = 10 [26.8 ± 5.2, 4M:6F]; HC = 10 [24.9 ± 7.8, 4M:6F]	One subject with comorbid GAD and BDD.	Sertraline (n=1).	Passive viewing task	Facial emotion recognition	Happiness, fear, neutral	SCID/Y-BOCS	Compared to HC, OCD patients exhibited attenuated activation in both left (p=0.008) and right amygdala (p=0.023) when contrasting all facial expressions with fixations.
	Cardoner et al. (39)	Case-control Outpatients fMRI	OCD = 21 [28.52 ± 5.9, 10M: 11F]; HC = 21 [26.2 ± 3.4, 10M: 11F]	Depression and ADs (n=7), MDD (n=2), GAD (n=2), SAD (n=2), PD (n=1).	Fluoxetine (n=4), fluvoxamine (n=2), citalopram (n=1), clomipramine (n=2), clomipramine with SSRI (n=11). Therapy not reported.	Emotional Face Matching Task: static matching task	Facial emotion recognition	Happiness, fear (and anger)	DSM-IV/Y-BOCS	OCD patients were less accurate in matching both emotional faces as well as nonemotional shapes compared to HC (p=0.04). OCD patients showed significantly enhanced activation of visual striate areas, right fusiform gyrus, left posterior thalamus, right amygdala and parahippocampal cortex as well as dorsolateral prefrontal and right premotor cortex when comparing trials with emotional faces versus nonemotional shapes (p < 0.005, whole–brain uncorrected).
	Corcoran et al. (40)	Case-control	OCD = 40; HC = 36. Overall mean age was 34.0 years ± 11.1), no group differences in age or gender (63% women).	Comorbidities: MDD (32.5%), AD (13.9%).	Not reported.	Hexagon labelling task	Facial emotion recognition	Sadness, anger, fear, disgust	ADIS-IV or SCID/Y-BOCS	OCD patients were significantly less accurate than HC in recognizing disgust (p < 0.01). Within the OCD group, 27 individuals were unimpaired in disgust recognition (MHR = 22.6, SD = 1.7), while 13 individuals were impaired (MHR = 12.9, SD = 3.4). Patients with impairments scored significantly higher on the Y-BOCS and lower on the GAF.

(Continued)

TABLE 1 | Continued

Domain	Author	Method	Participants	Comorbid diagnoses?	Concurrent medication/ therapy?	Task description	Subdomain	Emotions assessed	Diagnosis/ symptom assessment	Main results
Affective cues										
	Daros et al. (41)	Meta-analysis Case-control	OCD = 221 [30.4 ± 7.6, 102M:119F]; HC = 224 [30.9 ± 8.8, 102M: 122F]	Not reported in all studies included in the meta-analysis. Approximately 30% has at least one comorbid AD and approximately 13% had comorbid MDD.	Not reported in all studies included in the meta-analysis. Based on information from 3 studies, approximately 59% taking psychotropic medication, most commonly antidepressants.	Only studies using labelling tests were included. Studies using blended emotions were included only if they included stimuli at 100% intensity.	Facial emotion recognition	Happiness, surprise, sadness, anger, fear, disgust, neutral	DSM-III-R or DSM-IV diagnosed	Overall emotion recognition accuracy was lower in patients compared to controls (d=−0.55; N=11; 95% CI= −0.92 to −0.19,p=0.03) with larger effects for static (d=−0.77, N=7, 95% CI= −1.23 to −0.32, p=0.01) compared to morphed expressions (d=−0.14, N=4, 95% CI=−0.51 to 0.24, p=0.48). Recognition of overall negative emotions was also impaired l (d=−0.34, N=11, 95% CI=−0.56 to −0.11, p < 0.01), as were disgust (d=−0.59, N=11, 95% CI= −1.06 to −0.11, p=0.02), anger (d= −0.36, N=10, 95% CI=−0.67 to −0.05, p=0.02) and sadness (d=−0.31, N=10, 95% CI=−0.062 to 0.00, p=0.05) separately.
	Jhung et al. (42)	Case-control Outpatients	OCD = 41 [24.9 ± 5.3, 32M: 9F]; HC = 37 [26.0 ± 6.0, 28M: 9F]	Comorbid diagnoses were allowed but no specifics are provided.	Not reported.	Hexagon labelling task (incl. ambiguous faces)	Facial emotion recognition	Sadness, anger, fear, disgust	SCID/Y-BOCS	After adjusting for age, sex and depression, patients were significantly more likely to perceive ambiguous emotions as disgust (p=0.005) and less likely to perceive them as anger (p=0.008). Higher cleaning scores predicted lower perception of anger (p=0.01) and greater perception of disgust in ambiguous expressions before (p=0.003) and after controlling for covariates (p=0.005). Hoarding predicted poorer recognition of nonambiguous disgust before (p=0.049) but not after controlling for covariates (p=0.08).
	Kornreich et al. (43)	Case-control Outpatients	OC = 22 [37.3 ± 8.0, M/F =9/ 13]; NC = 22 [37.2 ± 9.0, M/ F = 9/13]	Not reported.	All OCD patients were being treated with SSRIs. Therapy not reported.	Labelling task with morphed expressions (30 or 70% neutral)	Facial emotion recognition	Happiness, surprise, sadness, anger, fear, disgust, shame, contempt	DSM-IV/Y-BOCS	No significant differences between patients and HC for accuracy nor intensity.
	Lawrence et al. (44)	Case-control 7 inpatients, 10 outpatients fMRI	OCD = 17 [34.9 ± 8.2, 10M: 7F]; HC = 19 [34.0 ± 9.4, 11M: 8F]	MDD (n=1 present, n=3 past), DD (n= 4), SP (n=1), PD (n=1), PDA (n=1), PTSS (n=1), BDD (n=1). Personality disorders: avoidant (n=5), obsessive-compulsive (n=3), depressive (n=1), paranoid (n=1),	Citalopram (n=2), clomipramine (n=1), fluoxetine (n=3), fluvoxamine (n= 1), paroxetine (n= 4), venlafaxine (n=1), zopiclone (n=1) and buspirone (n=1). Therapy not reported.	Static labelling task (behavior) + backward masking paradigm (fMRI)	Facial emotion recognition	Fear, disgust, neutral	SCID/Y-BOCS	No behavioral differences between OCD patients and HC nor between high- or low washing patients. Compared to HC, OCD patients showed enhanced activation in the left ventrolateral prefrontal cortex and reduced activation in the thalamus when contrasting facial expressions of disgust with neutral expressions (ps < 0.05). This pattern was especially pronounced for patients with more washing symptoms.

(Continued)

TABLE 1 | Continued

Domain	Author	Method	Participants	Comorbid diagnoses?	Concurrent medication/ therapy?	Task description	Subdomain	Emotions assessed	Diagnosis/ symptom assessment	Main results
Affective cues										
				and borderline (n=1).						
	Lochner et al. (45)	Randomized double-blind case-controlled crossover study	OCD = 20; [34.1 ± 11.0, 11M: 9F]; subgroups: OCD with SSRI treatment (n =11); OCD without SSRI treatment (n=9); HC = 20 [34.8 ± 10.8, 9M: 11F]	Specific phobia (n = 2).	Sertraline (n=3), fluoxetine (n=5), escitalopram (n=1), citalopram (n=1) and paroxetine (n=1). Therapy not reported.	Labelling task with morphing video clips modified from Montagne et al. (46)	Facial emotion recognition	Happiness, sadness, anger, fear, disgust	MINI-plus, ICD-10/Y-BOCS	OCD severity was marginally associated with decreased disgust recognition after adjusting for Y-BOCS and MADRS (p=0.06). On placebo, accuracy was similar across groups. OCD patients on SSRIs showed significantly increased disgust recognition after escitalopram challenge compared to when they were on placebo and compared to the other two groups.
	Mavrogiorgou et al. (47)	Case-control Outpatients	OCD = 20 [38.1 ± 10.6, 12M: 8F]; HC = 20 [38.2 ± 13.0, 12M: 8F]	Comorbid MDD and ADs not considered as exclusion criteria.	SSRIs (n=18), St. John's wort (n=1), SSRIs + antipsychotic drugs (n=13). CBT treatment were not considered as exclusion criteria.	Static labelling task.	Facial emotion recognition	Happiness, surprise, sadness, anger, fear, disgust	ICD-10, DSM-IV criteria/Y-BOCS	No significant difference between patients and HC in emotion recognition ($p > 0.5$).
	Montagne et al. (46)	Case-control	OCD = 21 (9M: 12F; Subgroups: HRAC [n=13; 36.6 ± 11.3, 5M:8F], CC [n= 5; 41.6 ± 9.1, 3M:2F] and PS [n=3; 24.3 ± 4.5, 1M:2F]; HC = 47 [40.6 ± 12.3, 24M:23F]	Not reported.	All patients were medication-free for at least 4 weeks prior to testing. Therapy not reported.	Labelling task with morphing video clips	Facial emotion recognition	Happiness, surprise, sadness, fear, disgust	MINI for DSM-IV/Y-BOCS	Patients from HRAC group needed less emotional intensity than HC to recognize facial expression of fear ($p < 0.02$) and happiness ($p < 0.04$) correctly.
	Parker et al. (48)	Case-control Outpatients	OCD = 15 [37.7 ± 10.2, 7M:8F]; HC = 15 [31.3 ± 12.2, 3M: 12F]	Not reported.	Most were receiving behavioral and/or psychopharmacologic treatment.	Hexagon labelling task	Facial emotion recognition	Happiness, surprise, sadness, anger, fear, disgust	DSM-IV criteria/Y-BOCS	For disgust recognition, there was no significant difference between OCD patients and HC, although one OCD subject showed markedly poor disgust recognition.
	Rector et al. (49)	Case-controlled cross-sectional study	OCD without CBT treatment = 20; PDA = 15; GSP= 10; OCD +	Exclusion criteria included concurrent diagnosis of a mood disorder,	Patients were on stable medication (no change in medication type or dose during 8 weeks prior to	Static labelling task	Facial emotion recognition	Happiness, surprise, sadness, anger, fear, disgust	SCID/Y-BOCS	Untreated OCD group performed significantly worse on disgust recognition than the PDA ($p < 0.05$), GSP ($p < 0.01$) and OCD group treated with CBT ($p < 0.05$). OCD group treated with CBT recognized anger significantly better than

(Continued)

TABLE 1 | Continued

Domain	Author	Method	Participants	Comorbid diagnoses?	Concurrent medication/ therapy?	Task description	Subdomain	Emotions assessed	Diagnosis/ symptom assessment	Main results
Affective cues										
		Tertiary care clinic	treatment responders to CBT = 11. Overall age was 33.6 ± 8.5 years), 55% women. Characteristics per group not reported.	SSDs, PDA or GSP.	testing). No specifics reported. Exclusion criteria included past treatment with CBT.					untreated OCD ($p < 0.05$) and PDA group ($p < 0.05$).
	Sprengelmeyer et al. (50)	Case-control	OCD = 12 [34.8 ± 10.1, 5M:7F]; HC (task 2) = 40 [42.9 ± 14.3, 19M:21F]	Not reported.	Not reported.	Both a hexagon and a static labelling task	Facial emotion recognition	Happiness, surprise, sadness, anger, fear, disgust	DSM-III-R	OCD group significantly less accurate in recognizing disgust in the emotional hexagon task than HC ($p < 0.001$) and somewhat less accurate in recognizing anger ($0.01 > p < 0.05$). Recognition of static expressions of disgust was also significantly impaired in the OCD group ($p < 0.01$).
	Toh et al. (51)	Case-control Outpatients	OCD = 19 [37.0 ± 10.4, 5M: 14F]; BDD = 21 [34.3 ± 11.9, 5M: 16F]; HC = 21 [35.7 ± 10.6, 8M: 13F]	SAD (n=2), MDD (n=6).	SSRIs (n=10), SNRIs (n=3), TCAs (n = 1), with some receiving atypical antipsychotic augmentation (n = 4). Therapy not reported.	Static labelling task.	Facial emotion recognition	Happiness, surprise, sadness, anger, fear, disgust, neutral	MINI500/Y-BOCS	BDD group were less accurate overall compared to the OCD and HC groups (comparison OCD and HC not mentioned). Severe OCD was associated with poorer emotion recognition.
	Via et al. (52)	Case-control fMRI	OCD = 67 [33.1 ± 8.5, 38M:29F]; HC = 67 [32.8 ± 10.2, 38M:29F]	MDD (n=4), DD (n=2), GAD (n=3), PD (n=4), SP (n=3).	Citalopram (n=2), clomipramine (n=29), clomipramine + SSRI (n=9), escitalopram (n=7), fluoxetine (n=7), fluoxetine + SSRI (n=1), fluvoxamine (n=4), fluvaoxamine + SSRI (n=3),phenelzine (n=1), sertraline (n=1), sertraline + SSRI (n=1), adjunct antipsychotica (n=12)	Modified Emotional Face Matching Task (static matching task)	Facial emotion recognition	Happiness, fear (and anger)	SCID/DY-BOCS	No behavioral differences between patients and HC in matching of emotional faces. Compared to HC, patients exhibited enhanced activation in bilateral amygdala, and secondary visual cortex extended to intraparietal sulcus, right anterior insula cortex, premotor cortex, right orbitofrontal cortex and right middle temporal gyrus ($ps < 0.05$) when matching fearful faces compared to matching shapes. Only left amygdala survived whole brain level correction.

(Continued)

TABLE 1 | Continued

Domain	Author	Method	Participants	Comorbid diagnoses?	Concurrent medication/ therapy?	Task description	Subdomain	Emotions assessed	Diagnosis/ symptom assessment	Main results
Nonaffective cues										
	Jung et al. (53)	Case-control fMRI	OCD = 15 [23.4 ± 4.7, 12M:3F]; HC = 15 [25.67 ± 3.46, 9M:6F]	Comorbid axis I diagnoses were considered exclusion criteria.	Monoamine oxidase inhibitors (n=2), SSRI + antianxiety (n=3), SSRI + antianxiety + anti-psychotics (n=3). Therapy not reported.	One-back task with biological and scrambled motion	Biological motion perception	Not applicable.	SCID for DSM-II/Y-BOCS	Compared to HC, patients exhibited increased activation in the right superior and middle temporal gyrus, the left inferior temporal and fusiform gyrus, and reduced activation in the right postcentral gyrus ($p < 0.001$, uncorrected).
	Kim et al. (54)	Case-control Outpatients	OCD = 20 [24.3 ± 6.2, 12M:8F]; HC = 16 [23.2 ± 5.8, 11M:5F]	Not reported.	Sertraline (n=4), citalopram (n=6), fluoxetine (n=5), fluvoxamine (n=2), risperidone (n=5), olanzapine (n=1), clonazepam (n=14), valproic acid (n=1), and lamotrigine (n=1). Therapy not reported.	Biological motion detection and discrimination tasks	Biological motion perception	Not applicable.	DSM-IV criteria/Y-BOCS	Patients found it more difficult to detect biological motion within noise dots ($p=0.003$) and to discriminate biological motion from scrambled motion ($p=0.034$), whereas their ability to perceive nonbiological global motion and static global form was comparable to HC.
	Shin et al. (55)	Case-control Outpatients	OCD = 54 [25.0 ± 6.5, 32M:22F]; HC = 42 [23.4 ± 4.6, 32M:10F]	Comorbid axis I diagnoses were considered exclusion criteria.	Medication-naïve (n=24), medication-free for 4 weeks (n=30). Therapy not reported.	Body and face discrimination task	Recognition of faces and bodies	Not applicable.	SCID/	Compared to HC, patients were less accurate in discriminating human bodily postures ($p < 0.001$), but not in discriminating faces or chairs.

OCD, obsessive-compulsive disorder; HC, healthy controls; SSRIs, selective serotonin reuptake inhibitors; EMODIFF, The Facial Emotion Intensity Differentiation Test; PEAT, Penn's Emotion Acuity Test; DSM, Diagnostic and Statistical Manual of Mental Disorders; SCID, Structured Clinical Interview for DSM Axis I Disorders; Y-BOCS, Yale–Brown Obsessive-Compulsive Scale; OAD, other anxiety disorders; AD, anxiety disorder; ODD, oppositional defiant disorder; SCL-90, Symptom Checklist-90; PD, panic disorder; GAD, generalized anxiety disorder; MDD, major depression disorder; ADHD, attention-deficit hyperactivity disorder; TCA, tricyclic antidepressants; KSADS-PL, Kiddie Schedule for Affective Disorders and Schizophrenia; YGTSS, the Yale Global Tic Severity Scale; CBT, cognitive-behavioral therapy; KAMT, Kinney's Affect Matching Test; MINI, Mini International Neuropsychiatric Interview; SAD, Social anxiety disorder; ADIS-IV, Anxiety Disorders Interview Schedule for DSM-IV; GAF, Global Assessment of Functioning; OR, Odds ratio; OCI-R, obsessive-compulsive inventory revised; MHR, mean hit rate; DD, dysthymic disorder; PDA, panic disorder with agoraphobia; SSDs, Schizophrenia spectrum disorders; PTSS, posttraumatic stress disorder; BDD, body dysmorphic disorder; ICD, International Statistical Classification of Diseases; MADRS, Montgomery–Asberg Depression Rating Scale; HRAC, High Risk Assessment and Checking; CC, contamination and cleaning; PS, Perfectionism and Symmetry; GSP, generalized social phobia; GTS, Gilles de la Tourette's syndrome; OBS, obsessive-compulsive symptoms; SNRIs, serotonin–norepinephrine reuptake inhibitors; SP, social phobia; DY-BOCS, Dimensional Yale-Brown Obsessive-Compulsive Scale; SGA, second-generation antipsychotic; MOCI, Maudsley Obsessive Compulsive Scale; HDRS, Hamilton Depression Rating Scale.

English)]. Based on a combined sample of 221 patients and 223 controls, the review concluded that OCD patients were significantly less accurate in identifying the six basic emotions overall compared with controls, showing a medium effect size (Cohen's d = −0.55), with larger effects for static (Cohen's d = −0.77) compared to morphed emotional expressions (Cohen's d = −0.14). OCD patients were also impaired in the recognition of negative emotions as a whole (Cohen's d = −0.34) and had particularly difficulties with the recognition of disgust (Cohen's d = −0.59) and anger (Cohen's d = −0.36). A marginally significant deficit in the recognition of sadness was also found (Cohen's d = −0.31), while fear recognition was not significantly impaired (Cohen's d = −0.09). Thus, based on these ten patients studies, OCD is associated with pronounced impairments in the recognition of facial expressions of disgust, while modest impairments in the recognition of other negative emotions, specifically anger and sadness, but not fear, are also observed.

The Role of Symptom Severity in Facial Emotion Recognition

Several studies additionally report on the relation between facial emotion recognition and symptom severity of patients. Although obtaining no significant emotion recognition deficits, Parker et al. (48) did show that the patient with the most severe symptoms as measured by the Yale-Brown Obsessive-Compulsive Scale [Y-BOCS; (62)] showed marked impairments in the recognition of disgust, and suggested that such impairments might only arise for severe cases. In the study by Corcoran et al. (40), most of the patients were as accurate in recognizing disgust as healthy controls. However, approximately one-third of the patient group showed marked impairments, which led to a significant overall difference between patients and controls. The authors found that those patients who were impaired on disgust recognition had higher Y-BOCS scores as well as significantly lower scores on a scale of global functioning. Lochner and colleagues (45) also report a marginally significant negative relation between symptom severity (Y-BOCS total) and disgust recognition accuracy in a morphing task after correcting for depression scores. Furthermore, a significantly negative correlation between total Y-BOCS scores and the recognition of fear was found in an emotional matching task by Bozikas and colleagues (36), but this effect did not survive Bonferroni correction. No correlation with any of the other emotions was obtained. A study by Toh, Castle, and Rossell (51) reports a negative correlation between symptom severity (Y-BOCS total) and overall facial affect recognition but do not provide any specifics since the focus of their study concerned patients with body dysmorphic disorder, for which patients with OCD served as a reference group. Other studies however, did not observe significant relations with symptom severity (47, 49, 52) and the review by Daros and colleagues (41) also was not able to detect a significant relation between symptom severity and overall emotion recognition, nor with anger or disgust individually, based on the ten studies included in their meta-analysis. Hence, overall, there does not seem to be very strong evidence for a relation between symptom severity and facial recognition impairments.

The Role of Symptom Subtype in Facial Emotion Recognition

So far, studies investigating the role of symptom subtype do not seem to provide clear differences in emotion recognition between different subdomains of OCD. One study specifically compared different subdomains of OCD (46). Patients were divided into three subgroups; high risk assessment and checking, contamination and cleaning, and perfectionism and symmetry. While no significant findings emerged for disgust, the study showed a significant difference between patients scoring high on risk assessment and checking and controls in sensitivity to fear and happiness, indicating that they were able to correctly identify these emotions at a lower intensity level than controls. Jhung et al. (42) showed that having more hoarding symptoms was associated with poorer disgust recognition, yet this relation did not remain after controlling for age, sex, and depression scores. Additionally, the studies by Corcoran et al. (40) and Rector et al. (49) showed no differences in disgust recognition between patients with and without primary contamination concerns.

Biases in Facial Emotion Recognition

Some studies have additionally demonstrated that OCS is associated with specific biases in facial emotion perception. Aigner et al. (35) used a task that required OCD patients to rate faces as neutral, happy or sad, and the degree of intensity of these emotions. Results showed that OCD patients displayed a bias to recognize neutral faces as sad, as well as a bias to recognize happy faces as neutral and happy faces as sad (35). Patients were also less accurate in identifying sad expressions, but only for female faces. One study also indicates that patients with OCD may have bias toward perceiving faces as disgusting (42). This study investigated how patients responded to ambiguous faces (e.g., 50% disgust and 50% anger). They found that, compared to controls, OCD patients were significantly more likely to perceive ambiguous facial expressions as disgust and less likely as anger.

Neural Correlates of Facial Emotion Processing

The processing of emotional faces is associated with a wide range of brain regions, including visual, limbic, temporoparietal, prefrontal, and subcortical areas, with some areas showing differential sensitivity to specific emotions (18). For example, the amygdala seems to be most specifically activated by fear, whereas the insula is particularly sensitive to expressions of disgust (18). A few functional magnetic resonance imaging (fMRI) studies have investigated how patients with OCD process facial emotions on a neural level, using passive or implicit viewing (38, 44) or active matching tasks (39, 52).

A study by Cannistraro et al. (38) indicates that the passive or implicit perception of faces or facial expressions in general, rather than emotional faces specifically, is associated with altered neural activity. The authors used a simple emotional faces paradigm consisting of the passive viewing of alternating blocks of fearful, happy and neutral faces. While both patients and healthy controls showed activity in left and right amygdala for fearful compared to neutral facial expressions, no between-group differences were observed for this contrast. The study did found that when contrasting all facial expressions with fixation, reactivity of the amygdala was attenuated in OCD patients compared to healthy controls.

Another study suggests altered neural processing of facial expressions of disgust in patients (44). In a backward masking paradigm that presented neutral, disgusted, and fearful facial expressions just above conscious awareness level, patients with OCD displayed increased activity in the left ventrolateral prefrontal cortex (an area involved in response inhibition and response modulation) and reduced activity in the thalamus (involved in memory, attention, and information processing) for disgusted compared to neutral expressions. Importantly, they found this effect to be driven by those patients scoring high on washing symptoms, suggesting this activity may be particularly characteristic for those who suffer from compulsions that relate to contamination concerns.

Two other studies focused on tasks that require more explicit attention to presented emotions as they involve active matching of emotional faces. Cardoner et al. (39) used a task involving the matching of a happy or fearful target face to two out of three possible emotional probe faces (happy, fearful, and angry). Results showed that matching emotional faces versus matching shapes resulted in increased activation in a distributed network of brain regions known to be involved in face processing, including the amygdala, fusiform gyrus, thalamus, and dorsolateral prefrontal cortex in OCD patients compared to controls. Patients also demonstrated significantly increased connectivity between these face-processing regions and greater activation of the right dorsolateral prefrontal cortex and the left anterior insula region for fearful compared to happy faces. In addition, the task-related activation and functional connectivity was found to be associated with symptom severity as measured by the Y-BOCS. Using a similar task, Via et al. (52) showed that matching fearful faces, compared to matching shapes, resulted in increased activation of the amygdala region in patients, as well as other regions that did not survive whole-brain level correction such as the right anterior insula cortex, premotor cortex, right orbitofrontal cortex, and right middle temporal gyrus. Amygdala activation for this contrast also significantly correlated with the severity of aggression/checking and sexual/religious dimensions. These studies suggest that when explicit emotional recognition is required, patients show increased neural reactivity in various brain regions involved in face and emotion processing, most consistently the amygdala, during the processing of fearful expressions, compared to controls.

Affective Prosody

Though many researchers have investigated the recognition of emotions from facial expressions, to our knowledge, only a single study has focused on the ability to identify emotions based on vocal information, i.e., prosodic intonation, in OCD (36). In this study, participants were presented with audio-recorded sentences expressing one of five basic emotions (happy, sad, surprise, fear, and anger) and were asked to identify the corresponding emotion. Results showed no significant group differences between patients and controls. The compulsion subscale of the Y-BOCS did show a significantly negative correlation with general affective prosody recognition and with the recognition of sadness specifically. These effects did however not survive Bonferroni correction. Therefore, this study indicates no deficits in the ability of individuals with OCD to recognize these five basic emotions. Yet, the sixth basic emotion of disgust, which seems especially relevant to the symptomatology of OCD, was not investigated here.

Nonaffective Social Cues

Only few studies have investigated how individuals with OCD perceive or process nonaffective social cues, i.e., the processing of nonemotional information by others. These studies provide some initial evidence that individuals with OCD have more difficulty in perceiving social cues such as biological motion and body poses. A study focusing on the perception of biological motion, which refers to the ability to identify the movements of animate beings, showed that, compared to controls, patients were less accurate in perceiving biological motion within noise dots, and less able to discriminate between biological and nonbiological or scrambled motion (54). Their ability to perceive nonbiological motion however, was comparable to controls. A subsequent fMRI study found that during the observation of biological versus scrambled motion, patients showed aberrant activation in several brain regions, including increased activation in the right superior and middle temporal gyrus, the left inferior temporal, and fusiform gyrus, and reduced activation in the right postcentral gyrus compared to healthy controls (53). These regions have been implicated in the integration of form and motion, object and face recognition, and the visual imagery of objects (63), and the authors suggested that increased activity in these regions may reflect the exertion of additional effort or the recruitment of additional strategies in patients, whereas healthy controls have a more automatic, reflexive perception of motion. A later study investigating body and face perception, reported that patients with OCD were significantly less accurate in discriminating static pairs of bodily postures implying actions, whereas their ability to discriminate faces and chairs was unimpaired (55).

Section Summary and Discussion: Social Cue Perception

To summarize, there is support for altered processing of both affective and nonaffective social cues in OCD, from both behavioral and neuroimaging studies. Multiple behavioral studies show specific facial emotion recognition deficits (39, 40, 49, 50), mainly with regard to expressions of disgust (40, 49, 50). Additionally, outcomes from a meta-analysis by Daros et al. (41)—including ten patient studies—also point to the presence of emotion recognition deficits in OCD, specifically for negative emotions such as disgust and, to a lesser extent, anger. Such a specific deficit in the recognition of facial expressions of disgust might represent an important marker of OCD and seems in line with studies highlighting the relevance of disgust in the symptomology of OCD, due to the role of this expression in the appraisal of potential contamination [see, e.g., (56)]. Yet, studies investigating the possible role of symptom subtype indicate no clear relation between specific symptom subtypes and facial emotion recognition deficits (40, 46, 49). It seems possible that disgust is involved in the symptomatology of OCD patients in a more general sense, as the emotion does not only convey possible contamination but also for example the violations of moral rules and interpersonal norms, to which individuals with OCD are thought to be particularly sensitive (56). Bhikram and colleagues suggest that patients with OCD learn to associate a broader range of stimuli and facial expressions with disgust due to an increased propensity to perceive them as disgusting, which might in turn decrease their ability to realistically identify stimuli expressing disgust. This is in line with the finding by Jhung et al. (42) that patients with OCD displayed a bias toward perceiving ambiguous faces as expressing disgust rather than anger. It should be noted however, that sample sizes in the studies investigating the role of subtypes were very small (N between 3 and 15), which hinders the ability to detect reliable effects.

Despite evidence for a disgust recognition deficit on a meta-analytic level, a great number of individual studies did not observe any deficits in facial emotion recognition [e.g., (36, 37, 42, 43, 46, 47)], which may suggest that deficits are associated with specific subgroups of patients or task characteristics. Although some studies show a positive relation between symptom severity and disgust recognition impairment (40, 45, 48), many studies did not and the meta-analysis by Daros et al. (41) was not able to detect such a relation based on the studies included in their review. Some studies additionally show that disgust recognition impairments are present in some but not all patients (40, 48). Interestingly, recognition of facial expressions of disgust also seem to be enhanced or restored by cognitive behavioral therapy and SSRI treatment (45, 49), suggesting that treatment status may play a role. Clearly, more research into possible moderating variables is required.

Besides initial evidence for a bias toward perceiving ambiguous faces as expressing disgust (42), individuals with OCD may be characterized by a bias to perceive facial expressions as more negatively valenced than they actually are (35). Such a bias is often also present in depression [see (64) for a review], and future studies are therefore needed to investigate to what extent the presence of depressive symptoms may account for this. Interestingly, biases toward threat-related stimuli have not been reported so far in OCD, which is remarkable given that this is commonly reported in anxiety disorders (57).

Neuroimaging studies demonstrate altered activation in various brain areas during the processing of facial emotions in OCD patients (38, 39, 44, 52), even in the absence of behavioral differences in facial emotion recognition. This seems to suggest that patients with OCD process emotional information differently, perhaps because they recruit compensatory mechanisms. Interestingly, reduced or similar amygdala activation was found in patients compared to healthy controls during the passive viewing or indirect perception of facial expressions in general (38, 44) while enhanced activation of this area was observed in tasks that required active recognition of emotional expressions (39, 52). The amygdala is involved in many different processes, and responds to a variety of emotional stimuli, but has been most consistently implicated in mediating fear and anxiety reactions, and heightened amygdala responses have often been observed in disorders of anxiety (65). Increased amygdala reactivity during situations in which OCD patients have to pay active attention to facial emotions and label or match them, and during the perception of fear specifically, therefore seems consistent with a heightened emotion or threat responsiveness, yet the finding of reduced activity during passive or indirect viewing of facial emotions deserves further exploration. In addition, patients showed altered neural activity in several other regions, such as the ACC, insula and ventro- and dorsolateral prefrontal cortex. These regions have also been implicated in neurobiological and neurocognitive accounts of the disorder [e.g., (16, 56, 66)] and increased activity in these regions may for example represent altered affective responsiveness and increased emotion regulation attempts during emotion processing (67). Moreover, altered activity in the thalamus was observed during the processing of facial emotions, an area which is thought to represent a key node in the disturbed fronto-striatal feedback loops thought to be involved in the pathogenesis of the disorder (16). Additionally, there are some indications that the specific neural alterations seem to depend on obsessive-compulsive subtype (44, 52), which highlights the importance of further elucidating the role of symptom subtypes.

The single study investigating the processing of nonfacial affective cues in OCD (36) showed no significant differences in the recognition of affective prosody between patients and healthy controls, although more severe compulsions did appear to be associated with decreased performance on the affective prosody task. Clearly, more research is needed to further explore possible deficits in the recognition of emotions from other cues than facial expressions in OCD, such as vocal, auditory or bodily cues.

There is also a scarcity of studies in the domain of nonaffective social cue perception. The few studies that do exist indicate that OCD patient seem to have difficulties identifying biological motion and body poses but not faces implying action (54, 55). Jung et al. (53) additionally showed that the perception of biological motion was associated with altered activity in several brain regions associated with the representation of visual information. These results suggest that it is possible that OCD patients already experience impairments at very basic, visual levels of social cognition.

MENTALIZING/TOM

The terms mentalizing and ToM are often used interchangeable and refer to the ability to infer the mental states of others (68). ToM is often divided in the ability to infer the feelings and emotions of others (affective ToM) and the ability to infer other people's intentions and beliefs [cognitive ToM; (69)]. ToM has been found to involve many brain regions, most consistently the temporoparietal junction extending to the superior temporal sulcus, and the medial prefrontal cortex (dorsomedial- and ventromedial prefrontal cortex), but also regions thought to be engaged in a more task-specific manner such as the precuneus, anterior temporal lobes, inferior frontal gyrus including the orbitofrontal cortex, amygdala, insula, and ACC (29, 70). Research generally distinguishes first-order (e.g., what is that person thinking)? and more complex second-order (e.g., what is he/she thinking that another person is thinking)? levels of ToM (71). A more recent division additionally separates social-cognitive and social-perceptual components (72, 73). Social-cognitive ToM involves inferring mental states of others based on their behavior, and reflects "reasoning" processes. Social-perceptual ToM, on the other hand, refers to the ability to infer other's mental states based on perceptual features. The current section will focus on studies investigating ToM abilities in OCD patients (*Mentalizing/ToM in OC*) and on the role of symptom severity and level of insight into one's own mental illness (*The Role of Symptom Severity and Level of Insight in ToM*). No studies investigating the neural correlates of mentalizing/ToM in OCD were identified. **Table 2** contains an overview of the studies discussed in this section.

Mentalizing/ToM in OCD

The Reading the Mind in the Eyes Task (RMET) represents a measure of affective, social-perceptual ToM, whereby individuals are required to infer emotional and mental states of others based on only the eye region of the face (81). Two studies in patients report lower RMET scores (73, 80), although after controlling for general neurocognitive functioning, between-group differences in the study by Misir and colleagues (73) were not significant anymore. Yet, two other studies report scores similar in patients and controls (77, 78).

Other studies focused on more social-cognitive aspects of ToM in OCD. Sayın, Oral, Utku, Baysak, and Candansayar (79) used a number of different tasks. An adapted version of the cartoon picture story based on Brüne (82) was used to assess first- and second-order false beliefs. A story of the so-called hinting task (83, 84) was used to assess the ability to infer real intentions behind indirect statements. To assess more advanced, "third-order" ToM (e.g., he knows they think he will lie), the double-bluff story from the set of "Strange Stories" was used (85), which asks participants to identify why a character of the story said something that was not meant literally. Although patients performed worse on all ToM tasks, the difference with controls was significant only for the double-bluff task, which they found to be associated with reduced memory capacity: performance on this task was positively correlated with both immediate and delayed recall on a visual reproduction task. Tulacı et al. (80) employed the same tasks along with a faux pas test (86) and demonstrated significant group differences, with patients performing worse on all tasks. Misir et al. (73) also showed significant social-cognitive ToM deficits in patients compared to controls in all measures of a test battery called the Dokuz Eylül ToM Index (DEToMI), which remained significant after controlling for general neurocognitive functioning. The DEToMI consists of a series of verbal or visual tasks assessing social-cognitive aspects of ToM and includes first- and second-order false belief tasks, as well as irony, metaphor, and faux pas recognition tasks (73). In contrast, Mavrogiorgou et al. (47) found no significant impairments compared to controls on the hinting task, multiple sets from "Strange Stories" nor on the faux pas test. The authors did find a marginally significant deficit on a proverb test (87), which assesses the ability to recognize the hidden meaning behind indirect speech and which has been found to be strongly related to ToM (88). Thus, most but not all studies show deficient social-cognitive ToM in OCD patients.

Liu et al. (76) specifically compared affective and cognitive components of ToM using the so-called Yoni task (89). In this task, a cartoon face was presented in the middle of the screen with four colored pictures in each corner of the screen. Participants had to identify the picture that the cartoon was referring to based on an incomplete sentence at the top of the screen and cues such as the eye gaze and expression of the cartoon face and the facial expressions of the corner images. The study demonstrated impairments in OCD patients specifically on second-order, cognitive levels of ToM, which remained significant after controlling for general neurocognitive abilities, while first-order and affective levels of ToM were not significantly different from controls. A single study by Buhlmann, Wacker, and Dziobek (74) employed a multimodal task called the Movie for the Assessment of Social Cognition (90) to assess general ToM skills in OCD patients. In this task, participants watched a short movie and were instructed to answer questions about the characters' thoughts, intentions and emotions at set time points during the movie. No differences between OCD patients and controls were found, suggesting that patients with OCD do not show impairments during more integrated assessments of ToM.

The Role of Symptom Severity and Level of Insight in ToM

İnanç and Altıntaş (75) observed a negative relation between symptom severity and RMET performance in patients, while Misir and colleagues (73) observed a moderate negative correlation between symptom severity and DEToMI total score. Yet, other patient studies did not demonstrate significant relations between symptom severity and ToM (47, 76, 78, 79). There is however evidence to suggest that the extent to which patients are aware of the irrationality of their obsessions and/or compulsions, i.e., their level of insight, is related to ToM abilities (73, 75, 80). Tulacı et al. (80) found significant negative correlations between insight level and all ToM tasks, with ToM performance significantly lower in patients with poor compared to good insight. Interestingly, patients with good insight did not differ from healthy controls on the RMET and first- and second-order false belief task, but did score significantly lower on the double bluff, faux pass and hinting task. Misir et al. (73) also reported a negative correlation between the level of insight and the DEToMI total score. İnanç and Altıntaş (75) specifically investigated the role of insight within a sample of treatment-resistant and treatment-responding patients. They found a significant negative correlation between RMET performance and level of insight. RMET scores were also significantly lower in the treatment-resistant group. Thus, these studies suggest that ToM may be especially impaired in those OCD patients with poor illness insight, and to a lesser extent in patients with good insight.

TABLE 2 | Overview of studies investigating theory of mind in obsessive-compulsive disorder.

Author	Method	Participants	Comorbid diagnosis?	Concurrent medication/ therapy?	Task	ToM domain	Diagnosis or symptom assessment	Main results
Bozikas et al. (36)	Case-control Outpatients	OCD = 25 [32.7 ± 9.0, 10M:15F]; HC = 25 [33.4 ± 7.3, 14M:11F]	Depression (n=4), PD (n=2).	ATD without (n=11) and with (n=5) atypical antipsychotics, antipsychotics only (n=1). All patients were receiving CBT.	Fantie's Affective Cartoon Test	Social-perceptual, affective	DSM-IV, MINI/Y-BOCS	No significant differences between OCD patients and HC.
Buhlmann et al. (74)	Case-control	OCD = 35 [34.0 ± 9.1, 18M:17F]; HC = 35 [32.7 ± 11.0, 14M:21F]	MDD (n=7), panic disorder (n=2), specific phobia (n=2), AA (n=1), CTD (n=1), dysthymia (n=1), hypochondriasis (n=1).	Not reported.	Movie for the Assessment of Social Cognition	Multimodal assessment	SCID	No significant differences between OCD patients and HC.
İnanç and Altıntaş (75)	Patients only (in- and outpatients) Correlational study	OCD = 71 (subgroups: treatment resistant = 30 [32.8 ± 9.0, 8M: 22F], treatment responders = 41 [32.4 ± 9.8, 12M:29F])	Exclusion criteria included several psychiatric conditions including active schizophrenia or psychosis, acute suicidality, and substance abuse.	Not reported.	RMET	Social-perceptual, affective	SCID/Y-BOCS	Significant negative correlation between the RMET and the level of insight ($p < 0.01$), and between the RMET and symptom severity ($p < 0.01$). RMET scores were also significantly lower in the treatment-resistant group ($p=0.001$).
Liu et al. (76)	Case-control Outpatients	OCD = 40 [24.6 ± 4.1, 18M:22F]; HC = 38 [23.3 ± 2.7, 16M:22F]	Comorbid psychiatric disorder was considered an exclusion criterion.	Not reported.	Yoni task	First-order, second-order, cognitive + affective	SCID/Y-BOCS	OCD patients scored significantly lower than HC in second-order, affective mental state attributions ($p=0.002$), even after neurocognitive functioning was taken into account ($p=0.023$).
Mavrogiorgou et al. (47)	Case-control Outpatients	OCD = 20 [38.1 ± 10.6, 12M:8F]; HC = 20 [38.2 ± 13.0, 12M:8F]	Comorbid MDD or ADs were not considered exclusion criteria.	SSRIs (n=18), St. John's wort (n=1), SSRIs plus antipsychotic drugs (n=13). CBT was not consider an exclusion criteria.	Hinting Task (double-bluff, persuasion, mistakes, and white lies stories), faux pas test, proverb test	First-order, second-order, social-cognitive	ICD-10 and DSM-IV criteria/Y-BOCS	No significant difference between OCD patients and HC with regard to ToM tasks. However, patients with OCD performed marginally worse on the proverb task ($p=0.053$).
Misir et al. (73)	Case-control Outpatients	OCD = 34 [32,4 ± 10.0, 13M:21F]; HC = 30 [34,4 ± 9,7, 17M:13F].	Comorbidities not reported, but many psychiatric conditions served as exclusion criteria.	SSRI's (n=29). Therapy not reported.	DEToMI (includes first- and second-order false belief tasks, irony, metaphor and faux pas recognition tasks), RMET.	First- and second-order, social-cognitive + social-perceptual, affective	SCID/Y-BOCS	Patients' DEToMI ($p=0.002$) and RMET total scores ($p=0.005$) were significantly lower than HC. When controlled for neurocognitive functioning, between-group difference for RMET was no longer significant ($p=0.087$). There also was a moderate negative correlation between symptom severity and DEToMI total score ($r= -0.376$; $p=0.026$).
Pertusa et al. (77)	Case-control	OCD (n=31), AD (n=19), and HC (n=55).	GAD (n=8), PD +/- agoraphobia (n=5), SP (n=5), MDD (n=2), ED	Not reported.	RMET	Social-perceptual, affective	SCID/DY-BOCS	No significant differences between OCD patients and HC.

(Continued)

TABLE 2 | Continued

Author	Method	Participants	Comorbid diagnosis?	Concurrent medication/ therapy?	Task	ToM domain	Diagnosis or symptom assessment	Main results
			(n=2), dysthymia (n=1).					
Pino et al. (78)	Case-control	OCD = 24 [39.1 ± 12.9, 12M:11F]; HC = 23 [38.7 ± 11.9,13M:11F].	Comorbidities: axis I disorders were considered as exclusion criteria.	Not reported.	RMET	Social-perceptual, affective	SCID/Y-BOCS	No significant differences between OCD patients and HC.
Sayin et al. (79)	Case-control Outpatients	OCD = 30 [34.3 ± 11.5, 10M:20F]; HC = 30 [33.0 ± 10.6, 10M:20F].	Not reported.	ATD only (n = 18), ATD + antipsychotics, (n = 6), ATD, antipsychotics + benzodiazepines (n=6). Therapy not reported.	First- and second-order false belief tasks, hinting task, double-bluff story from "Strange Stories" set.	First- and second-order, social-cognitive	SCID/Y-BOCS	Patients scored significantly worse on the double-bluff task compared to HC ($p < 0.01$). Performance on double-bluff task was positively correlated with visual reproduction immediate recall ($r=0.411$, $p <0.05$) and visual reproduction-delayed recall ($r=0.478$, $p < 0.05$), while the hinting task was positively correlated with verbal memory ($r=0.481$, $p < 0.05$).
Tulacı et al. (80)	Case-control	OCD = 80 (subgroups: PI [n=24, 31.2 ± 11.3, 9M:15F], GI [n=56, 28.8 ± 9.0, 19M: 37F]); HC = 80 (no demographics provided).	Presence of comorbidities (PI: n=13, GI: n=33).	Single ATD (PI: n=8, GI: n=39), > 1 ATD (PI: n=1, GI: n=3), 1 ATD and 1 antipsychotic (PI: n=12, GI: n=6), > 1 ATD and antipsychotic (PI: n=2, GI: n=0). Therapy not reported.	First-order and second-order false-belief tasks, hinting test, Faux Pas test, double-bluff story from "Strange Stories" set, RMET.	First- and second-order, social-cognitive + social-perceptual, affective	SCID/Y-BOCS	Scores were significantly lower in patients than HC for all ToM tasks ($p < 0.05$). Scores were also significantly lower in the PI compared to GI group ($p < 0.05$). No significant differences between good insight group and HC for first- and second-order false-belief or RMET scores ($p > 0.05$). When comparing GI patients with HC, only faux pas, and double-bluff test scores were significantly lower in patients ($p < 0.05$).

ToM, Theory of mind; OCD, obsessive-compulsive disorder; HC, healthy controls; RMET, Reading the Mind in the Eyes Task; PD, panic disorder; ATD, antidepressant; K-SADS, Kiddie-Schedule for Affective Disorders and Schizophrenia; DSM, Diagnostic and Statistical Manual of Mental Disorders; MINI, Mini International Neuropsychiatric Interview; MDD, major depression disorder; AA, alcohol abuse; CTD, chronic tic disorder; SCID, Structured Clinical Interview for DSM Axis I Disorders; OCI-R, obsessive-compulsive inventory revised; SSRIs, selective serotonin reuptake inhibitors; Ads, anxiety disorders; CBT, cognitive-behavioral therapy; ICD, International Statistical Classification of Diseases; DEToMI, Dokuz Eylül Theory of Mind Index; HD, hoarding disorder; GAD, generalized anxiety disorder; SP, social phobia; ED, eating disorder; PI, poor insight; GI, good insight.

Section Summary and Discussion: Mentalizing/ToM

In summary, there is some evidence for deficient mentalizing or ToM in OCD. Some of these studies find deficits in both affective and cognitive ToM (73, 80) whereas in other studies deficits are limited to (social-)cognitive and higher-order domains (76, 79). Yet other studies, however, show no clear deficits (36, 47, 74, 77, 78). The observed ToM deficits seem to depend in part on more general cognitive abilities (73, 79), which is unsurprising as ToM tasks draw upon general cognitive and verbal abilities to a much greater extent than lower-level processes such as emotion recognition [see, e.g., (91)]. These studies thus indicate that the cognitive deficits that patients with OCD experience may also impact on social cognitive abilities such as ToM. However, ToM deficits in OCD do not seem to be explained by more general cognitive deficits alone (73, 76), highlighting the importance of investigating social cognition in the disorder as a separate construct.

While most studies do not indicate a significant relation between ToM and symptom severity (47, 76, 78, 79), level of illness insight of patients does appear to be an important moderator of ToM deficits (73, 75, 80). Poor insight in OCD is associated with several clinical characteristics, such as higher comorbidity rates, specifically depression and schizophrenia spectrum disorders, poorer treatment response, more severe symptoms, and longer illness duration (92, 93). Notably, obsessive-compulsive symptoms are highly prevalent in schizophrenia and patients with first-episode psychosis with prevalence rates up to 64% (94), and the presence of these symptoms have been associated with poorer social cognitive abilities in patients with schizophrenia, specifically for higher-order ToM (95). Approximately 22%–25% of patients are characterized by poor insight (92, 93). As such, it seems possible that these patients represent a subgroup of OCD with greater ToM disturbances. However, more general factors related to poor insight such as poorer global, cognitive, and intellectual functioning may also play a role (94).

To our knowledge, no studies have investigated the neural correlates of ToM in relation to OCD. Given the observed deficits in ToM inferences, regions involved in ToM such as the temporoparietal junction and the medial prefrontal cortex may be affected. Furthermore, several brain regions implicated in the psychopathology of OCD [see, e.g., (16)] have been linked to ToM as well. For example, it has been suggested that more affective or implicit ToM assessments involve regions such as the orbitofrontal cortex, (dorsal) ACC, and insula, whereas cognitive and explicit assessments depend on brain areas related to more general cognitive resources such as the rostral ACC and medial and lateral PFC (29). Future studies may provide important insights into the underlying neural mechanisms of disturbed ToM inferences.

EXPERIENCE SHARING AND EMPATHY

Experience sharing refers to the vicarious experience and brain activity that is triggered by observing behavior of others. Green et al. (4) divide this concept in "motor resonance" and "affect sharing." Motor resonance is defined as the functional correspondence between the motor state in others and the self and is believed to represents a bottom-up process involving the so-called mirror neuron system [MNS; (4)]. This system consists of a group of neurons that are thought to be involved in the recognition and understanding of others actions by imitating or "mirroring" the actions or behaviors performed by others as they are activated by both the execution and observation of actions (95). It involves a network of brain regions including the inferior frontal gyrus, dorsal, and ventral premotor cortex, and the inferior and superior parietal lobule as well as other regions depending on sensory modality (96). For example, the execution and observation of emotional expressions demonstrates vicarious activity in regions such as the insula, amygdala, and cingulate gyrus (96).

The second aspect of experience sharing is "affect sharing," which refers to the observation of emotional expressions in others and the corresponding experience of these emotions as well as the activation of emotion-related brain areas in the self (4). Affect sharing is thought to represent a bottom-up process depending on the coupling of perception and action which possibly involves the MNS, and is considered a crucial subcomponent of empathy (97, 98). Empathy is considered a multifaceted construct including both bottom-up affect sharing processes as well as more top-down executive processes such as perspective taking skills and emotion regulation, which are mostly thought to involve prefrontal brain regions (99, 100). Many researchers also distinguish between affective empathy (the ability to share others' emotional states) and cognitive empathy [the ability to understand others' emotions; see, e.g., (69)]. By this definition, cognitive empathy is equated with affective ToM. Yet other researchers narrow down the concept of empathy to the isomorphic state (knowingly) elicited by the affective state of others [e.g., (101)]. The following section will focus on motor resonance (*Motor Resonance*) and affect sharing and empathy (*Affect Sharing and Empathy*). Research on emotion regulation, which constitutes a critical subcomponent of empathy, will be discussed below in the section *Emotion Experience and Regulation*. **Table 3** contains an overview of the studies discussed in this section.

Motor Resonance

Although no studies have directly investigated how the actions of others are represented in the brain of patients with OCD, there is some indirect evidence to suggest that patients with OCD may show deficient motor resonance. A study by Rounis, Banca, and Voon (104) for example showed that patients with OCD scored significantly lower than healthy controls on a task that required them to imitate meaningless hand and finger gestures performed by an experimenter. In addition, previously discussed studies (*Nonaffective Social Cues*) on the recognition of biological motion (53, 54) and body poses implying action (55) may likewise indicate a deficiency in representing the actions of others in the brain. Besides behavioral reports of impairments in motion or action recognition (54, 55), the study by Jung et al. (53) showed that patients demonstrated increased activity in several brain regions that are thought to be part of the MNS during the perception of biological motion, and have proposed that this activation may reflect increased effort or neural inefficiency of this system. However, since their study concerned moving black dots rather than real human beings performing actions, direct evidence for altered motor resonance and MNS functioning in OCD is still missing.

Affect Sharing and Empathy

Current measures of affect sharing and empathy in OCD are limited to self-report questionnaires such as the Interpersonal reactivity index [IRI; (105)]. The IRI represents a widely used measure of empathy containing four subscales, of which two scales measure affective components of empathy (empathic concern and personal distress) and two scales measure cognitive components (perspective taking and fantasy). Empathic concern refers to feelings of concern and sympathy for others, whereas the personal distress scale focuses on self-oriented feelings of anxiety and distress intense interpersonal situations. Empathic concern is thought to promote prosocial behavior toward others (105), whereas the experience of interpersonal distress is often considered maladaptive, and has been found to be elevated in mood and anxiety disorders (106). The perspective taking subscale refers to one's more cognitive tendency or ability to spontaneously adapt the viewpoint of others, whereas the fantasy scale measures the tendency to identify oneself with fictitious characters in books, movies, or plays.

Using the IRI, Fontenelle et al. (102) demonstrated that patients with OCD displayed greater self-reported levels of empathic concern and personal distress compared to healthy controls. Within patients, higher neutralizing and hoarding symptoms as measured by the obsessive-compulsive inventory–revised (OCI-R) were associated with high scores on the fantasy dimension. Patients with higher symptoms of checking, ordering, washing, and hoarding also showed more empathic concern, whereas all symptom dimensions were related to higher personal distress. However, after correcting for comorbid depression and anxiety, only the relation between hoarding symptoms and fantasy remained. In another sample of OCD patients, Kang, Namkoong, Yoo, Jhung, and Kim (103)

TABLE 3 | Overview of studies investigating experience sharing and empathy in obsessive-compulsive disorder.

Domain	Author	Method	Participants	Comorbid diagnosis?	Concurrent medication/ therapy?	Task/ questionnaire	Subdomain	Diagnosis/ symptom assessment	Main results
Empathy									
	Fontenelle et al. (102)	Case-control	OCD = 53 [39.3 ± 13.8, 29M:36F]; HC = 53 [35.5 ± 13.0, 24M:46F]	MDD (n=19), SP (n=3), DD (n=3).	SSRIs (n=42), benzodiazepine (n=21), antipsychotic (n=17). Therapy: CBT (n=17).	IRI	Cognitive empathy (PT and FT) + affective empathy (EC and PD)	SCID/OCI-R	Compared to HC, patients showed higher levels of EC (p=0.006) and PD (p < 0.001). Within patients, hoarding symptoms correlated with EC (r=0.39; p < 0.001), FT (r=0.36; p < 0.01), and PD (r=0.39; p < 0.001). After adjusting for covariates, only the association between hoarding and FT remained (r=0.41; p < 0.001).
	Kang et al. (103)	Case-control	OCD = 107 [27.5 ± 9.22, 72M:35F]; HC = 130 [26.0 ± 4.8, 82M/48F]	MDD (n=20), SP (n=5), BDD (n=20, panic disorder (n=1).	All patients were taking medications. Therapy not reported.	IRI	Cognitive empathy (PT and FT) + affective empathy (EC and PD)	SCID/Y-BOCS	Patients with OCD showed significantly lower PT (p=0.003) and higher PD (p=0.001) compared to HC. PD correlated significantly with forbidden thoughts symptoms (r=0.254, p=0.017) after correcting for gender, anxiety and depression levels.
	Pino et al. (78)	Case-control	OCD = 24 [39.1 ± 12.9, 12M:11F]; HC = 23 [38.7 ± 11.9,13M:11F]	Comorbid disorders were considered as exclusion criteria.	Not reported.	BES, EQ, EAT	Cognitive (BES cognitive, EQ, EAT) and affective empathy (BES affective)	SCID/Y-BOCS	OCD patients scored lower than controls on the EQ (p < 0.001), cognitive subscale of the BES (p=0.020) and attribution of negative emotions except disgust in the EAT (ps <0.005). There also was a positive relation between the cognitive BES subscale and Y-BOCS obsessions (r=−0.423, p=0.002) and compulsions (r= −0.420, p=0.003).subscales. No differences were found between patients and HC on the affective empathy subscale of the BES.
Motor resonance									
	Kim et al. (54)	Case-control Outpatients	OCD = 20 [24.3 ± 6.2, 12M:8F]; HC = 16 [23.2 ± 5.8, 11M:5F]	Not reported.	Sertraline (n=4), citalopram (n=6), fluoxetine (n=5), fluvoxamine (n=2), risperidone (n=5), olanzapine (n=1), clonazepam (n=14), valproic acid (n=1), and lamotrigine (n=1). Therapy not reported.	Biological motion detection and discrimination tasks	Biological motion perception	DSM-IV criteria/Y-BOCS	Patients found it more difficult to detect biological motion within noise dots (p=0.003) and to discriminate biological motion from scrambled motion (p=0.034), whereas their ability to perceive nonbiological global motion and static global form was comparable to HC.
	Jung et al. (53)	Case-control fMRI	OCD = 15 [23.4 ± 4.7, 12M:3F]; HC = 15 [25.67 ± 3.46, 9M:6F]	Comorbid axis I diagnoses were considered exclusion criteria.	Monoamine oxidase inhibitors (n=2), SSRI + antianxiety (n=3), SSRI + antianxiety + anti-psychotics	One-back task with biological and scrambled motion	Biological motion perception	SCID for DSM-II/Y-BOCS	Compared to HC, patients exhibited increased activation in the right superior and middle temporal gyrus, the left inferior temporal and fusiform gyrus and reduced activation in the right postcentral gyrus (p < 0.001, uncorrected).

(Continued)

TABLE 3 | Continued

Domain	Author	Method	Participants	Comorbid diagnosis?	Concurrent medication/ therapy?	Task/ questionnaire	Subdomain	Diagnosis/ symptom assessment	Main results
					(n=3). Therapy not reported.				
	Rounis et al. (104)	Case-control Outpatients	OCD = 24 [37.9 ± 14.7; 14M:10F] HC = 22 [37.4 ± 13.5; 12M:10F]	Comorbid psychiatric disorders were considered exclusion criteria.	SSRI (n=15) and SSRI + antipsychotic (n=4).	Meaningless gesture imitation task, extracted from the Birmingham Cognitive Screen	Action imitation	MINI/Y-BOCS	Scores on hand and finger imitation gestures were significantly lower for patients compared to HC (p=0.001). There were no significant correlations of imitation scores with the Y-BOCS.
	Shin et al. (55)	Case-control Outpatients	OCD = 54 [25.0 ± 6.5, 32M:22F]; HC = 42 [23.4 ± 4.6, 32M:10F]	Comorbid axis I diagnoses were considered exclusion criteria.	Medication-naïve (n=24), medication-free for 4 weeks (n=30). Therapy not reported.	Body and face discrimination task	Recognition of faces and bodies	SCID	Compared to HC, patients were less accurate in discriminating human bodily postures (p < 0.001), but not in discriminating faces or chairs.

OCD, obsessive-compulsive disorder; HC, healthy controls; MDD, major depressive disorder; SP, social phobia; DD, dysthymic disorder; SSRIs, selective serotonin reuptake inhibitors; CBT, cognitive-behavioral therapy; IRI, Interpersonal reactivity index; PT, Perspective Taking; FT, Fantasy; EC, Empathic Concern; PD, Personal Distress; SCID, Structured Clinical Interview for DSM Axis I Disorders; OCI-R, Obsessive-compulsive Inventory Revised; BDD, Body dysmorphic disorder; BES, Basic Empathy Scale; EQ, Empathy Quotient; EAT, Emotion Attribution Task; Y-BOCS, Yale–Brown Obsessive-Compulsive Scale; Diagnostic and Statistical Manual of Mental Disorders; MINI, Mini International Neuropsychiatric Interview.

showed increased personal distress and decreased perspective taking compared to healthy controls, with no differences for empathic concern or fantasy. When taking symptoms of depression and anxiety into account, the personal distress scale was also positively related to the forbidden thoughts dimension of the Y-BOCS measure of OCD symptoms, which refers to the presence of obsessions related to aggression, sex, and religion. These studies suggest that patients may be characterized by increased affective levels of empathy, especially with regard to empathic distress, and possibly decreased cognitive empathic abilities, as indicated by poorer perspective taking skills. However, these differences may be in part explained by comorbid levels of anxiety and depression, rather than specific symptom dimensions of OCD, as correlations with specific symptom dimensions often disappeared after including depression and anxiety levels as covariate.

In a study using different empathy measures (78), patients with OCD had lower scores than controls on the cognitive empathy subscale of the Basic Empathy Scale [BES; (107)] and on the Empathy Quotient (108), a questionnaire focusing mostly on cognitive empathy. Pino et al. (78) also showed a negative relation between scores on the cognitive BES subscale and the presence of obsessions and compulsions (as assessed by the Y-BOCS). Participants in this study also performed an emotion attribution task, in which the ability to identify the emotions of other's based on short stories was assessed (109). Here, patients scored lower than controls on the attribution of all negative emotions except disgust. However, Pino et al. (78) found no differences were compared to controls on the affective empathy subscale of the BES. Thus, this study indicates that OCD patients are characterized by specific deficits in cognitive, but not affective components of empathy.

Section Summary and Discussion: Experience Sharing and Empathy

Few studies have been conducted on experience sharing and empathy in patients with OCD. There are some indirect indications that patients with OCD may show deficient motor resonance or impaired MNS functioning as they have been shown to display poorer imitation of other's actions (104), impaired recognition and neural processing of biological motion (53, 54) and deficient perception of body poses implying actions (55), yet direct evidence for altered motor resonance from neuroimaging studies are missing. Likewise, there are no neuroimaging or experimental studies on affect sharing in patients with OCD. Evidence from self-report questionnaires does indicate that patients experience a heightened affective responsiveness to emotions of others (102, 103) or a similar emotional congruence with others compared to controls (78). Increased affective distress may be linked to more general levels of anxiety or depression, as most correlations with specific symptom dimensions did not remain after taking this into account. With regard to more top-down, cognitive aspects of empathy, some studies indicate a decreased self-reported ability to understand the emotions of others (78, 103), with scores on the emotion attribution task providing more experimental evidence for this (78). These findings seems in line with previously discussed experimental studies on affective ToM showing a decreased ability to identify the emotions of others in patients using the RMET (73, 80), which has also been considered as an index of cognitive empathy. Importantly however, research on experience sharing and empathic functioning in OCD is still in its infancy. Future studies using experimental as well as neuroimaging methods may shed more light on the specificity and origin of empathic alterations in the disorder.

EMOTION EXPERIENCE AND REGULATION

The term "emotion experience" refers to the emotion reactions (on either a subjective, observable, or neurophysiological level) that individuals experience in response to positive or negative stimuli (4). The ability to exert control over how and when these emotions are experienced and expressed is called emotion regulation (67). Whereas emotional reactivity is known to involve the dorsal anterior cingulate, insula, amygdala, and periaqueductal grey (PAG), explicit or conscious (top-down) regulation of emotion is associated with brain activity in the dorso- and ventro lateral prefrontal cortex, (pre)supplementary motor area and parietal cortex. Emotion regulation can however also be an automatic (bottom-up) process, and more implicit or unconscious emotion regulation has been linked to the ventral anterior cingulate and the ventromedial prefrontal cortex (67).

Given that OCD was until recently defined as an anxiety disorder, it has long been recognized that abnormal experience and regulation of emotions plays a crucial role in the symptomatology of OCD [see, e.g., (110)]. It has even been argued that the mental and behavioral compulsions that characterize OCD patients represent a maladaptive coping or emotion regulation mechanism of dealing with aversive and unwanted emotions triggered by obsessional thoughts (111). However, emotional disturbances may also importantly impact how we deal with social situations. For example, an influential framework by Decety and Meyer (100) suggests that emotion regulation is an important cognitive skill which helps control one's own arousal or distress. Individuals who become overaroused by other's distress due to problems with emotion regulation, might therefore be unable to deal with others emotions in a prosocial or adaptive fashion due to the cognitive resources that are used up too regulate their own emotions (112). Emotion regulation is thus considered a crucial subcomponent for adaptive empathic responding. Given that the way we experience and regulate our emotions is of critical importance for successful social interaction, the following section will describe existing research on the experience (*Emotion Experience*) and regulation (*Emotion Regulation*) of emotions in patients with OCD. **Table 4** contains an overview of the studies discussed in this section.

Emotion Experience

There is an abundance of evidence from neuroimaging studies demonstrating that patients with OCD show altered reactivity to emotional stimuli in nonsocial contexts. For example, a recent meta-analysis, including 25 studies with a total of 571 patients and 564 controls, showed that, compared to controls, patients experience increased activation in limbic, frontal, and temporal areas (bilateral amygdala, right putamen, orbitofrontal cortex, ACC, ventromedial prefrontal cortex, middle temporal, and left inferior occipital cortices) during the processing of aversive or symptom-provoking (versus neutral) stimuli (129), indicating heightened emotional reactivity.

Additionally, several studies indicate decreased neural sensitivity to rewarding stimuli, and increased sensitivity to stimuli indicating loss, using gambling (120), risky choice (117), monetary incentive delay (121, 123–125), probabilistic learning (128), or other incentive paradigms (126). For example, studies have shown reduced neural sensitivity in the nucleus accumbens (119, 121) and ACC (125) in response to anticipated rewards, and increased activity in the insula (120, 123) and lateral and medial frontal cortex during anticipated loss (123, 125). Decreased functional connectivity between the nucleus accumbens and limbic areas such as the amygdala during the anticipation of gain and loss has also been observed (124). Additionally, the direct processing of rewarding outcomes has been associated with decreased responsiveness in right medial and lateral orbitofrontal cortex (128) as well as in the caudate nucleus (119, 128). More widespread activation in the frontostriatal circuit including the putamen, precentral cortex, posterior insula, and ACC as well as cerebellum, in response to rewards has been reported as well (123). The processing of positive feedback and monetary reward has also been associated with decreased activation in frontal regions and the posterior cingulate [PCC; (126)]. In addition, the processing of rewards has been related to increased functional connectivity between the left PCC and the right ventromedial prefrontal cortex as well as between left and right PCC (126) and decreased connectivity between frontal and limbic regions (119).

Other studies using probabilistic learning tasks have demonstrated increased prediction error-related activation in the ACC (122, 127) and right putamen (122) during the omission of expected reward, while the unexpected receipt of reward has been associated with increased activity in the nucleus accumbens of patients (127). Studies on performance monitoring in OCD patients have also consistently shown enhanced amplitudes of the ERN during the commission of errors [see (13)], which may also be considered as aversive, negative stimuli or events. This ERP component has been suggested to represent a prediction error signal as it is generated in the ACC and likewise reflects a worse-than-expected outcome [see (136)] that has been found to scale with the emotional significance of the outcome [see (137)]. This suggests that increased ERNs in OCD patients are indicative of an increased affective reactivity to errors.

Despite clear indications for altered emotion experience in OCD in individual contexts, less is known about the emotional reactions of individuals with OCD in response to social emotion-inducing stimuli. Several studies have investigated the experience of basic emotions in patients with OCD as indexed by their facial expressions in response to emotion-inducing video clips of social scenarios (114, 117, 118). Mergl et al. (117) showed that patients with OCD demonstrated significantly slower initial velocity of involuntary laughing movements in response to a humorous movie clip of Mr. Bean. Studies by Bersani et al. (114) and Valeriani et al. (118) showed video clips of social scenarios to patients with OCD to elicit specific emotions (amusement, fear, surprise, anger, sadness, disgust). In both studies, patients with OCD generally displayed fewer concordant and more discordant emotions in response to the clips and also showed less facial

TABLE 4 | Overview of studies investigating emotion experience and emotion regulation in obsessive-compulsive disorder.

Domain	Author	Methods	Participants	Comorbid diagnosis?	Concurrent medication/ therapy	Task/ questionnaire	Emotions assessed/ stimulus-type	Diagnosis/ symtom assessment	Main results
Social emotion experience									
	Basile et al. (113)	Case-control fMRI	OCD = 13 [37.0 ± 11.1; 10M:3F] HC = 19 [26.2 ± 2.1; 11M:8F]	Comorbid MDD and ADs not considered as exclusion criteria.	SSRI or tricycles (n=6). Therapy: CBT (n=9).	Guilt-judgement task	Deontological guilt, altruistic guilt, anger, sadness	DSM-IV-TR criteria/PI/Y-BOCS	Compared to HC, OCD patients felt significantly more guilt in both the deontological guilt ($p < 0.02$) and altruistic guilt condition ($p < 0.009$). When experiencing guilt compared to nonmoral emotions (anger and sadness), patients exhibited reduced activation in the ACC, superior and medial frontal gyri ($p < 0.001$).
	Bersani et al. (114)	Case-control Outpatients	OCD = 10 [40.22 ± 13.49; 5M:5F] Schizophrenia = 10 [40.88 ± 12.97; 5M:5F] HC = 10 [40.20 ± 10.49; 5M:5F]	Comorbid axis I diagnoses were considered exclusion criteria.	OCD: clomipramine (n = 7), fluvoxamine (n = 4) sertraline (n = 1), escitalopram (n = 1), citalopram (n = 1), valproic acid (n = 3), gabapentin (n = 1), alprazolam (n = 3), lorazepam (n = 1), and zolpidem (n = 1). Schizophrenia: paliperidone (n = 3), aripiprazole (n = 4), olanzapine (n = 1), quetiapine (n = 1), clozapine (n = 1), risperidone (n = 1), valproic acid (n = 4), and lithium (n = 1). Therapy not reported.	Emotion-eliciting videoclip of social scenarios while facial activity was videotaped	Amusement, fear, surprise, anger, sadness, disgust, neutral	SCID/BPRS/ Y-BOCS	Compared to HC, OCD patients showed significantly less concordant responses ($p=0.004$), more discordant responses ($p=0.003$) and less facial expressions ($p < 0.001$). No differences were found between OCD and schizophrenia patients.
	Fontenelle et al. (115)	Case-control fMRI	OCD = 18 [34.8 ± 11.5; 11M:7F] HC = 18 [32.4 ± 9.2; 11M:7F]	Borderline and antisocial personality disorders, alcohol or substance abuse and suicidality were considered as exclusion criteria.	Almost all OCD were medicated with SSRI, with the exception of one with SNRI. Also with: antipsychotics (n=7), benzodiazepines (n=6), tricyclic antidepressant (n=1), topiramate (n=1), memantine (n=1). Therapy not reported.	Moral sentiments association task	Guilt, compassion, anger, disgust, neutral	SCID/Y-BOCS/ DOCS	During guilt provocation, OCD showed higher activity in postcentral gyrus and reduced activity in angular gyrus compared to HC ($p < 0.005$). During compassion provocation, OCD showed higher activity in dorsal anterior cingulate compared to HC ($p < 0.005$). During anger provocation, OCD showed higher activity in caudate nucleus, paracingulate and precentral gyri, and reduced activity in angular gyrus compared to HC ($p < 0.005$). During disgust provocation, OCD showed higher activity in medial frontal/paracingulate cortex and decreased activity in left NAcc compared to HC ($p < 0.005$). The combined emotion analysis revealed that OCD showed higher

(Continued)

TABLE 4 | Continued

Domain	Author	Methods	Participants	Comorbid diagnosis?	Concurrent medication/ therapy	Task/ questionnaire	Emotions assessed/ stimulus-type	Diagnosis/ symtom assessment	Main results
									activity in lingual gyrus and decreased activity in left NAcc and middle temporal gyri compared to HC.
	Hennig-Fast et al. (116)	Case-control fMRI	OCD = 20 [31.10 ± 8.58; 10M:10F] HC = 20 [29.70 ± 4.75; 10M:10F]	None of the participants received any additional comorbid axis I diagnoses.	Not reported.	Imaginative emotion-inducing task	Shame, guilt, neutral	DSM-IV criteria/SCID/ Y-BOCS	Patients reported higher levels of shame and guilt on the questionnaires administered, but not during the experimental task, compared to HC. In the shame compared to neutral condition, OCD showed increased activation in bilateral middle temporal gyrus, left uncus, left parahippocampal gyrus and hypothalamus, and decreased activation in middle frontal gyrus and inferior parietal lobule, compared to HC ($p < 0.001$). In the guilt compared to neutral condition, OCD showed increased activation in left superior frontal gyrus, right precentral gyrus, bilateral cingulate gyrus, right superior temporal gyrus and right sub-gyral region, and decreased activation in left anterior cingulate, compared to HC ($p < 0.001$). In the OCD group, Y-BOCS scores correlated positively with activation of left middle, bilateral superior, left medial frontal gyri, bilateral parahippocampal gyrus and left posterior cingulate, and negatively with activation of precuneus during shame condition. Y-BOCS scores correlated positively with activation of left middle frontal gyrus and temporo-parietal junction during guilt condition.
	Mergl et al. (117)	Case-control Outpatients	OCD = 34 [35.8 ± 11.5; 19M:15F] HC = 34 [37.5 ± 13.1; 19M:15F]	Not reported.	Studied in unmedicated state and after a 10-week treatment with the SSRI sertraline and semi-standardized behavioral therapy.	Emotion-inducing (humorous) videoclip of Mr. Bean	Laughter	Y-BOCS/ CGI	Compared to HC, patients showed slower initial velocities of involuntary facial movements in left eye ($p=0.007$), right eye ($p=0.014$), left angle of the mouth ($p=0.003$) and right angle of the mouth ($p=0.013$). Patients and HC rated the videoclips as

(Continued)

TABLE 4 | Continued

Domain	Author	Methods	Participants	Comorbid diagnosis?	Concurrent medication/ therapy	Task/ questionnaire	Emotions assessed/ stimulus-type	Diagnosis/ symtom assessment	Main results
									equally humorous, however the frequency of laughing reactions was significantly lower in OCD ($p < 0.001$). Higher Y-BOCS scores were associated with lower laughing frequencies (p=0.011).
	Valeriani et al. (118)	Case-control Outpatients	OCD severe = 10 [40.61 ± 6.12; 5M:5F] OCD mild-moderate = 11 [37.77 ± 8.21; 5M:6F] HC = 15 [41.71 ± 12.53; 7M:8F]	Comorbid axis I diagnoses were considered exclusion criteria.	Valproate (severe=6, mild=3), SSRI (severe=9, mild=10), aripiprazole (severe=4), benzodiazepines (severe=7, mild=7), clomipramine (severe=6, mild=1).	Emotion-eliciting videoclip of social scenarios	Surprise, fear, happy, disgust, anger, sadness	SCID/Y-BOCS	HC reported more concordant responses compared to both severe ($p < 0.01$) and mild OCD (p=0.02). Severe OCD showed less concordant facial expressions compared to mild OCD (p=0.03) and HC ($p < 0.01$), and mild OCD showed less concordant facial expressions compared to HC ($p < 0.01$). Compared to mild, severe OCD showed significantly poorer performance in response to happiness- and disgust-eliciting videoclips.
Nonsocial emotion experience									
	Admon et al. (119)	Case-control Outpatients fMRI and DTI	OCD = 13 HC = 13	None of the participants met criteria for additional Axis I disorders. 3 patients met criteria for Axis II cluster A personality disorders. 3 patients had a history of MDD and 3 of social phobia.	All patients were treated with serotonergic agents (sertraline, paroxetine, escitalopram, clomipramine), 4 patients received in addition a low-dose antipsychotic agent (risperidone, haloperidol). Therapy not reported.	Interactive risky choice game	Threat, reward	DSM-IV criteria/ SCID-P/Y-BOCS	Compared to HC, patients chose significantly fewer nonmatch risky choices (p=0.02). OCD showed higher activation of the amygdala in response to threat (p=0.02) and lower activation of the NAcc in response to reward compared to HC (p=0.02). Amygdala-dACC (p=0.03) and NAcc-OFC (p=0.01) were more weakly functionally connected in patients compared to HC, and stronger functional connections between these regions were related to lower severity of OCD symptoms.
	Choi et al. (120)	Case-control fMRI	PG = 15M [27.93 ± 3.59] OCD = 13M [24.92 ± 6.92] HC = 15M [26.60 ± 4.29]	OCD: tic disorder (n=1), OC personality disorder (n=1), schizotypal personality disorder (n=1).	Not reported.	Monetary incentive delay task	Reward, loss-avoidance, neutral	SCID/Y-BOCS	No statistically significant differences in BOLD response between HC and OCD during anticipation of gain. During anticipation of loss, OCD showed increased activation in the anterior insula, putamen and caudate nucleus compared to HC ($p < 0.005$ uncorrected).

(Continued)

TABLE 4 | Continued

Domain	Author	Methods	Participants	Comorbid diagnosis?	Concurrent medication/ therapy	Task/ questionnaire	Emotions assessed/ stimulus-type	Diagnosis/ symtom assessment	Main results
	Figee et al. (121)	Case-control Outpatients fMRI	OCD = 18 [34 ± 8.3; 5M:13F] HC = 19 [32 ± 6.6; 6M:13F]	MDD (n=2), additional disorders on Axis I (n=4), OC personality disorder (n=2).	SSRI (n=5), tricyclic antidepressant (n=3), combined noradrenergic and serotoninergic antidepressant (n=1).	Monetary incentive delay task	Reward, no reward	MINI/Y-BOCS	Compared to HC, OCD showed reduced activation of the NAcc (bilateral) and the left insula during anticipation of monetary gain ($p < 0.05$ corrected). No statistically significant correlations were found between Y-BOCS scores and BOLD responses during reward anticipation.
	Hauser et al. (122)	fMRI Adults and children	OCD = 33 [23.4 ± 9.5; 21M:12F] HC = 34 [24.5 ± 11.2; 13M:21F]	MDD (n=3), panic disorder with agoraphobia (n=2), social phobia (n=4), specific phobia (n=4), GAD (n=2), body dysmorphic disorder (n=1), pain disorder (n=1), AN (n=2), ADHD (n=2), CD (n=1), other childhood emotional disorders (n=2), chronic tic disorder (n=1).	SSRI (n=13), neuroleptics (n=4), SSNRI (n=3), benzodiazepine (n=2), levothyroxin (n=2), NaSSA (n=1), anticholinergics (n=1), tricyclic antidepressant (n=1).	Probabilistic reversal learning task	Reward, punishment	SCID or K-SADS-PL/Y-BOCS or CY-BOCS/ DSM-5 criteria	OCD showed increased reward prediction error-related activation in the ACC and right putamen ($p < 0.05$ corrected), also after controlling for age. Neither ACC nor putamen correlated with Y-BOCS total, obsessions subscale or compulsion subscale.
	Jung et al. (123)	Case-control Outpatients fMRI	OCD = 20 [25.70 ± 6.99; 13M:7F] HC = 20 [24.75 ± 3.68; 13M:7F]	Tic disorder (n=1), OC personality disorder (n=2), schizotypal personality disorder (n=1).	Medication-naïve (n=15), medication-free for 4 weeks (n=5).	Monetary incentive delay task	Gain, loss, neutral	SCID/Y-BOCS	During gain anticipation, there were no statistically significant differences between OCD and HC. During loss anticipation, OCD showed reduced activation of lateral PFC including the superior frontal cortex and postcentral cortex, and reduced activation of anterior insula, compared to HC ($p < 0.001$ uncorrected). In the gain outcome contrast, patients showed increased activation of putamen, precentral cortex, posterior insula, ACC and cerebellum compared to HC ($p < 0.001$). In the loss avoidance contrast, patients showed increased activation of ventral striatal, midbrain, superior temporal cortex and inferior parietal cortex compared to HC ($p < 0.001$). Ventral striatal activation in patients was significantly correlated with Y-BOCS ($p=0.045$).

(Continued)

TABLE 4 | Continued

Domain	Author	Methods	Participants	Comorbid diagnosis?	Concurrent medication/ therapy	Task/ questionnaire	Emotions assessed/ stimulus-type	Diagnosis/ symtom assessment	Main results
	Jung et al. (124)	Case-control Outpatients Functional connectivity analysis	OCD = 19 [25.84 ± 7.15; 12M:7F] HC = 18 [24.83 ± 3.88; 11M:7F]	Not reported.	Medication-naïve (n=15), medication-free for 4 weeks (n=4).	Monetary incentive delay task	Gain, loss, neutral	SCID	During gain anticipation, OCD showed increased functional connectivity of the NAcc with the posterior insula and occipital regions, and reduced functional connectivity of the NAcc with the left amygdala positioned adjacent to the anterior insula, middle frontal cortex and midbrain ($p < 0.01$ corrected). During loss anticipation, OCD showed increased functional connectivity of the NAcc with the occipital cortex and reduced functional connectivity of the NAcc with the bilateral amygdala compared to HC ($p < 0.01$ corrected). OCD patients' overall symptom severity was positively correlated with functional connectivity between NAcc and medial OFC and negatively correlated with functional connectivity between NAcc and lateral OFC ($p < 0.001$).
	Kaufmann et al. (125)	Case-control Outpatients fMRI	OCD = 19 [34.8 ± 11.0; 8M:11F] HC = 19 [34.9 ± 11.8; 8M:11F]	Affective disorder (n=7), phobic disorders (n=3), impulse control disorder (n=1), personality disorder (n=3).	Clomipramine (n=1), venlafaxine (n=1), clomipramine + paroxetine (n=1). None of the patients took benzodiazepines within 4 weeks before the scanning session. Patients were currently under treatment (CBT).	Monetary incentive delay task	Reward, loss-avoidance, neutral	DSM-IV criteria/SCID/ Y-BOCS/ OCI-R	OCD showed fewer delayed responses in loss-avoidance than in reward trails, whereas the opposite was true in HC ($p=0.05$). No statistically significant differences were found in activation of brain regions of the reward circuitry between HC and OCD. Patients showed higher activation of superior/medial frontal and cingulate region in loss-avoidance condition compared to HC, but less activation in reward condition ($p=0.018$). Y-BOCS ratings did not correlate with BOLD responses.
	Koch et al. (126)	Case-control fMRI	OCD = 44 [32.7 ± 9.3; 17M:27F] HC = 37 [32.0 ± 8.0; 15M:22F]	MDD (n=16), AD (n=1), MDD + AD (n=5), personality disorder (n=2), impulse control (n=1).	SSRI (n=20), SNRI (n=4), tricyclic antidepressant (n=4), benzodiazepines (n=1), atypical antipsychotic (n=1). Therapy not reported.	Monetary reward task	Reward, punishment	DSM-IV criteria/Y-BOCS	No activation differences between HC and OCD in punishment trials. In reward trials, patients showed reduced activation in the frontal cortex bilaterally and the posterior cingulate extending into the left precuneus ($p < 0.05$ corrected). Patients showed a

(Continued)

TABLE 4 | Continued

Domain	Author	Methods	Participants	Comorbid diagnosis?	Concurrent medication/ therapy	Task/ questionnaire	Emotions assessed/ stimulus-type	Diagnosis/ symtom assessment	Main results
									significantly increased connectivity between the left PCC/precuneus and the left vmPFC and the right PCC, compared to HC ($p < 0.05$ corrected). No significant correlation between Y-BOCS and connectivity patterns were found.
	Murray et al. (127)	Case-control fMRI	OCD = 18 [35.6 ± 10.1; 11M:7F] HC = 18 [32.1 ± 6.5; 15M:3F]	Comorbid axis I diagnoses were considered exclusion criteria.	Most patients were taking SSRIs.	Probabilistic learning task	Reward, punishment, neutral	DSM-IV-TR criteria/SCID	During negative prediction error processing, OCD showed higher activation of ACC compared to HC ($p=0.006$). During positive prediction error processing, OCD showed increased activation of NAcc compared to HC ($p=0.031$). There were no correlations between Y-BOCS scores and either ACC or NAcc activation.
	Remijnse et al. (128)	fMRI	OCD = 20 [34 (19-54); 5M:15F] HC = 27 [32 (22-53); 8M:19F]	PTSD (n=1), panic disorder (n=2), GAD (n=4), SAD (n=4), opioid abuse in sustained full remission (n=1), Tourette disorder (n=1).	Patients were free from psychotropic medication for at least 2 weeks, and in case of fluoxetine or antipsychotic medication for at least 1 month.	Probabilistic reversal learning task	Positive, negative, neutral feedback	SCID/Y-BOCS/PI-R	Compared to HC, OCD patients showed reduced activation of in lateral and medial orbitofrontal cortex ($ps < 0.005$) during reward processing.
	Riesel et al. (13)	Meta-analysis EEG	OCD = 1007 HC = 1100	Not reported.	Not reported.	Performance monitoring tasks	Not applicable.	Y-BOCS	Compared to HC, patients showed a robust increase of ERN in conflict-response tasks ($p < 0.001$), that was not modulated by symptom severity, depressive symptoms, medication and age.
	Thorsen et al. (129)	Meta-analysis Case-control fMRI, PET or SPECT	OCD = 571 [33.44 ± 5.91] HC = 564 54.35% of subjects were males	Comorbidities: anxiety and mood disorders in some studies.	68% of studies included medicated patients. Studies with treated patients were excluded.	Emotional processing tasks	E.g., fear, disgust, neutral, distress, urges to ritualize	Y-BOCS	Compared to HC, patients showed significantly increased activation in the right OFC extending into the sgACC and vmPFC, right putamen, bilateral amygdala, left inferior occipital gyrus, and right middle temporal gyrus during emotional processing, across all paradigms ($p < 0.005$). The percentage of patients using medication correlated negatively with activation in the right amygdala and left inferior occipital gyrus in patients compared to HC ($p < 0.005$). Patients with higher symptom severity showed

(Continued)

TABLE 4 | Continued

Domain	Author	Methods	Participants	Comorbid diagnosis?	Concurrent medication/ therapy	Task/ questionnaire	Emotions assessed/ stimulus-type	Diagnosis/ symtom assessment	Main results
									significantly increased activation in the right rostral sgACC, the left medial prefrontal cortex and the right precuneus ($p < 0.005$). Studies with a higher rate of comorbidity with anxiety and mood disorders also found more pronounced activation in the right putamen, amygdala, and insula as well as decreased activation in the left amygdala and right vmPFC in patients compared with HC ($p < 0.005$).
Emotion Regulation									
	De Wit et al. (130)	Case-control fMRI	OCD = 43 [38.4 ± 10.0; 21M:22F] HC = 38 [39.6 ± 11.4; 18M:20F]	Current or past psychosis was considered as exclusion criteria. 56% of patients met criteria for current comorbid Axis I diagnosis.	Medication-free for at least 4 weeks. Therapy not reported.	Emotion regulation task + ERQ	Fear, neutral, OCD-related	SCID/Y-BOCS/PI	Compared to HC, patients showed higher distress ratings for fear and OCD-related stimuli ($p < 0.001$). HC and OCD did not differ in fear regulation, but patients had a significantly larger regulation effect on OCD-related stimuli ($p < 0.01$). In patients, Y-BOCS score correlated with ERQ reappraisal ($p=0.001$). During emotion provocation patients compared with HC showed an increased amplitude and/or altered timing of the BOLD response in the right amygdala ($p_{FWE-SVC}=0.004$) and occipital cortex at the uncorrected level. During emotion regulation, patients showed decreased activity in left dlPFC ($p_{FWE-SVC}=0.009$) in fear regulation, and increased dmPFC activity ($p_{FWE-SVC}=0.001$) in OCD-related regulation. In patients regulation success did not correlate with brain activity. Disease severity correlated inversely with regulation-related activity in bilateral dmPFC ($p_{FWE-SVC}=0.002$) and thalamus ($p_{FWE-SVC}=0.04$).
	Fernández de la Cruz et al. (131)	Case-control Outpatients	HD = 24 HD + OCD = 19	Psychosis, bipolar I disorder or	Not reported.	DERS	Not applicable.	MINI/DY-BOCS/OCI-R	All three clinical groups obtained higher scores on the DERS compared with

(Continued)

TABLE 4 | Continued

Domain	Author	Methods	Participants	Comorbid diagnosis?	Concurrent medication/ therapy	Task/ questionnaire	Emotions assessed/ stimulus-type	Diagnosis/ symtom assessment	Main results
			OCD = 17 HC = 20	substance abuse were considered as exclusion criteria.					HC (p < 0.001). Patients obtained higher scores in the domains 'nonacceptance of emotional responses', 'impulse control difficulties', 'limited access to strategies for regulation' and 'lack of emotional clarity' compared with HC (p < 0.05). In the entire clinical sample there were significant positive correlations between measures of OCD and DERS (p < 0.001).
	Fink et al. (132)	Case-control	C-OCD = 30 [33.27 ± 11.39; 13M:17F] HC = 30 [32.8 ± 11.9; 13M:17F]	Tic disorder, psychotic or bipolar disorder, and substance abuse were considered as exclusion criteria. Comorbidities: MDD (n=4), MDD with partial remission (n=7), dysthymia (n=1), panic disorder (n=1).	SSRI (n=12), SNRI (n=2), tricyclic antidepressant (n=4). Therapy: outpatient treatment (n=1), inpatient treatment (n=28).	ERQ	Disgust	DSM-IV criteria/Y-BOCS/SCID	Compared to HC, patients scored significantly lower on ERQ subscale cognitive reappraisal (p < 0.001) and significantly higher on expressive suppression (p=0.001).
	Paul et al. (133)	Case-control Outpatients EEG	OCD = 24 [31.7 ± 9.1; 11M:13F] HC = 24 [31.2 ± 8.2; 11M:13F]	Presence of comorbid disorders other than anxiety or Axis II disorders (apart from borderline personality disorder) was considered as exclusion criteria. Comorbidities: agoraphobia with panic disorder (n=1), specific phobia (n=1), social phobia (n=1), adjustment disorder (n=1), OC personality disorder (n=2).	SSRI (n=9). Therapy: CBT (n=9).	ERQ and CERQ + emotion regulation task	Aversive, OCD-related, neutral	Y-BOCS/Y-BOCS Symptom Checklist/ OCI-R	Patients scored significantly lower in the CERQ subscale positive refocusing (p < 0.001) and in the ERQ subscale reappraisal (p < 0.001), and higher in the CERQ subscale catastrophizing (p=0.001) than HC. OCD showed a significant LPP enhancement for OCD-related relative to neutral pictures (p=0.003), which was not present in HC. While HC showed significantly reduced LPP amplitudes during both distraction and reappraisal, patients showed a LPP reduction during distraction at trend level (p=0.08), but no significant LPP attenuation during reappraisal (p > 0.99).
	Picò-Pérez et al. (134)	Case-control	OCD = 73 [37.74 ± 10.19;	MDD (n=10), GAD (n=3), eating disorder	Fluoxetine (n=13), escitalopram (n=5), sertraline	ERQ	Not applicable.	Y-BOCS	OCD scored significantly higher in suppression (p < 0.005) and lower in

(Continued)

TABLE 4 | Continued

Domain	Author	Methods	Participants	Comorbid diagnosis?	Concurrent medication/ therapy	Task/ questionnaire	Emotions assessed/ stimulus-type	Diagnosis/ symtom assessment	Main results
		Resting-state fMRI	43M:30F] HC = 42 [39.43 ± 9.79; 22M:20F]	(n=3), tics (n=3), panic disorder (n=2), dysthymia (n=2), OC personality disorder (n=2), ADHD (n=1), agoraphobia (n=1), gambling disorder (n=1).	(n=3), fluvoxamine (n=2), paroxetine (n=1), clomipramine (n=8), SSRI + clomipramine (n=12), SSRIs combinations (n=1), antipsychotic augmentations (n=22).				reappraisal ($p < 0.0005$) compared to HC. Compared to patients, HC showed higher connectivity between the right amygdala and the right postcentral gyrus ($p < 0.05$ FWE-cluster corrected). The connectivity between these two regions was significantly correlated with Y-BOCS scores in the patient group ($p=0.009$). In the OCD group there was a negative association between suppression and functional connectivity between the left amygdala and the precuneus and the bilateral angular gyri ($p < 0.05$ FEW-cluster corrected).
	Yap et al. (135)	Case-control	OCD = 59 [32.88 ± 10.45; 26M:33F]; HC = 59 [32.81 ± 10.34; 26M:33F]	More than one comorbid condition (n=11), depressive disorders (n=28), AD (n=15), hoarding disorder (n=2), bipolar disorder (n=2), autism (n=2), schizoaffective disorder (n=1), alcohol use disorder (n=1).	Not reported.	DERS	Not applicable.	DOCS/DSM-5 criteria/Y-BOCS	OCD scored significantly higher on DERS total ($p < 0.001$) and subscales of nonacceptance ($p=0.014$), goals ($p < 0.001$), impulse control ($p=0.007$) and strategies ($p < 0.001$), compared to HC. Significant group differences were found also for DERS-aware ($p=0.004$) and DERS-clarity ($p < 0.001$), but these differences did not remain significant after controlling for depression and anxiety. There were no significant associations between any DERS subscale and Y-BOCS.

OCD, obsessive-compulsive disorder; HC, healthy controls; SSRI, selective serotonin reuptake inhibitor; CBT, cognitive-behavioral therapy; MDD, major depressive disorder; AD, anxiety disorder; DSM, Diagnostic and Statistical Manual of Mental Disorders; PI, Padua Inventory; Y-BOCS, Yale-Brown Obsessive Compulsive Scale; SCID, Structured Clinical Interview for DSM Axis I Disorders; BPRS, Brief Psychiatric Rating Scale; OCI-R, Obsessive-Compulsive Inventory Revised; DASS, Depression Anxiety Stress Scale; DOCS, Dimensional Obsessive-Compulsive Scale; SNRI, serotonin norepinephrine reuptake inhibitor; NAcc, nucleus accumbens; CGI, Clinical Global Impressions severity and improvement scores; MOCI, Maudsley Obsessive-Compulsive Inventory; ADIS-R, Anxiety Disorders Interview Schedule Revised; ERN, error-related negativity; sgACC, subgenual anterior cingulate cortex; vmPFC, ventromedial prefrontal cortex; OFC, orbitofrontal cortex; MINI, Mini International Neuropsychiatric Interview; DY-BOCS, Dimensional Yale-Brown Obsessive Compulsive Scale; DERS, Difficulties in Emotion Regulation Scale; ERQ, Emotion Regulation Questionnaire; dlPFC, dorsolateral prefrontal cortex; dmPFC, dorsomedial prefrontral cortex; C-OCD, contamination-related subtype of OCD; ERC, Emotion Regulation Checklist; CERQ, Cognitive Emotion Regulation Questionnaire; LPP, late positive potential; GAD, generalized anxiety disorder; ADHD, attention deficit hyperactivity disorder; NDRI, norepinephrine-dopamine reuptake inhibitor; PG, pathological gambling; SSNRI, selective serotoninergic and noradrenergic reuptake inhibitors; NaSSA, noradrenergic and specific serotoninergic antidepressants; AN, anorexia nervosa; CD, conduct disorder; PFC, prefrontal cortex; BOLD, blood oxygenation level dependent; SAD, social anxiety disorder; PTSD, post-traumatic stress disorder; Dacc, dorsal anterior cingulate cortex.

mimicry of emotions than healthy controls. These responses were similar to those of patients with schizophrenia (114) and the expression of happiness and disgust was especially poor in those with severe compared to mild-to-moderate OCD symptoms (118). Together, these studies indicate that individuals with OCD show less facial expressivity and less appropriate emotional experiences in response to social scenarios eliciting various basic emotions.

Some other studies have focused on social stimuli inducing more complex emotional responses, specifically the subjective experience and neural processing of guilt and shame, two inherently-social emotions, elicited by depicted scenarios of moral transgressions. In a study by Basile, Mancini, Macaluso, Caltagirone, and Bozzali (113), patients with OCD reported to experience more guilt than controls while processing guilt-inducing sentences, especially for sentences indicating guilt derived from transgressing an inner moral rule (deontological guilt) compared to altruistic guilt, which is defined as guilt of having disregarded a personal altruistic goal. The experience of guilt versus nonmoral, basic emotions (anger and sadness) was accompanied by reduced activation in the ACC extending to superior/medial frontal gyrus. According to the authors, the increased rather than decreased activity in this region previously associated with the experience of guilt could be explained by cerebral efficiency, as feelings of guilt are more frequently experienced in patients with OCD. In a comparable task, patients with OCD showed higher activation than controls in various regions including the superior frontal- and precentral gyrus, cingulate gyrus, superior temporal gyrus and decreased activation in anterior cingulate while processing guilt-inducing compared to neutral sentences (116). Symptom severity (Y-BOCS) was positively associated with activation of left middle frontal gyrus and temporo-parietal junction during the experience of guilt. Shame on the other hand was associated with increased activation in the uncus, parahippocampal gyrus, and middle temporal gyrus, as well as the hypothalamus, and decreased activity in the middle frontal gyrus and inferior parietal lobe in patients compared to controls. Thus, the authors showed that the experience of shame and guilt was associated with increased reactivity in a widespread neural network. On the behavioral level, patients did not report to experience more guilt and shame in the experimental task, although self-report questionnaires did demonstrate generally higher levels of guilt and shame in patients, which the authors suggest may indicate an increased sensitivity to social norms. Fontenelle et al. (115) used multivariate pattern analysis to identify brain regions that discriminate OCD patients from controls across different moral emotions evoked while reading different scripts. They showed that several brain regions including the nucleus accumbens, lingual gyrus, and middle temporal gyrus, were able to discriminate patients from controls across distinct moral emotions (guilt, compassion, anger, and disgust). Together, these studies suggest that patients with OCD tend to experience more guilt in response to (moral) emotion-evoking stimuli (113), and show altered neural processing of such stimuli (113, 115, 116).

Emotion Regulation

Several studies have investigated emotion regulation skills in OCD, all of which are limited to nonsocial contexts. These studies have largely focused on self-report or observer-reported measures, such as the Emotion Regulation Questionnaire [ERQ; (138)]. The ERQ focuses specifically on cognitive reappraisal, which refers to the tendency to change the interpretation of an emotion-eliciting situation so that it diminishes its negative impact, and expressive suppression, which refers to a more maladaptive emotion regulation strategy that consists of the inhibition of emotion-expressive behavior. Fink, Pflugradt, Stierle, and Exner (132) and Picó-Pérez et al. (134) showed that OCD patients make less use of reappraisal and more use of suppression techniques. Picó-Pérez and colleagues additionally demonstrated using resting-state functional connectivity analyses with the left and right amygdala as seed regions, that within patients, suppression was negatively related to connectivity between the left amygdala, the precuneus and the bilateral angular gyri. These findings thus suggest that impaired parietolimbic connectivity may be associated with the preferential use of maladaptive emotion regulation techniques.

Other studies likewise demonstrated self-reported emotion regulation impairments in OCD patients using the Difficulties in Emotion Regulation Scale (DERS), a questionnaire that focuses not only on the modulation of emotions but also more generally on the awareness, understanding, and acceptance of emotions (139). The DERS consist of six subscales: (1) nonacceptance of emotional responses; (2) difficulty engaging in goal-directed behavior when distressed; (3) impulse control difficulties when distressed; (4) lack of awareness of emotions; (5) limited access to (adaptive) strategies for regulation; and (6) lack of emotional clarity. Fernández de la Cruz et al. (131) showed that patients compared to controls had significantly higher scores on all subscales except for the "lack of emotional awareness scale." Similarly, Yap et al. (135) found that OCD patients scored significantly higher than controls on all DERS subscales, and group differences remained significant after correcting for depression and anxiety on all scales except for the lack of emotional awareness and emotional clarity scales. These findings indicate that patients with OCD have difficulties regulating their emotions, specifically expressed in the tendency to show a nonacceptance of emotions, experienced difficulties in goal-directed behavior and impulse control when distressed, and the use of maladaptive regulation strategies. Additionally, these difficulties seem at least partly independent of more general depressive or anxious symptoms.

Two studies employed emotion-provocation paradigms to assess the neural correlates of emotion regulation in patients, and indicate that patients show altered neural activity during emotion regulation (130, 133). In an fMRI study by De Wit et al. (130), patients and controls viewed general- and disorder-specific emotion-provoking stimuli, and were instructed to either attend these stimuli or to regulate their emotions through cognitive reappraisal. OCD patients gave higher ratings of distress after viewing emotion-provoking stimuli, which was accompanied by amygdala-hyper responsiveness, but comparable distress reduction as control after instructed emotion regulation. During emotion regulation, OCD patients showed diminished left dorsolateral prefrontal cortex activity and increased left dorsomedial prefrontal activity compared to controls, which may indicate the use of alternative or compensatory emotion regulation mechanisms. They also showed less frontal-amygdala connectivity than controls, which the authors proposed may be reflective of a generally diminished ability to effectively regulate pathological anxiety. Using a similar task, Paul et al. (133) assessed the electrophysiological correlates of emotion regulation. Compared to controls, OCD patients had higher arousal ratings after viewing symptom-provoking stimuli as well as enhanced amplitudes of an event-related potential called the late positive potential (LPP) while viewing these images. The LPP is thought to reflect facilitated attention to emotional stimuli, and has been found to be modulated by emotion regulation strategies (140). Indeed, healthy controls showed reduced LPP amplitudes after instructed emotion regulation. However, patients with OCD did not show a reduction in the LPP during cognitive reappraisal, despite the fact that subjective arousal ratings were successfully reduced. Self-reported emotion regulation skills were also assessed, using the ERQ and the Cognitive Emotion Regulation Questionnaire [CERQ; (141)]. The CERQ focusses on cognitive (i.e., explicit) emotion regulation strategies, and consists of nine different scales, of which four focus on more maladaptive or dysfunctional strategies (self-blame, focusing on thought/rumination, catastrophizing, blaming others), and of which five are thought to represent somewhat more adaptive methods (acceptance, positive refocusing, refocus on planning, positive reappraisal, putting in perspective). Here too, patients indicated poorer self-reported emotion regulation skills as indicated by lower scores on the reappraisal subscale of the ERQ as well as lower scores on the positive refocusing subscale and higher scores on the catastrophizing subscale of the CERQ.

Section Summary and Discussion: Emotion Experience and Regulation

Research clearly indicates that the experience of emotions in patients with OCD is altered. Patients with OCD show heightened affective reactivity and altered neural processing of various emotion-inducing and emotion-provoking stimuli, show decreased neural sensitivity to reward and heightened (prediction) error responses. Less is known about emotion experience in social contexts. Some studies indicate that patients show less appropriate emotional experiences and facial expressivity in response to emotion-inducing social scenarios. These studies may for example suggest that patients with OCD experience less emotional contagion, which is the automatic mimicking and synchronizing of facial expressions, vocalizations, postures, and movements with others leading to similar emotions (100). Alternatively, it has also been put forward that these incongruent responses could reflect an increased effort to suppress or resist unpleasant emotions (142) and may therefore reflect emotion regulation attempts. Yet, still alternative explanations are possible. The use of medication such as antidepressants has for example been associated with alterations in emotion experience, such as emotional blunting (143). The impact of different kinds of medications should therefore be explored further. Nevertheless, these studies suggest that observable basic emotional responses to various social situations are disturbed in OCD. Additionally, studies have

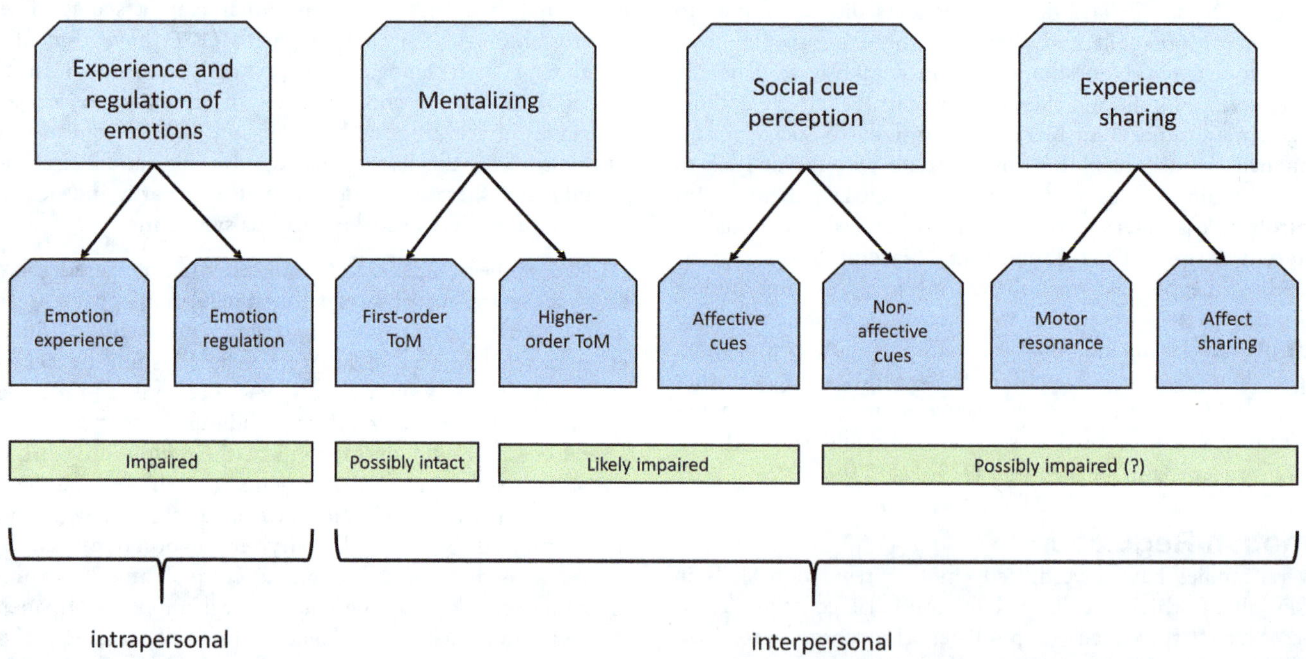

FIGURE 1 | Schematic overview of social cognitive alterations in obsessive-compulsive disorder with regard to the domains discussed in the current review, based on Green et al. (4). These domains can be divided in intrapersonal and interpersonal domains. Much research has been conducted on the intrapersonal domain, providing strong evidence from neuroimaging studies for altered emotion experience and impaired emotion regulation. Evidence with regard to the interpersonal domain however is limited and less consistent. Affective cue perception is likely impaired, specifically with regard to the recognition of facial expressions of disgust. Similarly, there is evidence for theory-of-mind (ToM) impairments especially with regard to higher-order inferences. There is also some evidence for impaired perception of nonaffective cues, although research is scarce. Studies on experience sharing are lacking, though there are some indirect indications that these domains may be affected as well.

indicated that patients experience increased levels of more complex social emotions such as guilt and altered neural processing of various moral emotions compared to healthy controls, which seems in line with theories of OCD that highlight the role of responsibility, guilt and shame in the etiology of the disorder. For example, the cognitive theory of OCD suggests that patients misinterpret intrusive thoughts as indicating that they are responsible for preventing harm coming to others or oneself, which in turn triggers actions such as compulsions to prevent feared events (144). Similarly, it has been argued that patients are characterized by a fear of guilt resulting from behaving irresponsibly and/or from not behaving responsibly, which in turn triggers compulsive symptoms (145).

Many studies additionally show that OCD patients employ more maladaptive emotion regulation skills, and that these effects seem largely independent of comorbid depression and anxiety levels. There is also evidence for altered neural activity during emotion regulation in patients (130, 133), which may point to the use of compensatory or (inefficient) alternative emotion regulation strategies.

To conclude, studies indicate that patients with OCD are characterized by increased emotional reactivity and poor emotion regulation abilities. These emotional disturbances may be triggered by external factors or stimuli, such as in the studies discussed. However, patients with OCD often also experience emotions that are not specifically triggered by the social context but which are rather elicited by more internal processes such as obsessive thoughts. If patients are unable to effectively regulate these emotions, this will unequivocally impact how individuals with OCD interact with their environment. Yet, currently, research on the experience and regulation of emotions in various social contexts is still lacking.

DISCUSSION

In the current review, we aimed to offer an overview of the relation between social cognition in patients with OCD. Overall, these studies indicate that patients are characterized by social cognitive alterations in almost all domains suggested by Green et al. (4). Evidence indicates that OCD patients show deficits in the perception of social cues, specifically with regard to the recognition of facial expressions of disgust, and also show altered neural processing of facial emotions. There are also indications that patients are characterized by deficits in nonaffective social cues, such as deficits in the recognition and perception of nonaffective social cues, such as biological motion and body poses implying action in OCD patients. However, studies in this domain are scarce and may be subjected to publication bias. Furthermore, there is support for deficient ToM or mentalizing abilities in patients with OCD, which may be particularly pronounced in those with poor illness insight. Studies on motor resonance and affect sharing OCD are lacking. Impaired imitation of other's actions has been reported, which, together with observed deficits in the perception of biological motion or action, may point to deficient motor resonance and impaired functioning of the MNS, yet this remains to be investigated. Additionally, self-report studies indicate that patients with OCD experience increased empathic distress when confronted with the distress of others, or similar emotional congruence, suggesting that affect sharing is intact, and possibly exaggerated. On a more intrapersonal level, there is convincing evidence that patients with OCD show heightened affective and altered neural reactivity to emotional stimuli, and have poor emotion regulation skills, which may also have important repercussions for social interactions. Following the example of Green et al. (4), **Figure 1** provides a schematic overview of the social cognitive disturbances in OCD as discussed in this review. A word of caution is necessary however, as findings are inconsistent and many social cognitive domains remain underexplored, which makes it difficult to draw firm conclusions with regard to a social cognitive profile associated with obsessive-compulsive symptomatology. It should also be noted here that the current review addressed only a limited range of domains relevant for daily-life social functioning, and there may be many more processes relevant to OCD that could affect social functioning. However, in this review we decided to focus specifically on the domains as demarcated by Green et al. (4).

Nevertheless, the social cognitive deficits that were found may in part explain why patients with OCD experience such poor quality of life on social domains. Problems in the ability to recognize basic social cues such as facial expressions and biological motion and the ability to understand more advanced mental states carry obvious implications for social functioning, as these abilities are critical in order to navigate the social environment in an adaptive manner. The current review additionally demonstrated that on a more intrapersonal level, patients with OCD are characterized by heightened emotional and neural reactivity as well as by problems in emotion regulation, which may directly contribute to the development and maintenance of obsessions and compulsions [see, e.g., (111)], but which may also importantly hinder the enjoyment of social relations and contribute to maladaptive social behavior. For example, the elevated scores on empathic personal distress indicate that patients with OCD also display a heightened emotional reactivity to social stimuli and situations. Indeed, emotion regulation is critical in order to show adaptive empathic or prosocial reactions to experiences of others and is thus considered a critical component of relationship formation and maintenance. Given that emotions are often regulated with the goal of influencing social situations and interaction partners within a social context (146), regulation of emotions in a social context is arguably much more complex than when one does not have to deal with this context. Until now, however, the experience and regulation of emotions has mainly been investigated in nonsocial contexts. This is surprising as the social context can be an important source of emotions. This seems particularly true for individuals with OCD, who experience difficulties in managing their daily lives due to the invalidating and time-consuming nature of their symptoms. This can also put a huge strain or burden on family members and loved ones, who sometimes engage in symptom accommodation in order to help patients with their anxiety and/or in order to avoid conflict, which may in turn contribute to worsening of symptoms [e.g., (147)]. Perceived or experienced stigmatization may likewise represent an important social trigger of feelings of shame or embarrassment (148). Additionally, there is evidence indicating that the obsessions and compulsions from which patients with OCD suffer often have a social component in itself. Patients with OCD often show increased feelings of responsibility or guilt for how their actions may affect others (149). They might for example have intrusions about hurting someone they love, resulting in feelings of guilt and avoidance of this loved one to prevent harm. Moreover, patients might be afraid that something bad will happen to a loved one if a certain ritual is not carried out, even though they recognize the irrationality of this behavior. The cognitive theory of OCD highlights this inflated sense of responsibility for other's harm as it suggests that patients misinterpret intrusive thoughts as indicating that they are responsible for preventing harm coming to others or oneself, which in turn triggers actions such as compulsions to prevent feared events (144). Importantly, these symptoms are thought to form an important obstacle for enjoyable and successful social interactions. Moreover, anxiety or distress triggered by symptoms itself rather than the social context, can also impact how patients deal with their social environment if patients are unable to effectively regulate these emotions. Extending investigations on the symptomatology of OCD from an individual to a social context is therefore highly important for future investigations as it may importantly contribute to our understanding of the symptomatology and social difficulties in daily life of patients.

The fact that several individual studies do not indicate any social cognitive deficits, such as facial emotion recognition and ToM impairments, suggests that these deficits may only be present or are more pronounced in a specific subset of patients, although in some cases statistical power may also play a role. An important target for future studies is therefore to unravel which characteristics of patients are associated with poorer social cognitive functioning. A promising factor in this respect is level of illness insight of patients, as several studies show deficient ToM abilities only in those with less insight (73, 75, 80). However, the role of factors related to poor insight, such as increased comorbidity with schizophrenia, or poorer overall cognitive, emotional or intellectual functioning, needs to be investigated as well. Deficits in more general cognitive abilities often found in patients with OCD may also contribute to social cognitive difficulties. For example, cognitive skills such as reasoning and problem solving are thought to be necessary in order to make accurate ToM inferences, and impairments herein may thus also affect social cognitive processes (14). It is therefore possible that ToM impairments in OCD patients are primarily an indirect result of more prominent deficits in general cognitive abilities. Relatedly, medication or treatment status may also help explain incongruent findings. Studies by Lochner et al. (45) and Rector et al. (49) indicate that medication or psychological treatment might affect (i.e. improve) the ability to recognize facial expressions of disgust, as these studies showed higher recognition scores after SSRI and CBT treatment. Yet, many studies including OCD patients did not report whether they were receiving any concurrent medications or treatment, and it is currently unknown how different types of medication may impact emotion recognition. The use of medication could also affect other social cognitive processes, as antidepressants are for example known to have an effect on more general cognitive functioning, such as attention, executive functioning and memory (150). These results stress the importance of taking treatment status into account when assessing emotion recognition as well as social cognitive skills in general. Lastly, given that OCD is a heterogeneous disorder with many different manifestations, different subtypes may be associated with different social cognitive profiles. Yet, current investigations of subdimensions have been rather inconclusive. This may be explained by the fact that these studies have been largely limited to small samples and a focus on overt symptoms (e.g., checking or cleaning) of the disorder rather than on underlying reasons for these behaviors. Importantly, underlying motivational dimensions such as "harm avoidance" and "incompleteness" may be a more fruitful approach to clarify heterogeneous findings in OCD (151). Whereas "harm avoidance" seems to represent a more anxiety-focused motivation to prevent harm, "incompleteness" refers to a more sensory-affective motivation where individuals feel that actions are incompletely achieved that are more closely related to perfectionism and obsessive-compulsive spectrum disorders. Such motivational and orthogonal dimensions of OCD might represent a more valuable approach to explain social cognitive heterogeneity than more categorical, behaviorally driven subtype characterizations. In summary, important moderating factors that might help unravel heterogeneity in findings include level of illness insight, comorbidities (e.g., schizophrenia, depression), nonsocial neurocognitive functioning, medication or treatment status, and symptom dimensions.

Besides characteristics related to patients, characteristics of the tasks may also contribute to the inconsistencies in results. A wide variety of different tasks have been used to assess the same social cognitive domain, which makes comparison across studies difficult. For example, emotion recognition tasks differed with regard to the nature of the expressions (e.g., static versus morphed), the stimuli set, and the specific task instructions (e.g., labelling versus matching). The number of trials presented also varied considerably. For example, Kornreich et al. (43) presented only 12 trials with facial expressions whereas Jhung et al. (42) and Kang et al. (103) presented as much as 360 trials. Factors like this not only limit the comparability of results between studies but also raise questions with regard to the validity and reliability of the tasks employed. More standardized test batteries are needed to draw out a clear social cognitive profile across the various subdomains of social cognition, which will allow for better comparisons across studies and disorders.

While it has been shown that several social cognitive tasks, especially assessments of ToM, have high test-retest or interrater reliability [see, e.g., (152)], the extent to which impairments on

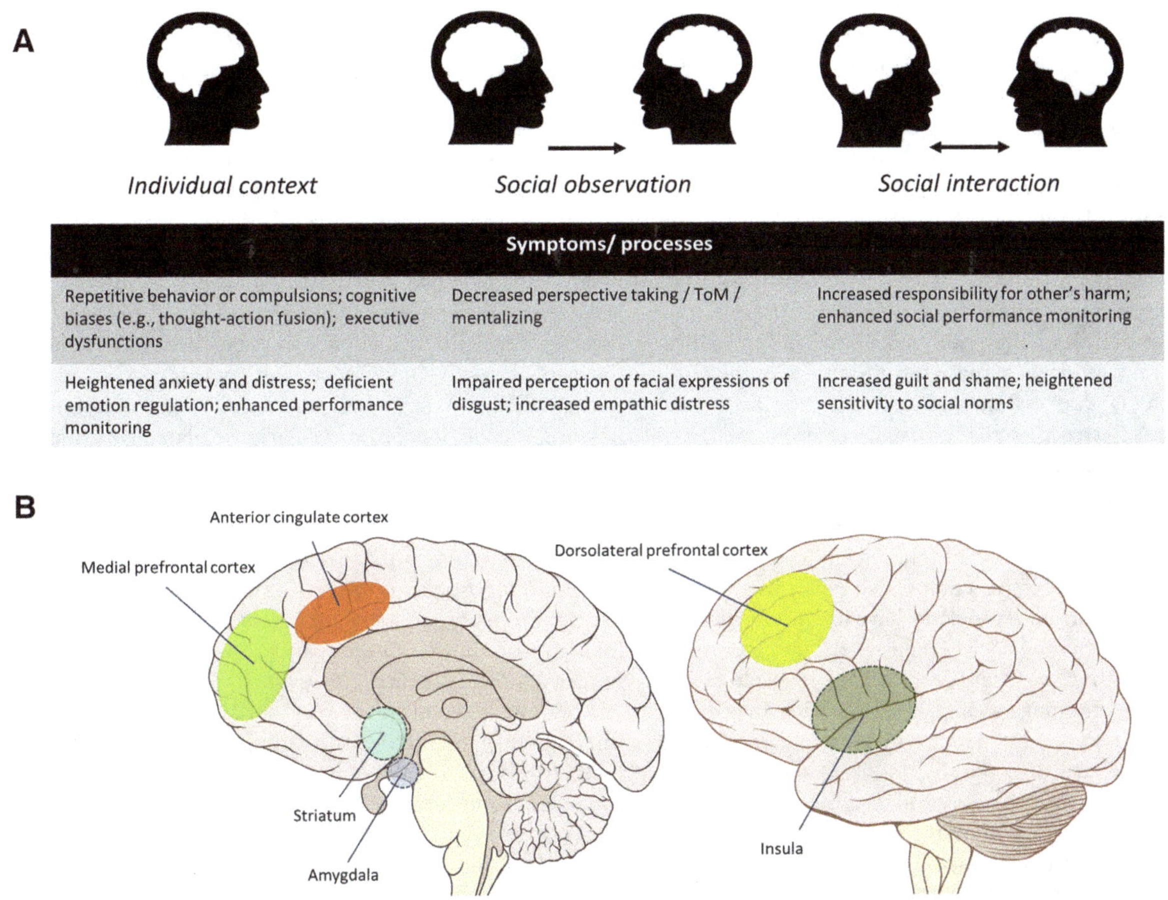

Adapted from original picture by Patrick J. Lynch, medical illustrator [CC BY 2.5 (https://creativecommons.org/licenses/by/2.5)]

FIGURE 2 | Overview of symptoms and processes of obsessive-compulsive disorder discussed in this review **(A)**, from an individual context *via* a social observational and finally toward an interactive context, as well as hypothesized brain regions primarily implicated in these social alterations based on the current review **(B)**. Increased activity in the anterior cingulate cortex and insula in patients has been reported during the processing of the negative or aversive stimuli, as well as during negative prediction errors and error processing more generally. Reduced responsiveness of the striatum (specifically nucleus accumbens) has been demonstrated during the processing of positive prediction errors and rewards. Altered amygdala activity has been reported during the processing of emotional stimuli and fearful or threatening facial expressions. Reduced activation of the dorsolateral prefrontal cortex has been observed during emotion regulation. Although studies on the neural correlates of mentalizing/theory of mind (ToM) are lacking, studies in healthy volunteers have consistently implicated the medial prefrontal cortex in this process. Given that deficits in ToM have been observed in obsessive-compulsive disorder, this region may also be affected in the disorder.

the various social cognitive tasks that OCD patients exhibit are valid indications of social cognitive problems in daily life is currently unclear. Notably, effect sizes for disgust recognition deficits in OCD patients were much smaller for tasks employing morphed compared to static facial expressions (41), whereas the first can be seen as the most ecologically valid and subtle assessment of emotion recognition. Furthermore, many tasks focus on a specific aspect of social cognition (e.g., the ability to identify emotions from either facial expression or vocal or narrative information), whereas in real life individuals need to integrate all these different modalities (e.g., facial, bodily, paralinguistic, auditory and contextual cues) to make sense of others and to function in a socially appropriate way. Only one study used such a multimodal task in OCD patients (74). Interestingly, this study showed no differences in performance between patients and healthy controls. On the one hand, the integration of different processes or modalities may result in higher complexity and cognitive load, such as during higher-order ToM inferences. On the other hand, it possible that the availability of cues from multiple modalities helps compensate for deficits in specific modalities, due to an increased richness of the environment. There are several other multimodal tasks available [see, e.g., (152)], which could help assess social cognitive functioning in a more ecologically valid manner.

The extent to which observed social cognitive deficits are specific to OCD or can be seen as more transdiagnostic deficits that contribute to psychopathology in general should also be investigated in more detail. For example, a recent meta-analysis of 30 different clinical disorders demonstrated social cognitive deficits across practically all these disorders (153). A more standardized test battery covering multiple social cognitive domains may help more clearly elucidate differences and communalities across disorders. The observed bias of OCD patients to assign more negative valence to faces may well be related to comorbid mood disturbances as this is something also commonly found in depression (64). Likewise, problems with mentalizing and altered emotion experience and regulation have been reported in many other disorders as well (153, 154). Importantly, only a subset of the reviewed studies included comorbid diagnoses or symptoms as covariate in their analysis or considered the presence of comorbidities as an exclusion criterion (see **Tables 1–3**). On the other hand, some of these deficits, such as problems in emotion regulation, were found to remain after taking comorbid symptoms such as depression and anxiety into account, suggesting that they form a unique part of the symptomatology of the disorder. In addition, specific deficits in the recognition of disgusted faces and a bias to perceive ambiguous faces as expressing disgust, for example, have not been reported in other disorders, and thus seem to represent a rather unique aspect of obsessive-compulsive symptomatology.

Findings from the current review may have important clinical implications as the identified social cognitive deficits represent important targets for intervention. There are for example facial emotion recognition trainings available (155) which may help remediate disgust recognition deficits in patients. Similarly, trainings exist with regard to ToM (156, 157) and emotion regulation [e.g., (158)], and there is evidence that compassion training may help overcoming empathic personal distress (159). Whether such interventions may also effectively reduce symptomatology and daily life problems in social functioning in OCD remains to be investigated. Tackling social (cognitive) problems in OCD is of critical importance, as poor social functioning has been associated with, among other things, poorer quality of life, and poorer functional outcomes including more severe symptoms, and a higher number of psychiatric comorbidity (10). The social aspects and impact of OCD are therefore not something to be ignored.

TOWARD A SOCIAL NEUROCOGNITIVE INTERACTIVE ACCOUNT OF OCD

Available measures of social cognition have been criticized as they are limited to a "spectator" account of social cognition, whereby individuals merely observe others while thinking about their mental states, instead of interacting with them (1, 160). Schilbach et al. (160) argue that social interactions importantly contribute to our understanding of the mental states of others and that social cognition might be fundamentally different when we are in active interaction with others compared to when we are solely observing others. In social interaction, we might depend on more implicit, automatic, and spontaneous emotional processes rather than explicit cognitive inferences to understand others and there is evidence for a dissociation between such implicit and explicit levels of social cognition (1, 161). Patients with high-functioning autism, for example, generally show reduced implicit or spontaneous inferences of others mental states, despite showing intact explicit cognitive mental attributions [e.g., (162, 163)], suggesting that they are mainly characterized by a problem of social interaction (1). This seems relevant to patients with OCD as well. More often than during observation, social interactions involve an emotional component, and in an interactive context it is essential to regulate these emotions in such a way that relations with others are facilitated. Given that patients with OCD show heightened affective reactivity and social emotions such as inflated feelings of responsibility and guilt, as well as poor emotion regulation skills, this may be particularly challenging for patients with OCD. Moreover, during social interaction, many different cognitive processes need to be integrated in an ongoing fashion in order to behave in an adaptive manner, as one does not only need to take own actions, thoughts and emotions into account, but also the actions, thoughts and emotions of others, as well as their effect on the self, and vice versa. To get a better perspective on daily-life disturbances in OCD, it is therefore important to not only study social cognition in these patients from an observer's perspective, but to additionally start focusing on more implicit and interactive paradigms (see **Figure 2A** for a schematic overview).

Neuroimaging methods may aid the investigation of more implicit and interactive social cognitive processes, as such methods do not require explicit prompting or responding. For example, recent advances in the field of virtual reality provide exciting new opportunities for mimicking realistic social interactions in the MRI scanner [see, e.g., (164)]. However, although recent studies have started using neuroimaging techniques to investigate social cognition in OCD, most studies so far have focused on behavioral assessments. Future studies using neuroimaging techniques are needed to gain more insight into the neural mechanisms underlying altered social cognitive processes. Results from the current review demonstrate that patients with OCD show altered neural activity in- and connectivity between brain regions associated with the recognition, experience, and regulation of emotions, such as the amygdala, insula, nucleus accumbens, ACC, and dorsolateral prefrontal areas (see also **Figure 2B**). Importantly, these results show that those brain areas known to be affected in OCD during nonsocial cognitive and affective processes, also seem to be affected during social variants of these processes. Yet, to date, neuroimaging studies on OCD have mainly been limited to nonsocial cognitive processes, while incorporating the social context in cognitive neuropsychiatric investigations may importantly advance our understanding of the social and functional impairments that characterize OCD patients. A promising candidate in this respect is performance monitoring. As mentioned in the introduction, research has consistently shown enhanced ERN amplitudes in OCD. This has led to the suggestion that this enhancement reflects a possible biomarker of the disorder [see e.g., (165)]. However, increased amplitudes of the ERN are not limited to OCD, but are also found in other anxiety disorders as well as in depression [see (13)]. Importantly, with the integration of social context in performance monitoring research, a more disorder- or symptom-specific marker of OCD may be identified. For instance, the heightened feelings of responsibility for harm and interpersonal guilt that characterize patients suggests that patients with OCD might show specifically enhanced monitoring of their own performance in interactive social responsibility contexts, i.e., when their actions directly have consequences for someone else (166). Such enhancements might not be expected for other disorders with more self-focused symptoms such as health anxiety. So-called social performance monitoring paradigms [see e.g., (166–168)] therefore represent a relevant example of an interactive and implicit measure of social cognition that may substantially inform us on possible alterations in social interactive behavior in patients with OCD.

CONCLUSION

To conclude, the reviewed studies indicate that OCD seems to be associated with alterations in social cue perception, specifically impaired recognition of facial expressions of disgust and biological motion and actions, poorer mentalizing or ToM skills, possibly suboptimal motor resonance, heighted or altered affective and neural responding, and poorer emotion regulation abilities, all of which are processes that may contribute to deficient social functioning in patients with OCD. This review provides an important first step to drawing out a unique social cognitive profile of OCD. However, findings are somewhat inconsistent, and the number of studies in the various subdomains of social cognition are scarce and difficult to compare due to heterogeneity in participant and task characteristics. Future studies should aim to further explore the role of social cognition in OCD using multimodal and ecologically valid paradigms, with a focus on potential moderating factors and developmental pathways. Finally, investigating social interactive behavior in OCD from a cognitive neuropsychiatric perspective remains an essential endeavor as it may importantly advance our understanding of the symptomatology and daily-life disturbances in this intricate and burdensome disorder.

AUTHOR CONTRIBUTIONS

MJ wrote the first version of the manuscript. SO and ED provided feedback and revised the manuscript. All authors approved of the final version.

ACKNOWLEDGMENTS

We would like to thank Francesca Casetta for her help in generating the tables for this article.

REFERENCES

1. Schilbach L. Towards a second-person neuropsychiatry. *Philos Trans R Soc B (- Biol Sci)* (2016) 371:1686. doi: 10.1098/rstb.2015.0081
2. Happé F, Cook JL, Bird G. The structure of social cognition: In(ter) dependence of sociocognitive processes. *Annu Rev Psychol* (2017) 68:243–67. doi: 10.1146/annurev-psych-010416-044046
3. Schneider D, Klimecki O, Burgmer P, Kessler T. Social Cognition. In: Zeigler-Hill V, Shackelford TK, editors. *Encyclopedia of Personality and Individual Differences*. Cham: Springer International Publishing (2019).
4. Green MF, Horan WP, Lee J. Social cognition in schizophrenia. *Nat Rev Neurosci* (2015) 16(10):620–31. doi: 10.1038/nrn4005
5. Fett AK, Viechtbauer W, Dominguez MD, Penn DL, van Os J, Krabbendam L. The relationship between neurocognition and social cognition with functional outcomes in schizophrenia: a meta-analysis. *Neurosci Biobehav Rev* (2011) 35 (3):573–88. doi: 10.1016/j.neubiorev.2010.07.001
6. Ruscio AM, Stein DJ, Chiu WT, Kessler RC. The epidemiology of obsessive-compulsive disorder in the National Comorbidity Survey Replication. *Mol Psychiatry* (2010) 15(1):53–63. doi: 10.1038/mp.2008.94
7. American Psychiatric Association. *Diagnostic and statistical manual of mental disorders (5th ed.)*. Arlington, VA: American Psychiatric Association (2013).
8. Macy AS, Theo JN, Kaufmann SCV, Ghazzaoui RB, Pawlowski PA, Fakhry HI, et al. Quality of life in obsessive compulsive disorder. *CNS Spectrums* (2013) 18:21–33. doi: 10.1017/S1092852912000697
9. Mavrogiorgou P, Akyol. M, Siebers F, Kienast T, Juckel. G. Low psychosocial functioning in obsessive-compulsive disorder and its clinical implications. *J Obsessive-Compulsive Relat Disord* (2015) 5:87–92. doi: 10.1016/j.jocrd.2015.03.004
10. Rosa AC, Diniz JB, Fossaluza V, Torres AR, Fontenelle LF, De Mathis AS, et al. Clinical correlates of social adjustment in patients with obsessive-compulsive disorder. *J Psychiatr Res* (2012) 46(10):1286–92. doi: 10.1016/j.jpsychires.2012.05.019
11. Hezel DM, McNally RJ. A Theoretical review of cognitive biases and deficits in obsessive-compulsive disorder. *Biol Psychol* (2016) 121:221–32. doi: 10.1016/j.biopsycho.2015.10.012
12. Abramovitch A, Cooperman A. The cognitive neuropsychology of obsessive-compulsive disorder: a critical review. *J Obsessive-Compulsive Relat Disord* (2015) 5:24–36. doi: 10.1016/j.jocrd.2015.01.002
13. Riesel A. The erring brain: error-related negativity as an endophenotype for OCD—a review and meta-analysis. *Psychophysiology* (2019) 56(4):e13348. doi: 10.1111/psyp.13348
14. Ventura J, Wood RC, Hellemann GS. Symptom domains and neurocognitive functioning can help differentiate social cognitive processes in schizophrenia: a meta-analysis. *Schizophr Bull* (2013) 39(1):102–11. doi: 10.1093/schbul/sbr067
15. Melloni M, Urbistondo C, Sedeño L, Gelormini C, Kichic R, Ibanez A. The extended fronto-striatal model of obsessive-compulsive disorder: convergence from event-related potentials, neuropsychology and neuroimaging. *Front Hum Neurosci* (2012) 6:259. doi: 10.3389/fnhum.2012.00259
16. Milad MR, Rauch SL. Obsessive-compulsive disorder: beyond segregated cortico-striatal pathways. *Trends Cogn Sci* (2012) 16(1):43–51. doi: 10.1016/j.tics.2011.11.003
17. Nakao T, Okada K, Kanba S. Neurobiological model of obsessive-compulsive disorder: evidence from recent neuropsychological and neuroimaging findings. *Psychiatry Clin Neurosci* (2014) 68:587–605. doi: 10.1111/pcn.12195

18. Fusar-Poli P, Placentino A, Carletti F, Landi P, Allen P, Surguladze S, et al. Functional atlas of emotional faces processing: a voxel-based meta-analysis of 105 functional magnetic resonance imaging studies. *J Psychiatry Neurosci* (2009) 34:418–32. doi: 2010-01016-002
19. Nakao T, Nakagawa A, Yoshiura T, Nakatani E, Nabeyama M, Yoshizato C, et al. Brain activation of patients with obsessive-compulsive disorder during neuropsychological and symptom provocation tasks before and after symptom improvement: a functional magnetic resonance imaging study. *Biol Psychiatry* (2005) 57:901–10. doi: 10.1016/j.biopsych.2004.12.039
20. Schienle A, Schäfer A, Stark R, Walter B, Vaitl D. Neural responses of OCD patients towards disorder-relevant, generally disgust-inducing and fear-inducing pictures. *Int J Psychophysiol* (2005) 57:69–77. doi: 10.1016/j.ijpsycho.2004.12.013
21. Stein DJ, Arya M, Pietrini P, Rapoport JL, Swedo SE. Neurocircuitry of disgust and anxiety in obsessive-compulsive disorder: a positron emission tomography study. *Metab Brain Dis* (2006) 21:255–65. doi: 10.1007/s11011-006-9021-6
22. Pitman RK. A cybernetic model of obsessive-compulsive psychopathology. *Compr Psychiatry* (1987) 28(4):334–43. doi: 10.1016/0010-440X(87)90070-8
23. Falkenstein M, Hohnsbein J, Hoormann J, Blanke L. Effects of errors in choice reaction tasks on the ERP under focused and divided attention. In: Brunia CHM, Gaillard AWK, Kok A, editors. *Psychophysiological Brain Research*. Tilburg: Tilburg University Press (1990). p. 192–5.
24. Gehring WJ, Goss B, Coles MG, Meyer DE, Donchin E. A neural system for error detection and compensation. *Psychol Sci* (1993) 4:385–90. doi: 10.1111/j.1467-9280.1993.tb00586.x
25. Debener S, Ullsperger M, Siegel M, Fiehler K, von Cramon DY, Engel AK. Trial-by-trial coupling of concurrent electroencephalogram and functional magnetic resonance imaging identifies the dynamics of performance monitoring. *J Neurosci* (2005) 25(50):11730–7. doi: 10.1523/JNEUROSCI.3286-05.2005
26. Forbes CE, Grafman J. The role of the human prefrontal cortex in social cognition and moral judgment. *Annu Rev Neurosci* (2010) 33:299–324. doi: 10.1146/annurev-neuro-060909-153230
27. Lavin C, Melis C, Mikulan E, Gelormini C, Huepe D, Ibañez A. The anterior cingulate cortex: an integrative hub for human socially-driven interactions. *Front Neurosci* (2013) 7:64. doi: 10.3389/fnins.2013.00064
28. Lindquist KA. The brain basis of emotion: a meta-analytic review. *Behav Brain Sci* (2012) 35(3):121–43. doi: 10.1017/S0140525X11000446
29. Molenberghs P, Johnson H, Henry JD, Mattingley JB. Understanding the minds of others: a neuroimaging meta-analysis. *Neurosci Biobehav Rev* (2016) 65:276–91. doi: 10.1016/j.neubiorev.2016.03.020
30. Koban L, Pourtois G. Brain systems underlying the affective and social monitoring of actions: an integrative review. *Neurosci Biobehav Rev* (2014) 46(1):71–84. doi: 10.1016/j.neubiorev.2014.02.014
31. Kurtz MM, Richardson CL. Social cognitive training for schizophrenia: a meta-analytic investigation of controlled research. *Schizophr Bull* (2012) 38 (5):1092–104. doi: 10.1093/schbul/sbr036
32. Penton-Voak I, Munafo M, Looi CY. Biased facial emotion perception in mental health disorders: a possible target for psychological intervention? *Curr Dir Psychol Sci* (2017) 26(3):294–301. doi: 10.1177/0963721417704405
33. Tan BL, Lee SA, Lee J. Social cognitive interventions for people with schizophrenia: a systematic review. *Asian J Psychiatry* (2018) 35:115–31. doi: 10.1016/j.ajp.2016.06.013
34. Plana I, Lavoie M, Battaglia M, Achim AM. A meta-analysis and scoping review of social cognition performance in social phobia, posttraumatic stress disorder and other anxiety disorders. *J Anxiety Disord* (2014) 28(2):169–77. doi: 10.1016/j.janxdis.2013.09.005
35. Aigner M, Sachs G, Bruckmuller E, Winklbaur B, Zitterl W, Kryspin-Exner I, et al. Cognitive and emotion recognition deficits in obsessive–compulsive disorder. *Psychiatry Res* (2007) 149:121–8. doi: 10.1016/j.psychres.2005.12.006
36. Bozikas VP, Kosmidis MH, Giannakou M, Saitis M, Fokas K, Garyfallos G. Emotion perception in obsessive–compulsive disorder. *J Int Neuropsychol Soc* (2009) 15:148–53. doi: 10.1017/S1355617708090097
37. Buhlmann U, McNally RJ, Etcoff NL, Tuschen-Caffier B, Wilhelma S. Emotion recognition deficits in body dysmorphic disorder. *J Psychiatr Res* (2004) 38:201–6. doi: 10.1016/S0022-3956(03)00107-9
38. Cannistraro PA, Wright CI, Wedig MM, Martis B, Shin LM, Wilhelm S, et al. Amygdala responses to human faces in obsessive-compulsive disorder. *Biol Psychiatry* (2004) 56:916–20. doi: 10.1016/j.biopsych.2004.09.029
39. Cardoner N, Harrison BJ, Pujol J, Soriano-Mas C, Hernandez-Ribas R, Lopez- Sola M, et al. Enhanced brain responsiveness during active emotional face processing in obsessive compulsive disorder. *World J Biol Psychiatry* (2011) 12:349–63. doi: 10.3109/15622975.2011.559268
40. Corcoran KM, Woody SR, Tolin DF. Recognition of facial expressions in obsessive–compulsive disorder. *J Anxiety Disord* (2008) 22:56–66. doi: 10.1016/j.janxdis.2007.01.003
41. Daros AR, Zakzanis KK, Rector NA. A quantitative analysis of facial emotion recognition in obsessive–compulsive disorder. *Psychiatry Res* (2014) 215:514–21. doi: 10.1016/j.psychres.2013.11.029
42. Jhung K, Namkoong K, Kang JI, Ha RY, An SK, Kim CH, et al. Perception bias of disgust in ambiguous facial expressions in obsessive–compulsive disorder. *Psychiatry Res* (2010) 178:126–31. doi: 10.1016/j.psychres.2009.11.023
43. Kornreich C, Blairy S, Philippot P, Dan B, Foisy M, Hess U, et al. Impaired emotional facial expression recognition in alcoholism compared with obsessive-compulsive disorder and normal controls. *Psychiatry Res* (2001) 102(3):235–48. doi: 10.1016/S0165-1781(01)00261-X
44. Lawrence NS, An SK, Mataix-Cols D, Ruths F, Speckens A, Phillips ML. Neural responses to facial expressions of disgust but not fear are modulated by washing symptoms in OCD. *Biol Psychiatry* (2007) 61(9):1072–80. doi: 10.1016/j.biopsych.2006.06.033
45. Lochner C, Simmons C, Kidd M, Chamberlain SR, Fineberg NA, van Honk J, et al. Differential effects of escitalopram challenge on disgust processing in obsessive-compulsive disorder. *Behav Brain Res* (2012) 226(1):274–80. doi: 10.1016/j.bbr.2011.09.029
46. Montagne B, de Geus F, Kessels RP, Denys D, de Haan EH, Westenberg HG. Perception of facial expressions in obsessive-compulsive disorder: a dimensional approach. *Eur Psychiatry* (2008) 23(1):26–8. doi: 10.1016/j.eurpsy.2007.07.007
47. Mavrogiorgou P, Bethge M, Luksnat S, Nalato F, Juckel G, Brüne M. Social cognition and metacognition in obsessive-compulsive disorder: an explorative pilot study. *Eur Arch Psychiatry Clin Neurosci* (2016) 266 (3):209–16. doi: 10.1007/s00406-016-0669-6
48. Parker HA, McNally RJ, Nakayama K, Wilhelm S. No disgust recognition deficit in obsessive-compulsive disorder. *J Behav Ther Exp Psychiatry* (2004) 35(2):183–92. doi: 10.1016/j.jbtep.2004.04.008
49. Rector NA, Daros AR, Bradbury CL, Richter MA. Disgust recognition in obsessive–compulsive disorder: Diagnostic comparisons and posttreatment effects. *Can J Psychiatry* (2012) 57(3):177–83. doi: 10.1177/070674371205700307
50. Sprengelmeyer R, Young AW, Pundt I, Sprengelmeyer A, Calder AJ, Berrios G, et al. Disgust implicated in obsessive–compulsive disorder. *Proc R Soc B: Biol Sci* (1997) 264:1767–73. doi: 10.1098/rspb.1997.0245
51. Toh WL, Castle DJ, Rossell SL. Facial affect recognition in body dysmorphic disorder versus obsessive-compulsive disorder: an eye-tracking study. *J Anxiety Disord* (2015) 35:49–59. doi: 10.1016/j.janxdis.2015.08.003
52. Via E, Cardoner N, Pujol J, Alonso P, López-Solà M, Real E, et al. Amygdala activation and symptom dimensions in obsessive-compulsive disorder. *Br J Psychiatry* (2014) 204(1):61–8. doi: 10.1192/bjp.bp.112.123364
53. Jung WH, Gu BM, Kang DH, Park JY, Yoo SY, Choi CH, et al. BOLD response during visual perception of biological motion in obsessive-compulsive disorder: an fMRI study using the dynamic point-light animation paradigm. *Eur Arch Psychiatry Clin Neurosci* (2009) 259(1):46–54. doi: 10.1007/s00406-008-0833-8
54. Kim J, Blake R, Park S, Shin YW, Kang DH, Kwon JS. Selective impairment in visual perception of biological motion in obsessive-compulsive disorder. *Depression Anxiety* (2008) 25(7):15–25. doi: 10.1002/da.20402
55. Shin NY, Jang JH, Kim HS, Shim G, Hwang JY, Kim SN, et al. Impaired body but not face perception in patients with obsessive-compulsive disorder. *J Neuropsychol* (2013) 7(1):58–71. doi: 10.1111/j.1748-6653.2012.02035.x
56. Bhikram T, Abi-Jaoude E, Sandor P. OCD: obsessive–compulsive … disgust? *The role disgust obsessive–compulsive Disord J Psychiatry Neurosci* (2017) 42 (5):300–6. doi: 10.1503/jpn.160079

57. Armstrong T, Olatunji BO. Eye tracking of attention in the affective disorders: a meta-analytic review and synthesis. *Clin Psychol Rev* (2012) 32:704–23. doi: 10.1016/j.cpr.2012.09.004
58. Surcinelli P, Codispoti M, Montebarocci O, Rossi N, Baldaro B. Facial emotion recognition in trait anxiety. *J Anxiety Disord* (2006) 20:110–7. doi: 10.1016/j.janxdis.2004.11.010
59. Pittenger C, Bloch MH. Pharmacological treatment of obsessive-compulsive disorder. *Psychiatr Clinics North America* (2014) 37(3):375–91. doi: 10.1016/j.psc.2014.05.006
60. Allen J, Abbott M, Rapee R, Coltheart M. Ew gross! Recognition of expressions of disgust by children with obsessive-compulsive disorder. *Behav Change* (2006) 23(4):239–49. doi: 10.1375/bech.23.4.239
61. Amiri A, Ghasempour A, Fahimi S, Abolghasemi A, Akbari E, Agh A, et al. Recognition of facial expression of emotion in patients with obsessive-compulsive disorder and average people. *Armaghane-danesh Yasuj Univ Med Sci J* (2012) 17:30–8.
62. Goodman WK, Price LH, Rasmussen SA, Mazure C, Fleischmann RL, Hill CL, et al. The yale-brown obsessive-compulsive scale: I. Development, use, and reliability. *Arch Gen Psychiatry* (1989) 46:1006–11. doi: 10.1001/archpsyc.1989.01810110048007
63. Grossman E, Donnelly M, Price R, Pickens D, Morgan V, Neighbor G, et al. Brain areas involved in perception of biological motion. *J Cogn Neurosci* (2000) 12:711–20. doi: 10.1162/089892900562417
64. Weightman MJ, Air TM, Baune BT. A review of the role of social cognition in major depressive disorder. *Front Psychiatry* (2014) 5:179. doi: 10.3389/fpsyt.2014.00179
65. Duval ER, Javanbakht A, Liberzon I. Neural circuits in anxiety and stress disorders: a focused review. *Ther Clin Risk Manage* (2015) 11:115–26. doi: 10.2147/TCRM.S48528
66. Endrass T, Ullsperger M. Specificity of performance monitoring changes in obsessive-compulsive disorder. *Neurosci Biobehav Rev* (2014) 46(1):124–38. doi: 10.1016/j.neubiorev.2014.03.024
67. Etkin A, Büchel C, Gross JJ. The neural bases of emotion regulation. *Nat Rev Neurosci* (2015) 16:693–700. doi: 10.1038/nrn4044
68. Premack D, Woodruff G. Does the chimpanzee have a theory of mind? *Behav Brain Sci* (1978) 1:515–26. doi: 10.1017/S0140525X00076512
69. Walter H. Social cognitive neuroscience of empathy: concepts, circuits, and genes. *Emotion Rev* (2012) 4(1):9–17. doi: 10.1177/1754073911421379
70. Schurz M, Radua J, Aichhorn M, Richlan F, Perner J. Fractionating theory of mind: a meta-analysis of functional brain imaging studies. *Neurosci Biobehav Rev* (2014) 42:9–34. doi: 10.1016/j.neubiorev.2014.01.009
71. Baron-Cohen S. (1995). *Mindblindness. An Essay on Autism and Theory of Mind.* Retrieved from http://books.google.com.
72. McGlade N, Behan C, Hayden J, O'Donoghue T, Peel R, Haq F. Mental state decoding vs mental state reasoning as a mediator between cognitive and social function in psychosis. *Br J Psychiatry* (2008) 193:77–8. doi: 10.1192/bjp.bp.107.044198
73. Mısır E, Bora E, Akdede BB. Relationship between social-cognitive and social-perceptual aspects of theory of mind and neurocognitive deficits, insight level and schizotypal traits in obsessive-compulsive disorder. *Compr Psychiatry* (2018) 83:1–6. doi: 10.1016/j.comppsych.2018.02.008
74. Buhlmann U, Wacker R, Dziobek I. Inferring other people's states of mind: comparison across social anxiety, body dysmorphic, and obsessive-compulsive disorders. *J Anxiety Disord* (2015) 34:107–13. doi: 10.1016/j.janxdis.2015.06.003
75. İnanç L, Altıntaş M. Are mentalizing abilities and insight related to the severity of obsessive-compulsive disorder. *Psychiatry Invest* (2018) 15 (9):843–51. doi: 10.30773/pi.2018.05.02.2
76. Liu W, Fan J, Gan J, Lei H, Niu C, Chan RCK, et al. Disassociation of cognitive and affective aspects of theory of mind in obsessive-compulsive disorder. *Psychiatry Res* (2017) 255:367–72. doi: 10.1016/j.psychres.2017.06.058
77. Pertusa A, Bejerot S, Eriksson J, Fernández de la Cruz L, Bonde S, Russell A, et al. Do patients with hoarding disorder have autistic traits? *Depression Anxiety* (2012) 29(3):210–8. doi: 10.1002/da.20902
78. Pino MC, De Berardis D, Mariano M, Vellante F, Serroni N, Valchera A, et al. Two systems for empathy in obsessive-compulsive disorder: mentalizing and experience sharing. *Braz J Psychiatry* (2016) 38(4):307–13. doi: 10.1590/1516-4446-2015-1679
79. Sayin A, Oral N, Utku C, Baysak E, Candansayar S. Theory of mind in obsessive-compulsive disorder: comparison with healthy controls. *Eur Psychiatry* (2010) 25:116–22. doi: 10.1016/j.eurpsy.2009.09.002
80. Tulacı R G, Cankurtaran EŞ, Özdel K, Öztürk N, Kuru E, Özdemir İ. The relationship between theory of mind and insight in obsessive-compulsive disorder. *Nordic J Psychiatry* (2018) 72(4):273–80. doi: 10.1080/08039488.2018.1436724
81. Baron-Cohen S, Wheelwright S, Hill J, Raste Y, Plumb I. The "Reading the mind in the eyes" test revised version: a study with normal adults, and adults with Asperger syndrome or high-functioning autism. *J Child Psychol Psychiatry* (2001) 42:241–51. doi: 10.1111/1469-7610.00715
82. Brüne M. Theory of mind and the role of IQ in chronic disorganize schizophrenia. *Schizophr Res* (2003) 60:57–64. doi: 10.1016/S0920-9964(02)00162-7
83. Değirmencioğlu B, Alptekin K, Akdede BB, Erdil N, Aktener A, Mantar A, et al. The validity and reliability study of the Dokuz Eylül theory of mind index in patients with schizophrenia. *Turkish J Psychiatry* (2018) 29(3):193–201. doi: 10.5080/u18268
84. Corcoran R, Mercer G, Frith CD. Schizophrenia, symptomatology and social inference: investigating "theory of mind" in people with schizophrenia. *Schizophr Res* (1995) 17:5–13. doi: 10.1016/0920-9964(95)00024-G
85. Happé FGE. An advanced test of theory of mind: understanding of story characters' thoughts and feelings by able autistic, mentally handicapped and normal children and adults. *J Autism Dev Disord* (1994) 24:129–54. doi: 10.1007/BF02172093
86. Baron-Cohen S, O'Riordan M, Stone V, Jones R, Plaisted K. Recognition of faux pas by normally developing children and children with Asperger syndrome or high-functioning autism. *J Autism Dev Disord* (1999) 29:407–18. doi: 10.1023/A:1023035012436
87. Barth A, Küfferle B. Die Entwicklung eines Sprichworttests zur Erfassung konkretistischer Denkstörungen bei schizophrenen Patienten. *Nervenarzt* (2001) 72:853–8. doi: 10.1007/s001150170019
88. Brüne M, Bodenstein L. Proverb comprehension reconsidered–'theory of mind' and the pragmatic use of language in schizophrenia. *Schizophr Res* (2005) 75(2-3):233–9. doi: 10.1016/j.schres.2004.11.006
89. Shamay-Tsoory SG, Aharon-Peretz J. Dissociable prefrontal networks for cognitive and affective theory of mind: a lesion study. *Neuropsychologia* (2007) 45:3054–67. doi: 10.1016/j.neuropsychologia.2007.05.021
90. Dziobek I, Fleck S, Kalbe E, Rogers K, Hassenstab J, Brand M, et al. Introducing MASC: a movie for the assessment of social cognition. *J Autism Dev Disord* (2006) 36:623–36. doi: 10.1007/s10803-006-0107-0
91. Ahmed FS, Miller SL. Executive function mechanisms of theory of mind. *J Autism Dev Disord* (2011) 41:667–78. doi: 10.1007/s10803-010-1087-7
92. Kishore VR, Samar R, Reddy YCJ, Chandrasekhar CR, Thennaras K. Clinical characteristics and treatment response in poor and good insight obsessive-compulsive disorder. *Eur Psychiatry* (2004) 19:202–8. doi: 10.1016/j.eurpsy.2003.12.005
93. Catapano F, Perris F, Fabrazzo M, Cioffi V, Giacco D, De Santis V, et al. Obsessive-compulsive disorder with poor insight: A three-year prospective study. *Prog Neuro Psychopharmacol Biol Psychiatry* (2010) 34(2):323–30. doi: 10.1016/j.pnpbp.2009.12.007
94. Buckley PF, Miller BJ, Lehrer DS, Castle DJ. Psychiatric comorbidities and schizophrenia. *Schizophr Bull* (2009) 35:383–402. doi: 10.1093/schbul/sbn135
95. Ntouros E, Bozikas VP, Andreou C, Kourbetis D, Lavrentiadis G, Garyfallos G. Emotional perception and theory of mind in first episode psychosis: the role of obsessive-compulsive symptomatology. *Psychiatry Res* (2014) 220:112–7. doi: 10.1016/j.psychres.2014.07.058
96. Lewin AB, Bergman RL, Peris TS, Chang S, McCracken JT, Piacentini J. Correlates of insight among youth with obsessive-compulsive disorder. *J Child Psychol Psychiatry* (2010) 51(5):603–11. doi: 10.1111/j.1469-7610.2009.02181.x
97. Rizzolatti G, Craighero L. The mirror-neuron system. *Annu Rev Neurosci* (2004) 27:169–92. doi: 10.1146/annurev.neuro.27.070203.144230
98. Molenberghs P, Cunnington R, Mattingley JB. Brain regions with mirror properties: a meta-analysis of 125 human fMRI studies. *Neurosci Biobehav Rev* (2012) 36:341–9. doi: 10.1016/j.neubiorev.2011.07.004
99. Decety J, Jackson PL. A social-neuroscience perspective on empathy. *Curr Dir Psychol Sci* (2006) 15(2):54–8. doi: 10.1111/j.0963-7214.2006.00406.x

100. Decety J, Meyer M. From emotion resonance to empathic understanding: a social developmental neuroscience account. *Dev Psychopathol* (2008) 20:1053–80. doi: 10.1017/S0954579408000503
101. De Vignemont F, Singer T. The empathic brain: how, when and why? *Trends Cogn Sci* (2006) 10(10):435–41. doi: 10.1016/j.tics.2006.08.008
102. Fontenelle LF, Soares ID, Miele F, Borges MC, Prazeres AM, Rangé BP, et al. Empathy and symptoms dimensions of patients with obsessive-compulsive disorder. *J Psychiatr Res* (2009) 43:455–63. doi: 10.1016/j.jpsychires.2008.05.007
103. Kang JI, Namkoong K, Yoo SW, Jhung K, Kim SJ. Abnormalities of emotional awareness and perception in patients with obsessive–compulsive disorder. *J Affect Disord* (2012) 141:286–93. doi: 10.1016/j.jad.2012.04.001
104. Rounis E, Banca P, Voon V. Deficits in limb praxis in patients with obsessive-compulsive disorder. *J Neuropsychiatry Clin Neurosci* (2016) 28:232–5. doi: 10.1176/appi.neuropsych.15090233
105. Davis MH. Measuring individual differences in empathy: evidence for a multidimensional approach. *J Pers Soc Psychol* (1983) 44(1):113–26. doi: 10.1037/0022-3514.44.1.113
106. Schreiter S, Pijnenborg GH, Aan Het Rot M. Empathy in adults with clinical or subclinical depressive symptoms. *J Affect Disord* (2013) 150:1–16. doi: 10.1016/j.jad.2013.03.009
107. Jolliffe D, Farrington DP. Development and validation of the basic empathy Scale. *J Adol* (2006) 29:589–611. doi: 10.1016/j.adolescence.2005.08.010
108. Baron-Cohen S, Wheelwright S. The empathy quotient: an investigation of adults with Asperger syndrome or high functioning autism, and normal sex differences. *J Autism Dev Disord* (2004) 34:163–75. doi: 10.1023/B:JADD.0000022607.19833.00
109. Blair RJ, Cipolotti L. Impaired social response reversal. *Case 'acquired Sociopathy'. Brain* (2000) 123:1122–41. doi: 10.1093/brain/123.6.1122
110. Robinson LJ, Freeston MH. Emotion and internal experience in obsessive-compulsive disorder: reviewing the role of alexithymia, anxiety sensitivity and distress tolerance. *Clin Psychol Rev* (2014) 34:256–71. doi: 10.1016/j.cpr.2014.03.003
111. Calkins AW, Berman NC, Wilhelm S. Recent advances in research on cognition and emotion in OCD: a review. *Curr Psychiatry Rep* (2013) 15:357. doi: 10.1007/s11920-013-0357-4
112. Nielsen L. The simulation of emotion experience: on the emotional foundations of theory of mind. *Phenomenol Cogn Sci* (2002) 1:255–86.
113. Basile B, Mancini F, Macaluso E, Caltagirone C, Bozzali M. Abnormal processing of deontological guilt in obsessive–compulsive disorder. *Brain Struct Funct* (2014) 219:1321–31. doi: 10.1007/s00429-013-0570-2
114. Bersani G, Bersani FS, Valeriani G, Robiony M, Anastasia A, Colletti C, et al. Comparison of facial expression in patients with obsessive-compulsive disorder and schizophrenia using the facial action coding system: a preliminary study. *Neuropsychiatr Dis Treat* (2012) 8:537–47. doi: 10.2147/NDT.S37174
115. Fontenelle LF, Frydman I, Hoefle S, Oliveira-Souza R, Vigne P, Bortolinia TS, et al. Decoding moral emotions in obsessive-compulsive disorder. *NeuroImage: Clin* (2018) 19:82–9. doi: 10.1016/j.nicl.2018.04.002
116. Hennig-Fast K, Michl P, Müller J, Niedermeier N, Coates U, Müller N, et al. Obsessive-compulsive disorder–a question of conscience?An fMRI study of behavioural and neurofunctional correlates of shame and guilt. *J Psychiatr Res* (2015) 68:354–62. doi: 10.1016/j.jpsychires.2015.05.001
117. Mergl. R, Vogel M, Mavrogiorgou P, Göbel. C, Zaudig. M, Hegerl. U, et al. Kinematical analysis of emotionally induced facial expressions in patients with obsessive–compulsive disorder. *Psychol Med* (2003) 33(8):1453–62. doi: 10.1017/S0033291703008134
118. Valeriani G, Bersani FS, Liberati D, Polli E, Girolami MT, Zullo D, et al. Generalized and specific emotion impairments as potential markers of severity in obsessive-compulsive disorder: a preliminary study using Facial Action Coding System (FACS). *Psychiatria Danubina* (2015) 27(2):159–67.
119. Admon R, Bleich-Cohen M, Weizmant R, Poyurovsky M, Faragian S, Hendler T. Functional and structural neural indices of risk aversion in obsessive-compulsive disorder (OCD). *Psychiatry Res* (2012) 203:207–13. doi: 10.1016/j.pscychresns.2012.02.002
120. Choi JS, Shin YC, Jung WH, Jang JH, Kang DH, Choi CH, et al. Altered brain activity during reward anticipation in pathological gambling and obsessive-compulsive disorder. *PloS One* (2012) 7(9):e45938. doi: 10.1371/journal.pone.0045938
121. Figee M, Vink M, de Geus F, Vulink N, Veltman DJ, Westenberg H, et al. Dysfunctional reward circuitry in obsessive-compulsive disorder. *Biol Psychiatry* (2011) 69:867–74. doi: 10.1016/j.biopsych.2010.12.003
122. Hauser TU, Iannaccone R, Dolan RJ, Ball J, Hättenschwiler J, Drechsler R, et al. Increased fronto-striatal reward prediction errors moderate decision making in obsessive–compulsive disorder. *Psychol Med* (2017) 47(7):1246–58. doi: 10.1017/S0033291716003305
123. Jung WH, Kang DH, Han JY, Jang JH, Gu BM, Choi JS, et al. Aberrant ventral striatal responses during incentive processing in unmedicated patients with obsessive-compulsive disorder. *Acta Psychiatrica Scand* (2011) 123:376–86. doi: 10.1111/j.1600-0447.2010.01659.x
124. Jung WH, Kang DH, Kim E, Shin KS, Jang JH, Kwon JS. Abnormal corticostriatal-limbic functional connectivity in obsessive-compulsive disorder during reward processing and resting-state. *NeuroImage: Clin* (2013) 3:27–38. doi: 10.1016/j.nicl.2013.06.013
125. Kaufmann C, Beucke JC, Preusse F, Endrass T, Schlagenhauf F, Heinz A, et al. Medial prefrontal brain activation to anticipated reward and loss in obsessive-compulsive disorder. *NeuroImage: Clin* (2013) 2:212–20. doi: 10.1016/j.nicl.2013.01.005
126. Koch K, Reeß TJ, Rus OG, Gürsel DA, Wagner G, Berberich G, et al. Increased default mode network connectivity in obsessive–compulsive disorder during reward processing. *Front Psychiatry* (2018) 9:254. doi: 10.3389/fpsyt.2018.00254
127. Murray GK, Knolle F, Ersche KD, Craig KJ, Abbott S, Shabbir SS, et al. Dopaminergic drug treatment remediates exaggerated cingulated prediction error responses in obsessive-compulsive disorder. *Psychopharmacology* (2019) 236(8):2325–36. doi: 10.1007/s00213-019-05292-2
128. Remijnse PL, Nielen MM, van Balkom AJ, Hendriks GJ, Hoogendijk WJ, Uylings HB, et al. Differential frontal-striatal and paralimbic activity during reversal learning in major depressive disorder and obsessive-compulsive disorder. *Psychol Med* (2009) 39(9):1503–18. doi: 10.1017/S0033291708005072
129. Thorsen AL, Hagland P, Radua J, Mataix-Cols D, Kvale G, Hansen B, et al. Emotional processing in obsessive-compulsive disorder: A systematic review and meta-analysis of 25 functional neuroimaging studies. *Biol Psychiatry: Cogn Neurosci Neuroimaging* (2018) 3:563–71. doi: 10.1016/j.bpsc.2018.01.009
130. De Wit SJ, van der Werf YD, Mataix-Cols D, Trujillo JP, van Oppen P, Veltman DJ, et al. Emotion regulation before and after transcranial magnetic stimulation in obsessive compulsive disorder. *Psychol Med* (2015) 45:3059–73. doi: 10.1017/S0033291715001026
131. Fernández de la Cruz L, Landau D, Iervolino AC, Santo S, Pertusa A, Singh S, et al. Experiential avoidance and emotion regulation difficulties in hoarding disorder. *J Anxiety Disord* (2013) 27(2):204–9. doi: 10.1016/j.janxdis.2013.01.004
132. Fink J, Pflugradt E, Stierle C, Exner C. Changing disgust through imagery rescripting and cognitive reappraisal in contamination-based obsessive-compulsive disorder. *J Anxiety Disord* (2018) 54:36–48. doi: 10.1016/j.janxdis.2018.01.002
133. Paul. S, Simon D, Endrass T, Kathmann N. Altered emotion regulation in obsessive-compulsive disorder as evidenced by the late positive potential. *Psychol Med* (2016) 46:137–47. doi: 10.1017/S0033291715001610
134. Picó-Pérez M, Ipser J, Taylor P, Alonso P, López-Solà C, Real E, et al. Intrinsic functional and structural connectivity of emotion regulation networks in obsessive-compulsive disorder. *Depression Anxiety* (2019) 36 (2):110–20. doi: 10.1002/da.22845
135. Yap K, Mogan C, Moriarty A, Dowling N, Blair-West S, Gelgec C, et al. Emotion regulation difficulties in obsessive-compulsive disorder. *J Clin Psychol* (2017) 74:695–709. doi: 10.1002/jclp.22553
136. Ullsperger M, Fischer AG, Nigbur R, Endrass T. Neural mechanisms and temporal dynamics of performance monitoring. *Trends Cogn Sci* (2014) 18 (5):259–67. doi: 10.1016/j.tics.2014.02.009
137. Proudfit GH, Inzlicht M, Mennin DS. Anxiety and error monitoring: the importance of motivation and emotion. *Front Hum Neurosci* (2013) 7:636. doi: 10.3389/fnhum.2013.00636
138. Gross JJ, John OP. Individual differences in two emotion regulation processes: implications for affect, relationships, and well-being. *J Pers Soc Psychol* (2003) 85(2):348–62. doi: 10.1037/0022-3514.85.2.348

139. Gratz KL, Roemer L. Multidimensional assessment of emotion regulation and dysregulation: development, factor structure, and initial validation of the difficulties in emotion regulation scale. *J Psychopathol Behav Assess* (2004) 26:41–54. doi: 10.1023/B:JOBA.0000007455.08539.94
140. Hajcak G, MacNamara A, Olvet DM. Event-related potentials, emotion, and emotion regulation: an integrative review. *Dev Neuropsychol* (2010) 35:129–55. doi: 10.1080/87565640903526504
141. Garnefski N, Kraaij V, Spinhoven P. Negative life events, cognitive emotion regulation and emotional problems. *Pers Individ Dif* (2001) 30:1311–27. doi: 10.1016/S0191-8869(00)00113-6
142. Oltmanns TF, Gibbs NA. Emotional responsiveness and obsessive-compulsive behavior. *Cogn Emotion* (1995) 9(6):563–78. doi: 10.1080/02699939508408983
143. Price J, Cole V, Goodwin GM. Emotional side-effects of selective serotonin reuptake inhibitors: qualitative study. *Br J Psychiatry* (2009) 195:211–7. doi: 10.1192/bjp.bp.108.051110
144. Salkovskis P, Shafrana R, Rachman S, Freeston MH. Multiple pathways to inflated responsibility beliefs in obsessional problems: possible origins and implications for therapy and research. *Behav Res Ther* (1999) 37:1055–72. doi: 10.1016/S0005-7967(99)00063-7
145. Mancini F, Gangemi A. Fear of guilt from behaving irresponsibly in obsessive–compulsive disorder. *J Behav Ther Exp Psychiatry* (2004) 35 (2):109–20. doi: 10.1016/j.jbtep.2004.04.003
146. Shuman V. Studying the social dimension of emotion regulation. *Front Psychol* (2013) 4:6–8. doi: 10.3389/fpsyg.2013.00922
147. Wu MS, McGuire JF, Martino C, Phares V, Selles RR, Storch EA. A meta-analysis of family accommodation and OCD symptom severity. *Clin Psychol Rev* (2016) 45:34–44. doi: 10.1016/j.cpr.2016.03.003
148. Fennell D, Liberato ASQ. learning to live with OCD: labeling, the self, and stigma. *Deviant Behav* (2007) 28(4):305–31. doi: 10.1080/01639620701233274
149. Foa EB, Amir N, Bogert KVA, Molnar C, Przeworski A. Inflated perception of responsibility for harm in obsessive–compulsive disorder. *J Anxiety Disord* (2001) 15(4):259–75. doi: 10.1016/S0887-6185(01)00062-7
150. Prado CE, Watt. S, Crowe SF. A meta-analysis of the effects of antidepressants on cognitive functioning in depressed and non-depressed samples. *Neuropsychol Rev* (2018) 28(1):32–72. doi: 10.1007/s11065-018-9369-5
151. Summerfeldt LJ, Kloosterman PH, Antony MM, Swinson RP. Examining an obsessive-compulsive core dimensions model: structural validity of harm avoidance and incompleteness. *J Obsessive-Compulsive Relat Disord* (2014) 3:83–94. doi: 10.1016/j.jocrd.2014.01.003
152. Henry J, Cowana DG, Lee T, Sachdev PS. Recent trends in testing social cognition. *Curr Opin Psychiatry* (2015) 28(2):133–40. doi: 10.1097/YCO.0000000000000139
153. Cotter J, Granger K, Backx R, Hobbs M, Looi CY, Barnett JH. Social cognitive dysfunction as a clinical marker: a systematic review of meta-analyses across 30 clinical conditions. *Neurosci Biobehav Rev* (2018) 84:92–9. doi: 10.1016/j.neubiorev.2017.11.014
154. Aldao A, Nolen-Hoeksema S, Schweizer S. Emotion-regulation strategies across psychopathology: a meta-analytic review. *Clin Psychol Rev* (2010) 30:217–37. doi: 10.1016/j.cpr.2009.11.004
155. Statucka M, Walder DJ. Efficacy of social cognition remediation programs targeting facial affect recognition deficits in schizophrenia: a review and consideration of high-risk samples and sex differences. *Psychiatry Res* (2013) 206(2–3):125–39. doi: 10.1016/j.psychres.2012.12.005
156. Hofmann SG, Doan SN, Sprun M, Wilson A, Ebesutani C, Andrews LA, et al. Training children's theory-of-mind: a meta-analysis of controlled studies. *Cognition* (2016) 150:200–12. doi: 10.1016/j.cognition.2016.01.006
157. Vass E, Fekete Z, Simon V, Simon L. Interventions for the treatment of theory of mind deficits in schizophrenia: systematic literature review. *Psychiatry Res* (2018) 267:37–47. doi: 10.1016/j.psychres.2018.05.001
158. Allen LB, Barlow DH. Relationship of exposure to clinically irrelevant emotion cues and obsessive-compulsive symptoms. *Behav Mod* (2009) 33:743–62. doi: 10.1177/0145445509344180
159. Klimecki OM, Leiberg S, Ricard M, Singer T. Differential pattern of functional brain plasticity after compassion and empathy training. *Soc Cogn Affect Neurosci* (2014) 9:873–9. doi: 10.1093/scan/nst060
160. Schilbach L, Timmermans B, Reddy V, Costall A, Bente G, Schlicht T, et al. Toward a second-person neuroscience. *Behav Brain Sci* (2013) 36(4):393–414. doi: 10.1017/S0140525X12000660
161. Schneider D, Slaughter VP, Dux PE. Current evidence for automatic theory of mind processing in adults. *Cognition* (2017) 162:27–31. doi: 10.1016/j.cognition.2017.01.018
162. Callenmark B, Kjellin L, Rönnqvist L, Bölte S. Explicit versus implicit social cognition testing in autism spectrum disorder. *Autism* (2014) 18(6):684–93. doi: 10.1177/1362361313492393
163. Schneider D, Slaughter VP, Bayliss AP, Dux PE. A temporally sustained implicit theory of mind deficit in autism spectrum disorders. *Cognition* (2013) 129:410–7. doi: 10.1016/j.cognition.2013.08.004
164. Parsons TD, Gaggioli A, Riva G. Virtual reality for research in social neuroscience. *Brain Sci* (2017) 7(4):42. doi: 10.3390/brainsci7040042
165. Riesel A, Goldhahn S, Kathmann N. Hyperactive performance monitoring as a transdiagnostic marker: results from health anxiety in comparison to obsessive–compulsive disorder. *Neuropsychologia* (2017) 96:1–8. doi: 10.1016/j.neuropsychologia.2016.12.029
166. De Bruijn ERA, Jansen M, Overgaauw S. Enhanced error-related brain activations for mistakes that harm others: ERP evidence from a novel social performance-monitoring paradigm. *NeuroImage* (2020) 204:116238. doi: 10.1016/j.neuroimage.2019.116238
167. De Bruijn ERA, de Lange FP, von Cramon DY, Ullsperger M. When errors are rewarding. *J Neurosci* (2009) 29:12183–6. doi: 10.1523/JNEUROSCI.1751-09.2009
168. De Bruijn ERA, Ruissen MI, Radke S. Electrophysiological correlates of oxytocin induced enhancement of social performance monitoring. *Soc Cogn Affect Neurosci* (2017) 12:1668–77. doi: 10.1093/scan/nsx094

16

Frequency-Tagging Electroencephalography of Superimposed Social and Non-Social Visual Stimulation Streams Reveals Reduced Saliency of Faces in Autism Spectrum Disorder

Sofie Vettori[1,2*], *Milena Dzhelyova*[2,3], *Stephanie Van der Donck*[1,2], *Corentin Jacques*[1,3], *Jean Steyaert*[1,2], *Bruno Rossion*[3,4,5] *and Bart Boets*[1,2]

[1] *Center for Developmental Psychiatry, Department of Neurosciences, KU Leuven, Leuven, Belgium,* [2] *Leuven Autism Research (LAuRes), KU Leuven, Leuven, Belgium,* [3] *Institute of Research in Psychological Science, Institute of Neuroscience, University of Louvain, Louvain-La-Neuve, Belgium,* [4] *Université de Lorraine, CNRS, CRAN-UMR 7039, Nancy, France,* [5] *Université de Lorraine, CHRU-Service de Neurologie, Nancy, France*

***Correspondence:**
Sofie Vettori
sofie.vettori@kuleuven.be

Individuals with autism spectrum disorder (ASD) have difficulties with social communication and interaction. The social motivation hypothesis states that a reduced interest in social stimuli may partly underlie these difficulties. Thus far, however, it has been challenging to quantify individual differences in social orientation and interest, and to pinpoint the neural underpinnings of it. In this study, we tested the neural sensitivity for social versus non-social information in 21 boys with ASD (8-12 years old) and 21 typically developing (TD) control boys, matched for age and IQ, while children were engaged in an orthogonal task. We recorded electroencephalography (EEG) during fast periodic visual stimulation (FPVS) of social versus non-social stimuli to obtain an objective implicit neural measure of relative social bias. Streams of variable images of faces and houses were superimposed, and each stream of stimuli was tagged with a particular presentation rate (i.e., 6 and 7.5 Hz or *vice versa*). This frequency-tagging method allows disentangling the respective neural responses evoked by the different streams of stimuli. Moreover, by using superimposed stimuli, we controlled for possible effects of preferential looking, spatial attention, and disengagement. Based on four trials of 60 s, we observed a significant three-way interaction. In the control group, the frequency-tagged neural responses to faces were larger than those to houses, especially in lateral occipito-temporal channels, while the responses to houses were larger over medial occipital channels. In the ASD group, however, faces and houses did not elicit significantly different neural responses in any of the regions. Given the short recording time of the frequency-tagging paradigm with multiple simultaneous inputs and the robustness of the individual responses, the method could be used as a sensitive marker of social preference in a wide range of populations, including younger and challenging populations.

Keywords: frequency tagging, autism spectrum disorder (ASD), EEG, social attention, faces

INTRODUCTION

Individuals with autism spectrum disorder (ASD) are characterized by impairments in social communication and interaction, and the presence of restricted and repetitive patterns of interests and behavior. They often struggle with social interactions in daily life (1). Several developmental accounts [e.g., (2–4)] propose a developmental cascade in which early-onset impairments in social attention deprive children of adequate social learning experiences necessary for the development of successful social interactions (5). As a result, the classical preference for social over non-social stimuli (e.g., faces over artefacts) that is observed in early life and throughout development [e.g., (6–9)] might not arise, further disrupting the development of social skills and social cognition, and ultimately social functioning and interaction. Due to differences in neural reward processing, autistic people may not experience social stimuli as rewarding as neurotypical people do [e.g., (10–12)]. However, findings on this matter have not been entirely consistent. While Zeeland et al. (12), find that the response to social rewards is particularly decreased in children with ASD in relation to social reciprocity, reward responses to non-social stimuli were also reduced. Therefore, whether aberrant reward processing in ASD is confined to social stimuli or reflects a more general deficit in stimulus-reward associations remains unclear. Likewise, whether attentional processing is particularly impaired for social stimuli or for more complex stimuli in general, remains inconclusive (13).

Empirical evidence from eye-tracking studies confirms that the classical attentional preference for social versus non-social stimuli in the general population is reduced or even absent in individuals with ASD. While evidence is mixed during the first months of life, infants who later develop autism symptoms show reduced social orienting by the end of the first year (14, 15). Recently, a large cohort study (16) with toddlers (12–48 months old) reported enhanced preference for visual stimuli displaying geometric repetition as compared to social stimuli (e.g., videos of playing children) in children later diagnosed with ASD, in particular for an ASD subtype with more severe symptoms. These results suggest that perhaps, the decreased social engagement observed by the end of the first year of life is the developmental *consequence* of impairments in a different functional system during infancy. Hence, an alternative hypothesis is that decreased social orienting and motivation could, for example, be a consequence of difficulties in processing the incoming social information, rather than their cause (14, 15).

In a meta-analysis, Frazier and colleagues (17) analyzed and integrated results of 122 independent studies investigating gaze patterns in infants, children, and adults with ASD as compared to TD individuals. They concluded that individuals with ASD show a basic difficulty selecting socially relevant versus socially irrelevant information. Moreover, gaze abnormalities persist across age and worsen during the perception of human interactions. Other meta-analyses of eye-tracking studies report similar evidence for decreased visual attention to social stimuli in individuals with ASD (18, 19), and demonstrate that an increase in social load, either by including child directed speech or by including several persons interacting with each other, further results in decreased attention to social stimuli in participants with ASD. Thus, generally, eye-tracking research supports a reduced preferential looking bias for social stimuli in ASD. However, effect sizes are moderate and vary across studies, stimuli, and designs (18, 19).

Eye-tracking, often the methodology of choice to study social preference, conveys information about overt orienting processes. However, covert attention is not assessed by eye-tracking studies, possibly resulting in an underestimation of the social bias in studies comparing individuals with and without ASD. The covert processing of social information in ASD has been mostly studied *via* event-related potentials (ERPs) extracted from electroencephalography (EEG) [e.g., (20–26)]. The vast majority of studies focused on the N170, a negative ERP peaking at about 170 ms over occipito-temporal sites following the sudden onset of a face stimulus (27). This component is particularly interesting since it differs reliably between faces and other stimuli in neurotypical individuals (see 28 for review) and reflects the interpretation of a stimulus as a face, beyond the physical characteristics of the visual input (29–31). An extensive amount of research has investigated how the N170 may be different in individuals with ASD versus TD controls. A recent meta-analysis pointed to a small but significant delay in N170 latency in response to faces in ASD compared to TD controls (32). However, the effect is not systematically found and does not relate to behavioral measures of social functioning in ASD (33). Moreover, its specificity is questionable, since it may reflect the generally slower processing of meaningful, even non-social, visual stimuli (34). Neural processing of social and nonsocial stimuli has also been studied through functional near-infrared spectroscopy (fNIRS). Atypicalities in the neural processing of social information in 4–6 month old infants at high familial risk for ASD were demonstrated (35) and replicated in an independent sample (36). While these methods provide information about the covert processing of social and nonsocial information, they are limited by the need to present social and nonsocial stimuli *at different times*, in order to isolate and compare neural responses to each of them.

To address this limitation, our recent study (37) relied on an EEG frequency-tagging approach [(38), see (39) for review] to investigate to what extent school-aged boys with and without ASD show a bias toward social stimuli. Specifically, we *simultaneously* presented two stimulation streams of widely varying images of faces or houses, tagged at different frequency rates, next to each other. With eye-tracking, we measured the fixations within specific areas of interest spanning each stimulus type, thereby offering an index of the overt attentional preference. With EEG, we measured the amplitude of the frequency-tagged electroencephalographic response to each of the stimulus types, thereby offering an index of the neural saliency of each type of stimuli. Frequency-tagged EEG showed enhanced neural responses for faces versus houses in the TD group, and a significant reduction of this social bias in boys with ASD as compared to TD boys. Importantly, this reduced social bias in ASD, as indexed by a group by stimulus type interaction, was already significant after only 5 s of stimulus presentation. Frequency-tagging EEG responses and eye tracking results (i.e., proportional looking times) were highly correlated, implying that individuals who looked relatively more at the stream of faces also showed higher face-tagged EEG responses. However, solely based on the eye-tracking results, we could not conclude that social preference was significantly reduced in the ASD group. Thus, the eye-tracking preferential looking data did not differentiate significantly between both groups, whereas the frequency-tagging EEG data did. Moreover, and unfortunately, participants looked in between both streams of stimuli for a large proportion of time. Another issue is that individual differences in spatial attention and attentional disengagement might also have affected the amplitude of the neural responses, and individuals with ASD have been reported to present alterations in both these domains. Indeed, orienting to a visual stimulus outside the current focus of attention requires two (potentially separable) components: First, one must disengage from whatever currently occupies one's attention, and, second, one must shift to the peripheral stimulus (40, 41). Pertaining to visuo-spatial attention, individuals with ASD have been reported to present a sharper focus of attention (42) and they may benefit less and more slowly from a spatial cue in a Posner task (43). Pertaining to attentional disengagement, and in line with the restricted and repetitive behaviors and the characteristic difficulties in flexibility in ASD, a systematic review (41) concluded that there is robust behavioral and electrophysiological evidence from infants, children, and adults that autistic individuals have difficulties with disengagement. Mo *et al.* (44) further showed that this difficulty with attentional disengagement is rather domain-general and not specific to social stimuli.

Based on these considerations, the present study aims at improving our measures and strengthen our previous observations by spatially superimposing the two types of stimulus streams, so that differences in looking patterns, spatial attention, and disengagement cannot influence the processing saliency of each stimulus category. More precisely, while recording EEG signals, we present two streams of widely varying images of faces and houses, tagged at different frequency rates, simultaneously and superimposed at exactly the same position (**Figure 1**; **Movie S1**). Combining frequency-tagging with EEG allows disentangling neural responses to each of the stimulation streams, even when they are superimposed. Previous frequency-tagging EEG research with superimposed stimuli has shown that attention can modulate neural processing in a nonspatial manner. Enhanced processing (indicated by increased frequency-tagging EEG responses) of particular visual features (e.g., color, orientation, or direction of motion) or objects has been reported when those are attended, even when they are spatially overlapping [e.g., (45–49)]. In particular, one study presented spatially overlapping frequency-tagged face and house images while magnetoencephalography (MEG) responses were monitored as participants attended to the overlapping streams for cued targets. By combining the frequency-tagged MEG responses with functional ROIs defined from functional MRI (fMRI), the researchers found that attention to faces resulted in enhanced sensory responses in a face-selective region of the fusiform

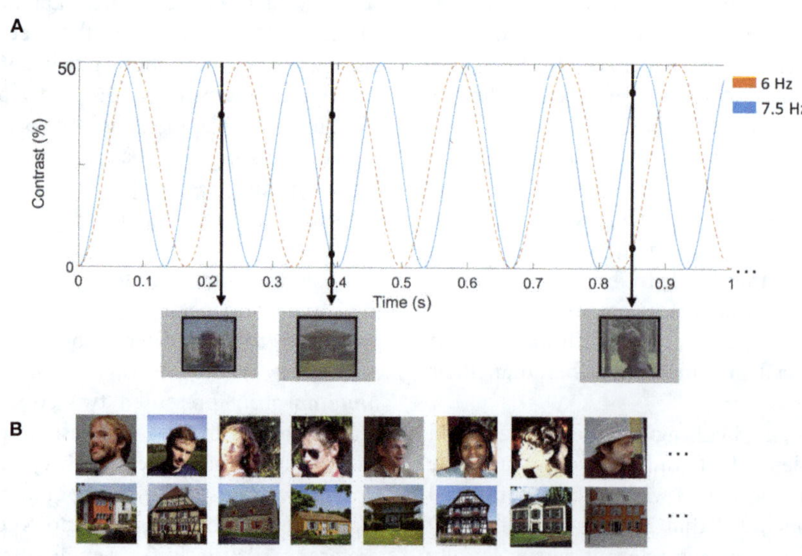

FIGURE 1 | (A) Illustration of a stimulation sequence. The total experiment consisted of four sequences of 60 s. We counterbalanced frequencies (6 and 7.5 Hz) of the stimuli. In the illustrated example, images of houses were presented at 6 Hz, while images of faces were presented at 7.5 Hz. In the other two trials, faces were presented at 6 Hz and houses at 7.5 Hz. Images were contrast-modulated from 0 to 50%. The first black arrow depicts what was presented at 0.22 s. At this time point, the second face is presented at approximately 30% contrast, while the second house is also presented at 30% contrast. **(B)** Examples of face and house stimuli. Written informed consent was obtained from the individuals for the publication of the images.

gyrus, whereas attention to houses resulted in increased responses in a place-selective region of the parahippocampal gyrus (50).

In the current study, images of natural faces (highly varying across viewpoint, luminance etc ...) were used as a prototype of the social category. Pictures of houses were used as the non-social category, as often used in neuroimaging and electrophysiology research to compare to faces, including recent studies in ASD (33). Pictures of houses are typically associated with responses in medial regions of the ventral occipitotemporal cortex, such as the collateral sulcus and the parahippocampal gyrus (50–54) whereas faces typically elicit responses in the lateral parts of the middle fusiform gyrus (latFG) and in the inferior occipital gyrus (IOG) of the ventral occipito-temporal cortex (VOTC) (55–58) [see (59) for a direct comparison using human intracerebral recording data]. Moreover, faces and houses evoke quantitatively and qualitatively different category-selective responses in scalp EEG (60).

In general, we expect to find a strong social bias in TD children, as indicated by larger frequency-tagged EEG amplitudes in response to face stimuli as compared to house stimuli. Based on the literature and in accordance with our previous study (37), we expect that children with ASD will show a reduced social bias compared to TD children, or even that the social bias may be absent.

MATERIAL AND METHODS

Participants

We recruited 47 boys, aged 8-to-12 years old. To match the groups on verbal and performance IQ (VIQ, PIQ) five participants (two from the TD group, three from the ASD group) were *a priori* excluded from the reported analyses, resulting in a sample of 21 typically developing (TD) boys (mean age = 11.0 years ± SD = 1.2) and 21 boys with ASD (mean age = 10.9 ± 1.5, **Table 1**). However, inclusion of these participants did not change any results of the analyses. The sample in this study is identical to the one in the previous study (37), where social and non-social stimuli were presented side-by-side. All participants had normal or corrected-to-normal vision, and had a verbal and performance IQ above 80. Thirty-nine participants were right-handed. Participants with ASD were recruited through the Autism Expertise Center of the University Hospitals Leuven, Belgium. TD participants were recruited through elementary schools and sports clubs.

TABLE 1 | Participant characteristics.

	ASD (mean ± SD)	TD (mean ± SD)	*t(df)*	*p*
Verbal IQ	107 ± 12	112 ± 12	t(40) = −1.41	0.18
Performance IQ	104 ± 15	110 ± 14	t(40) = −1.44	0.21
Age	10.8 ± 1.6	11 ± 1.2	t(40) = 0.80	0.43
Social Responsiveness Scale (*T*-score)	85 ± 12	42 ± 6	t(40) = 14.57	<.0001

Participant exclusion criteria were the presence or suspicion of a psychiatric, neurological, learning, or developmental disorder [other than ASD or comorbid attention deficit hyperactivity disorder (ADHD) in ASD participants] in the participant or in a first- or second-degree relative. This was assessed with a checklist filled out by the parents. Inclusion criteria for the ASD group were a formal diagnosis of ASD made by a multidisciplinary team in a standardized way according to DSM-IV-TR or DSM-5 criteria (1) and a total *T*-score above 60 on the Social Responsiveness Scale [SRS parent version (61)]. Seven participants with ASD took medication to reduce symptoms related to ASD and/or ADHD (Rilatine, Concerta, Aripiprazol). The TD sample comprised healthy volunteers, matched on age, verbal and performance IQ. Parents of the TD children also completed the SRS questionnaire to exclude the presence of substantial ASD symptoms. Descriptive statistics for both groups are displayed in **Table 1**, showing that they did not differ for age and IQ. Evidently, both groups differed highly significantly on SRS scores.

The Medical Ethical Committee of the university hospital approved the study, and the participants as well as their parents provided informed consent according to the Declaration of Helsinki. All participants received a monetary reward and a small present of their choice. The experiment was embedded in a larger research project consisting of three testing sessions. Intellectual abilities were assessed in a separate session. The current frequency-tagging experiment was included in the third session.

IQ Measures

An abbreviated version of the Dutch Wechsler Intelligence Scale for Children, Third Edition [WISC-III-NL; (62, 63)] was administered. Performance IQ was estimated by the subtests Block Design and Picture Completion, verbal IQ by the subtests Vocabulary and Similarities (64).

Frequency Tagging Experiment

Stimuli

Forty-eight color images of faces and 48 images of houses were used, all within their original background, making the images widely variable. Stimuli were selected from (65) and (60). Amplitude spectra of the face and house stimuli are available in supplementary material (**Figure S1** and **Figure S2, Supplementary Material**). The spectral analyses show that house stimuli have more energy in higher spatial frequencies and cardinal orientations. Faces and houses were presented superimposed on the screen, with a broad rectangular outline around them (**Figure 1**): one stimulation stream presented faces, and the other stream presented houses. All images differed highly in terms of viewpoint, lighting conditions and background. All stimuli were resized to 250 x 250 pixels, had equal pixel luminance and root-mean-square contrast on the whole image. Shown at a distance of 60 cm, and at a resolution of 1,920 x 1,200, the stimuli subtended approximately 13° of visual angle. Both the face and the object images were presented in a random order.

Procedure

After electrode-cap placement, participants were seated at a viewing distance of 60 cm and were instructed to maintain a constant distance. Stimuli were displayed on the screen [24-in. light-emitting diode (LED)-backlit liquid crystal display (LCD) monitor] through sinusoidal contrast modulation on a light grey background using Java. We used a screen with a refresh rate of 60 Hz, ensuring that the refresh rate was an integer multiple of the presentation frequencies. A sequence lasted 64 s, including 60 s of stimulation at full contrast, flanked by 2 s of fade-in and fade-out, with contrast gradually increasing and decreasing between 0 and 50%. Fade-in and fade-out were used to avoid abrupt eye movements and eye blinks due to the sudden appearance or disappearance of flickering stimuli. In total, there were four sequences, hence the total duration of the stimulus presentation was about 4 minutes.

Figure 1 and **Movie S1** (**Supplementary Material**) illustrate a sequence, consisting of two streams of simultaneously presented series of images. In each sequence, images of one stimulus category were presented at 6 Hz and images of the other category at 7.5 Hz. The two streams of images were superimposed to one another and shown at the center of the screen. All images were drawn randomly from their respective categories, cycling through all available images before any image repetition. The presentation rate (6 *vs.* 7.5 Hz) was counterbalanced across both stimulus types (faces *vs.* houses), resulting in two conditions presented in a randomized order. The presentation frequencies were selected so that they are close to each other, in order to minimize differences in absolute EEG response (39, 66, 67).

Participants were instructed to look freely at the images on the screen and to press a key whenever they detected brief (300 ms) changes in the color of the rectangular outline surrounding the images. These color changes occurred randomly, 15 times per sequence. This task was orthogonal to the effect/manipulation of interest and ensured that participants maintained a constant level of attention throughout the entire experiment.

Electroencephalography Recording

EEG was recorded using a BioSemi ActiveTwo amplifier system with 64 Ag/AgCl electrodes. During recording, the system uses two additional electrodes for reference and ground (CMS, common mode sense, and DRL, driven right leg). Horizontal and vertical eye movements were recorded using four electrodes placed at the outer canthi of the eyes and above and below the right orbit. The EEG was sampled at 512 Hz.

Electroencephalography Analysis

Preprocessing

All EEG processing was performed using Letswave 6 (https://www.letswave.org/) and MATLAB 2017 (the MathWorks). EEG data was segmented in 67-s segments (2s before and 5s after each sequence), bandpass filtered (0.1 to 100 Hz) using a fourth-order Butterworth filter, and downsampled to 256 Hz. Next, noisy electrodes were linearly interpolated from the three spatially nearest electrodes (not more than 5% of the electrodes, -i.e., three electrodes, were interpolated). All data segments were re-referenced to a common average reference. While in frequency-tagging studies we typically apply blink correction (using ICA) for any participant blinking more than 2 SD above the mean [e.g., (68–70)], in the present study we did not perform any blink correction as none of the participants blinked excessively, i.e., more than two standard deviations above the mean across all participants (0.36 times per second). Note that frequency-tagging yields responses with a high SNR at specific frequency bins, while blink artefacts are broadband and thus do not generally interfere with the responses at the predefined frequency (67). Hence, blink correction (or removal of trials with many blinks) is not systematically performed in such studies [e.g., (71–73)].

Frequency-Domain Analysis

Preprocessed segments were further cropped to contain an integer number of 1.5 Hz cycles (i.e., largest common divisor of both 6 and 7.5 Hz), beginning after fade-in and until 59.38 s (15,203 time bins). The resulting segments were averaged per condition (i.e., segments with the same combination of stimulus category and presentation rate) in the time domain to preserve the complex phase of the response and reduce EEG activity out-of-phase with the stimulation (i.e., noise). The averaged waveforms were transformed into the frequency domain using a Fast Fourier transform (FFT), and the amplitude spectrum was computed with a high spectral resolution (0.017 Hz, 1/59.38 s) resulting in a very high signal-to-noise ratio (SNR) (39, 67).

The recorded EEG contains signal at harmonics frequencies (i.e., integer multiples) of the frequencies at which images are presented (6 and 7.5 Hz) (39, 67). We used two measures to describe the response in relation to the noise level: signal-to-noise ratio (SNR) to better visualize the data [e.g., (74)] and baseline-corrected amplitudes to quantify the response across harmonics (65). SNR spectra were computed for each electrode by dividing the value at each frequency bin by the average value of the 20 neighboring frequency bins (12 bins on each side, i.e., 24 bins, but excluding the 2 bins directly adjacent and the 2 bins with the most extreme values). **Figure 2** displays the SNR spectra. We computed baseline-corrected amplitudes in a similar way by subtracting the average amplitude of the 20 surrounding bins. For group visualization of topographical maps (**Figure 3**), we computed across-subjects averages of the baseline-corrected amplitudes for each condition and electrode separately.

Since the response is inherently distributed over multiple harmonics and all the harmonic frequencies represent some aspect of the periodic response, we combine the response amplitudes across all those harmonics whose response amplitude is significantly higher than the amplitude of the surrounding noise bins [as recommended in (65)]. To define the harmonics that were significantly above noise level, we computed Z-score spectra on group-level data for each stimulation frequency (60, 68, 74, 75). We averaged the FFT amplitude spectra across electrodes in the relevant regions-of-

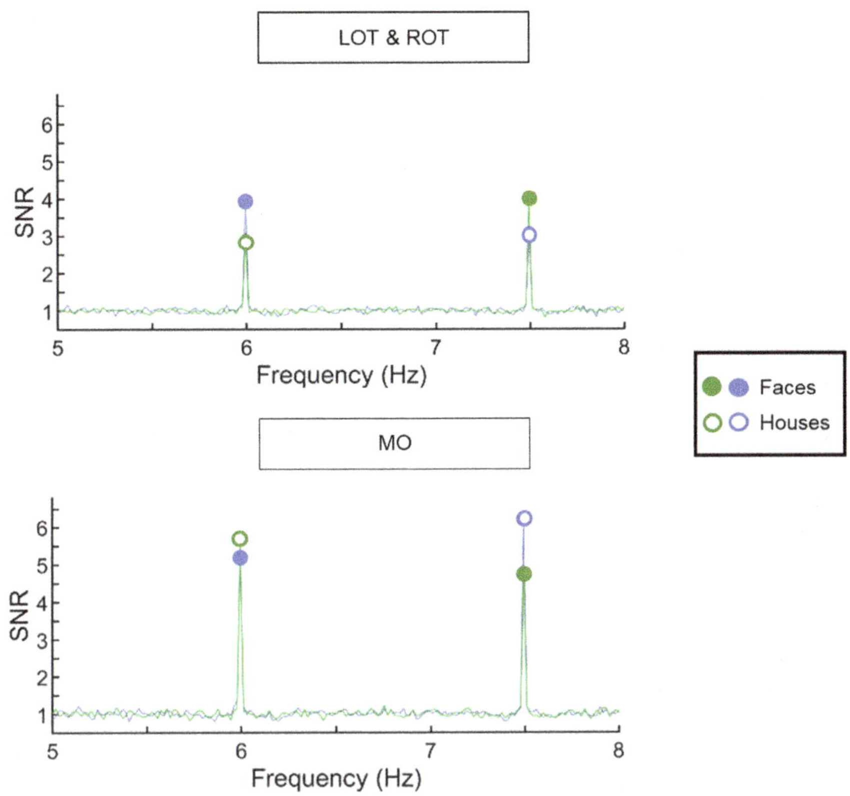

FIGURE 2 | Signal-to-noise ratio (SNR) spectra averaged across all participants (across the two groups) show clear responses at the first harmonic frequencies of interest. Data are plotted for the left and right occipito-temporal region (upper panel) and the medial occipital region (lower panel). The frequency spectrum is plotted from 5 to 8 Hz. In green, images of houses are presented at 6 Hz, while images of faces were presented at 7.5 Hz. In blue, the frequencies were reversed. Full circles display the neural response for faces, empty circles display the neural response for houses. In left and right occipito-temporal ROIs, the response to faces is larger than to houses. In the medial occipital ROI, the response to houses is larger than the response to faces.

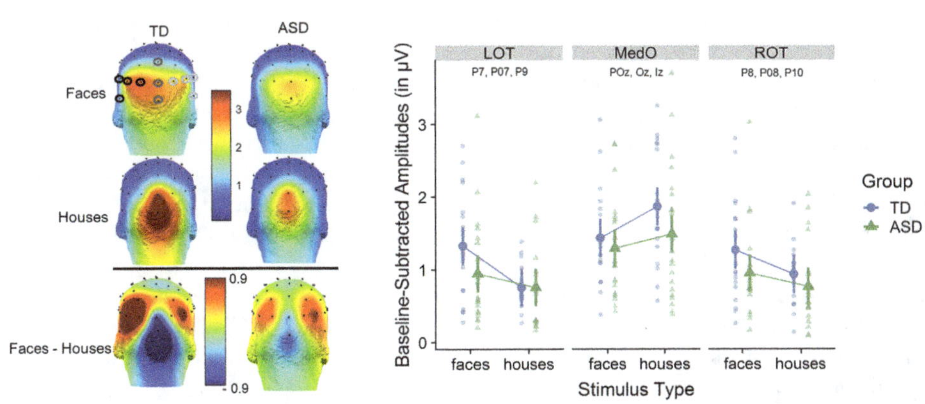

FIGURE 3 | Left: scalp distribution of the electroencephalography (EEG) signal during fast periodic visual stimulation (baseline subtracted amplitudes in µV). Frequency-tagged neural responses to the streams of periodically presented faces and houses are shown for each participant group, as well as the differential response for faces minus houses. The analysis of the response to both types of stimuli focused on three regions of interests (ROIs): medial occipital (MO: Iz, Oz, POz), left occipito-temporal (LOT: O1, PO7, P7, P9), and right occipito-temporal (ROT: O2, PO8, P8, P10). Right: averaged baseline-subtracted amplitudes for each stimulus condition (faces or houses) for each group and for each ROI. The individual subject data is displayed in the background. Statistical analysis shows an interaction between group, stimulus type and ROI.

interest (ROIs) based on topographical maps, and transformed these values into Z-scores (i.e., the difference between the amplitude at each frequency bin and the mean amplitude of the corresponding 20 surrounding bins, divided by the SD of the amplitudes in these 20 surrounding bins). For 6 Hz, Z-scores were significant (i.e., $Z > 2.32$ or $p < 0.01$) until the 5th harmonic (30 Hz) and for 7.5 Hz, Z-scores until the fourth harmonic (30 Hz) were significant. To include an equal number of harmonics for both stimulation frequencies and to exclude shared harmonics (30 Hz), we selected the first three harmonics for both frequencies and summed the baseline-corrected amplitudes of those for each frequency and each condition separately. Hence, we quantified neural responses to faces and houses at 6 Hz and at 7.5 Hz by summing the baseline-subtracted responses for 3 harmonics: 6, 12, and 18 Hz for the 6 Hz stimulation frequency; and 7.5, 15, and 22.5 Hz for the 7.5 Hz stimulation frequency. Therefore, we obtained an index of neural saliency per stimulus type (i.e., houses versus faces) and per presentation rate.

Based on *a priori* knowledge, in accordance with previous studies and confirmed by visual inspection of the topographical maps of both groups (**Figure 3**), we identified regions of interest (ROI) in which the signal was maximal and averaged the signal at these nearby electrodes. The analysis of the response to both types of stimuli focused on three ROIs: medial occipital (MO: Iz, Oz, POz), left occipito-temporal (LOT: O1, PO7, P7, P9) and right occipito-temporal (ROT: O2, PO8, P8, P10) (**Figure 3**).

Statistical Analysis

We statistically analyzed the baseline-corrected amplitudes in each ROI and at each presentation frequency for each stimulus type at the group-level using general linear mixed-effects models (LMEMs) using the AFEX package v0.22-1 (76) in R v3.4.3 (R Core Team, 2012). In particular, we examined the neural responses (i.e., baseline-subtracted amplitudes) with *stimulus type* (houses *vs.* faces) and *ROI* (MO, LOT, ROT) as within-subject factors, and *group* (ASD *vs.* TD) as a between-subject factor. We included a random intercept per participant in the model. *Post-hoc* T-tests were performed on the fitted model using the emmeans package (77). Tukey-corrected p-values were used to compare means and unstandardized effect sizes are reported [cf. (78, 79)].

In addition, we determined the significance of responses for each individual participant and each stimulus type as follows [e.g., (66, 69, 71)]: 1) the raw FFT amplitude spectrum was averaged across electrodes per ROI, and 2) cut into segments centered on the target frequency bin and harmonics (i.e., 6, 12, 18 Hz or 7.5, 15, 22.5 Hz), surrounded by 20 neighboring bins on each side; 3) the amplitude values across the segments of FFT spectra were summed; 4) the summed FFT spectrum was transformed into a *z*-score using the 20 surrounding bins (see above). Responses of a given participant were considered significant if the z-score at the target frequency bin exceeded 1.64 (i.e., $p < 0.05$ one-tailed: signal > noise). Finally, we computed spearman correlations between the neural measures and the scores on the Social Responsiveness Scale (SRS). To this end, we used the corrplot package in R (78).

RESULTS

No Group Difference in Orthogonal Task Performance

Both groups performed equally on the behavioral color change detection task, suggesting a similar level of attention throughout the experiments. Both groups showed accuracies between 97 (SD = 6%) and 97.1% (SD = 3.9%) with mean response times between 0.47 (SD = 0.07) and 0.46 (SD = 0.04) seconds, for ASD and TD respectively. Statistical analyses (two-sided t-tests) showed no significant differences between the ASD group and the TD group [accuracy: t(36) = -0.03, p = 0.49; response times t (36)= 0.71, p = 0.24].

Electroencephalography Responses in Autism Spectrum Disorder Participants Are Not Modulated by Social Versus Non-Social Stimulation

We observed robust frequency-tagged responses, in the three regions of interest (ROI) and for the two stimulus types (see **Figure 2** for SNR spectrograms and **Figure 3** for scalp distributions and averaged response amplitudes). Analyses at the individual level indicated that, despite the short recording time, all participants showed significant responses to houses and to faces in the pre-specified ROIs.

At the group level, statistical analyses showed a main effect of *stimulus type* [$F(1,441) = 5.02$; $p = 0.026$] [faces (1.20 μV) larger than houses (1.08 μV) and a main effect of *ROI* (F(2,441)= 58.10, $p < 0.0001$] [larger responses in MO (1.51 μV) than in LOT (0.94 μV) and ROT (0.97 μV)]. These effects were qualified by a significant interaction effect between *stimulus type* and *ROI* [$F(2,441) = 19.10$, $p < 0.0001$] and, most importantly a significant three-way interaction between *group, stimulus type,* and *ROI* [$F(2,441) = 3.40$, $p = 0.034$)]. *Post-hoc* testing revealed that over the left occipito-temporal channels, the response for faces (1.32 μV) was larger than for houses (0.75 μV) in the TD group [$T(441) = 4.73$, $p = 0.0002$)]. While over the ROT channels the responses were also higher to faces (1.26 μV) than to houses (0.91 μV) in the TD group, this effect did not reach significance [$T(441) = 2.75$, $p = 0.207$]. Over medial occipital channels, responses to houses (1.82 μV) were significantly higher than to faces (1.44 μV) in the TD group [$T(441) = -3.54$, $p = 0.0226$]. In contrast, in the ASD group, the responses to faces were not significantly different from responses to houses, in none of the ROIs [LOT: $T(441) = 1.6$, $p = 0.91$, ROT: $T(441) = 1.56$, $p = 0.92$, MO: T(441) = −1.64, $p = 0.89$)]. Mean amplitude values for the ASD group in LOT were 0.95 μV (faces) and 0.76 μV (houses); in ROT 0.95 μV (faces) and 0.77 μV (houses); and in MO 1.30 μV (faces) and 1.49 μV (houses).

Taken together, the three-way interaction indicates that the neural organization of the TD participants is more differentiated and specialized in terms of anatomically localized stimulus-specific responses, whereas the response pattern of the ASD group is not modulated by the social versus non-social character of the stimulation.

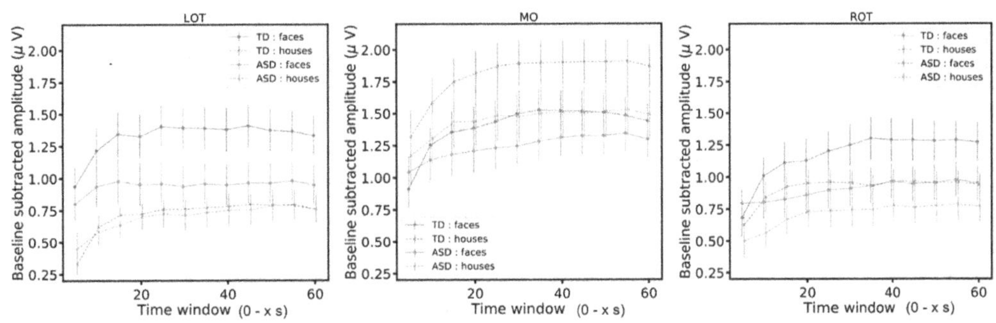

FIGURE 4 | The figure shows the baseline subtracted amplitudes of the responses for segments of increasing length (5 to 60 s in steps of 5 s: 5, 10, 15,..., 60 s). The mean amplitudes (± SEM) are displayed.

In addition, we considered how the neural responses evolved over the course of a stimulation sequence, as this could also inform about the minimal sequence length needed to observe an interaction effect. To do so, we cut the original data in segments of increasing length (5 to 60 s in steps of 5 s: 5, 10, 15,..., 60 s). For all segments, we plotted the evolution of the signal relative to the sequence duration (**Figure 4**). Overall, after an initial buildup period, mean amplitudes remain stable over the trial duration and reflect the findings described above. More specifically, in left and right OT channels, the *group* x *stimulus type* interaction (indicative of a differential social bias in ASD *vs.* TD) is significant from 25 s onwards [$F(1,285) = 4.61$, $p = 0.03$)] and remains significant during the entire trial ($p < .05$).

No Associations Between Neural Responses and Social Responsivity

Spearman correlations showed that individual differences in the amplitude of the neural responses were not significantly related to individual differences in social responsivity as reported by the parents on the SRS questionnaire. Neither the difference between faces and houses, nor the amplitudes of faces and houses separately were correlated with the SRS. This was the case within the two groups and across the groups.

DISCUSSION

Individuals with autism spectrum disorder (ASD) have difficulties with social communication and interaction. Here, we quantified the saliency of processing social versus non-social information by frequency-tagging superimposed streams of widely variable images of faces and houses while recording EEG. This approach allows monitoring brain responses to simultaneously presented stimuli, and, importantly, changes in response amplitude represent dynamic neural changes related to the intensity of processing the driving stimulus. Whereas a recent study showed reduced social bias in ASD using a frequency-tagging EEG approach with streams of social and non-social stimuli presented side-by-side (37), here we extend and specify these findings by presenting the stimulation streams superimposed. By doing so, we can specifically measure the neural processing and saliency of each stimulus category, while ruling out potential confounds related to looking patterns, spatial attention and attentional disengagement.

Within a short amount of time (i.e., four trials of 60 s), we observed significant responses for each participant and each stimulus type. These responses were implicit in the sense that they did not require any active behavior of the participant, apart from looking at the screen. Importantly, they were determined in an objective manner since they were locked to the stimulation frequencies (39, 67) and did not require any subjective interpretation on the part of the researcher. The stimulation-tagged brain responses were located over medial occipital and occipito-temporal regions. Results showed a significant interaction between stimulus type, group and regions of interest (ROI). In the TD group, faces elicited larger responses than houses over occipito-temporal channels, while houses evoked stronger responses than faces over medial occipital channels. Conversely, in the ASD group, the differences between faces and houses were not significant in any of the ROIs. In other words, TD participants showed a differentiated localization and tuning of the neural responses toward social versus non-social stimuli, whereas the response pattern of the ASD group was not modulated by the social versus non-social character of the stimulation.

Reduced interest in social stimuli in ASD might result in less frequent engagement with faces. Accordingly, developing neural systems devoted to face processing may lack experience-expectant visual input, which may be necessary for establishing the neural architecture for expert face processing competency (2). Here, we show that even when individuals with ASD show similar spatial attention to the stream of faces, EEG frequency-tagging still evokes lower face-selective neural activity in occipito-temporal areas as compared to TD individuals. We observed that in the TD group, faces elicited larger responses than houses over occipito-temporal channels, while houses evoked stronger responses than faces over medial occipital channels. This result is in line with previous observations, indicating that lateral ventral occipito-temporal brain regions (i.e., inferior occipital gyrus, lateral fusiform gyrus) respond preferentially to face stimuli while medial occipito-temporal structures (medial temporal gyrus, collateral sulcus, and parahypocampal gyrus) display a preference for house stimuli (51, 53, 54, 80). Likewise, previous research combining frequency-tagging MEG with functional ROIs defined from fMRI showed that attention allocation selectively modulated the amplitude of the frequency-tagged responses to superimposed stimuli: attention to faces resulted in selectively enhanced responses in the fusiform area, whereas attention to houses increased the neural responses in the parahippocampal place area (50). In addition, the medial occipital brain topography in response to the houses may be particularly driven by particular low-level characteristics of the houses, such as rectangular features (81) and cardinal orientation (82, 83). Indeed, in general, houses have more energy in higher spatial frequencies and cardinal orientation, as was also confirmed by the amplitude spectra of the face and house stimuli used in this study (**Figure S1, Supplementary Material**). Along these lines, previous ERP studies have shown larger amplitudes in early visual ERPs over medial occipital electrodes for images with more high spatial frequency content (84).

In the TD group, significantly increased responses to faces versus houses were found only in the left ROI. At first glance, this observation appears inconsistent with the typical right lateralization of the human cortical face network (57, 59, 85). Nevertheless, other studies in children within this age range have not found the right lateralization pattern for face preference that is typically observed in adults [e.g., (86)]. Moreover, studies using a frequency-tagging oddball EEG paradigm across different ages suggest a non-linear development of the right hemispheric specialization for human face perception (87). In 5 year old children (87) and 8–12 year old children (70), face-selective responses did not differ across hemispheres, while the same paradigm in adults [e.g., (76)] and in infants (88) elicits right lateralized electrophysiological occipito-temporal face-selective responses.

Strikingly, in the ASD group, the neural responses for faces and houses were not significantly different from each other in any of the ROIs. Previous observations already indicated altered sensitivity to face stimuli in the fusiform face area (FFA) of ASD (89–93), although this finding has not always been replicated (94–98). One possibility is that less frequent engagement with faces might have resulted in altered specialization of the FFA in ASD participants.

In a previous study (37), we presented streams of social and non-social stimuli side-by-side and we showed that frequency-tagging is a sensitive method allowing us to observe a reduced social bias in boys with ASD. Here, by superimposing both streams of stimuli, we showed that even in the absence of explicit looking behavior, frequency-tagging allows measuring the relative neural saliency of faces and houses. As a result, we quantified the implicit social bias in children with and without ASD, while controlling for potential influences of visuo-spatial attention and/or attentional disengagement. Against this background, our findings suggest that in children with ASD, as compared with TD children, the face-sensitive areas are less preferentially responsive for faces compared to houses and that the typical social bias in these areas is reduced. Our findings generally corroborate developmental accounts that relate social experiences to the specialized neural wiring of the face processing network.

Unexpectedly, however, children with ASD also show less differentiated responses to the house stimulation in the medial occipital region. Taken together, this suggests that, generally, the neural wiring in children with ASD is less differentiated and specialized, and less modulated by the social versus non-social character of the stimulation, which may possibly point toward a more general developmental delay in social and non-social visual sensory processing. This finding might echo broader predictive coding accounts of ASD, suggesting a generally atypical attentional information processing style that is manifested most clearly in the social domain—possibly to the high complexity inherent to social situations (13).

We did not observe significant correlations between the SRS and the face or house-related neural responses. The SRS measures the severity of ASD symptoms over a variety of domains, based on evaluations by the parents. Hence, while it gives a clear idea of the perceived symptoms in daily life, this measure does not purely reflect the actual behavior and performance, and is also determined by several other parent-related processes (e.g., whether there are other children in the family with an ASD diagnosis) (99). Second, the variation of amplitude of the EEG response across individuals also reflects general factors such as skull thickness and cortical folding (see the discussion in (100). While these factors should be neutralized when comparing relatively large groups of participants or when comparing different paradigms in the same participants, they add variance to amplitude differences within a group of individuals, reducing the significance of correlation measures [see (33, 101)]

Further studies are required to replicate this finding in a larger and more heterogeneous and representative sample. Given the short recording time of the frequency-tagging paradigm with multiple simultaneous inputs and the robustness of the individual responses, the method could be used as a fast marker of social preference in a wide range of populations, including low-functioning individuals with ASD, and young children and infants (87, 88). Therefore, the approach has potential to pinpoint developmental trajectories in longitudinal research, from infancy onwards. Moreover, implicit objective measures can help overcome the difficulty of interpreting behavioral findings (which may be influenced by many factors such as motivation, task understanding, etc.). Since in the current study no positional counterbalancing is needed, few trials are required in order to obtain robust data. This is especially an advantage when testing challenging populations, where testing time is limited.

AUTHOR CONTRIBUTIONS

SVe, MD, SVa, BR, and BB conceived and designed the study. SVa and JS contributed to participant recruitment. SVe and SVa collected the data. SVe, CJ, and MD statistically analyzed and interpreted the data, and all authors discussed the results. SVe and BB drafted the manuscript. All authors provided feedback and approved the final version.

ACKNOWLEDGMENTS

We want to thank the participants and their parents for participating in our study.

REFERENCES

1. American Psychiatric Association. *Diagnostic and statistical manual of mental disorders (DSM-5).* (2013).
2. Chevallier C, Kohls G, Troiani V, Brodkin ES, Schultz RT. The social motivation theory of autism. *Trends Cognit Sci* (2012) 16(4):231–9. doi: 10.1016/j.tics.2012.02.007
3. Klin A, Jones W, Schultz R, Volkmar F. The enactive mind, or from actions to cognition: lessons from autism. *Philos Trans R Soc Lond B Biol Sci* (2003) 358 (1430):345–60. doi: 10.1098/rstb.2002.1202
4. Klin A, Shultz S, Jones W. Social visual engagement in infants and toddlers with autism: early developmental transitions and a model of pathogenesis. *Neurosci Biobehav Rev* (2015) 50:189–203. doi: 10.1016/j.neubiorev.2014.10.006
5. Happé F, Cook JL, Bird G. The Structure of Social Cognition: In(ter) dependence of Sociocognitive Processes. *Annu Rev Psychol* (2017) 68 (1):243–67. doi: 10.1146/annurev-psych-010416-044046
6. Crouzet SM, Kirchner H, Thorpe SJ. Fast saccades toward faces: face detection in just 100 ms. *J Vis* (2010) 10(4):16.1–17. doi: 10.1167/10.4.16
7. Goren CC, Sarty M, Wu PY. Visual following and pattern discrimination of face-like stimuli by newborn infants. *Pediatrics.* (1975) 56(4):544–9.
8. Johnson MH, Dziurawiec S, Ellis H, Morton J. Newborns' preferential tracking of face-like stimuli and its subsequent decline. *Cognition.* (1991) 40(1–2):1–19. doi: 10.1016/0010-0277(91)90045-6
9. Purcell DG, Stewart AL. The face-detection effect: configuration enhances detection. *Percept Psychophy* (1988) 43(4):355–66. doi: 10.3758/BF03208806
10. Kohls G, Schulte-Rüther M, Nehrkorn B, Müller K, Fink GR, Kamp-Becker I, et al. Reward system dysfunction in autism spectrum disorders. *Soc Cognit Affect Neurosci* (2013) 8(5):565–72. doi: 10.1093/scan/nss033
11. Stavropoulos KKM, Carver LJ. Reward anticipation and processing of social versus nonsocial stimuli in children with and without autism spectrum disorders. *J Child Psychol Psychiatry* (2014) 55(12):1398–408. doi: 10.1111/jcpp.12270
12. Zeeland AAS-V, Dapretto M, Ghahremani DG, Poldrack RA, Bookheimer SY. Reward processing in autism. *Autism Res* (2010) 3(2):53–67. doi: 10.1002/aur.122
13. Van de Cruys S, Evers K, Van der Hallen R, Van Eylen L, Boets B, de-Wit L, et al. Precise minds in uncertain worlds: Predictive coding in autism. *Psychol Rev* (2014) 121(4):649–75. doi: 10.1037/a0037665
14. Gliga T, Jones EJH, Bedford R, Charman T, Johnson MH. From early markers to neuro-developmental mechanisms of autism. *Dev Rev* (2014) 34 (3):189–207. doi: 10.1016/j.dr.2014.05.003
15. Jones EJH, Gliga T, Bedford R, Charman T, Johnson MH. Developmental pathways to autism: A review of prospective studies of infants at risk. *Neurosci Biobehav Rev* (2014) 39:1–33. doi: 10.1016/j.neubiorev.2013.12.001
16. Moore A, Wozniak M, Yousef A, Barnes CC, Cha D, Courchesne E, et al. The geometric preference subtype in ASD: identifying a consistent, early-emerging phenomenon through eye tracking. *Mol Autism* (2018) 9:19. doi: 10.1186/s13229-018-0202-z
17. Frazier TW, Strauss M, Klingemier EW, Zetzer EE, Hardan AY, Eng C, et al. A Meta-Analysis of Gaze Differences to Social and Nonsocial Information Between Individuals With and Without Autism. *J Am Acad Child Adolesc Psychiatry* (2017) 56(7):546–55. doi: 10.1016/j.jaac.2017.05.005
18. Chita-Tegmark M. Social attention in ASD: A review and meta-analysis of eye-tracking studies. *Res Dev Disabil* (2016) 48:79–93. doi: 10.1016/j.ridd.2015.10.011
19. Guillon Q, Hadjikhani N, Baduel S, Rogé B. Visual social attention in autism spectrum disorder: Insights from eye tracking studies. *Neurosci Biobehav Rev* (2014) 42:279–97. doi: 10.1016/j.neubiorev.2014.03.013
20. Benning SD, Kovac M, Campbell A, Miller S, Hanna EK, Damiano CR, et al. Late Positive Potential ERP Responses to Social and Nonsocial Stimuli in Youth with Autism Spectrum Disorder. *J Autism Dev Disord* (2016) 46 (9):3068–77. doi: 10.1007/s10803-016-2845-y
21. Dawson G, Carver L, Meltzoff AN, Panagiotides H, McPartland J, Webb SJ. Neural correlates of face and object recognition in young children with autism spectrum disorder, developmental delay, and typical development. *Child Dev* (2002) 73(3):700–17. doi: 10.1111/1467-8624.00433
22. Gunji A, Goto T, Kita Y, Sakuma R, Kokubo N, Koike T, et al. Facial identity recognition in children with autism spectrum disorders revealed by P300 analysis: a preliminary study. *Brain Dev* (2013) 35(4):293–8. doi: 10.1016/j.braindev.2012.12.008
23. McCleery JP, Akshoomoff N, Dobkins KR, Carver LJ. Atypical Face Versus Object Processing and Hemispheric Asymmetries in 10-Month-Old Infants at Risk for Autism. *Biol Psychiatry* (2009) 66(10):950–7. doi: 10.1016/j.biopsych.2009.07.031
24. Monteiro R, Simões M, Andrade J, Castelo Branco M. Processing of Facial Expressions in Autism: a Systematic Review of EEG/ERP Evidence. *Rev J Autism Dev Disord* (2017) 4(4):255–76. doi: 10.1007/s40489-017-0112-6
25. O'Connor K, Hamm JP, Kirk IJ. Neurophysiological responses to face, facial regions and objects in adults with Asperger's syndrome: an ERP investigation. *Int J Psychophysiol Off J Int Organ Psychophysiol* (2007) 63 (3):283–93. doi: 10.1016/j.ijpsycho.2006.12.001
26. Webb SJ, Jones EJH, Merkle K, Murias M, Greenson J, Richards T, et al. Response to familiar faces, newly familiar faces, and novel faces as assessed by ERPs is intact in adults with autism spectrum disorders. *Int J Psychophysiol Off J Int Organ Psychophysiol* (2010) 77(2):106–17. doi: 10.1016/j.ijpsycho.2010.04.011
27. Bentin S, Allison T, Puce A, Perez E, McCarthy G. Electrophysiological Studies of Face Perception in Humans. *J Cognit Neurosci* (1996) Nov8 (6):551–65. doi: 10.1162/jocn.1996.8.6.551
28. Rossion B, Jacques C. The N170: understanding the time-course of face perception in the human brain. *The Oxford handbook of ERP components,* (2011) 115–42.
29. Caharel S, Leleu A, Bernard C, Viggiano M-P, Lalonde R, Rebaï M. Early holistic face-like processing of Arcimboldo paintings in the right occipito-temporal cortex: evidence from the N170 ERP component. *Int J Psychophysiol Off J Int Organ Psychophysiol* (2013) 90(2):157–64. doi: 10.1016/j.ijpsycho.2013.06.024
30. Churches O, Nicholls M, Thiessen M, Kohler M, Keage H. Emoticons in mind: an event-related potential study. *Soc Neurosci* (2014) 9(2):196–202. doi: 10.1080/17470919.2013.873737
31. Rossion. Understanding face perception by means of human electrophysiology. *Trends Cognit Sci* (2014) 18(6):310–8. doi: 10.1016/j.tics.2014.02.013
32. Kang E, Keifer CM, Levy EJ, Foss-Feig JH, McPartland JC, Lerner MD. Atypicality of the N170 Event-Related Potential in Autism Spectrum Disorder: A Meta-analysis. *Biol Psychiatry Cognit Neurosci Neuroimaging* (2018) 3(8):657–66. doi: 10.1016/j.bpsc.2017.11.003
33. Key AP, Corbett BA. The Unfulfilled Promise of the N170 as a Social Biomarker. *Biol Psychiatry Cognit Neurosci Neuroimaging* (2020) Mar5 (3):342–53. doi: 10.1016/j.bpsc.2019.08.011
34. Vettori S, Jacques C, Boets B, Rossion B. Can the N170 be used as an electrophysiological biomarker indexing face processing difficulties in autism spectrum disorder?. *Biol. Psychiatry Cogn Neurosci Neuroimaging* (2019) 4(3):321–3.
35. Lloyd-Fox S, Blasi A, Elwell CE, Charman T, Murphy D, Johnson MH. Reduced neural sensitivity to social stimuli in infants at risk for autism. *Proc R Soc B Biol Sci* (2013) 280(1758):20123026. doi: 10.1098/rspb.2012.3026
36. Braukmann R, Lloyd-Fox S, Blasi A, Johnson MH, Bekkering H, Buitelaar JK, et al. Diminished socially selective neural processing in 5-month-old infants at high familial risk of autism. *Eur J Neurosci* (2018) 47(6):720–8. doi: 10.1111/ejn.13751

37. Vettori S, Dzhelyova M, Van der Donck S, Jacques C, Van Wesemael T, Steyaert J, et al. Combined frequency-tagging EEG and eye tracking reveal reduced social bias in boys with autism spectrum disorder. *Cortex.* (2020) 125:135–48. doi: 10.1016/j.cortex.2019.12.013
38. Regan D, Heron JR. Clinical investigation of lesions of the visual pathway: a new objective technique. *J Neurol Neurosurg Psychiatry* (1969) 32(5):479–83. doi: 10.1136/jnnp.32.5.479
39. Norcia AM, Appelbaum LG, Ales JM, Cottereau BR, Rossion B. The steady-state visual evoked potential in vision research: A review. *J Vis* (2015) May 115(6):4–4. doi: 10.1167/15.6.4
40. Posner MI, Cohen. Components of visual orienting. In: . *Attention and performance.* Hillsdale, NJ: Erlbaum; (1984).
41. Sacrey L-AR, Armstrong VL, Bryson SE, Zwaigenbaum L. Impairments to visual disengagement in autism spectrum disorder: A review of experimental studies from infancy to adulthood. *Neurosci Biobehav Rev* (2014) 47:559–77. doi: 10.1016/j.neubiorev.2014.10.011
42. Robertson CE, Kravitz DJ, Freyberg J, Baron-Cohen S, Baker CI. Tunnel Vision: Sharper Gradient of Spatial Attention in Autism. *J Neurosci* (2013) 33(16):6776–81. doi: 10.1523/JNEUROSCI.5120-12.2013
43. Townsend J, Courchesne E, Covington J, Westerfield M, Harris NS, Lyden P, et al. Spatial Attention Deficits in Patients with Acquired or Developmental Cerebellar Abnormality. *J Neurosci* (1999) 19(13):5632–43. doi: 10.1523/JNEUROSCI.19-13-05632.1999
44. Mo S, Liang L, Bardikoff N, Sabbagh MA. Shifting visual attention to social and non-social stimuli in Autism Spectrum Disorders. *Res Autism Spectr Disord* (2019) 65:56–64. doi: 10.1016/j.rasd.2019.05.006
45. Pei F, Pettet MW, Norcia AM. Neural correlates of object-based attention. *J Vis* (2002) 2(9):1–1. doi: 10.1167/2.9.1
46. Chen Y, Seth AK, Gally JA, Edelman GM. The power of human brain magnetoencephalographic signals can be modulated up or down by changes in an attentive visual task. *Proc Natl Acad Sci* (2003) 100(6):3501–6. doi: 10.1073/pnas.0337630100
47. Müller MM, Andersen S, Trujillo NJ, Valdés-Sosa P, Malinowski P, Hillyard SA. Feature-selective attention enhances color signals in early visual areas of the human brain. *Proc Natl Acad Sci U S A.* (2006) 103(38):14250–4. doi: 10.1073/pnas.0606668103
48. Andersen SK, Fuchs S, Müller MM. Effects of feature-selective and spatial attention at different stages of visual processing. *J Cognit Neurosci* (2011) 23 (1):238–46. doi: 10.1162/jocn.2009.21328
49. Störmer VS, Winther GN, Li S-C, Andersen SK. Sustained multifocal attentional enhancement of stimulus processing in early visual areas predicts tracking performance. *J Neurosci Off J Soc Neurosci* (2013) 33 (12):5346–51. doi: 10.1523/JNEUROSCI.4015-12.2013
50. Baldauf D, Desimone R. Neural mechanisms of object-based attention. *Science.* (2014) 344(6182):424–7. doi: 10.1126/science.1247003
51. Epstein R, Kanwisher N. A cortical representation of the local visual environment. *Nature.* (1998) 392(6676):598–601. doi: 10.1038/33402
52. Jacques C, Witthoft N, Weiner KS, Foster BL, Rangarajan V, Hermes D, et al. Corresponding ECoG and fMRI category-selective signals in human ventral temporal cortex. *Neuropsychologia.* (2016) 83:14–28. doi: 10.1016/j.neuropsychologia.2015.07.024
53. Kadipasaoglu CM, Conner CR, Whaley ML, Baboyan VG, Tandon N. Category-selectivity in human visual cortex follows cortical topology: a grouped icEEG study. *PloS one* (2016) 11(6).
54. Weiner KS, Grill-Spector K. Sparsely-distributed organization of face and limb activations in human ventral temporal cortex. *NeuroImage.* (2010) Oct 152(4):1559–73. doi: 10.1016/j.neuroimage.2010.04.262
55. Grill-Spector K, Weiner KS, Kay K, Gomez J. The Functional Neuroanatomy of Human Face Perception. *Annu Rev Vis Sci* (2017) 153:167–96. doi: 10.1146/annurev-vision-102016-061214
56. Haxby null, Hoffman null, Gobbini null. The distributed human neural system for face perception. *Trends Cognit Sci* (2000) 4(6):223–33. doi: 10.1016/S1364-6613(00)01482-0
57. Kanwisher N, McDermott J, Chun MM. The fusiform face area: a module in human extrastriate cortex specialized for face perception. *J Neurosci Off J Soc Neurosci* (1997) 17(11):4302–11. doi: 10.1523/JNEUROSCI.17-11-04302.1997
58. Puce A, Allison T, Gore JC, McCarthy G. Face-sensitive regions in human extrastriate cortex studied by functional MRI. *J Neurophysiol* (1995) 74 (3):1192–9. doi: 10.1152/jn.1995.74.3.1192
59. Hagen S, Jacques C, Maillard L, Colnat-Coulbois S, Rossion B, Jonas J. Spatially dissociated intracerebral maps for face- and house-selective activity in the human ventral occipito-temporal cortex. *Cereb Cortex* (in press).
60. Jacques C, Retter TL, Rossion B. A single glance at natural face images generate larger and qualitatively different category-selective spatio-temporal signatures than other ecologically-relevant categories in the human brain. *NeuroImage.* (2016) 137:21–33. doi: 10.1016/j.neuroimage.2016.04.045
61. Constantino JN, Gruber CP. *Social responsiveness scale (SRS).* CA;: Western Psychological Services Torrance (2012).
62. Kort W, Schittekatte M, Dekker PH, Verhaeghe P, Compaan EL, Bosmans M, et al. *WISC-III NL wechsler intelligence scale for children.* (2005).
63. Wechsler D. *The Wechsler intelligence scale for children (3rd ed.).* San Antonio, TX: The Psychological Corporation (1991).
64. Sattler JM. *Assessment of children: Cognitive applications.* (2001).
65. Retter TL, Rossion B. Uncovering the neural magnitude and spatio-temporal dynamics of natural image categorization in a fast visual stream. *Neuropsychologia.* (2016) 91:9–28. doi: 10.1016/j.neuropsychologia.2016.07.028
66. Boremanse A, Norcia AM, Rossion B. Dissociation of part-based and integrated neural responses to faces by means of electroencephalographic frequency tagging. *Eur J Neurosci* (2014) 40(6):2987–97. doi: 10.1111/ejn.12663
67. Regan D. *Human brain electrophysiology: Evoked potentials and evoked magnetic fields in science and medicine.* Amsterdam, The Netherlands: Elsevier; (1989).
68. Dzhelyova M, Jacques C, Rossion B. At a Single Glance: Fast Periodic Visual Stimulation Uncovers the Spatio-Temporal Dynamics of Brief Facial Expression Changes in the Human Brain. *Cereb Cortex.* (2017) 27 (8):4106–23. doi: 10.1093/cercor/bhw223
69. Van der Donck S, Dzhelyova M, Vettori S, Thielen H, Steyaert J, Rossion B, et al. Fast Periodic Visual Stimulation EEG Reveals Reduced Neural Sensitivity to Fearful Faces in Children with Autism. *J Autism Dev Disord* (2019) 49(11):4658–73. doi: 10.1007/s10803-019-04172-0
70. Vettori S, Dzhelyova M, Van der Donck S, Jacques C, Steyaert J, Rossion B, et al. Reduced neural sensitivity to rapid individual face discrimination in autism spectrum disorder. *NeuroImage Clin* (2019) 21:101613. doi: 10.1016/j.nicl.2018.101613
71. Hemptinne C, Liu-Shuang J, Yuksel D, Rossion B. Rapid Objective Assessment of Contrast Sensitivity and Visual Acuity With Sweep Visual Evoked Potentials and an Extended Electrode Array. *Invest Ophthalmol Vis Sci* (2018) 59(2):1144–57. doi: 10.1167/iovs.17-23248
72. Rossion BA. Robust sensitivity to facial identity in the right human occipito-temporal cortex as revealed by steady-state visual-evoked potentials. *J Vis* (2011) 11(2):16–6. doi: 10.1167/11.2.16
73. Zimmermann FGS, Yan X, Rossion B. An objective, sensitive and ecologically valid neural measure of rapid human individual face recognition. *R Soc Open Sci* (2019) 6(6):181904. doi: 10.1098/rsos.181904
74. Rossion, Torfs K, Jacques C, Liu-Shuang J. Fast periodic presentation of natural images reveals a robust face-selective electrophysiological response in the human brain. *J Vis* (2015) 15(1):18–8. doi: 10.1167/15.1.18
75. Liu-Shuang J, Norcia AM, Rossion B. An objective index of individual face discrimination in the right occipito-temporal cortex by means of fast periodic oddball stimulation. *Neuropsychologia.* (2014) 52:57–72. doi: 10.1016/j.neuropsychologia.2013.10.022
76. Singmann H, Bolker B, Westfall J, Aust F. (2018). *afex: Analysis of Factorial Experiments [Internet].* Available from: https://CRAN.R-project.org/package=afex.
77. Lenth R, Singmann H, Love J, Buerkner P, Herve M. (2019). *emmeans: Estimated Marginal Means, aka Least-Squares Means [Internet].* Available from: https://CRAN.R-project.org/package=emmeans.
78. Wei T, Simko V. (2017). *R package "corrplot": Visualization of a Correlation Matrix [Internet].* Available from: https://github.com/taiyun/corrplot.
79. Pek J, Flora DB. Reporting effect sizes in original psychological research: A discussion and tutorial. *Psychol Methods* (2018) 23(2):208–25. doi: 10.1037/met0000126
80. Epstein RA, Bar M, Kveraga K. Neural systems for visual scene recognition. *Scene Vision* (2014), 105–34. doi: 10.7551/mitpress/9780262027854.003.0006

81. Nasr S, Echavarria CE, Tootell RBH. Thinking outside the box: rectilinear shapes selectively activate scene-selective cortex. *J Neurosci Off J Soc Neurosci* (2014) 34(20):6721–35. doi: 10.1523/JNEUROSCI.4802-13.2014
82. Furmanski CS, Engel SA. An oblique effect in human primary visual cortex. *Nat Neurosci* (2000) 3(6):535–6. doi: 10.1038/75702
83. Nasr S, Tootell RBH. A cardinal orientation bias in scene-selective visual cortex. *J Neurosci Off J Soc Neurosci* (2012) 32(43):14921–6. doi: 10.1523/JNEUROSCI.2036-12.2012
84. Hansen BC, Johnson AP, Ellemberg D. Different spatial frequency bands selectively signal for natural image statistics in the early visual system. *J Neurophysiol* (2012) 108(8):2160–72. doi: 10.1152/jn.00288.2012
85. Sergent J, Signoret JL. Functional and anatomical decomposition of face processing: evidence from prosopagnosia and PET study of normal subjects. *Philos Trans R Soc Lond B Biol Sci* (1992) 335(1273):55–61; discussion 61-62. doi: 10.1098/rstb.1992.0007
86. Dundas EM, Plaut DC, Behrmann M. An ERP investigation of the co-development of hemispheric lateralization of face and word recognition. *Neuropsychologia.* (2014) 61:315–23. doi: 10.1016/j.neuropsychologia.2014.05.006
87. Lochy A, de Heering A, Rossion B. The non-linear development of the right hemispheric specialization for human face perception. *Neuropsychologia.* (2019) 18126:10–9. doi: 10.1016/j.neuropsychologia.2017.06.029
88. de Heering A, Rossion B. Rapid categorization of natural face images in the infant right hemisphere. *eLife.* (2015) 4:e06564. doi: 10.7554/eLife.06564
89. Dalton KM, Nacewicz BM, Johnstone T, Schaefer HS, Gernsbacher MA, Goldsmith HH, et al. Gaze fixation and the neural circuitry of face processing in autism. *Nat Neurosci* (2005) 8(4):519–26. doi: 10.1038/nn1421
90. Deeley Q, Daly EM, Surguladze S, Page L, Toal F, Robertson D, et al. An event related functional magnetic resonance imaging study of facial emotion processing in Asperger syndrome. *Biol Psychiatry* (2007) 62(3):207–17. doi: 10.1016/j.biopsych.2006.09.037
91. Hubl D, Bölte S, Feineis-Matthews S, Lanfermann H, Federspiel A, Strik W, et al. Functional imbalance of visual pathways indicates alternative face processing strategies in autism. *Neurology.* (2003) 61(9):1232–7. doi: 10.1212/01.WNL.0000091862.22033.1A
92. Pierce K, Müller RA, Ambrose J, Allen G, Courchesne E. Face processing occurs outside the fusiform "face area" in autism: evidence from functional MRI. *Brain J Neurol* (2001) 124(Pt 10):2059–73. doi: 10.1093/brain/124.10.2059
93. Schultz RT, Gauthier I, Klin A, Fulbright RK, Anderson AW, Volkmar F, et al. Abnormal ventral temporal cortical activity during face discrimination among individuals with autism and Asperger syndrome. *Arch Gen Psychiatry* (2000) 57(4):331–40. doi: 10.1001/archpsyc.57.4.331
94. Bird G, Catmur C, Silani G, Frith C, Frith U. Attention does not modulate neural responses to social stimuli in autism spectrum disorders. *NeuroImage.* (2006) 31(4):1614–24. doi: 10.1016/j.neuroimage.2006.02.037
95. Hadjikhani N, Joseph RM, Snyder J, Chabris CF, Clark J, Steele S, et al. Activation of the fusiform gyrus when individuals with autism spectrum disorder view faces. *NeuroImage.* (2004) 22(3):1141–50. doi: 10.1016/j.neuroimage.2004.03.025
96. Hadjikhani N, Joseph RM, Snyder J, Tager-Flusberg H. Abnormal activation of the social brain during face perception in autism. *Hum Brain Mapp* (2007) 28(5):441–9. doi: 10.1002/hbm.20283
97. Kleinhans NM, Richards T, Sterling L, Stegbauer KC, Mahurin R, Johnson LC, et al. Abnormal functional connectivity in autism spectrum disorders during face processing. *Brain J Neurol* (2008) 131(Pt 4):1000–12. doi: 10.1093/brain/awm334
98. Pierce K, Haist F, Sedaghat F, Courchesne E. The brain response to personally familiar faces in autism: findings of fusiform activity and beyond. *Brain J Neurol* (2004) 127(Pt 12):2703–16. doi: 10.1093/brain/awh289
99. De la Marche W, Noens I, Kuppens S, Spilt JL, Boets B, Steyaert J. Measuring quantitative autism traits in families: informant effect or intergenerational transmission? *Eur Child Adolesc Psychiatry* (2015) 24(4):385–95. doi: 10.1007/s00787-014-0586-z
100. Xu B, Liu-Shuang J, Rossion B, Tanaka J. Individual Differences in Face Identity Processing with Fast Periodic Visual Stimulation. *J Cognit Neurosci* (2017) Mar 3029(8):1368–77. doi: 10.1162/jocn_a_01126
101. Rossion. Biomarkers of Face Perception in Autism Spectrum Disorder: Time to Shift to Fast Periodic Visual Stimulation With Electroencephalography? *Biol Psychiatry Cognit Neurosci Neuroimaging* (2020) 5(3):258–60. doi: 10.1016/j.bpsc.2020.01.008

17

Disturbing Dreams and Psychosocial Maladjustment in Children: A Prospective Study of the Moderating Role of Early Negative Emotionality

Aline Gauchat[1,2], *Antonio Zadra*[2], *Mira El-Hourani*[2,3], *Sophie Parent*[4], *Richard E. Tremblay*[2,3,5,6] *and Jean R. Séguin*[3,7*]

[1] *Clinique de Consultation Conjugale et Familiale Poitras-Wright, Côté, Longueuil, QC, Canada,* [2] *Department of Psychology, Université de Montréal, Montreal, QC, Canada,* [3] *CHU Ste-Justine Research Center, Montreal, QC, Canada,* [4] *School of Psychoeducation, Université de Montréal, Montreal, QC, Canada,* [5] *Department of Pediatrics, Université de Montréal, Montreal, QC, Canada,* [6] *School of Public Health, University College Dublin, Dublin, Ireland,* [7] *Department of Psychiatry and Addictology, Université de Montréal, Montreal, QC, Canada*

***Correspondence:**
Jean R. Séguin
jean.seguin@umontreal.ca

Although frequent disturbing dreams, including bad dreams and nightmares, have been repeatedly associated with poor psychological well-being in adults, considerably less information exists on their psychosocial correlates in children. Recent empirical and theoretical contributions suggest that the association between disturbing dream frequency and psychosocial adaptation in children may differ as a function of children's negative emotionality. The current study assessed the moderating effect of very early negative emotionality (17 months of age) in the relation between disturbing dream frequency and psychosocial maladjustment (i.e., externalizing + internalizing behaviors) in a sample of 173 11-year-old children. Mixed-model analyses revealed that disturbing dream frequency was associated with some internalizing behaviors but that the association between disturbing dream frequency and most externalizing behaviors was moderated by early negative emotionality. The latter result indicates that the relation between disturbing dream frequency and externalizing behaviors was significant in 11-year-old children showing moderate negative emotionality early in life, but particularly strong in those children with high early negative emotionality. Whereas, a moderating effect of early negative emotionality was not found between disturbing dream frequency and internalizing behaviors, the findings highlight the more specific role of early emotional negativity as a developmental moderator for the link between disturbing dreams and externalizing behaviors in children. The results are discussed in light of recent models of disturbed dreaming production.

Keywords: disturbing dreams, nightmares, bad dreams, dreaming, psychosocial maladjustment, temperament, negative emotionality

INTRODUCTION

Up to 20% of children experience psychosocial adjustment difficulties (1, 2) which are typically divided between externalizing and internalizing problems (3, 4), although both categories evince common and unique risk factors (5). Studies show that while good sleep quality is associated with optimal behavior development, poor sleep is related to both externalizing and internalizing problems (6–17). Even after controlling for other risk factors, sleep problems appear to explain a small but significant proportion of the variance in both externalizing and internalizing behaviors (15, 18). However, different sleep problems appear to be associated with different externalizing or internalizing problems (6, 19).

Among these sleep problems, disturbing dreams (DDs; vivid dreams marked by intense negative emotions such as fear, anxiety, and anger) are frequently experienced by children (20–24). DDs may be associated with a wide range of psychosocial difficulties as they may signal problems with emotional regulation processes that normally occur during sleep as well as in dreams (for more details about this hypothesis, see (22, 25–28). While frequent DDs, including bad dreams and nightmares, have been repeatedly associated with poor psychological well-being and increased psychopathology in clinical and non-clinical adult populations (27), considerably less information exists on their psychosocial maladjustment correlates in children.

A recent review of the literature suggests that the occurrence of frequent DDs during childhood and adolescence is associated with a range of difficulties (21). First, DD frequency is associated with other sleep-related problems including insomnia, sleepwalking, bruxism, sleep talking, sleep terrors, nighttime awakenings, and unwillingness to go to bed (29–37). Second, DDs have also been linked to a range of specific mental health symptoms and psychosocial problems, including low prosociality (37, 38), academic problems (33), emotional excitability and being easily emotionally hurt (39), emotional symptoms (37, 38, 40), psychotic experiences (41, 42), borderline personality disorder (40), other mental health disorders (43), as well as suicidal ideation and suicide attempts (44–46). A prospective study found that DD frequency at 12 years of age was related to symptoms of psychosis during adulthood (47).

Moreover, DD frequency has been associated with internalizing problems in childhood and adolescence and repeatedly linked to anxiety (6, 48–54). Prospective studies of adolescents and late teenagers have similarly revealed links between parent-rated DDs at 10–19 years of age and later symptoms of anxiety and depression at 18–32 years of age (55). Moreover, DD frequency has also been linked to externalizing problems. Indeed, some studies of children show that DDs are associated with conduct disorders (37), rule-breaking, aggression, impulsivity (56), and hyperactivity (37, 57, 58). However, other studies did not find these associations (38, 59). Some studies also reported significant associations between DD frequency and attention deficit hyperactivity disorder (ADHD) (60) as well as with ADHD subtypes (61, 62), and one prospective study found that parent-rated DDs at 10–19 years of age predicted symptoms of inattention and direct/indirect aggression at 18–32 years of age (55).

Finally, some studies reviewed above combine sleep-related difficulties into one construct, thus not taking into account the differential relations of each sleep problem with unique measures of daytime functioning (16, 63, 64). Thus, whether or not DDs are related equally across internalizing and externalizing problems remains to be determined.

To further clarify inconsistencies in the literature, the construct of "affect distress," defined as a trait-like disposition to react to emotional stressors with heightened negative affect and distress (27, 65) should be taken into account as it may play a role in the association between DDs and psychosocial adjustment difficulties. First, Levin and Nielsen's (27) model of DD production proposes that DDs occur out of an interaction between "affect load," or day-to-day variations in emotional stress, and the aforementioned construct of affect distress, which can be viewed as a temperament subtype. Affect distress would fall under the negative emotionality dimension of temperament (66, 67). In the developmental literature, negative emotionality encompasses individual differences in typical reactions to negative emotional experiences, which can be readily observed from birth (68, 69). In fact, negative emotionality was found to be stable from early childhood to early adolescence (70) and was found to have a moderate continuity 17 years later (3–20 years old) (71).

Second, negative emotionality or difficultness, which refers to the tendency to experience negative emotions (fear, anger, sadness, discomfort) and high emotional distress when confronted to novel, ambiguous, and intense situations (66), has been related to psychosocial maladjustment throughout infancy and childhood (72–74). Recently, it is its moderating effect that has been mainly reported in the literature. Indeed, difficultness is already known to moderate relations between a variety of risk factors and children's behavior, such as the associations between cumulative contextual risk and children's externalizing, internalizing, and sleep problems (75–78). Some early temperamental characteristics may indeed predispose children to develop later behavior problems, particularly when other risk factors are present (79–82).

Taken together, Nielsen and Levin's (22) model of DD production and developmental literature on temperament suggests that the link between the frequency of DDs and psychosocial adaptation may differ as a function of a child's negative emotionality. This hypothesized moderator effect of negative emotionality has never been empirically tested. Furthermore, there is a lack of data on the relation between DDs and externalizing problems, and most studies of DDs in children suffer from one of the following three methodological limitations. First, DD frequency in children is often assessed through parent reports, despite the fact that this method has been shown to underestimate DD frequency and distress in comparison to child self-reports (37, 48, 50, 83). Second, many studies did not include any adjustment for possible confounding factors, such as risk factors common to both psychopathology and DDs (e.g., socio-economic status or comorbid sleep problems), despite the fact that taking such factors into account has been shown to attenuate observed associations (84). Third, and finally, although it is important to measure children's psychosocial maladjustment through multiple informants due to differences in child behavior across contexts (58, 85), multiple informants have rarely been used in the reviewed studies (21).

The goal of the present study was to first investigate the relationship between DD frequency and psychosocial maladjustment in children across a wide range of internalizing and externalizing behaviors and, second, to take into account the possible moderator effect of early emotional negativity. Methodological shortcomings characteristic of many studies in the field were also addressed: (a) measures of DD frequency were obtained from the children themselves, (b) socio-economic status and co-morbid sleep disorders were taken into account in the analyses, and (c) children's psychosocial maladjustment was assessed through multiple informants.

Two main and complementary predictions were tested: (1) DD frequency will be positively associated with psychosocial maladjustment across several internalizing and externalizing behavioral domains; and (2) negative emotionality will moderate this relation between measures of DD frequency and psychosocial maladjustment across several internalizing and externalizing behavioral domains. Specifically, we tested the hypothesis that the association between DD frequency and internalizing and externalizing problems would be strengthened with increasing levels of negative emotionality. These hypotheses will be tested separately for each internalizing (anxiety, social withdrawal, and emotional problems) and externalizing (opposition, physical aggression, reactive, proactive aggression, indirect aggression, and ADHD) symptoms.

MATERIALS AND METHODS

Participants

Participants were part of a longitudinal study focusing on the social, psychological, and cognitive development of children from urban socio-economic backgrounds in the province of Québec, Canada. At the study's inception, 1,000 families were randomly selected from the Québec 1996–1997 birth register (86). Of these, 572 consented to participate in the original study and were then assessed annually in French (~82%) or English (Canada's two official languages) from the age of 5 months. Due to annual attrition, variability in the participants' year to year availability for data collection, and funding constraints which limited the capacity to follow-up all families, a total of 173 children (comprised equally of boys and girls) completed the present study (mean age = 11.4 years, SD = 0.1). These 173 children did not differ from the remainder of the original 572 5-month-old children in terms of their socio-economic level, including family income (p = 0.68), family type (single parent or not; p = 0.57), maternal level of education (p = 0.33), or negative emotionality at 17 months of age (p = 0.54). They did not differ on other behavioral measures at 17 months in term of hyperactivity (p = 0.73); inattention (p = 0.89); emotional troubles (p = 0.77); anxiety (p = 0.74); physical aggression (p = 0.71), except for opposition with children in the current sample being a little less oppositional (M = 3.2; SD = 1) than the remainder of the sample (M = 3.5; SD = 1.1); t = 2.8; $p < 0.05$.

Measures

Assessment of Disturbing Dreams

Participants from this longitudinal sample self-reported about their DDs for the first time at 11 years of age. The instructions to children referred to DDs using the expression "bad dreams" (defined as very disturbing dreams) because the term DD was too unfamiliar to them given their age. Children were required to answer the question: "On average, how frequently do you have bad dreams?" using the following choices: "Never," "Sometimes," "Often," "Always," or "Don't know." Participants reporting bad dreams were also asked to estimate the number of bad dreams experienced over the past month. For children who reported "never" in the previous question, the number of bad dreams was coded as 0 while maximum frequency was set at 30 (i.e., 1 DD/day) to limit the impact of potential outliers. Thus, values for monthly DD frequency ranged between 0 and 30. A 1-month retrospective frequency estimate was used instead of a 1-year estimate as it has been shown to correspond more closely to prospectively collected log-based frequency measures of DDs from the same individuals (87, 88).

Measures of Psychosocial Maladjustment

Psychosocial maladjustment was measured using a battery of validated scales (89–91) drawn from various instruments. Some scales from the Preschool Behavior Questionnaire (92), the Child Behavior Checklist (93), and the Reactive and Proactive Aggression Questionnaire (94) were used to create the questionaire. The scales (and mean Cronbach alpha across informants) included measures of both internalizing problems: anxiety (4 items, Mα = 0.72, e.g., being nervous, high-strung or tense), social withdrawal (3 items, Mα = 0.68, e.g., prefers to play alone rather than with other children), and emotional problems (3 items, Mα = 0.69, e.g., has trouble enjoying him or herself); and externalizing problems: opposition (3 items, Mα = 0.51, e.g., punishment doesn't change the child's behavior), physical aggression (4 items, Mα = 0.75, e.g., physically aggresses people), reactive aggression (4 items, Mα = 0.75, e.g., reacts aggressively when someone takes a personal belonging, for example by hitting, pushing, or slapping another child), proactive aggression (3 items, Mα = 0.55, e.g., scares other children to get what is wanted), indirect aggression (3 items, Mα = 0.69, e.g., when angry at someone, tries to get others to dislike the other person), and ADHD symptoms (7 items, Mα = 0.86, e.g., cannot settle on anything for more than a few moments; is impulsive/acts without thinking; is inattentive). These validated scales (89, 91) have been shown to be sensitive to various environmental, familial, and perinatal risk and protective factors (95–99) as well as to early sleep patterns (100). The instrument was completed by the participants themselves at 11 years of age as well as by each child's father and teacher in order to get a complete description of their difficulties across the social context. Questions for the child version were read to them by the research assistant but they could record answers confidentially.

Covariables

Socio-Economic Status

Three variables were used to evaluate each family's socio-economic status: family income (continuous variable), level of maternal education (dichotomous variable, with a high level being defined as having a secondary school diploma or higher), and whether or not the child was in a single-parent family (dichotomous variable).

Sleep

Two sleep-related variables were included: sleepwalking, since this sleep disorder has been repeatedly associated with DDs (29, 33, 34, 39, 57) and daytime somnolence because poor sleep quality (which usually leads to daytime somnolence) is associated with poor mood and behaviors (6, 100, 101). Two questions to the mother were "Does your child sleepwalk in his/her sleep?" and "In general, is your child sleepy during the day?" Both could be answered with "Never," "Sometimes," "Often," or "Always."

Negative Emotionality

Negative emotionality was assessed at 17 months using a shortened scale developed by Vitaro and colleagues (102) of the original fussy/difficult temperament scale developed by Bates and colleagues (103) (example of item: intensity of the child's protest). This seven-item scale was completed by the mother, in order to avoid a shared-method variance problem with the informants who completed the psychosocial adjustment measures for our analyses (102). The measure of negative emotionality used in the present study showed good internal consistency with a Cronbach alpha of 0.71.

Procedure

Each parent, or legal guardian responsible for the child, and teacher received an invitation by mail to participate in the study. Consent was obtained from parents or legal guardians and assent was obtained from the child. The study was approved by the Research Ethics Committee of the CHU Ste-Justine Research Center, and the study protocol also complied with the ethical guidelines of the American Psychological Association ("Ethical Principles of Psychologists and Code of Conduct," 2017).

Analyses

Model used: Mixed-effects model analyses were estimated using the "Statistical Package for the Social Sciences" (Version 18) (104) to investigate relationships between DDs and dimensions of psychosocial maladjustment. Nine models were tested, one for each measure of psychosocial maladjustment, three for internalizing problems, and six for externalizing problems. Specifically, responses provided by the three informants (child, teacher, and father) were included for each psychosocial maladjustment scale within the mixed-effects models where each of the informants represents a repeated component. A mixed-effects model as opposed to a traditional repeated-measure ANOVA allows for an unbalanced design. This model is also adapted for situations with unequal covariance as it does not assume equal correlations across informants. In a mixed-effects model, if one or two informants are missing, the other informants are still included in the analyses, whereas traditional repeated-measures ANOVA requires data from all three informants for each participant entered in the analyses. Thus, the mixed-effect model actually uses all the available information for parameter estimation (105). Responses were available from all three informants for 78 participants (42.6%)—from the child and teacher for 38 participants (22%), from the child and father for 32 participants (18.6%), and only from the child in 32 cases (18.6%). There was no systematic pattern of missing responses related to child behavior outcomes.

Preliminary Analyses

Sex differences on DD frequency measures were assessed with T-tests. Potential a priori covariates were selected for inclusion in the analyses on an empirical basis in order to enter only meaningful variables and avoid loss of power (106) as it has been done in other studies (81). This was done by first computing correlations or ANOVAs between potential control variables (socioeconomic status; SES, sleepwalking, somnolence) and outcome variables to determine which control variables should be entered as fixed effects for which outcome measures. If a potential control variable was related to an outcome variable (at $p \leq 0.05$) assessed by at least one of the informants, it was entered in the analysis. Maternal level of education was thus entered in the analyses for anxiety, physical aggression, ADHD symptoms, and opposition, whereas family income was entered in the analyses for anxiety, ADHD symptoms, and opposition (for all those variables, a higher socio-economic status was linked to less psychosocial maladjustment). The family type and sleep disorder variables were not related to any of the psychosocial maladjustment measures. Whenever interactions between two variables were not significant, the interaction term was removed from the analytical model and only the main effect was tested.

Our two overarching hypotheses were tested using the mixed-effects model for each psychosocial maladjustment problem within internalizing and externalizing problems. Informant source and child sex were always entered as fixed effects. Interactions between DD measures and child sex or informant source were tested since children's behaviors can be perceived differently at school vs. at home and because behavioral difficulties differ between boys and girls (85, 107, 108), resulting in differences in observed associations between DDs and behavioral difficulties as a function of context and sex.

Interactions between DDs and early negative emotionality were investigated to test the second hypothesis which proposed that early negative emotionality moderates the relationship between DD frequency and psychosocial maladjustment. DD frequency and early negative emotionality were centered.

RESULTS

Descriptive Statistics

Of the 173 children that completed the questionnaires, 129 (82.7%) reported experiencing at least one DD per month. The mean frequency of DDs reported per month by the entire sample was 3.6 ($SD = 5.3$), with 12% of the sample having 10 or more DD per month. A significantly greater proportion of girls (88.7%)

TABLE 1 | Main effects of DD frequency on internalizing problems.

Variables	F	df(v1, v2)	p	d
Social withdrawal	5.26	1,141.75	0.02	0.39
Emotional problems	9.17	1,175.91	0.003	0.45
Anxiety	2.89	1,131.75	0.09	0.30

reported having at least one DD in the last month than did boys (76.3%), $\chi^2 = 4.21, p < 0.05$. However, there were no significant sex differences in the actual number of DDs experienced in the past month. Using the MIXED models, none of the DDs by informant interactions were significant, and early negative emotionality was not correlated to DDs ($r = 0.04$; $p = 0.58$). Correlations between each informant for a given variable vary between $r = 0.03$ for opposition and $r = 0.28$ for anxiety with a mean of $Mr = 0.17$.

Before testing the moderating effect of early negative emotionality on each childhood-dependent variable, we examined its correlation with DDs to determine if it met the criteria for moderation analysis. DDs and early negative emotionality were not correlated ($r = 0.04$; $p = 0.58$). We also examined associations between early negative emotionality and dependent variables. Correlations ranged from $r = 0.03$ to $r = 0.07$ with a mean of $Mr = 0.05$ for internalizing behaviors, and they ranged from $r = 0.05$ to $r = 0.20$ with a mean of $Mr = 0.09$ for externalizing behaviors. None of those correlations were significant except the one between early emotional negativity and physical aggression ($r = 0.19$; $p \leq 0.05$).

Associations Between DD Frequency and Internalizing Behaviors

When considering internalizing behaviors, none of the interactions between DDs and temperament were significant (all $p_s > 0.50$). They were therefore removed from the models. **Table 1** shows main effects and effect sizes for the association between DD frequency and internalizing problems once control variables were included in the statistical models. DD frequency was positively related to 2 of the 3 measures of internalizing behaviors (social withdrawal and emotional problems), with Cohen's d statistics of effect size for continuous variables in the small to medium range (109). This only partially supports the first hypothesis, as no moderating effect of early negative emotionality was found.

Associations Between DD Frequency and Externalizing Behaviors

The interaction term between early emotional negativity and DDs was kept in all models examining externalizing behaviors because p-values were consistently below 0.13 (ranging from 0.001 for proactive aggression and 0.13 for opposition), suggesting that this pattern was not random. **Table 2** presents results of the analyses of main effects and interactions for each externalizing behavior. **Figure 1** plots these interactions using the method proposed by Aiken and West (110) by showing the strength of the association between DD frequency and each dimension of externalizing behaviors plotted as a function of early negative emotionality level [low (−1 SD), average or high (+1 SD)]. As can be seen in **Figure 1**, the pattern of interactions was highly consistent across dimensions of externalizing behaviors, where associations between frequency of DDs and externalizing behaviors were systematically positive and significant for children with moderate to high levels of early negative emotionality. For these children, effect sizes were medium to large, ranging from $d = 0.41$ to $d = 0.85$ (109). This pattern of interactions and absence of main effects only partially supports the second hypothesis.

DISCUSSION

The results of the present study partially support our predictions that DD frequency would be positively associated with psychosocial maladjustment in children and that early emotional negativity would moderate this relationship. In line with previous adult and childhood literature, DD frequency was positively related to psychosocial maladjustment of the internalizing type: across informants, children with higher DD frequency scored higher on two of the three measures of internalizing problems (i.e., emotional problems and social withdrawal) without moderation by early emotional negativity. For psychosocial maladjustment of the externalizing type, there was a moderation effect of early emotional negativity: the association between DDs and externalizing difficulties was stronger with increasing levels of early emotional negativity.

The associations between DD frequency and internalizing behaviors remained significant even after adjusting for socio-economic and sleep-related variables. That DDs in children were associated with a range of internalizing problems (e.g., emotional problems and social withdrawal) is consistent with findings reported in children and adult populations (21, 27, 40, 56). However, unlike some reports, DD frequency in the present study was not significantly related to anxiety. The effect size for this relation ($d = 0.30$) was too small to reach statistical significance given our sample size. By comparison, effect sizes in previous studies have ranged between 0.20 and 0.72 ($Md = 0.53$) (49, 51, 53). Differences in measures of anxiety themselves (e.g., source of informant, symptoms scale vs. clinical diagnosis) may also partially account for this. The fact that none of the interactions with informants were significant shows that despite contextual differences in behaviors, the association between DDs and psychosocial maladjustment is robust and did not differ as a function of informant source.

The absence of the hypothesized moderator effect of early emotional negativity on internalizing problems may have been related to the measure used in the present study. Specifically, our measure of early emotional negativity at 17 months may not have been sensitive to the complete spectrum of manifestations of affect distress. For example, in contrast to observations in infants, studies have shown that toddlers high in emotional reactivity are more likely to manifest their reactivity through inhibition

TABLE 2 | Main effects of DD frequency and interactions with early negative emotionality for each externalizing behavior problem.

	Main effects of DDs				Main effects of negative emotionality				Interaction between DDs and negative emotionality			
Variables	*F*	*df(v1, v2)*	*p*	*d*	*F*	*df(v1, v2)*	*p*	*d*	*F*	*df(v1, v2)*	*p*	*d*
Indirect aggression	0.85	1,160.9	0.36	0.14	0.59	1,160.1	0.44	0.12	6.64	1,154.8	0.01	0.41
Physical aggression	0.68	1,136.9	0.41	0.14	0.48	1,125.1	0.49	0.12	6.21	1,129.1	0.01	0.44
Reactive aggression	0.42	1,160.2	0.52	0.10	0.36	1,154.7	0.55	0.09	4.25	1,152	0.04	0.33
Proactive aggression	0.10	1,140.8	0.33	0.05	1.69	1,138.2	0.19	0.22	9.41	1,134.1	0.003	0.53
Hyperactivity, impulsivity and attention symptoms (HIA)	1.03	1,129.9	0.31	0.17	0.51	1,118.2	0.48	0.13	5.69	1,120.1	0.02	0.44
Opposition	0.01	1,127.9	0.97	0.02	0.34	1,114.9	0.56	0.10	2.34	1,117.5	0.13	0.28

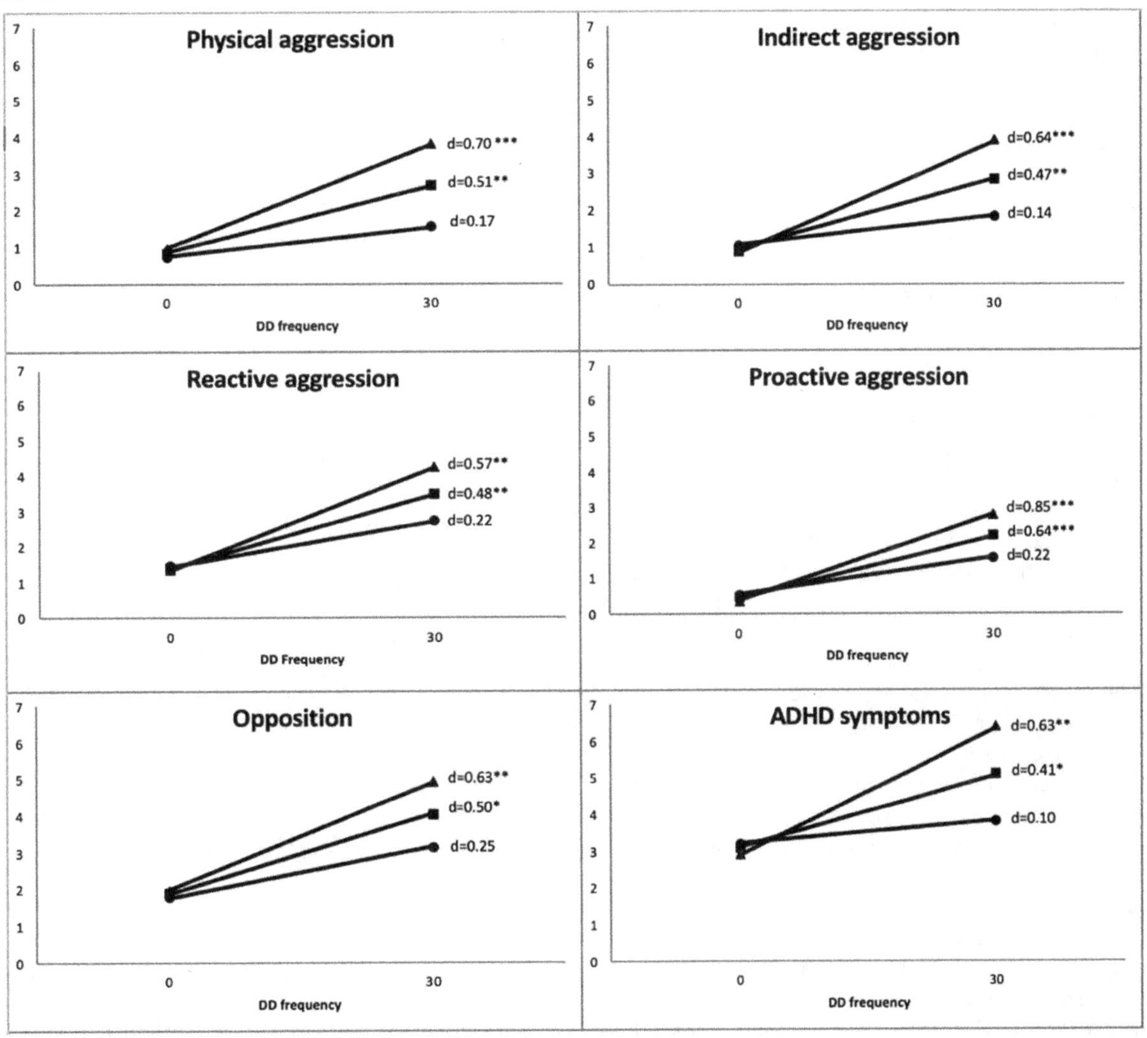

FIGURE 1 | Strength of association between monthly DD frequency (x-axis) and externalizing behaviors (y-axis) as a function of averaged negative emotionality and ± 1 SD. $^*p < 0.05$; $^{**}p < 0.01$; $^{***}p < 0.001$. Externalizing behaviors were standardized across a range from 0 to 7. Monthly DD frequency ranged from 0 to 30.

or withdrawal (111–114). These behavioral manifestations have been associated with later proneness to internalizing difficulties (79, 115–117). By contrast, our measure did not include items specifically formulated to detect these behavioral manifestations of early emotional reactivity, which might explain why it did not correlate with, or moderate, later internalizing difficulties.

Thus, our measure may be more sensitive to behavioral manifestations of toddlers' "affect distress," like aggression, that are linked to later externalizing problems than to subsequent internalizing problems.

The finding that early negative emotionality specifically moderated the relationship between DDs and externalizing behaviors is new. In fact, this is the first study to document that DDs in children with early moderate to high early emotional negativity are strongly associated with externalizing behaviors (with corresponding ds ranging between 0.60 and 0.90). The consistency of results across externalizing problems may be due to a common underlying factor (3, 118). How the relation between frequent DDs and externalizing behaviors in children with a history of moderate to elevated negative early emotionality evolves over time remains to be clarified. However, some studies have shown that early emotional negativity may moderate other associations implicating later externalizing behaviors, such as the relation between early child care and externalizing behaviors during adolescence (119). Another study (76) found that low early negative emotionality at 18 months emerged as a protective factor in children experiencing a cumulative risk of developing internalizing and sleep problems at 24 months. Consequently, and in the absence of a concurrent measure of negative emotionality, this long-term effect noted across several studies also supports the hypothesis that negative emotionality is a relatively stable developmental characteristic.

The correlational nature of our study does not allow us to draw conclusions about the direction of the link between DDs and psychosocial adjustment. On the one hand, it is possible that DDs have an impact on psychosocial adjustment as it has been shown that DDs could influence the dreamer's mood the following day (120). Frequent DDs in children could similarly result in negative emotions and distress during wakefulness much like the nightmare-related distress documented in adults (27, 121–123). Thus, it is possible that repeated and negative experiencing of DDs elicits negative reactive emotions during wakefulness.

On the other hand, it is also possible that psychosocial adjustment problems and related perceived stress may have an impact on the frequency of DDs (27, 124, 125). In this case, DDs would reflect issues and concerns experienced during wakefulness. Alternatively, it is possible that a third variable explains the relation between DDs and psychosocial adjustment. This would be consistent with suggestions that DDs represent a failure in the emotional regulation function believed to occur during normal dreaming (126–128). Psychosocial maladjustment problems are also known to be related to problems in emotional regulation (74, 129–131). As discussed earlier, this interpretation would be consistent with the hypothesis of a moderator effect of emotional negativity and DDs on psychosocial adjustment. While our study has some key strengths including the use of an early measure of negative emotionality, control variables, and multiple informants for the assessment of psychosocial maladjustment, it also has some shortcomings. With the exception of the children's early emotional negativity measure, this was essentially a cross-sectional correlational study, and as such, it cannot address the developmental sequence with regard to DDs and psychosocial maladjustment.

Longitudinal studies are needed to clarify the nature and time course of DDs in relation to psychosocial maladjustment. Also, as has been done in adults, the inclusion of measures of potentially more severe forms of maladjustment such as suicidality (which emerges in early adolescence) may be helpful as suicidal ideation has been linked to both internal distress and externalizing behaviors such as impulsivity and conduct disorders (132–134). In fact, one review found that impulsivity and emotional dysregulation could explain the link between sleep disturbances and suicidality (135). More studies should investigate these associations specifically with DDs. In addition, the study of other moderator variables could further our understanding of these complex developmental issues. Disorganized attachment, for instance, is a promising candidate as it has been related to both externalizing behaviors and DDs and could play a moderator role in these relations (136–139).

In sum, the present study highlights the role of early emotional negativity as a developmental moderator for the link between DDs and externalizing behaviors in children and points to the need to consider temperamental traits when investigating associations between DDs and internalizing and externalizing problems from a developmental perspective.

ETHICS STATEMENT

The studies involving human participants were reviewed and approved by Research Ethics Committee of the CHU Ste-Justine Research Center. Written informed consent to participate in this study was provided by the adult informants themselves, the study participants' parents or legal guardian, and assent was provided by the children themselves.

AUTHOR CONTRIBUTIONS

AG contributed to study design, analyzed the results, and wrote the manuscript draft. AZ obtained supporting grants, supervised the study, contributed to the statistical analyses, and reviewed the manuscript. ME-H reviewed the data collection and reviewed the manuscript. RT obtained supporting grants and contributed to the study design, data collection, and reviewed the manuscript. SP and JS obtained supporting grants, designed and supervised the study, contributed to the statistical analyses and their interpretation, and reviewed the manuscript. All authors contributed to the article and approved the submitted version.

FUNDING

This study was funded by the Canadian Institutes for Health Research via grant MOP 44072 to JS, grant MOP-97910 to JS and SP, and grant MOP 97865 to AZ; the Fonds de Recherche en Santé du Québec via the Réseau Santé Mentale du Québec (Québec Mental Health Network), fellowships to JS and grant 981055 to JS and RT, and grant 991027 to JS; the Social Sciences and Humanities Research Council of Canada, grants 839-2000-1008 to RT and JS and 410-2007-1957 to AZ; and the Fonds de Recherche du Québec - Société et Culture infrastructure grants 2002-RS-79238 (RT, JS, and SP), # 2009-RG-124779 and #2015-RG-178735 (both to RT and JS). ME-H was supported by the Fonds Maria et Georginia Daoussis and AG and JS were supported by the Fonds Monique Gaumond pour la recherche en maladies affectives.

ACKNOWLEDGMENTS

This article was adapted from a study contained in the first author's doctoral thesis entitled Rêves dysphoriques et rêves récurrents chez les enfants et les adolescents: investigations cliniques et corrélats psychosociaux. The authors are grateful to Charles-Édouard Giguère for data management and statistical analyses, and to our partner, the Institut de la Statistique du Québec. We thank all the parents and children for their generous participation in the study.

REFERENCES

1. Essex MJ, Kraemer HC, Slattery MJ, Burk LR, Boyce W, Woodward HR, et al. Screening for childhood mental health problems: outcomes and early identification. *J Child Psychol Psychiatry.* (2009) 50:562–70. doi: 10.1111/j.1469-7610.2008.02015.x
2. Fechete GL, Susa-Erdogan G, Benga O. Internalizing problems in a sample of Romanian preschool children. Contributions of both child and maternal temperament along with family functioning. *Early Child Dev Care.* (2018) 188:46–61. doi: 10.1080/03004430.2016.1266485
3. Castellanos-Ryan N, Brière FN, O'Leary-Barrett M, Banaschewski T, Bokde A, Bromberg U, et al. The structure of psychopathology in adolescence and its common personality and cognitive correlates. *J Abnormal Psychol.* (2016) 125:1039. doi: 10.1037/abn0000193
4. Cicchetti D, Toth LT (eds.). *Internalizing and Externalizing Expressions of Dysfunction, Vol. 2.* Hillsdale, NJ: Lawrence Erlbaum and Associates (1991).
5. Bayer JK, Ukoumunne OC, Lucas N, Wake M, Scalzo K, Nicholson JM. Risk factors for childhood mental health symptoms: National Longitudinal Study of Australian Children. *Pediatrics.* (2011) 128:e865–79. doi: 10.1542/peds.2011-0491
6. Alfano CA, Gamble AL. The role of sleep in childhood psychiatric disorders. *Child Youth Care Forum.* (2009) 38:327–40. doi: 10.1007/s10566-009-9081-y
7. Alfano CA, Ginsburg GS, Kingery JN. Sleep-related problems among children and adolescents with anxiety disorders. *J Am Acad Child Adolesc Psychiatry.* (2007) 46:224–32. doi: 10.1097/01.chi.0000242233.06011.8e
8. Aronen ET, Paavonen E, Fjallberg M, Soininen M, Torronen J. Sleep and psychiatric symptoms in school-age children. *J Am Acad Child Adolesc Psychiatry.* (2000) 39:502–8. doi: 10.1097/00004583-200004000-00020
9. Becker SP, Luebbe AM, Langberg JM. Attention-deficit/hyperactivity disorder dimensions and sluggish cognitive tempo symptoms in relation to college students' sleep functioning. *Child Psychiatry Hum Dev.* (2014) 45:675–85. doi: 10.1007/s10578-014-0436-8
10. El-Sheikh M, Saini EK, Gillis BT, Kelly RJ. Interactions between sleep duration and quality as predictors of adolescents' adjustment. *Sleep Health.* (2019) 5:180–6. doi: 10.1016/j.sleh.2018.11.004
11. Gregory AM, Caspi A, Eley TC, Moffitt TE, O'Connor TG, Poulton R. Prospective longitudinal associations between persistent sleep problems in childhood and anxiety and depression disorders in adulthood. *J Abnormal Child Psychol.* (2005) 33:157–63. doi: 10.1007/s10802-005-1824-0
12. Gregory AM, O'Connor TG. Sleep problems in childhood: A longitudinal study of developmental change and association with behavioral problems. *J Am Acad Child Adolesc Psychiatry.* (2002) 41:964–71. doi: 10.1097/00004583-200208000-00015
13. Gregory AM, Rijsdijk F, Lau JY, Dahl RE, Eley TC. The direction of longitudinal associations between sleep problems and depression symptoms: a study of twins aged 8 and 10 years. *Sleep.* (2009) 32:189–99. doi: 10.1093/sleep/32.2.189
14. Huhdanpää H, Klenberg L, Westerinen H, Fontell T, Aronen ET. Sleep and psychiatric symptoms in young child psychiatric outpatients. *Clin Child Psychol Psychiatry.* (2018) 23:77–95. doi: 10.1177/1359104517718366
15. Pieters S, Burk WJ, Van der Vorst H, Dahl RE, Wiers RW, Engels RC. Prospective relationships between sleep problems and substance use, internalizing and externalizing problems. *J Youth Adolesc.* (2015) 44:379–88. doi: 10.1007/s10964-014-0213-9
16. Quach JL, Nguyen CD, Williams KE, Sciberras E. Bidirectional associations between child sleep problems and internalizing and externalizing difficulties from preschool to early adolescence. *JAMA Pediatrics.* (2018) 172:e174363. doi: 10.1001/jamapediatrics.2017.4363
17. Rubens SL, Evans SC, Becker SP, Fite PJ, Tountas AM. Self-reported time in bed and sleep quality in association with internalizing and externalizing symptoms in school-age youth. *Child Psychiatry Hum Dev.* (2017) 48:455–67. doi: 10.1007/s10578-016-0672-1
18. Reid GJ, Hong RY, Wade TJ. The relation between common sleep problems and emotional and behavioral problems among 2-and 3-year-olds in the context of known risk factors for psychopathology. *J Sleep Res.* (2009) 18:49–59. doi: 10.1111/j.1365-2869.2008.00692.x
19. Gauchat A. *Rêves dysphoriques et rêves récurrents chez les enfants et les adolescents: corrélats psychosociaux et implications cliniques* (Doctoral dissertation), Université de Montréal. (2015). Available online at: https://papyrus.bib.umontreal.ca/xmlui/bitstream/handle/1866/11592/Aline_Gauchat_2014_these.pdf?sequence=2&isAllowed=y
20. Abdel-Khalek AM. Nightmares: prevalence, age and gender differences among kuwaiti children and adolescents. *Sleep Hypnosis.* (2006) 8:33–40. Available online at: http://www.sleepandhypnosis.org/ing/archivelist.aspx?SayiID=29
21. Gauchat A, Séguin JR, Zadra A. Prevalence and correlates of disturbed dreaming in children. *Pathol Biol.* (2014) 62:311–8. doi: 10.1016/j.patbio.2014.05.016
22. Nielsen T, Levin R. Nightmares: a new neurocognitive model. *Sleep Med Rev.* (2007) 11:295–310. doi: 10.1016/j.smrv.2007.03.004
23. Ophoff D, Slaats M, Boudewyns A, Glazemakers I, Van Hoorenbeeck K, Verhulst S. Sleep disorders during childhood: a practical review. *Eur J Pediatrics.* (2018) 177:641–8. doi: 10.1007/s00431-018-3116-z
24. Schredl M, Biemelt J, Roos K, Dunkel T, Harris N. Nightmares and stress in children. *Sleep Hypnosis.* (2008) 10:19–25. Available online at: https://www.sleepandhypnosis.org/ing/archivelist.aspx?SayiID=37
25. Ennis CR, Short NA, Moltisanti AJ, Smith CE, Joiner TE, Taylor J. Nightmares and nonsuicidal self-injury: the mediating role of emotional dysregulation. *Comprehens Psychiatry.* (2017) 76:104–12. doi: 10.1016/j.comppsych.2017.04.003
26. Kramer M. The selective mood regulatory function of dreaming: an update and revision. In: Moffitt A, Kramer M, Hoffmann R, editors. *The Functions of Dreaming.* Albany, NY: State University of New York Press. (1993). p. 139–95.

27. Levin R, Nielsen T. Disturbed dreaming, posttraumatic stress disorder, and affect distress: a review and neurocognitive model. *Psycholo Bull.* (2007) 133:482–528. doi: 10.1037/0033-2909.133.3.482
28. Nielsen T. The stress acceleration hypothesis of nightmares. *Front Neurol.* (2017) 8:201. doi: 10.3389/fneur.2017.00201
29. Hawkins C, Williams TI. Nigthmares, life events and behavior problems in preschool-children. *Child Care Health Dev.* (1992) 18:117–28. doi: 10.1111/j.1365-2214.1992.tb00346.x
30. Lebowitz ER, Shimshoni Y, Silverman WK. Family accommodation mediates nightmares and sleep-related problems in anxious children. *J Anxiety Disord.* (2019) 62:94–9. doi: 10.1016/j.janxdis.2019.01.004
31. Russell K, Rasmussen S, Hunter SC. Insomnia and nightmares as markers of risk for suicidal ideation in young people: investigating the role of defeat and entrapment. *J Clin Sleep Med.* (2018) 14:775–84. doi: 10.5664/jcsm.7104
32. Salzarulo P, Chevalier A. Sleep pronlems in children and their relationship with early disturbances of the waking-sleep rythms. *Sleep.* (1983) 6:47–51. doi: 10.1093/sleep/6.1.47
33. Schredl M, Blomeyer D, Görlinger M. Nigthmares in children: influencing factors. *Somnologie.* (2000) 4:145–9. doi: 10.1007/s11818-000-0007-z
34. Shang CY, Gau SSF, Soong WT. Association between childhood sleep problems and perinatal factors, parental mental distress and behavioral problems. *J Sleep Res.* (2006) 15:63–73. doi: 10.1111/j.1365-2869.2006.00492.x
35. Simonds JF, Parraga H. Prevalence of sleep disorders and sleep behaviors in children and adolescents. *J Am Acad Child Adolesc Psychiatry.* (1982) 21:383–8. doi: 10.1016/S0002-7138(09)60942-0
36. Stein MA, Mendelsohn J, Obermeyer WH, Amromin J, Benca R. Sleep and behavior problems in school-aged children. *Pediatrics.* (2001) 107:e60. doi: 10.1542/peds.107.4.e60
37. Schredl M, Fricke-Oerkermann L, Mitschke A, Wiater A, Lehmkuhl G. Longitudinal study of nightmares in children: stability and effect of emotional symptoms. *Child Psychiatry Hum Dev.* (2009) 40:439–49. doi: 10.1007/s10578-009-0136-y
38. Smedje H, Broman J, Hetta J. Associations between disturbed sleep and behavioural difficulties in 635 children aged six to eight years: a study based on parents' perceptions. *opean Child Adolesc Psychiatry.* (2001) 10:1–9. doi: 10.1007/s007870170041
39. Fisher BE, Wilson AE. Selected sleep disturbances in schoolchildren reported by parents - prevalence, interrlatonships, behavioral-correlates and parental attributions. *Perceptual Motor Skills.* (1987) 64:1147–57. doi: 10.2466/pms.1987.64.3c.1147
40. Lereya ST, Winsper C, Tang NK, Wolke D. Sleep problems in childhood and borderline personality disorder symptoms in early adolescence. *J Abnormal Child Psychol.* (2017) 45:193–206. doi: 10.1007/s10802-016-0158-4
41. Fisher HL, Lereya ST, Thompson A, Lewis G, Zammit S, Wolke D. Childhood parasomnias and psychotic experiences at age 12 years in a United Kingdom birth cohort. *Sleep.* (2014) 37:475–82. doi: 10.5665/sleep.3478
42. Koopman-Verhoeff ME, Bolhuis K, Cecil CA, Kocevska D, Hudziak JJ, Hillegers MH, et al. During day and night: Childhood psychotic experiences and objective and subjective sleep problems. *Schizophrenia Res.* (2019) 206:127–34. doi: 10.1016/j.schres.2018.12.002
43. Lemyre A, Bastien C, Vallières A. Nightmares in mental disorders: a review. *Dreaming.* (2019) 29:144. doi: 10.1037/drm0000103
44. Liu X. Sleep and adolescent suicidal behavior. *Sleep.* (2004) 27:1351–8. doi: 10.1093/sleep/27.7.1351
45. Pigeon WR, Pinquart M, Conner K. Meta-analysis of sleep disturbance and suicidal thoughts and behaviors. *J Clin Psychiatry.* (2012) 73:e1160–7. doi: 10.4088/JCP.11r07586
46. Roberts J, Lennings C. Personality, psychopathology and nightmares in young people. *Personal Individual Differ.* (2006) 41:733–44. doi: 10.1016/j.paid.2006.03.010
47. Thompson A, Lereya S, Lewis G, Zammit S, Fisher H, Wolke D. Childhood sleep disturbance and risk of psychotic experiences at 18: UK birth cohort. *Br J Psychiatry.* (2015) 207:23–9. doi: 10.1192/bjp.bp.113.144089
48. Floress MT, Kuhn BR, Bernas RS, Dandurand M. Nightmare prevalence, distress, and anxiety among young children. *Dreaming.* (2016) 26:280. doi: 10.1037/drm0000034
49. Gregory AM, Eley TC. Sleep problems, anxiety and cognitive style in school-aged children. *Infant Child Dev.* (2005) 14:435–44. doi: 10.1002/icd.409
50. Mindell JA, Barrett KM. Nightmares and anxiety in elementary-aged children: is there a relationship? *Child Care Health Dev.* (2002) 28:317–22. doi: 10.1046/j.1365-2214.2002.00274.x
51. Nielsen TA, Laberge L, Paquet J, Tremblay RE, Vitaro F, Montplaisir J. Development of disturbing dreams during adolescence and their relation to anxiety symptoms. *Sleep.* (2000) 23:727–36. doi: 10.1093/sleep/23.6.1
52. Reynolds KC, Alfano CA. Things that go bump in the night: frequency and predictors of nightmares in anxious and nonanxious children. *Behav Sleep Med.* (2016) 14:442–56. doi: 10.1080/15402002.2015.1017099
53. Schredl M, Pallmer R, Montasser A. Anxiety dreams in school-aged children. *Dreaming.* (1996) 6:265–70. doi: 10.1037/h0094461
54. Simard V, Nielsen TA, Tremblay RE, Boivin M, Montplaisir JY. Longitudinal study of bad dreams in preschool-aged children: prevalence, demographic correlates, risk and protective factors. *Sleep.* (2008) 31:62–70. doi: 10.1093/sleep/31.1.62
55. Gregory AM, Van der Ende J, Willis TA, Verhulst FC. Parent-reported sleep problems during development and self-reported anxiety/depression, attention problems, and aggressive behavior later in life. *Arch Pediatrics Adolesc Med.* (2008) 162:330–5. doi: 10.1001/archpedi.162.4.330
56. Wong MM, Brower KJ, Conroy DA, Lachance KA, Craun EA. Sleep characteristics and behavioral problems among children of alcoholics and controls. *Alcohol Clin Exp Res.* (2018) 42:603–12. doi: 10.1111/acer.13585
57. Li SX, Yu MWM, Lam SP, Zhang J, Li AM, Lai KYC, et al. Frequent nightmares in children: Familial aggregation and associations with parent-reported behavioral and mood problems. *Sleep.* (2011) 34:487–93. doi: 10.1093/sleep/34.4.487
58. Muratori P, Menicucci D, Lai E, Battaglia F, Bontempelli L, Chericoni N, et al. Linking sleep to externalizing behavioral difficulties: a longitudinal psychometric survey in a cohort of Italian school-age children. *J Primary Prev.* (2019) 40:231–41. doi: 10.1007/s10935-019-00547-2
59. Tsai F-J, Chiang H-L, Lee C-M, Gau SS-F, Lee W-T, Fan P-C, et al. Sleep problems in children with autism, attention-deficit hyperactivity disorder, and epilepsy. *Res Autism Spectrum Disord.* (2012) 6:413–21. doi: 10.1016/j.rasd.2011.07.002
60. Grünwald J, Schlarb AA. Relationship between subtypes and symptoms of ADHD. insomnia, and nightmares in connection with quality of life in children. *Neuropsychiatr Dis Treat.* (2017) 13:2341. doi: 10.2147/NDT.S118076
61. Chiang HL, Gau SSF, Ni HC, Chiu YN, Shang CY, Wu YY, et al. Association between symptoms and subtypes of attention-deficit hyperactivity disorder and sleep problems/disorders. *J Sleep Res.* (2010) 19:535–45. doi: 10.1111/j.1365-2869.2010.00832.x
62. Mayes SD, Calhoun SL, Bixler EO, Vgontzas AN, Mahr F, Hillwig-Garcia J, et al. ADHD subtypes and comorbid anxiety, depression, and oppositional-defiant disorder: differences in sleep problems. *J Pediatr Psychol.* (2008) 34:328–37. doi: 10.1093/jpepsy/jsn083
63. Wang B, Eastwood PR, Becker A, Isensee C, Wong JW, Huang R-C, et al. Concurrent developmental course of sleep problems and emotional/behavioral problems in childhood and adolescence as reflected by the dysregulation profile. *Sleep.* (2019) 42:zsy243. doi: 10.1093/sleep/zsy243
64. Zhang J, Xu Z, Zhao K, Chen T, Ye X, Shen Z, et al. Sleep habits, sleep problems, sleep hygiene, and their associations with mental health problems among adolescents. *J Am Psychiatr Nurses Assoc.* (2018) 24:223–34. doi: 10.1177/1078390317715315
65. Gieselmann A, Ait Aoudia M, Carr M, Germain A, Gorzka R, Holzinger B, et al. (2019) Aetiology and treatment of nightmare disorder: state of the art and future perspectives. *J Sleep Res.* 28:e12820. doi: 10.1111/jsr.12820
66. Rothbart MK, Ahadi SA, Hersey KL, Fisher P. Investigations of temperament at three to seven years: the children's behavior questionnaire. *Child Dev.* (2001) 72:1394–408. doi: 10.1111/1467-8624.00355
67. Rothbart MK, Jones LB. Temperament, self-regulation and education. *Sch Psychol Rev.* (1998) 27:479–91.
68. Gartstein MA, Rothbart MK. Studying infant temperament via the revised infant behavior questionnaire. *Infant Behav Dev.* (2003) 26:64–86. doi: 10.1016/S0163-6383(02)00169-8

69. Sanson A, Hemphill SA, Smart D. Connections between temperament and social development: a review. *Social Dev.* (2004) 13:142–70. doi: 10.1046/j.1467-9507.2004.00261.x
70. Kopala-Sibley DC, Olino T, Durbin E, Dyson MW, Klein DN. The stability of temperament from early childhood to early adolescence: a multi-method, multi-informant examination. *Eur J Personal.* (2018) 32:128–45. doi: 10.1002/per.2151
71. Pesonen A-K, Räikkönen K, Keskivaara P, Keltikangas-Järvinen L. Difficult temperament in childhood and adulthood: continuity from maternal perceptions to self-ratings over 17 years. *Personal Individual Differ.* (2003) 34:19–31. doi: 10.1016/S0191-8869(02)00021-1
72. Clark LA, Watson D, Mineka S. Temperament, personality, and the mood and anxiety disorders. *J Abnormal Psychol.* (1994) 103:103–16. doi: 10.1037/0021-843X.103.1.103
73. Rhee SH, Lahey BB, Waldman ID. Comorbidity among dimensions of childhood psychopathology: converging evidence from behavior genetics. *Child Dev Perspect.* (2015) 9:26–31. doi: 10.1111/cdep.12102
74. Uhl K, Halpern LF, Tam C, Fox JK, Ryan JL. Relations of emotion regulation, negative and positive affect to anxiety and depression in middle childhood. *J Child Family Stud.* (2019) 28:2988–99. doi: 10.1007/s10826-019-01474-w
75. Bush NR, Lengua LJ, Colder CR. Temperament as a moderator of the relation between neighborhood and children's adjustment. *J Appl Dev Psychol.* (2010) 31:351–61. doi: 10.1016/j.appdev.2010.06.004
76. Northerner LM, Trentacosta CJ, McLear CM. Negative affectivity moderates associations between cumulative risk and at-risk toddlers' behavior problems. *J Child Family Stud.* (2016) 25:691–9. doi: 10.1007/s10826-015-0248-x
77. Pluess M, Belsky J. Children's differential susceptibility to effects of parenting. *Family Sci.* (2010) 1:14–25. doi: 10.1080/19424620903388554
78. Veenstra R, Oldehinkel AJ, De Winter AF, Lindenberg S, Ormel J. Temperament, environment, and antisocial behavior in a population sample of preadolescent boys and girls. *Int J Behav Dev.* (2006) 30:422–32. doi: 10.1177/0165025406071490
79. Davis S, Votruba-Drzal E, Silk JS. Trajectories of internalizing symptoms from early childhood to adolescence: associations with temperament and parenting. *Social Dev.* (2015) 24:501–20. doi: 10.1111/sode.12105
80. Edwards RC, Hans SL. Infant risk factors associated with internalizing, externalizing, and co-occurring behavior problems in young children. *Dev Psychol.* (2015) 51:489. doi: 10.1037/a0038800
81. Jessee A, Mangelsdorf SC, Shigeto A, Wong MS. Temperament as a moderator of the effects of parental depressive symptoms on child behavior problems. *Social Dev.* (2012) 21:610–27. doi: 10.1111/j.1467-9507.2011.00639.x
82. Karreman A, van Tuijl C, van Aken MAG, Dekovic M. Predicting young children's externalizing problems interactions among effortful control, parenting, child gender. *Merrill Palmer Q J Dev Psychol.* (2009) 55:111–34. doi: 10.1353/mpq.0.0020
83. Schredl M, Fricke-Oerkermann L, Mitschke A, Wiater A, Lehmkuhl G. Factors affecting nightmares in children: parents' vs. children's ratings. *Eur Child Adolesc Psychiatry.* (2009) 18:20–5. doi: 10.1007/s00787-008-0697-5
84. Coulombe J, Reid GJ, Boyle MH, Racine Y. Concurrent associations among sleep problems, indicators of inadequate sleep, psychopathology, and shared risk factors in a population-based sample of healthy Ontario children. *J Pediatr Psychol.* (2010) 35:790–9. doi: 10.1093/jpepsy/jsp097
85. van der Ende J, Verhulst FC, Tiemeier H. Agreement of informants on emotional and behavioral problems from childhood to adulthood. *Psychol Assessment.* (2012) 24:293–300. doi: 10.1037/a0025500
86. Santé Québec JM, Desrosiers H, Tremblay RE. *"En 2001. J'aurai 5 ans", Enquête auprès des bébés de 5 mois: Rapport préliminaire de l'Étude longitudinale du développement des enfants du Québec (ÉLDEQ) [translation: "In 2001. I'll be 5 years old" Survey of 5 months old infants: Preliminary report from the Québec Longitudinal Study of Childhood Development (QLSCD)].* Montréal, QC: Ministère de la Santé et des Services sociaux, Gouvernement du Québec (1997).
87. Robert G, Zadra A. Measuring nightmare and bad dream frequency: impact of retrospective and prospective instruments. *J Sleep Res.* (2008) 17:132–9. doi: 10.1111/j.1365-2869.2008.00649.x
88. Zadra A, Donderi D. Nightmares and bad dreams: their prevalence and relationship to well-being. *J Abnormal Psychol.* (2000) 109:273–81. doi: 10.1037/0021-843X.109.2.273
89. Baillargeon RH, Normand CL, Séguin JR, Zoccolillo M, Japel C, Pérusse D, et al. The evolution of problem and social competence behaviors during toddlerhood: a prospective population-based cohort survey. *Infant Mental Health J.* (2007) 28:12–38. doi: 10.1002/imhj.20120
90. Gauchat A, Zadra A, Tremblay RE, Zelazo PD, Séguin JR. Recurrent dreams and psychosocial adjustment in preteenaged children. *Dreaming.* (2009) 19:75–84. doi: 10.1037/a0016549
91. Vaillancourt T, Miller JL, Fagbemi J, Côté S, Tremblay RE. Trajectories and predictors of indirect aggression: results from a nationally representative longitudinal study of Canadian children aged 2-10. *Aggress Behav.* (2007) 33:314–26. doi: 10.1002/ab.20202
92. Tremblay RE, Vitaro F, Gagnon C, Piché C, Royer N. A prosocial scale for the preschool behaviour questionnaire: concurrent and predictive correlates. *Int J Behav Dev.* (1992) 15:227–45. doi: 10.1177/016502549201500204
93. Achenbach TM. *The Child Behavior Checklist and Related Instruments.* Mahwah, NJ: Lawrence Erlbaum Associates Publishers (1999).
94. Dodge KA, Coie JD. Social-information-processing factors in reactive and proactive aggression in children's peer groups. *J Personal Social Psychol.* (1987) 53:1146–58. doi: 10.1037/0022-3514.53.6.1146
95. Charrois J, Côté SM, Paquin S, Séguin JR, Japel C, Vitaro F, et al. Maternal depression in early childhood and child emotional and behavioral outcomes at school age: examining the roles of preschool childcare quality and current maternal depression symptomatology. *Eur Child Adolesc Psychiatry.* (2019) 29:637–48. doi: 10.1007/s00787-019-01385-7
96. Huijbregts SCJ, Seguin JR, Zoccolillo M, Boivin M, Tremblay RE. Maternal prenatal smoking, parental antisocial behavior, and early childhood physical aggression. *Dev Psychopathol.* (2008) 20:437–53. doi: 10.1017/S0954579408000217
97. La Buissonnière-Ariza V, Séguin JR, Nassim M, Boivin M, Pine DS, Lepore F, et al. Chronic harsh parenting and anxiety associations with fear circuitry function in healthy adolescents: a preliminary study. *Biol Psychol.* (2019) 145:198–210. doi: 10.1016/j.biopsycho.2019.03.019
98. Paquin C, Castellanos-Ryan N, Vitaro F, Côté SM, Tremblay RE, Séguin JR, et al. Maternal depression symptoms, child behavior problems, and their transactional relations: Probing the role of formal childcare. *Dev Psychopathol.* (2019). doi: 10.1017/S0954579419000956. [Epub ahead of print].
99. Rioux C, Murray J, Castellanos-Ryan N, Séguin JR, Tremblay RE, Parent S. Moderation of parenting by inhibitory control in the prediction of the common and unique variance of hyperactivity-impulsivity and inattention. *Dev Psychopathol.* (2019). doi: 10.1017/S0954579419000774. [Epub ahead of print].
100. Touchette E, Petit D, Seguin JR, Boivin M, Tremblay RE, Montplaisir JY. Associations between sleep duration patterns and behavioral/cognitive functioning at school entry. *Sleep.* (2007) 30:1213–9. doi: 10.1093/sleep/30.9.1213
101. Touchette E, Petit D, Tremblay RE, Montplaisir JY. Risk factors and consequences of early childhood dyssomnias: New perspectives. *Sleep Med Rev.* (2009) 13:355–61. doi: 10.1016/j.smrv.2008.12.001
102. Vitaro F, Barker ED, Boivin M, Brendgen M, Tremblay RE. Do early difficult temperament and harsh parenting differentially predict reactive and proactive aggression? *J Abnormal Child Psychol.* (2006) 34:685–95. doi: 10.1007/s10802-006-9055-6
103. Bates JE, Freeland CA, Lounsbur ML. Measures of infant difficultness. *Child Dev.* (1979) 50:794–803. doi: 10.2307/1128946
104. IBM. *IBM SPSS Statistics for Windows (version 18).* Armonk, NY (2012).
105. Harrison XA, Donaldson L, Correa-Cano ME, Evans J, Fisher DN, Goodwin CED, et al. A brief introduction to mixed effects modelling and multi-model inference in ecology. *PeerJ.* (2018) 6:e4794. doi: 10.7717/peerj.4794
106. Tabachnick BG, Fidell LS. *Using Multivariate Statistics.* 6th ed. Boston, MA: Pearson Education (2013).
107. Carneiro A, Dias P, Soares I. Risk factors for internalizing and externalizing problems in the preschool years: systematic literature review based on the child behavior checklist 1½–5. *J Child Family Stud.* (2016) 25:2941–53. doi: 10.1007/s10826-016-0456-z

108. Costello E, Mustillo S, Erkanli A, Keeler G, Angold A. Prevalence and development of psychiatric disorders in childhood and adolescence. *Arch General Psychiatry.* (2003) 60:837–44. doi: 10.1001/archpsyc.60.8.837
109. Cohen J. A power primer. *Psychol Bull.* (1992) 112:155–9. doi: 10.1037/0033-2909.112.1.155
110. Aiken LS, West SG. *Multiple Regression: Testing and Interpreting Interactions.* Thousand Oaks, CA: Sage Publications, Inc; US (1991).
111. Kagan J, Snidman N. Infant predictors of inhibited and uninhibited profiles. *Psychol Sci.* (1991) 2:40–44. doi: 10.1111/j.1467-9280.1991.tb00094.x
112. Kagan J, Snidman N. Temperamental factors in human development. *Am Psychol.* (1991) 46:856–62. doi: 10.1037/0003-066X.46.8.856
113. Kagan J, Snidman N. *The Long Shadow of Temperament.* Cambridge; London: Belknap; Harvard Press (2004).
114. Putnam SP, Stifter CA. Behavioral approach–inhibition in toddlers: prediction from infancy, positive and negative affective components, and relations with behavior problems. *Child Dev.* (2005) 76:212–26. doi: 10.1111/j.1467-8624.2005.00840.x
115. Chronis-Tuscano A, Degnan KA, Pine DS, Perez-Edgar K, Henderson HA, Diaz Y, et al. Stable early maternal report of behavioral inhibition predicts lifetime social anxiety disorder in adolescence. *J Am Acad Child Adolesc Psychiatry.* (2009) 48:928–35. doi: 10.1097/CHI.0b013e3181ae09df
116. Fox NA, Henderson HA, Rubin KH, Calkins SD, Schmidt LA. Continuity and discontinuity of behavioral inhibition and exuberance: psychophysiological and behavioral influences across the first four years of life. *Child Dev.* (2001) 72:1–21. doi: 10.1111/1467-8624.00262
117. Prior M, Smart D, Sanson A, Oberklaid F. Does shy-inhibited temperament in childhood lead to anxiety problems in adolescence? *J Am Acad Child Adolesc Psychiatry.* (2000) 39:461–8. doi: 10.1097/00004583-200004000-00015
118. Krueger RF, Hicks BM, Patrick CJ, Carlson SR, Iacono WG, McGue M. Etiologic connections among substance dependence, antisocial behavior, and personality: modeling the externalizing spectrum. *J Abnormal Psychol.* (2002) 111:411–24. doi: 10.1037/0021-843X.111.3.411
119. Belsky J, Pluess M. Differential susceptibility to long-term effects of quality of child care on externalizing behavior in adolescence? *Int J Behav Dev.* (2012) 36:2–10. doi: 10.1177/0165025411406855
120. Lancee J, Schrijnemaekers NC. The association between nightmares and daily distress. *Sleep Biol Rhythms.* (2013) 11:14–9. doi: 10.1111/j.1479-8425.2012.00586.x
121. Belicki K. Nightmare frequency versus nightmare distress: relations to psychopathology and cognitive style. *J Abnormal Psychol.* (1992) 101:592–7. doi: 10.1037/0021-843X.101.3.592
122. Blagrove M, Farmer L, Williams E. The relationship of nightmare frequency and nightmare distress to well-being. *J Sleep Res.* (2004) 13:129–36. doi: 10.1111/j.1365-2869.2004.00394.x
123. Lee R, Suh S. Nightmare distress as a mediator between nightmare frequency and suicidal ideation. *Dreaming.* (2016) 26:308. doi: 10.1037/drm0000039
124. Kelly WE. Pathological and nonpathological worry: their relationships with nightmare frequency. *Psychiatry Behav Sci.* (2018) 8:1–6. doi: 10.5455/jmood.20180204033253
125. Secrist ME, Dalenberg CJ, Gevirtz R. Contributing factors predicting nightmares in children: trauma, anxiety, dissociation, emotion regulation. *Psychol Trauma Theory Res Pract Policy.* (2019) 11:114. doi: 10.1037/tra0000387
126. Cartwright R, Agargun MY, Kirkby J, Friedman JK. Relation of dreams to waking concerns. *Psychiatry Res.* (2006) 141:261–70. doi: 10.1016/j.psychres.2005.05.013
127. Hartmann E. *The Nature and Functions of Dreaming.* New York, NY: Oxford University Press (2010).
128. Scarpelli S, Bartolacci C, D'Atri A, Gorgoni M, De Gennaro L. The functional role of dreaming in emotional processes. *Front Psychol.* (2019) 10:459. doi: 10.3389/fpsyg.2019.00459
129. Aldao A, Nolen-Hoeksema S, Schweizer S. Emotion-regulation strategies across psychopathology: A meta-analytic review. *Clin Psychol Rev.* (2010) 30:217–37. doi: 10.1016/j.cpr.2009.11.004
130. Eisenberg N, Cumberland A, Spinrad TL, Fabes RA, Shepard SA, Reiser M, et al. The relations of regulation and emotionality to children's externalizing and internalizing problem behavior. *Child Dev.* (2001) 72:1112–34. doi: 10.1111/1467-8624.00337
131. Kim-Spoon J, Cicchetti D, Rogosch FA. A longitudinal study of emotion regulation, emotion lability-negativity, and internalizing symptomatology in maltreated and nonmaltreated children. *Child Dev.* (2013) 84:512–27. doi: 10.1111/j.1467-8624.2012.01857.x
132. Dougherty DM, Mathias CW, Marsh DM, Papageorgiou T, Swann AC, Moeller F. Laboratory measured behavioral impulsivity relates to suicide attempt history. *Suicide Life Threat Behav.* (2004) 34:374–85. doi: 10.1521/suli.34.4.374.53738
133. Gould MS, Greenberg T, Velting DM, Shaffer D. Youth suicide risk and preventive interventions: a review of the past 10 years. *J Am Acad Child Adolesc Psychiatry.* (2003) 42:386–405. doi: 10.1097/01.CHI.0000046821.95464.CF
134. Simon TR, Swann AC, Powell KE, Potter LB, Kresnow M-j, O'Carroll PW. Characteristics of impulsive suicide attempts and attempters. *Suicide Life Threat Behav.* (2001) 32:49–59. doi: 10.1521/suli.32.1.5.49.24212
135. Winsper C, Tang NKY. Linkages between insomnia and suicidality: prospective associations, high-risk subgroups and possible psychological mechanisms. *Int Rev Psychiatry.* (2014) 26:189–204. doi: 10.3109/09540261.2014.881330
136. Belfiore LA, Pietrowsky R. Attachment styles and nightmares in adults. *Dreaming.* (2017) 27:59. doi: 10.1037/drm0000045
137. Csoka S, Simor P, Szabo G, Kopp MS, Bodizs R. Early maternal separation, nightmares, and bad dreams: results from the hungarostudy epidemiological panel. *Attach Hum Dev.* (2011) 13:125–40. doi: 10.1080/14616734.2011.553991
138. van Ijzendoorn MH, Schuengel C, Bakermans-Kranenburg MJ. Disorganized attachment in early childhood: Meta-analysis of precursors, concomitants, and sequelae. *Dev Psychopathol.* (1999) 11:225–49. doi: 10.1017/S0954579499002035
139. Wang F, Willoughby M, Mills-Koonce R, Cox MJ. Infant attachment disorganization and moderation pathways to level and change in externalizing behavior during preschool ages. *Attach Hum Dev.* (2016) 18:534–53. doi: 10.1080/14616734.2016.1243139

18

Neuropsychiatric Symptoms and Quality of Life in Patients with Adult-Onset Idiopathic Focal Dystonia and Essential Tremor

Sangjin Lee [1], Sun Ju Chung [2] and Hae-Won Shin [1]*

[1] Department of Neurology, Chung-Ang University College of Medicine, Seoul, South Korea, [2] Department of Neurology, Asan Medical Center, Ulsan University College of Medicine, Seoul, South Korea

***Correspondence:**
Hae-Won Shin
shinhw@cau.ac.kr

Background: While idiopathic focal dystonia (IFD) and essential tremor (ET) have been considered pure movement disorders, they reportedly induce neuropsychiatric manifestations and may thus be more accurately described as network disorders.

Methods: The present multi-center, cross-sectional, case-control study evaluated the severity of depression and anxiety with the Beck Depression Inventory (BDI) and Beck Anxiety Inventory (BAI), respectively; the frequency of neuropsychiatric disorders with the Korean-Mini International Neuropsychiatry Interview; and QoL with the Short-Form 36 (SF-36).

Results: Seventy-four subjects participated in this study (IFD, 27; ET, 24; controls, 23). The BDI and BAI scores were higher in the IFD and ET groups than in the control group. Although the frequency of neuropsychiatric disorders diagnosed according to the Diagnostic and Statistical Manual of Mental Disorders, 4th Edition Axis I was comparable among the groups, the prevalence of major depressive disorder tended to be high among patients with IFD. QoL was correlated with the severity of depression and anxiety across the groups.

Conclusions: Depression and anxiety are more severe in patients with IFD and ET compared to healthy controls, while their severity is similar among patients with IFD and ET. Axis I major depressive disorder is relatively more prevalent in patients with IFD. Neuropsychiatric symptoms affect QoL regardless of the affected individual's condition, addressing neuropsychiatric symptoms in patients with movement disorders may be crucial to improving their QoL.

Keywords: focal dystonia, essential tremor, neuropsychiatry, non-motor manifestations, quality of life

INTRODUCTION

Dystonia has traditionally been classified as a movement disorder, caused by dysfunction in the motor system, particularly the basal ganglia (BG) (1, 2). As the BG are connected to the limbic system, its dysfunction induces consequent non-motor neuropsychiatric symptoms in patients with dystonia (3–5). Indeed, recent studies have shown that such neuropsychiatric manifestations, including depression, anxiety, and obsessive-compulsive traits, are observed in patients with focal or segmental dystonia (6–15). The recent finding that patients with essential tremor (ET), a common motor characterized dysfunction of the cerebellum and consequent isolated tremor, also present with neuropsychiatric symptoms, may implicate psychiatric manifestations as part of the primary pathophysiology of movement disorders (3, 16–20).

However, no study has considered this possibility or compared the prevalence of psychiatric symptoms between patients with different movement disorders. The increasing body of evidence has shown a close correlation between the QoL of patients with movement disorders and their presentation of neuropsychiatric symptoms (21, 22). Furthermore, evaluating differences in the presentation and prevalence of non-motor neuropsychiatric symptoms across movement disorders would help gain an insight into their pathophysiology and improve the patients' QoL. The present study thus evaluated the frequency and severity of neuropsychiatric manifestations in patients with idiopathic focal dystonia (IFD) and ET, relative to healthy controls, and whether the considered neuropsychiatric symptoms affect the QoL in these subjects.

MATERIALS AND METHODS

This prospective multi-center, cross-sectional, case-control study was approved by the Institutional Review Boards of Chung-Ang University Hospital (C2013231-1191) and Asan Medical Center (2014-0149). All participants provided written informed consent before participation.

Participants

The present study recruited patients with IFD, patients with ET, and age-matched, healthy controls without any neurological deficits. The sample sizes obtained using a power analysis were 43, 43, and 22 for patients with IFD, patients with ET, and controls, respectively. Diagnoses of IFD and ET were confirmed according to the Movement Disorder Society diagnostic criteria (23, 24). Specifically, among patients with ET, only those with tremor in both arms and without head tremor were enrolled to avoid the inclusion of patients with dystonic tremor. We excluded patients who presented with movement disorders other than dystonia or tremor or had a history of drug exposure to which the movement disorder could possibly be ascribed. None of the study subjects had been diagnosed with any psychiatric disorder, and all participants provided written informed consent prior to their enrollment in the study.

Clinical Measurements

All participants were interviewed to evaluate the severity of their depression and anxiety using the Beck Depression Inventory (BDI) and Beck Anxiety Inventory (BAI), respectively (25, 26). They were also asked to undergo the Korean-Mini International Neuropsychiatry Interview (MINI). MINI is a brief, reliable structured interview used for diagnosing Axis I psychiatric disorders according to the Diagnostic and Statistical Manual of Mental Disorders, 4th Edition (DSM-IV) (27). The cognitive function of all participants was tested with the Korean-Mini Mental Status Examination (K-MMSE). The health-related QoL of participants was evaluated with the 36-Item Short-Form Health Survey (SF-36) (28). The Burke-Fan-Marsden Dystonia Rating Scale (BFMDRS) was used to evaluate the severity of dystonia in patients with IFD (29).

TABLE 1 | Demographic and clinical characteristics of participants.

Group (number of subjects)	Idiopathic focal dystonia (27)	Essential tremor (24)	Controls (23)	*p*-value
Age (year)	58.79 ± 15.18	65.58 ± 10.96	55.82 ± 14.93	0.5712
Symptom duration (months)	100.21 ± 140.64	119.25 ± 91.14	–	0.5720
K-MMSE	27.21 ± 2.19	25.67 ± 4.74	26.93 ± 2.31	0.8508
BFMDRS	4.04 ± 3.71	–	–	–
- Movement score	3.75 ± 3.43	–	–	–
- Disability score	0.29 ± 0.71	–	–	–

Data are presented as mean ± SD unless stated otherwise. BFMDRS, Burke-Fahn-Marsden Dystonia Rating Scale; K-MMSE, Korean-Mini Mental Status Examination.

Statistical Analysis

The Kolmogorov-Smirnov and Shapiro-Wilk tests were used to test the normality of the variables; we found that the variables analyzed by analysis of variance did not follow a normal distribution. Accordingly, The Kruskal-Wallis H and Mann-Whitney *post-hoc* tests were used to compare parameters, including BDI, BAI, SF-36, K-MMSE, and age, among the three groups. The chi-square test was used to compare the frequency of psychiatric disorders between groups. Linear regression was performed to determine the correlation between the severity of non-motor scores, including BDI and BAI, and scores of SF-36. The correlation between BFMDRS and scores of SF-36 was also analyzed using linear regression. Data are expressed as mean ± SD, and $p < 0.05$ were considered to indicate statistical significance. The data were analyzed using SPSS 25.0 statistical software (IBM Corp., Armonk, NY, USA).

RESULTS

We recruited 27 patients with IFD, 24 patients with ET, and 23 healthy controls. Of the patients with IFD, 13 had cervical dystonia; 2, focal hand dystonia; and 11, cranial dystonia. The demographic and clinical characteristics of the subjects are described in **Table 1**. There were no significant differences in terms of age, sex, or K-MMSE score between the groups (**Table 1**). The mean BFMDRS in the IFD group was 7.04 ± 6.51 (mean movement score, 6.11 ± 5.33; mean disability score, 0.93 ± 1.63). Symptom duration was comparable between patients with IFD and ET (100.21 ± 140.64 and 119.25 ± 91.14 months, respectively).

The Kruskal-Wallis H-test showed that there was a significant difference in BDI and BAI among the groups (Kruskal-Wallis H-value = 13.018, 8.261; $df = 2, 2$; $p = 0.001, 0.016$, respectively). The Mann-Whitney *post-hoc* comparison revealed that patients with IFD and ET had higher BDI and BAI scores than healthy controls (IFD, ET, and control groups: 9.71 ± 6.85, 9.25 ± 7.40,

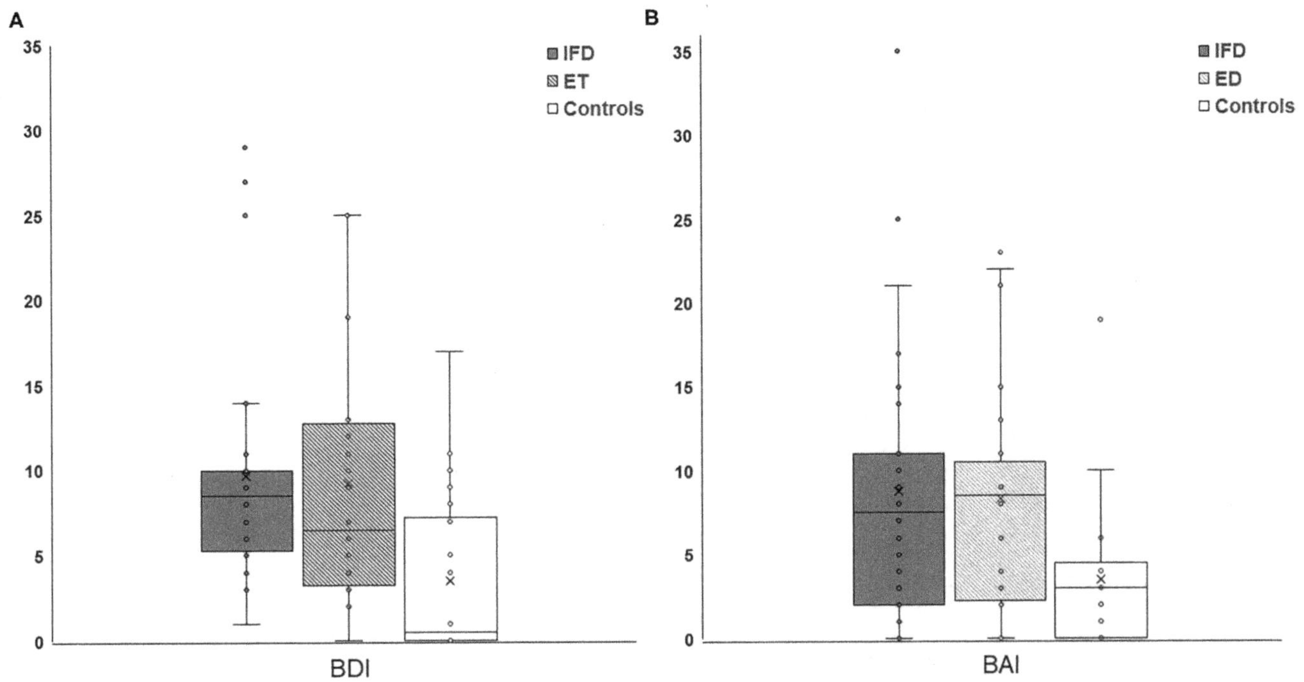

FIGURE 1 | Comparison of the severity of depression **(A)** and anxiety **(B)** between individuals with IFD and ET and controls. The depression and anxiety scores were higher among patients with IFD and ET than in controls but comparable between patients with IFD and ET. IFD, idiopathic focal dystonia; ET, essential tremor.

and 3.85 ± 4.96, respectively, for the BDI score; **Figure 1A**, $p = 0.001$ and $p = 0.013$; 8.79 ± 8.12, 8.33 ± 6.60, and 3.80 ± 4.40, respectively, for the BAI score; **Figure 1B**, $p = 0.004$ and $p = 0.010$). We found no significant difference in the BDI or BAI scores between the IFD and ET groups ($p = 0.525$ and 0.993, respectively; **Figure 1**). Additionally, no significant differences were found in either the BDI or BAI scores among IFD types.

The frequency of Axis-I psychiatric disorders was comparable across the groups ($p = 0.111$); however, patients with IFD tended to have a higher frequency of occurrence of psychiatric disorders (48, 33, and 17% in the dystonia, ET, and control groups, respectively; **Figure 2**).

There was significant difference in SF-36 score among groups (Kruskal-Wallis H-value = 13.918, $df = 2$, $p = 0.001$) Patients with IFD and ET showed lower SF-36 scores than those of healthy controls (110.21 ± 14.33, 109.04 ± 24.29, and 126.16 ± 12.89, respectively, $p < 0.05$). However, there was no significant difference in SF-36 scores between patients with IFD and ET ($p = 0.734$). The linear regression analysis showed that BDI and BAI scores were significantly correlated with SF-36 scores. Among patients with IFD, SF-36 scores were significantly correlated with both BDI and BAI scores but not with BFMDRS scores.

DISCUSSION

The principal findings of this study are as follows: (1) patients with IFD or ET presented higher levels of depression and anxiety than did healthy controls; (2) the severity of depression and anxiety did not differ significantly between patients with IFD and ET; (3) while psychiatric disorders were more common among patients with IFD, their prevalence did not significantly differ between patients with IFD and ET and healthy controls; (4) the severity of depression and anxiety was significantly correlated with QoL across all subjects; and (5) QoL was not correlated with motor symptoms in patients with IFD.

Our results replicate previous findings of a relatively higher prevalence and severity of anxiety and depression among patients with idiopathic dystonia or ET than in healthy controls (6, 8, 9, 11, 13–16, 18–20, 30). Although our study did not find a significant difference between the study groups in terms of the frequency of psychiatric disorders diagnosed according to the DSM-IV Axis I ($p = 0.11$), psychiatric disorders tended to be more prevalent among patients with IFD than among healthy controls. Along with higher depression and anxiety scores, the frequency of major depressive disorder tended to be higher in patients with IFD (8, 2, and 2 in IFD, ET, and healthy controls, respectively); however, on account of our limited sample size, statistical significance could not be confirmed.

The frequency with which Parkinson's disease (PD) induces depression and anxiety can be ascribed to the spread of neurodegeneration beyond the BG (31, 32), which is the key neural substrate of PD. Although dystonia is a movement disorder related to the BG, neuropsychiatric manifestations in dystonia have been overlooked because of the lack of a specific structural pathology in this condition (33, 34). Since sensory dysfunction was introduced in this motor system

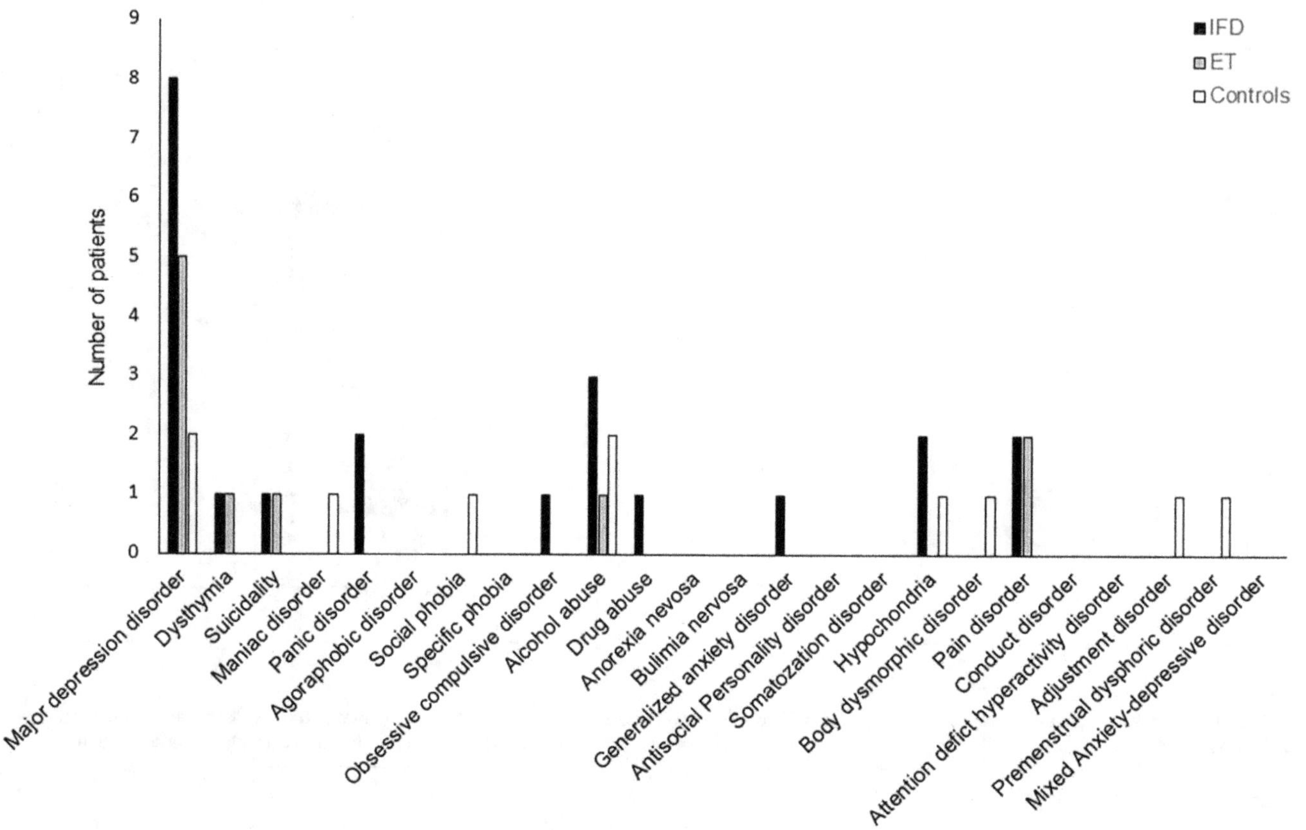

FIGURE 2 | The frequency of DSM-IV Axis I neuropsychiatric disorders among individuals with IFD and ET and controls. The overall frequency was comparable among the groups, but the incidence of major depressive disorder tended to be higher in patients with IFD.

disorder (35, 36), other neuropsychiatric manifestations have been highlighted as features of dystonia, particularly in the past decade (10–15). Furthermore, emerging evidence suggests that dystonia results from dysfunctional brain networks (37, 38). According to this hypothesis, the neuropsychiatric manifestations of dystonia can be considered primary consequences of the disrupted connection between the limbic and BG-motor symptoms in dystonia (7, 33, 39). ET could cause mood disorders and psychiatric symptoms by this same mechanism (4). Indeed, cross-sectional and longitudinal studies have reported an association between ET and non-motor symptoms (18). When ET is considered a neurodegenerative disorder such as PD, neuropsychiatric manifestations can be regarded as a consequence of pathological spread beyond the cerebellum, resulting in various symptoms besides tremor (40). On the other hand, the cerebellum is linked to the BG, and this thus provides a mechanism by which dysfunction of the cerebellum could affect the BG circuit (41). The disruption within the brain network could affect the function of remote regions connected with the cerebellum resulting in various symptoms other than tremor. Taken together, dysfunction in multiple nodes in the limbic system connecting the BG to the cerebellum may lead to the development of non-motor neuropsychiatric symptoms in patients with movement disorders. Future studies should use electrophysiological and neuroimaging methods to detect dysfunction in the brain network. This will elucidate the mechanisms of depression and anxiety in patients with IFD and ET. This may result in an alternative explanation to the one that states that depression and anxiety occur in patients with IFD and ET as a primary phenomenon due to disease-related disruption of neural networks. Considering that depression and anxiety are more common in patients with chronic illnesses and that the patients in our study had had IFD and ET for more than 100 months, the increased severity of depression and anxiety could be considered a secondary phenomenon due to the presence of a chronic condition (42, 43). Comparison of non-motor neuropsychiatric symptoms between *de novo* patients and healthy controls may clarify whether these symptoms have a direct relationship with the pathophysiology of IFD and ET. In our study, the severity of depression and anxiety as well as the frequency of Axis I psychiatric disorders were comparable between patients with IFD and ET, suggesting that the neuropsychiatric symptoms due to IFD and ET may share a pathophysiology attributable to dysfunctional neural networks.

We observed a significantly worse QoL in the IFD and ET groups than in the control group and a correlation between QoL and both anxiety and depression across all three groups.

Interestingly, in patients with IFD, the QoL was correlated with anxiety and depression, but not with the severity of dystonia. It suggests that the QoL in patients with IFD may be more affected by neuropsychiatric symptoms than motor symptoms due to dystonia itself.

This study was subject to several limitations. First, we could not recruit the optimal number of patients that was initially calculated in the power analysis. Accordingly, the results of this study should be considered preliminary. Larger studies are required to compare the presentation of neuropsychiatric symptoms across patients with different movement disorders to elucidate their exact pathophysiology. Second, unfortunately, we did not measure tremor scale to determine the tremor severity in patients with ET. Consequently, we could not evaluate the potential correlations between motor symptoms and depression and anxiety or QoL in patients with ET. Third, although MINI is useful as a tool for the assessment of psychiatric disorders, it would not be an optimal tool designed to specifically evaluate neuropsychiatric symptoms resulting from neurological and movement disorders.

In conclusion, patients with IFD and ET has more severe depression and anxiety than healthy controls, and the increased severity is similar among patients with IFD and ET. Axis I major depressive disorder is relatively more prevalent in patients with IFD. Neuropsychiatric symptoms affect QoL regardless of the affected individual's condition, suggesting that addressing neuropsychiatric symptoms in patients with movement disorders may be crucial to improving their QoL.

ETHICS STATEMENT

The studies involving human participants were reviewed and approved by the Institutional Review Boards of Chung-Ang University Hospital (C2013231-1191) and Asan Medical Center (2014-0149). The patients/participants provided their written informed consent to participate in this study.

AUTHOR CONTRIBUTIONS

SL contributed to the analysis, interpretation of the data, and drafting of the manuscript. SC contributed to the study's conception, data acquisition, and critical review. H-WS contributed to the study's conception, data acquisition, data analysis and interpretation, and critical review. All authors contributed to the article and approved the submitted version.

REFERENCES

1. Marsden CD. Motor disorders in basal ganglia disease. *Hum Neurobiol.* (1984) 2:245–50. doi: 10.1212/WNL.34.2.262-a
2. Hallett M. The neurophysiology of dystonia. *Arch Neurol.* (1998) 55:601–3. doi: 10.1001/archneur.55.5.601
3. Ring HA, Serra-Mestres J. Neuropsychiatry of the basal ganglia. *J Neurol Neurosurg Psychiatry.* (2002) 72:12–21. doi: 10.1136/jnnp.72.1.12
4. Marchand WR. Cortico-basal ganglia circuitry: a review of key research and implications for functional connectivity studies of mood and anxiety disorders. *Brain Struct Funct.* (2010) 215:73–96. doi: 10.1007/s00429-010-0280-y
5. Buot A, Yelnik J. Functional anatomy of the basal ganglia: limbic aspects. *Rev Neurol (Paris).* (2012) 168:569–75. doi: 10.1016/j.neurol.2012.06.015
6. Gundel H, Wolf A, Xidara V, Busch R, Ladwig KH, Jacobi F, et al. High psychiatric comorbidity in spasmodic torticollis: a controlled study. *J Nerv Ment Dis.* (2003) 191:465–73. doi: 10.1097/01.NMD.0000081667.02656.21
7. Lencer R, Steinlechner S, Stahlberg J, Rehling H, Orth M, Baeumer T, et al. Primary focal dystonia: evidence for distinct neuropsychiatric and personality profiles. *J Neurol Neurosurg Psychiatry.* (2009) 80:1176–9. doi: 10.1136/jnnp.2008.170191
8. Kuyper DJ, Parra V, Aerts S, Okun MS, Kluger BM. Nonmotor manifestations of dystonia: a systematic review. *Mov Disord.* (2011) 26:1206–17. doi: 10.1002/mds.23709
9. Stamelou M, Edwards MJ, Hallett M, Bhatia KP. The non-motor syndrome of primary dystonia: clinical and pathophysiological implications. *Brain.* (2012) 135(Pt 6):1668–81. doi: 10.1093/brain/awr224
10. Berardelli I, Ferrazzano G, Pasquini M, Biondi M, Berardelli A, Fabbrini G. Clinical course of psychiatric disorders in patients with cervical dystonia. *Psychiatry Res.* (2015) 229:583–5. doi: 10.1016/j.psychres.2015.07.076
11. Conte A, Berardelli I, Ferrazzano G, Pasquini M, Berardelli A, Fabbrini G. Non-motor symptoms in patients with adult-onset focal dystonia: sensory and psychiatric disturbances. *Parkinsonism Relat Disord.* (2016) 22(Suppl. 1):S111–4. doi: 10.1016/j.parkreldis.2015.09.001
12. Berman BD, Junker J, Shelton E, Sillau SH, Jinnah HA, Perlmutter JS, et al. Psychiatric associations of adult-onset focal dystonia phenotypes. *J Neurol Neurosurg Psychiatry.* (2017) 88:595–602. doi: 10.1136/jnnp-2016-315461
13. Yang J, Shao N, Song W, Wei Q, Ou R, Wu Y, et al. Nonmotor symptoms in primary adult-onset cervical dystonia and blepharospasm. *Brain Behav.* (2017) 7:e00592. doi: 10.1002/brb3.592
14. Novaretti N, Cunha ALN, Bezerra TC, Pena Pereira MA, de Oliveira DS, Macruz Brito MMC, et al. The prevalence and correlation of non-motor symptoms in adult patients with idiopathic focal or segmental dystonia. *Tremor Other Hyperkinet Mov.* (2019) 9:596. doi: 10.5334/tohm.466
15. Ospina-Garcia N, Escobar-Barrios M, Rodriguez-Violante M, Benitez-Valenzuela J, Cervantes-Arriaga A. Neuropsychiatric profile of patients with craniocervical dystonia: a case-control study. *Clin Neurol Neurosurg.* (2020) 193:105794. doi: 10.1016/j.clineuro.2020.105794
16. Chandran V, Pal PK, Reddy JY, Thennarasu K, Yadav R, Shivashankar N. Non-motor features in essential tremor. *Acta Neurol Scand.* (2012) 125:332–7. doi: 10.1111/j.1600-0404.2011.01573.x
17. Janicki SC, Cosentino S, Louis ED. The cognitive side of essential tremor: what are the therapeutic implications? *Ther Adv Neurol Disord.* (2013) 6:353–68. doi: 10.1177/1756285613489591
18. Louis ED. Non-motor symptoms in essential tremor: a review of the current data and state of the field. *Parkinsonism Relat Disord.* (2016) 22(Suppl. 1):S115–8. doi: 10.1016/j.parkreldis.2015.08.034
19. Aslam S, Zhang N, Adler CH, Caviness JN, Driver-Dunckley E, Mehta SH, et al. Essential tremor and depression. *Mov Disord Clin Pract.* (2017) 4:838–42. doi: 10.1002/mdc3.12530
20. Shalash AS, Mohamed H, Mansour AH, Elkady A, Elrassas H, Hamid E, et al. Clinical profile of non-motor symptoms in patients with essential tremor: impact on quality of life and age-related differences. *Tremor Other Hyperkinet Mov.* (2019) 9:1–8. doi: 10.5334/tohm.471

21. Lennox BR, Lennox GG. Mind and movement: the neuropsychiatry of movement disorders. *J Neurol Neurosurg Psychiatry.* (2002) 72(Suppl. 1):i28–31. doi: 10.1136/jnnp.72.suppl_1.i28
22. Lyketsos CG, Kozauer N, Rabins PV. Psychiatric manifestations of neurologic disease: where are we headed? *Dialogues Clin Neurosci.* (2007) 9:111–24.
23. Chouinard S, Louis ED, Fahn S. Agreement among movement disorder specialists on the clinical diagnosis of essential tremor. *Mov Disord.* (1997) 12:973–6. doi: 10.1002/mds.870120621
24. Albanese A, Bhatia K, Bressman SB, Delong MR, Fahn S, Fung VS, et al. Phenomenology and classification of dystonia: a consensus update. *Mov Disord.* (2013) 28:863–73. doi: 10.1002/mds.25475
25. Beck AT, Ward CH, Mendelson M, Mock J, Erbaugh J. An inventory for measuring depression. *Arch Gen Psychiatry.* (1961) 4:561–71. doi: 10.1001/archpsyc.1961.01710120031004
26. Beck AT, Epstein N, Brown G, Steer RA. An inventory for measuring clinical anxiety: psychometric properties. *J Consult Clin Psychol.* (1988) 56:893–7. doi: 10.1037/0022-006X.56.6.893
27. Sheehan DV, Lecrubier Y, Sheehan KH, Amorim P, Janavs J, Weiller E, et al. The Mini-International Neuropsychiatric Interview (M.I.N.I.): the development and validation of a structured diagnostic psychiatric interview for DSM-IV and ICD-10. *J Clin Psychiatry.* (1998) 59(Suppl. 20):22–33.
28. Ware JE, Jr., Sherbourne CD. The MOS 36-item short-form health survey (SF-36). I. conceptual framework and item selection. *Med Care.* (1992) 30:473–83. doi: 10.1097/00005650-199206000-00002
29. Comella CL, Leurgans S, Wuu J, Stebbins GT, Chmura T, Dystonia Study G. Rating scales for dystonia: a multicenter assessment. *Mov Disord.* (2003) 18:303–12. doi: 10.1002/mds.10377
30. Jhunjhunwala K, Pal PK. The non-motor features of essential tremor: a primary disease feature or just a secondary phenomenon? *Tremor Other Hyperkinet Mov.* (2014) 4:255. doi: 10.5334/tohm.230
31. Tan LC. Mood disorders in Parkinson's disease. *Parkinsonism Relat Disord.* (2012) 18(Suppl. 1):S74–6. doi: 10.1016/S1353-8020(11)70024-4
32. Schapira AHV, Chaudhuri KR, Jenner P. Non-motor features of Parkinson disease. *Nat Rev Neurosci.* (2017) 18:435–50. doi: 10.1038/nrn.2017.62
33. Neychev VK, Gross RE, Lehericy S, Hess EJ, Jinnah HA. The functional neuroanatomy of dystonia. *Neurobiol Dis.* (2011) 42:185–201. doi: 10.1016/j.nbd.2011.01.026
34. Standaert DG. Update on the pathology of dystonia. *Neurobiol Dis.* (2011) 42:148–51. doi: 10.1016/j.nbd.2011.01.012
35. Bara-Jimenez W, Shelton P, Hallett M. Spatial discrimination is abnormal in focal hand dystonia. *Neurology.* (2000) 55:1869–73. doi: 10.1212/WNL.55.12.1869
36. Abbruzzese G, Berardelli A. Sensorimotor integration in movement disorders. *Mov Disord.* (2003) 18:231–40. doi: 10.1002/mds.10327
37. Hendrix CM, Vitek JL. Toward a network model of dystonia. *Ann N Y Acad Sci.* (2012) 1265:46–55. doi: 10.1111/j.1749-6632.2012.06692.x
38. Schirinzi T, Sciamanna G, Mercuri NB, Pisani A. Dystonia as a network disorder: a concept in evolution. *Curr Opin Neurol.* (2018) 31:498–503. doi: 10.1097/WCO.0000000000000580
39. Jinnah HA, Neychev V, Hess EJ. The anatomical basis for dystonia: the motor network model. *Tremor Other Hyperkinet Mov.* (2017) 7:506. doi: 10.5334/tohm.383
40. Benito-León J. Essential tremor: a neurodegenerative disease? *Tremor Other Hyperkinet Mov.* (2014) 4:252. doi: 10.5334/tohm.227
41. Bostan AC, Strick PL. The basal ganglia and the cerebellum: nodes in an integrated network. *Nat Rev Neurosci.* (2018) 19:338–50. doi: 10.1038/s41583-018-0002-7
42. Katon W, Lin EH, Kroenke K. The association of depression and anxiety with medical symptom burden in patients with chronic medical illness. *Gen Hosp Psychiatry.* (2007) 29:147–55. doi: 10.1016/j.genhosppsych.2006.11.005
43. Kagee A. Symptoms of depression and anxiety among a sample of South African patients living with a chronic illness. *J Health Psychol.* (2008) 13:547–55. doi: 10.1177/1359105308088527

19

The Impact of COVID-19 on Psychological and Social Stigma for Indonesian Nurses

Mustikasari Mustikasari[1], Harif Fadhillah[2,3], Apri Sunadi[4], Nursalam Nursalam[3,5], Ati Surya Mediawati[3] and Muhammad Adam[1]*

[1] *Faculty of Nursing, Universitas Indonesia, Jakarta, Indonesia,* [2] *Faculty of Health Science, Muhammadiyah University of Jakarta, Jakarta, Indonesia,* [3] *Indonesian National Nursing Association, Jakarta, Indonesia,* [4] *Universitas Respati Indonesia, Yogyakarta, Indonesia,* [5] *Faculty of Nursing, Universitas Airlangga, Surabaya, Indonesia*

Correspondence:
Mustikasari Mustikasari
ns.mustikasari@gmail.com

Introduction: Nurses are on the front line and are at high risk of experiencing a mental health crisis during the pandemic due to the psychological impact and stigma. The aim of this study was to identify the role of psychological status and social stigma in anxiety, fear, depression, and mental health crises during the pandemic.

Materials and Methods: A cross-sectional design during December 2020–August 2021. A total of 2,156 nurses who work in health facilities, either hospitals, or communities based on the criteria of nurses who interact directly with COVID-19 patients, work at least 3 months, age 20–54 years, are literate, have internet access, and have the ability to access the electronic form. The eligible participants filled in online questionnaires that were sent to them via WhatsApp. Data were analyzed using Spearman rho correlation test with statistically significant p value < 0.05.

Results: A total of 2,156 respondents responded to the questionnaire, and the response rate was 100%. The psychological status of nurses was 78.4% moderate, 18.5% experienced social stigma, 44.0% showed an anxiety response, 53.5% fear, 64.5% depression in the very severe category, and 63.5% fell into a mental health crisis. The results of the inferential analysis showed that all $P < 0.05$ which indicated that psychological status and social stigma had a significant relationship with anxiety, fear, depression, and mental health crisis in nurses.

Conclusion: The psychological status and social stigma experienced by nurses during the COVID-19 pandemic indicate a bad situation and lead to a mental health emergency crisis.

Keywords: COVID-19, social stigma, mental health, anxiety, nursing

INTRODUCTION

Indonesia often faces infectious disease problems because Indonesia is a tropical country with the highest number of infectious diseases in the world (1, 2). However, at the end of 2019, Indonesia was still surprised by the emergence of a new infectious disease caused by the SARS-CoV-2, virus which was later known as coronavirus disease 2019 (COVID-19) (3, 4). Facing a pandemic that is also taking place in countries around the world, Indonesia is also experiencing the same crisis, both in the health sector as well as in all sectors of the country's structure. The impact that is felt the most is the health impact felt by the community, especially health workers (5, 6).

The existence of the COVID-19 pandemic at the beginning of the emergence of cases made Indonesia really keep tight so as not to cause transmission of the number of COVID-19 cases, so detailed analysis and in-depth tracing were applied to trace cases of close contact with COVID-19 spreaders, but public awareness which is still low and the information circulating about COVID-19 makes the tightness decrease (7). The result of not complying with the health protocol is the spike in COVID-19 cases in Indonesia, especially in the May–August 2020 period. The surge in COVID-19 cases had slowed down in Indonesia around February–May 2021, but the repatriation of Indonesian Health workers from abroad caused variants. The new COVID-19, namely the delta variant, spread to Indonesia and a second wave of COVID-19 emerged. The second wave caused a lot of health crises in Indonesia. Health facilities were full of patients, health workers were overwhelmed, and many died and fell ill with COVID-19 (8).

Health workers who have the highest mortality rate are nurses, nurses as staff who provide care for 24 h make them have to have close contact with patients (9, 10). Nurses who have used level 3 personal protective equipment in Indonesia still do not guarantee that they are not infected, because there are several other factors, such as decreased immunity, interaction with other health workers without a protocol when eating, and interaction with the community, that they are infected with COVID-19 are also very important allows. Based on the number of nurse deaths in Indonesia during January–July 2021, Indonesia has lost more than 300 nurses due to COVID-19 (11).

The pandemic atmosphere in Indonesia shows very tense conditions, especially during the spike period of the first wave and second wave of COVID-19. Feelings of fear of being infected, fear of sudden death, and fear of people who have had COVID-19 make people wary of each other (12, 13). This also creates conditions of anxiety, panic, fear, and even depression and mental health crises, due to stigma in society and psychological conditions (9, 10). It is very important to evaluate the psychological condition and social stigma felt by nurses, because nurses who are directly involved in care certainly feel a greater impact than just the physical impact, but also psychologically and socially. There are so many nurses who experience injustice in society, are ostracized, stigmatized, to experience discrimination and are expelled (7). Conditions like this in society make it easy for nurses to experience feelings of anxiety, fear, and mental health crises. Therefore, the purpose of this study was to determine the role of psychological conditions and social stigma on the incidence of anxiety, fear, depression and mental health crises in Indonesian nurses during the COVID-19 pandemic.

MATERIALS AND METHODS

This research has been conducted in Indonesia on nurses who provide direct care for COVID-19. The research was carried out from December 2020 to August 2021.

Study Design

We chose to use a quantitative study with a cross sectional approach to nurses in health facilities in Indonesia. The main reason for choosing the research design was to conduct a comprehensive survey by distributing questionnaires to find out the nurses' reactions to the COVID-19 pandemic. Ethical approval was obtained from the local Ethics Committee

TABLE 1 | Sociodemographic characteristics of respondents.

Characteristics of respondent	n (%)
Ages	
20–29 years	961 (44.6)
30–39 years	542 (25.1)
40–49 years	417 (19.3)
50 years and above	236 (10.9)
Gender	
Male	700 (32.5)
Female	1456 (67.5)
Marital status	
Married	677 (31.4)
Single	1455 (67.5)
Widow	24 (1.1)
Ethnic	
Javanese	1454 (67.5)
Sundanese	400 (18.6)
Cirebon	22 (1.0)
Betawi	185 (8.6)
Madura	73 (3.4)
Boyam	22 (1.0)
Religion	
Moeslem	2004 (92.9)
Buddhist	35 (1.6)
Hindu	31 (1.4)
Cristian	86 (4.0)
Educational background	
Diploma	662 (30.8)
Bachelor	1252 (58.1)
Master	242 (11.2)
Income	
< Minimum regional income	900 (41.7)
> Minimum regional income	1256 (58.3)

of the University of Indonesia with the number Ket-198/UN2.F12.D1.2.1/PPM.00.02/2021. Researchers in collecting data ensure that respondents voluntarily and without coercion are willing to fill out research questionnaires.

Participants and Settings

The sample included 2,156 nurses who worked in health facilities, either hospitals or communities, and were recruited from all nursing staff in Indonesia. Based on the respondent selection criteria, the main criteria in this study were nurses who interacted directly with COVID-19 patients, worked in health services, had worked for at least 3 months, aged 20–54 years, were willing to take part in the study, were literate, had internet access, and had the ability to access the electronic form. The following exclusion criteria were applied: immigrant nursing, being unwilling or unable to continue contributing to the study.

Recruitment

Patient recruitment was conducted between December 2020 and August 2021. The researcher, via online, informed the nurses about the purpose of the study and asked them whether they were willing to be contacted by the research and willing to fill out the questionnaire. The study coordinator contacted the interested nurses by online form and screened the eligible patients until the target number of 710 patients was reached. The eligible participants were informed about the voluntary nature of their participation, and online informed consent was obtained from them. After that, online questionnaires were sent to them via WhatsApp, and they were asked to fill out the questionnaires. The nurse who did not return the questionnaire was given the opportunity for 2 weeks. The researcher confirmed that if she was not willing to continue, the researcher did not force it. The research data was collected by giving initials without writing names, and the researchers also strictly maintained the confidentiality of the respondents.

Measures

Data were collected using an online questionnaire form. A socio-demographic form developed by the researchers was used to assess the patient's sociodemographic characteristics (age, gender, religion, marital status, and educational level). The questionnaire was developed by the researchers from the COVID-19 Social Psychological Survey to assess psychological condition and social stigma. This questionnaire consists of 27 items with a rating using a 4-point Likert scale starting from 1 (strongly disagree), 2 (disagree), 3 (agree), and 4 (strongly disagree), on unfavorable questions, the assessment is reversed. The result of score interpretation shows that < 56 has a low psychological condition,

TABLE 2 | Psychological condition, stigma, and crisis mental health during pandemic situation.

Psychological condition	n (%)
Psychological status	
Bad	271 (12.6)
Moderate	1690 (78.4)
Good	195 (9.0)
Social stigma	
Yes	399 (18.5)
No	1757 (81.5)
Anxiety	
Normal	505 (23.4)
Mild	256 (11.9)
Moderate	241 (11.2)
Severe	206 (9.6)
Very severe	948 (44.0)
Fear	
Normal	254 (11.8)
Mild	220 (10.2)
Moderate	340 (15.8)
Severe	188 (8.7)
Very severe	1154 (53.5)
Depression	
Normal	118 (5.5)
Mild	192 (8.9)
Moderate	215 (10.0)
Severe	236 (10.9)
Very severe	1395 (64.7)
Crisis mental health	
Mild	182 (8.4)
Moderate	604 (28.0)
Severe	1370 (63.5)

TABLE 3 | Predictors psychological condition caused anxiety, fear, depression, and crisis mental health during pandemic.

Variable	Psychological Status			*P*-value
	Bad	Moderate	Good	
Anxiety				0.000
Normal	51 (10.1)	416 (82.4)	38 (7.4)	
Mild	48 (18.8)	198 (77.3)	10 (3.9)	
Moderate	10 (4.1)	219 (90.9)	12 (5.0)	
Severe	47 (22.8)	139 (67.5)	20 (9.7)	
Very severe	115 (12.1)	718 (75.7)	115 (12.1)	
Fear				0.000
Normal	37 (14.6)	185 (72.8)	32 (12.6)	
Mild	12 (5.5)	202 (91.8)	6 (2.7)	
Moderate	56 (16.5)	270 (79.4)	14 (4.1)	
Severe	4 (2.1)	176 (93.6)	8 (4.3)	
Very severe	162 (14.0)	857 (74.3)	135 (11.7)	
Depression				0.000
Normal	16 (13.6)	76 (64.4)	26 (22.0)	
Mild	27 (14.1)	159 (82.8)	6 (3.1)	
Moderate	10 (4.7)	195 (90.7)	10 (4.7)	
Severe	46 (19.5)	184 (78.0)	6 (2.5)	
Very severe	172 (12.3)	1076 (77.1)	147 910.5)	
Crisis mental health				0.008
Normal	18 (9.9)	136 (74.7)	28 (15.4)	
Mild	64 (10.6)	516 (85.4)	24 (4.0)	
Moderate	189 (13.8)	1038 (75.8)	143 (10.4)	
Severe	271 (12.6)	1690 (78.4)	195 (9.0)	

56–65 has a moderate psychological condition and > 65 indicates a high psychological condition. While the social stigma is said to experience social stigma if the score obtained is < 24. Anxiety, fear, and depression were measured using a modified depression, anxiety, stress scale questionnaire which consisted of 21 questions using a 0–3 scale, namely a score of zero indicates never, a value of 1 is sometimes, a value of 2 is quite often and a value of 3 is very often. Interpretation score tNormal = 0–7, mild anxiety level = 8–9, moderate = 10–14, severe = 15–19 and very severe = 20, while the assessment for depression normal = 0–14, mild depression = 15–18, moderate = 19–25, severe = 26–33 and very severe 34. Measurement of the mental health crisis in Indonesian nurses during the COVID-19 pandemic was measured using a mental health questionnaire that had been developed by researchers. Question items consist of 9 questions with a Likert scale of 4 points; 0 points never, 1 point every day (1–7 days), 2 points more often (7–12 days), and 4 points almost every day (13–14 days). The result of the interpretation assessment is a score of 0–4: No referral is required at this time. 5–9: Clients may benefit from natural support or mental health services. 10–19: Clients should seek professional mental health services. 20–27: Clients should seek health crisis services as soon as possible. All questionnaires have been tested for validity first with 100 respondents, all questions show valid results, the calculated r value is between 0.772 and 0.985, so that it is greater than the r table value of 0.1638. While the questionnaire shows reliable with Cronbach's Alpha value between 0.875 and 0.995.

TABLE 4 | Predictors social stigma caused anxiety, fear, depression, and crisis mental health during pandemic.

Variable	Social Stigma		*p*-value
	Yes	No	
Anxiety			0.000
Normal	68 (13.5)	437 (86.5)	
Mild	32 (12.5)	224 (87.5)	
Moderate	38 (15.8)	203 (85.2)	
Severe	39 (18.9)	167 (81.1)	
Very severe	222 (23.4)	726 (76.6)	
Fear			0.000
Normal	37 (14.6)	217 (85.4)	
Mild	25 (11.4)	195 (88.6)	
Moderate	46 (13.5)	294 (86.5)	
Severe	30 (16.0)	158 (84.0)	
Very severe	261 (22.6)	893 (77.4)	
Depression			0.000
Normal	16 (13.6)	102 (86.4)	
Mild	28 (14.6)	164 (85.4)	
Moderate	26 (12.1)	189 (87.9)	
Severe	30 (12.7)	206 (87.3)	
Very severe	299 (21.4)	1096 (78.6)	
Crisis mental health			0.000
Normal	25 (13.7)	157 (86.3)	
Mild	94 (15.6)	510 (84.4)	
Moderate	280 (20.4)	1090 (79.6)	
Severe	399 (18.5)	1757 (81.5)	

Statistical Analysis

This study analyzed using descriptive and inferential analysis. A compliance test for normal distribution was applied using the Kolmogorov–Smirnov test. A descriptive value such as means, SDs, frequencies, and percentages was analyzed with frequent distribution. A Chi-square test was performed to compare the groups concerning demographic, independent, and dependent variables. The relationship between psychological condition and social stigma with anxiety, fear, depression, and crisis mental health was analyzed using Spearman rho correlation test with statistically significant p value < 0.05. The analyzes were conducted with SPSS® for Windows® version 22.0.

RESULTS

The total of 2,156 respondents responded to the questionnaire and the response rate was 100%. The results showed that the average nurse was 20–29 years old and the majority were women (67.5%). Most of the nurses were single (67.5%) and came from Java (67.5%). The religion of the majority of nurses is Islam (92.9%), the most educated level is at the undergraduate level (58.1%), and the income is above the minimum regional income (58.3%) (**Table 1**).

The psychological condition of nurses in a pandemic situation reflects the actual condition of nurses while providing care to patients, especially in the second wave of COVID-19. The psychological status of nurses based on the survey results showed moderate results (78.4%). Nurses who experienced social stigma were 399 (18.5%). The nurse showed a very severe anxiety response of 44.0%, as well as fear, which showed very severe (53.5%), and depression which showed very severe (64.5%). This condition allows nurses to experience a severe mental health emergency crisis of 63.5% (**Table 2**).

A bad psychological condition can lead to the emergence of accompanying psychological symptoms that worsen the nurse's condition and cause her to fall into a state of mental health crisis. Nurses with poor psychological status experienced severe anxiety (22.8%), very severe fear (14.0%), very bad depression (12.3%), and 12.6% of nurses who had fallen into a very bad mental health crisis (**Table 3**).

It is almost the same as psychological status conditions that can cause problems, including anxiety, fear, depression, and mental health crisis. This condition can also be exacerbated by the situation of social stigma shown by the community, the emergence of this stigma makes conditions facing a pandemic even more difficult. The results of a survey of Indonesian nurses showed that 23.4% of nurses who experienced social stigma showed a very poor anxiety response. Likewise, the fear experienced by nurses was also very high, namely, 22.6% who experienced stigma, they definitely showed very severe fear, and 21.4% experienced depression. Nurses who experienced social stigma also fell into a mental health crisis as much as 15.6% in mild conditions, 20.4% moderate, and 18.5% severe (**Table 4**).

DISCUSSION

Psychological status and social stigma have a high contribution to the incidence of anxiety, fear, depression, and mental health emergency crises in nurses who provide care in COVID-19 isolation rooms. Nurses revealed that carrying out their duties in isolation rooms is a challenge and vigilance that they must exercise caution, because it can cause various problems if they contract COVID-19 and the bad impact is on the health condition of each individual (11, 14). Nurses as the front line must not be afraid and retreat from the pandemic situation, nurses cannot choose to give up and must keep fighting because of the professionalism and professional oath that have been made (15, 16). Nurses in Indonesia and all countries are facing the same burden of problems, namely dealing with COVID-19, especially the psychological impact caused by the crisis during the pandemic (8).

The results showed that the average nurse was 20–29 years old and most were women, in line with several studies which stated that most of the nurses were women and the nurses who served in the isolation room were nurses who were young and did not have comorbidities (17, 18). Nurses in Indonesia who carry out their duties in isolation rooms are mostly single nurses, because the nurses on duty are volunteer nurses and fresh graduates who have been given the necessary training in the isolation room (8, 19, 20). Nurses who work in isolation rooms must be carefully considered and ensured that they still have excellent health to prevent transmission and worsening of the disease if infected with COVID-19 (9, 21).

The psychological condition of nurses in a pandemic situation reflects the actual condition of nurses while providing care to patients, especially in the second wave of COVID-19 (17, 19). The psychological status of nurses based on the survey results showed moderate results, also in line with several studies conducted in Indonesia. Indeed the pandemic situation caused an unfavorable psychological impact for nurses, especially in wave 2 of COVID-19 (5, 22). Nurses who experience social stigma also show high results, nurses are stigmatized because they are considered to be spreaders of the virus because they work in hospitals, there are lots of rejections given by the community, especially in the early stages of the emergence of COVID-19 (23, 24). As a result, this condition gave rise to symptoms in nurses such as responses to anxiety, fear, and depression which were in the very severe category (7, 20). Nurses who are on the front line in providing patient care, screening, tracing and becoming vaccination officers certainly create situations of excessive anxiety and fear, because COVID-19 can trigger a rapid worsening of the condition and death. Many nurses also fall into depression and need counseling with other health workers and psychiatrists (14, 25). If this condition makes it possible for nurses to experience a severe mental health emergency crisis, if left unchecked, health workers will become victims in a pandemic situation that continues.

It is almost the same as psychological status conditions that can cause problems including, anxiety, fear, depression, and mental health crisis (26, 27). This condition can also be exacerbated by the situation of social stigma shown by the community, the emergence of this stigma makes conditions facing a pandemic even more difficult. The results of a survey on Indonesian nurses who experienced social stigma showed a very bad response to anxiety, fear, and depression. Nurses who experience social stigma are also very many who fall into a mental health crisis, as a result, many nurses are traumatized and remember the extraordinary events of the pandemic (28, 29). The conditions of anxiety, fear, depression, and mental health crises not only occur due to the pandemic situation, nurses who have experienced the loss of their closest family members and sources of life support so far have also shown a very bad response, the deep trauma experienced by nurses is also felt to become a memorable memory. bad for him. Many nurses died as a result of battling the COVID-19 pandemic (7, 11).

The results of this study have research limitations, namely they have not measured the level of depth of the psychological feelings of nurses qualitatively, so that the results obtained are nurses expressing their hearts. So it is very important to pay attention to digging deeper into the psychological state of nurses, especially those who provide treatment in isolation rooms, nurses who have trauma from the pandemic and nurses who still have symptoms of long haul COVID-19. It is hoped that further researchers can continue and make innovations in resolving the psychological impact of the pandemic among nurses and other health workers.

CONCLUSION

The psychological status and social stigma experienced by nurses during the COVID-19 pandemic indicate a bad situation, many nurses are stigmatized in society, resulting in very bad anxiety, fear, depression, and causing a mental health emergency crisis.

ETHICS STATEMENT

The studies involving human participants were reviewed and approved by the Local Ethics Committee University of Indonesia with the number Ket-198/UN2.F12.D1.2.1/PPM.00.02/2021. Written informed consent to participate in this study was provided by the participants' legal guardian/next of kin.

AUTHOR CONTRIBUTIONS

MM, HF, AS, NN: study conception and design. NN, MA, AM: data collection, analysis, and interpretation of results. NN: manuscript preparation. All authors contributed to the article and approved the submitted version.

REFERENCES

1. Liberati A, Altman DG, Tetzlaff J, Mulrow C, Gøtzsche PC, Ioannidis JPA, et al. The PRISMA statement for reporting systematic reviews and meta-analyses of studies that evaluate health care interventions: explanation and elaboration. *PLoS Med.* (2009) 6:e1000100. doi: 10.1371/journal.pmed.1000100
2. Yao H, Chen JH, Xu YF. Rethinking online mental health services in China during the COVID-19 epidemic. *Asian J Psychiatr.* (2020) 50:102015. doi: 10.1016/j.ajp.2020.102015
3. Zulkipli ZN, Idris SH, Rahman NA. COVID-19 ANXIETY: MALAYSIAN REGULATORY MECHANISMS ON MENTAL HEALTH. *Int J Adv Sci Technol.* (2020) 29:2472–7.
4. Liu S, Yang L, Zhang C, Xiang YT, Liu Z, Hu S, et al. Online mental health services in China during the COVID-19 outbreak. *Lancet Psychiatry.* (2020) 7:e17–e18. doi: 10.1016/S2215-0366(20)30077-8
5. Peitl V, Zatezalo VG, Karlović D. Mental health issues and psychological crisis interventions during the COVID-19 pandemic and earthquakes in Croatia. *Arch Psychiatry Res.* (2020) 56:193— 8. doi: 10.20471/dec.2020.56.02.07
6. Zhu Z, Ph D, Xu S, Ph D, Wang H, Med M, et al. COVID-19 in Wuhan: immediate psychological impact on 5062 health workers. *medRxiv.* (2020) [Preprint]. doi: 10.1101/2020.02.20.20025338
7. Nursalam N, Sukartini T, Priyantini D, Mafula D, Efendi F. Risk factors for psychological impact and social stigma among people facing covid-19: a systematic review'. *Syst Rev Pharm.* (2020) 11:1022–8.
8. Priyantini D, Nursalam N, Sukartini T. Analysis of factors affecting the mental health crisis of coronavirus disease infection in Java Island. *J Ners.* (2021) 16:60–6. doi: 10.20473/jn.v16i1.23321
9. Gao Y, Li T, Han M, Li X, Wu D, Xu Y, et al. Diagnostic utility of clinical laboratory data determinations for patients with the severe COVID-19. *J Med Virol.* (2020) 92:791–6. doi: 10.1002/jmv.25770
10. Hu, B, Wang D. Clinical features of critically ill patients with COVID-19 infection in China. *Res Sq.* (2020) 8:1–21. doi: 10.21203/rs.3.rs-16250/v1
11. Priyantini D, Nursalam N, Sukartini T. The first psychological management intervention towards community resilience facing covid-19 infection. *Int J Pharm Res.* (2021) 13:4485–92. doi: 10.31838/ijpr/2021.13.01.654
12. Li Y, Xia L. Coronavirus disease 2019 (COVID-19): role of chest ct in diagnosis and management. *AJR Am J Roentgenol.* (2020) 214:1280–6. doi: 10.2214/AJR.20.22954
13. Liang H, Acharya G. Novel corona virus disease (COVID-19) in pregnancy: what clinical recommendations to follow? *Acta Obstet Gynecol Scand.* (2020) 99:439–42. doi: 10.1111/aogs.13836
14. Sohrabi C, Alsafi Z, O'Neill N, Khan M, Kerwan A, Al-Jabir A, et al. World health organization declares global emergency: a review of the 2019 novel coronavirus (COVID-19). *Int J Surg [Internet].* (2020) 76:71–6. doi: 10.1016/j.ijsu.2020.02.034
15. Metlay JP, Waterer GW, Long AC, Anzueto A, Brozek J, Crothers K, et al. Diagnosis and treatment of adults with community-acquired pneumonia. *Am J Respir Crit Care Med.* (2019) 200:E45— E67. doi: 10.1164/rccm.201908-1581ST
16. Zhou F, Yu T, Du R, Fan G, Liu Y, Liu Z, et al. Clinical course and risk factors for mortality of adult inpatients with COVID-19 in Wuhan, China: a retrospective cohort study. *Lancet.* (2020) 395:1054–62. doi: 10.1016/S0140-6736(20)30566-3
17. Percudani M, Corradin M, Moreno M, Indelicato A, Vita A. Mental health services in lombardy during COVID-19 outbreak. *Psychiatry Res.* (2020) 288:1–3. doi: 10.1016/j.psychres.2020.112980
18. Ping NPT, Shoesmith WD, James S, Nor Hadi NM, Yau EKB, Lin LJ. Ultra brief psychological interventions for covid-19 pandemic: introduction of a locally-adapted brief intervention for mental health and psychosocial support service. *Malaysian J Med Sci.* (2020) 27:51–6. doi: 10.21315/mjms2020.27.2.6
19. Li S, Wang Y, Xue J, Zhao N, Zhu T. The impact of covid-19 epidemic declaration on psychological consequences: a study on active weibo users. *Int J Environ Res Public Health.* (2020) 17:2032. doi: 10.3390/ijerph17062032
20. Mafula D, Nursalam N, Tintin S. Quality of nursing worklife based on caring model for improving nurse performance in hospitals. *Indones Nurs J Educ Clin.* (2020) 5:172–84. doi: 10.24990/injec.v5i2.339
21. Wang S, Guo L, Chen L, Liu W, Cao Y, Zhang J, et al. A case report of neonatal COVID-19 infection in China. *Clin Infect Dis.* (2020) 71:853–7. doi: 10.1093/cid/ciaa225
22. Lupe SE, Keefer L, Szigethy E. Gaining resilience and reducing stress in the age of COVID-19. *Curr Opin Gastroenterol.* (2020) 36:295–303. doi: 10.1097/MOG.0000000000000646
23. Mukhtar S. Mental health of medical workers in Pakistan during the pandemic COVID- 19 outbreak. *Asian J Psychiatr.* (2020) 51:19–21. doi: 10.1016/j.ajp.2020.102080
24. Stankovska G, Memedi I, Dimitrovski D. Coronavirus Covid-19 disease, mental health and psychosocial support. *Soc Regist.* (2020) 4:33–48. doi: 10.14746/sr.2020.4.2.03
25. Covid-19 National Emergency Response Center, Epidemiology and Case Management Team, Korea Centers for Disease Control and Prevention. Early epidemiological and clinical characteristics of 28 cases of coronavirus disease in South Korea. *Osong Public Heal Res Perspect.* (2020) 11:8–14. doi: 10.24171/j.phrp.2020.11.1.03
26. Oikarainen A, Mikkonen K, Kenny A, Tomietto M, Tuomikoski A, Meriläinen M. Educational interventions designed to develop nurses' cultural competence: a systematic review. *Int J Nurs Stud.* (2019) 98:75–86. doi: 10.1016/j.ijnurstu.2019.06.005
27. Guo Y-R, Cao Q-D, Hong Z-S, Tan Y-Y, Chen S-D, Jin H-J, et al. The origin, transmission and clinical therapies on coronavirus disease 2019 (COVID-19) outbreak – an update on the status. *Mil Med Res.* (2020) 7:11. doi: 10.1186/s40779-020-00240-0
28. Li W, Yang Y, Liu ZH, Zhao YJ, Zhang Q, Zhang L, et al. Progression of mental health services during the COVID-19 outbreak in China. *Int J Biol Sci.* (2020) 16:1732–8. doi: 10.7150/ijbs.45120
29. De Sousa A, Mohandas E, Javed A. Psychological interventions during COVID-19: challenges for low and middle income countries. *Asian J Psychiatr.* (2020) 51:102128. doi: 10.1016/j.ajp.2020.102128

Permissions

All chapters in this book were first published by Frontiers; hereby published with permission under the Creative Commons Attribution License or equivalent. Every chapter published in this book has been scrutinized by our experts. Their significance has been extensively debated. The topics covered herein carry significant findings which will fuel the growth of the discipline. They may even be implemented as practical applications or may be referred to as a beginning point for another development.

The contributors of this book come from diverse backgrounds, making this book a truly international effort. This book will bring forth new frontiers with its revolutionizing research information and detailed analysis of the nascent developments around the world.

We would like to thank all the contributing authors for lending their expertise to make the book truly unique. They have played a crucial role in the development of this book. Without their invaluable contributions this book wouldn't have been possible. They have made vital efforts to compile up to date information on the varied aspects of this subject to make this book a valuable addition to the collection of many professionals and students.

This book was conceptualized with the vision of imparting up-to-date information and advanced data in this field. To ensure the same, a matchless editorial board was set up. Every individual on the board went through rigorous rounds of assessment to prove their worth. After which they invested a large part of their time researching and compiling the most relevant data for our readers.

The editorial board has been involved in producing this book since its inception. They have spent rigorous hours researching and exploring the diverse topics which have resulted in the successful publishing of this book. They have passed on their knowledge of decades through this book. To expedite this challenging task, the publisher supported the team at every step. A small team of assistant editors was also appointed to further simplify the editing procedure and attain best results for the readers.

Apart from the editorial board, the designing team has also invested a significant amount of their time in understanding the subject and creating the most relevant covers. They scrutinized every image to scout for the most suitable representation of the subject and create an appropriate cover for the book.

The publishing team has been an ardent support to the editorial, designing and production team. Their endless efforts to recruit the best for this project, has resulted in the accomplishment of this book. They are a veteran in the field of academics and their pool of knowledge is as vast as their experience in printing. Their expertise and guidance has proved useful at every step. Their uncompromising quality standards have made this book an exceptional effort. Their encouragement from time to time has been an inspiration for everyone.

The publisher and the editorial board hope that this book will prove to be a valuable piece of knowledge for researchers, students, practitioners and scholars across the globe.

List of Contributors

Yael Apter-Levy, Orna Zagoory-Sharon and Ruth Feldman
The Center for Developmental Social Neuroscience, Interdisciplinary Center Herzliya, Herzliya, Israel

Jack J. Blanchard, Christina L. G. Savage, Ryan D. Orth and Anyela M. Jacome
Department of Psychology, University of Maryland, College Park, College Park, MD, United States

Melanie E. Bennett
Department of Psychiatry, University of Maryland, Baltimore, Baltimore, MD, United States
Department of Psychiatry, Baltimore VA Medical Center, Baltimore, MD, United States

Łukasz Okruszek
Social Neuroscience Lab, Institute of Psychology, Polish Academy of Sciences, Warsaw, Poland

Marta Chrustowicz
Faculty of Psychology, University of Warsaw, Warsaw, Poland

Karina S. Blair, Johannah Bashford-Largo, Niraj Shah, Jennie Lukoff, Jaimie Elowsky, Steven Vogel, Ru Zhang, Matthew Dobbertin and James R. Blair
Center for Neurobehavioral Research, Boys Town National Research Hospital, Boys Town, NE, United States

Amanda Emmert
Department of Psychiatry, Creighton University School of Medicine, Omaha, NE, United States

Seth Pollak
Department of Psychology, University of Wisconsin, Madison, WI, United States

Ilaria Cataldo
Affiliative Behavior and Physiology Lab, Department of Psychology and Cognitive Science, University of Trento, Trento, Italy
Mobile and Social Computing Lab, Bruno Kessler Foundation, Trento, Italy

Bruno Lepri
Mobile and Social Computing Lab, Bruno Kessler Foundation, Trento, Italy

Michelle Jin Yee Neoh
Social and Affective Neuroscience Lab, Psychology Program, School of Social Sciences, Nanyang Technological University, Singapore, Singapore

Gianluca Esposito
Affiliative Behavior and Physiology Lab, Department of Psychology and Cognitive Science, University of Trento, Trento, Italy
Social and Affective Neuroscience Lab, Psychology Program, School of Social Sciences, Nanyang Technological University, Singapore, Singapore
Lee Kong Chian School of Medicine, Nanyang Technological University, Singapore, Singapore

Max J. Rolison, Adam J. Naples, Helena J. V. Rutherford and James C. McPartland
Child Study Center, Yale School of Medicine, New Haven, CT, United States

Yonat Rum and Anat Perry
Psychology Department, The Hebrew University of Jerusalem, Jerusalem, Israel

Valeria Lucarini and Carlo Marchesi
Psychiatry Unit, Department of Medicine and Surgery, Medical Faculty, University of Parma, Parma, Italy

Martine Grice and Francesco Cangemi
IfL-Phonetics, University of Cologne, Cologne, Germany

Juliane T. Zimmermann
Department of Psychiatry and Psychotherapy, Medical Faculty, University of Cologne, Cologne, Germany

Kai Vogeley
Department of Psychiatry and Psychotherapy, Medical Faculty, University of Cologne, Cologne, Germany
Cognitive Neuroscience (INM-3), Institute of Neuroscience and Medicine, Research Center Jülich, Jülich, Germany

Matteo Tonna
Department of Mental Health, Azienda Unità Sanitaria Locale di Parma, Parma, Italy

Yafeng Pan
School of Psychology, Shenzhen University, Shenzhen, China
Department of Clinical Neuroscience, Karolinska Institutet, Stockholm, Sweden

Xiaojun Cheng
School of Psychology, Shenzhen University, Shenzhen, China

Lars O. White, Margerete J. S. Schoett and Jan Keil
Department of Child and Adolescent Psychiatry, University of Leipzig, Leipzig, Germany

Charlotte C. Schulz
Department of Child and Adolescent Psychiatry, University of Leipzig, Leipzig, Germany
Department of Neurology, Max Planck Institute for Human Cognitive and Brain Sciences, Leipzig, Germany

Melanie T. Kungl
Department of Psychology, University of Erlangen-Nuremberg, Erlangen, Germany

Jessica L. Borelli
THRIVE Laboratory, Psychology and Social Behavior, University of California, Irvine, Irvine, CA, United States

Pascal Vrtička
Research Group "Social Stress and Family Health", Max Planck Institute for Human Cognitive and Brain Sciences, Leipzig, Germany
Department of Psychology, Centre for Brain Science, University of Essex, Colchester, United Kingdom

Ville Renvall
Department of Neuroscience and Biomedical Engineering, Aalto University School of Science, Espoo, Finland
Advanced Magnetic Imaging Centre, Aalto University School of Science, Espoo, Finland

Jaakko Kauramäki and Sanna Malinen
Department of Neuroscience and Biomedical Engineering, Aalto University School of Science, Espoo, Finland

Riitta Hari
Department of Neuroscience and Biomedical Engineering, Aalto University School of Science, Espoo, Finland
Department of Art, Aalto University School of Arts, Design and Architecture, Espoo, Finland

Lauri Nummenmaa
Department of Neuroscience and Biomedical Engineering, Aalto University School of Science, Espoo, Finland
Turku PET Centre and Department of Psychology, University of Turku, Turku, Finland

Leanna M. Hernandez, Shulamite A. Green, Katherine E. Lawrence, Janelle Liu and Mirella Dapretto
Ahmanson-Lovelace Brain Mapping Center, University of California, Los Angeles, Los Angeles, CA, United States
Department of Psychiatry and Biobehavioral Sciences, University of California, Los Angeles, Los Angeles, CA, United States

Marisa Inada
Ahmanson-Lovelace Brain Mapping Center, University of California, Los Angeles, Los Angeles, CA, United States

Susan Y. Bookheimer
Ahmanson-Lovelace Brain Mapping Center, University of California, Los Angeles, Los Angeles, CA, United States
Staglin IMHRO Center for Cognitive Neuroscience, University of California, Los Angeles, Los Angeles, CA, United States

Kathryn M. Hauschild and Cara M. Keifer
Social Competence and Treatment Laboratory, Department of Psychology, Stony Brook University, Stony Brook, NY, United States

Peter Felsman
Social Competence and Treatment Laboratory, Department of Psychology, Stony Brook University, Stony Brook, NY, United States
Alan Alda Center for Communicating Science, Stony Brook University, Stony Brook, NY, United States

Matthew D. Lerner
Social Competence and Treatment Laboratory, Department of Psychology, Stony Brook University, Stony Brook, NY, United States
Department of Psychology, University of Virginia, Charlottesville, VA, United States

Florence Baillin, Aline Lefebvre and Richard Delorme
Human Genetics and Cognitive Functions, Institut Pasteur, UMR3571 CNRS, Université de Paris, Paris, France
Child and Adolescent Psychiatry Department, Robert Debré Hospital, Paris, France

Amandine Pedoux, Anna Maruani and Frédérique Amsellem
Child and Adolescent Psychiatry Department, Robert Debré Hospital, Paris, France

Yann Beauxis and Thomas Bourgeron
Human Genetics and Cognitive Functions, Institut Pasteur, UMR3571 CNRS, Université de Paris, Paris, France

Denis A. Engemann
Parietal Project-Team, INRIA Saclay – Île de France, Palaiseau, France

J. A. Scott Kelso
Human Brain and Behavior Laboratory, Center for Complex Systems and Brain Sciences, Florida Atlantic University, Boca Raton, FL, United States
Intelligent Systems Research Centre, University of Ulster, Derry Londonderry, United Kingdom

Guillaume Dumas
Human Genetics and Cognitive Functions, Institut Pasteur, UMR3571 CNRS, Université de Paris, Paris, France
Human Brain and Behavior Laboratory, Center for Complex Systems and Brain Sciences, Florida Atlantic University, Boca Raton, FL, United States
Department of Psychiatry, Université de Montréal, Montreal, QC, Canada
CHU Sainte-Justine Centre de Recherche, Precision Psychiatry and Social Physiology Laboratory, Montreal, QC, Canada

Myrthe Jansen, Sandy Overgaauw and Ellen R. A. De Bruijn
Department of Clinical Psychology, Institute of Psychology, Leiden University, Leiden, Netherlands
Leiden Institute for Brain and Cognition (LIBC), Leiden University, Leiden, Netherlands

Sofie Vettori, Stephanie Van der Donck, Jean Steyaert and Bart Boets
Center for Developmental Psychiatry, Department of Neurosciences, KU Leuven, Leuven, Belgium
Leuven Autism Research (LAuRes), KU Leuven, Leuven, Belgium

Milena Dzhelyova
Leuven Autism Research (LAuRes), KU Leuven, Leuven, Belgium
Institute of Research in Psychological Science, Institute of Neuroscience, University of Louvain, Louvain-La-Neuve, Belgium

Corentin Jacques
Center for Developmental Psychiatry, Department of Neurosciences, KU Leuven, Leuven, Belgium,
Institute of Research in Psychological Science, Institute of Neuroscience, University of Louvain, Louvain-La-Neuve, Belgium

Bruno Rossion
Institute of Research in Psychological Science, Institute of Neuroscience, University of Louvain, Louvain-La-Neuve, Belgium
Université de Lorraine, CNRS, CRAN-UMR 7039, Nancy, France
Université de Lorraine, CHRU-Service de Neurologie, Nancy, France

Aline Gauchat
Clinique de Consultation Conjugale et Familiale Poitras-Wright, Côté, Longueuil, QC, Canada
Department of Psychology, Université de Montréal, Montreal, QC, Canada

Antonio Zadra
Department of Psychology, Université de Montréal, Montreal, QC, Canada

Mira El-Hourani
Department of Psychology, Université de Montréal, Montreal, QC, Canada
CHU Ste-Justine Research Center, Montreal, QC, Canada

Sophie Parent
School of Psychoeducation, Université de Montréal, Montreal, QC, Canada

Richard E. Tremblay
Department of Psychology, Université de Montréal, Montreal, QC, Canada
CHU Ste-Justine Research Center, Montreal, QC, Canada
Department of Pediatrics, Université de Montréal, Montreal, QC, Canada
School of Public Health, University College Dublin, Dublin, Ireland

Jean R. Séguin
CHU Ste-Justine Research Center, Montreal, QC, Canada
Department of Psychiatry and Addictology, Université de Montréal, Montreal, QC, Canada

Sangjin Lee and Hae-Won Shin
Department of Neurology, Chung-Ang University College of Medicine, Seoul, South Korea

Sun Ju Chung
Department of Neurology, Asan Medical Center, Ulsan University College of Medicine, Seoul, South Korea

Mustikasari Mustikasari and Muhammad Adam
Faculty of Nursing, Universitas Indonesia, Jakarta, Indonesia

Harif Fadhillah
Faculty of Health Science, Muhammadiyah University of Jakarta, Jakarta, Indonesia
Indonesian National Nursing Association, Jakarta, Indonesia

Apri Sunadi
Universitas Respati Indonesia, Yogyakarta, Indonesia

Nursalam Nursalam
Indonesian National Nursing Association, Jakarta, Indonesia
Faculty of Nursing, Universitas Airlangga, Surabaya, Indonesia

Ati Surya Mediawati
Indonesian National Nursing Association, Jakarta, Indonesia

Index

S

T

U

V

www.ingramcontent.com/pod-product-compliance
Lightning Source LLC
LaVergne TN
LVHW081017210926
848485LV00004B/882